Body Fat Distri...

Moderate amount...
However, excess fa... lth
risk than fat on or l... ...e'
than an 'apple-shape.

Abdominal obesity greatly increases the risk of developing diabetes, heart disease, high blood fats, hypertension, stroke, sleep apnea, arthritis and some cancers. So-called 'cellulite' carries no extra health risk.

Waist Circumference directly reflects the increased health risk of abdominal obesity. Waist size associated with a high health risk:

Men ~ Over 40 inches   **Women** ~ Over 35 inches

Body Mass Index (BMI)

BMI is a general (but not specific) indicator of body fatness. Although BMI alone is not diagnostic, the higher the BMI, the greater the health risk of developing diabetes, high blood pressure and heart disease. BMI does not apply to heavily muscled persons. BMI is used in a different way for children.

Abdominal obesity greatly increases the risk of ill-health and earlier death.

Check Your BMI: Find your height (no shoes) - look across the row to the weight nearest your own. Then track down to BMI.

Ht	WEIGHT (LBS) ~ ADULTS													
5'1"	100	106	111	116	122	127	132	137	143	148	153	158	185	211
5'2"	104	109	115	120	126	131	136	142	147	153	158	164	191	218
5'3"	107	113	118	124	130	135	141	146	152	158	163	169	197	225
5'4"	110	116	122	128	134	140	145	151	157	163	169	174	204	232
5'5"	114	120	126	132	138	144	150	156	162	168	174	180	210	240
5'6"	118	124	130	136	142	148	155	161	167	173	179	186	216	247
5'7"	121	127	134	140	146	153	159	166	172	178	185	191	223	255
5'8"	125	131	138	144	151	158	164	171	177	184	190	197	230	262
5'9"	128	135	142	149	155	162	169	176	182	189	196	206	236	270
5'10"	132	139	146	153	160	167	174	181	188	195	202	207	243	278
5'11"	136	143	150	157	165	172	179	186	193	200	208	215	250	286
6'0"	140	147	154	162	169	177	184	191	199	206	213	221	258	294
6'1"	144	151	159	166	174	182	189	197	204	212	219	227	265	302
6'2"	148	155	163	171	179	186	194	202	210	218	225	233	272	311
6'3"	152	160	168	176	184	192	200	208	216	224	232	240	279	319
6'4"	156	164	172	180	189	197	205	213	221	230	238	246	287	328

| BMI | 19 | 20 | 21 | 22 | 23 | 24 | 25 | 26 | 27 | 28 | 29 | 30 | 35 | 40 |

BMI Classification:

BMI Below 19
Underweight

BMI 19-24.9
Healthy Weight
(Low Health Risk)

BMI 25-29.9
Overweight
(Moderate Health Risk)

BMI 30-40
Obese (High Health Risk)

BMI Over 40
Morbid Obesity
(Very High Risk)

Interactive BMI Calculator
www.calorieking.com

D0126612

Calories in Food

Calories in food are derived from protein, fat and carbohydrate. Alcohol also provides calories. Vitamins, minerals and water provide no calories.

Calorie Values Per Gram

Fat/Oil	~ 9 Calories
Carbohydrate	~ 4 Calories
Protein	~ 4 Calories
Alcohol	~ 7 Calories

Note that fats have over double the calories of protein and carbohydrate. The higher the fat content of food, the higher the calories.

Sample Calculation

QUARTER POUNDER®
WITH CHEESE
has 510 calories
derived from:

26g Fat (x 9 cals/gram)	= 234
40g Carbohyd.(x 4 cals/gram)	= 160
29g Protein (x 4 cals/gram)	= 116
Total Calories	= 510

Calorie Levels for Weight Loss

Start with a calorie-controlled diet that allows a moderate weight loss of ½ - 1 pound per week. Weight loss is usually much greater in the first few weeks due to extra fluid losses.

Note: It is better to increase exercise rather than lessen food calories too drastically.

Suggested Calories for Weight Loss

Women:	Non-active 1000 - 1200
	Active 1200 - 1500
Men:	Non-active 1200 - 1500
	Active 1500 - 1800
Teenagers:	1200 - 1800

ChooseMyPlate.gov

The MyPlate symbol represents the recommended proportion of foods from each food group. It focuses on the importance of making smart food choices in every food group, every day. Daily physical activity is also important. (More info: www.ChooseMyPlate.gov)

Examples of Single Serving Sizes

Grains (Eat 6 servings per day):
- 1 slice wholegrain bread (1 oz)
- ½ bun, small bagel or English muffin
- 4 small crackers or 1 tortilla
- 1 oz ready-to-eat wholegrain cereal
- ½ cup cooked cereal, rice or pasta

Vegetables (Eat 3-5 servings per day):
- 1 cup raw leafy vegetables
- 1½ cups raw chopped vegetables
- ½ cup cooked vegetables
- ½ - ¾ cup vegetable juice

Fruit (Eat 3-5 servings per day):
- 1 medium apple, orange, banana
- ½ cup canned fruit (in own juice)
- ¼ cup dried fruit
- ½ cup fruit juice (unsweetened)
- ¼ medium avocado

Protein (2-3 servings per day):
- 2-3 oz (cooked) lean meat/poultry/fish
- 2 eggs or 6 oz tofu or ¼ cup nuts
- 1 cup (cooked) dried beans or chickpeas

Dairy (2-3 servings per day):
- 1 cup (8 fl.oz) milk/soy (enriched)/yogurt
- 1½ oz cheese or ½ cup cottage cheese

Portion Size Counts!

Food portion size is critical to controlling calorie intake for weight control.

Super-sized food servings have become more common when eating out and in the home. This can mean a day's worth of calories being consumed in one meal; or a snack being equivalent to a full meal.

It is easy to underestimate portion size of foods and drinks, and unwittingly consume excess calories – even if the fat content is low or even zero!

To more accurately estimate portion size of different foods, weigh and measure your food with food scales, measuring spoons and cups. Better control of calories will result.

For a visual idea of portion sizes, visit **www.CalorieKing.com** See examples (fries and cola) on this page.

Allow for Extra Calories in Packaged Food

The actual weight of packaged foods is usually 5-10% more than the label net weight (the minimum legal weight) – and in some cases up to 50% more. However, manufacturers calculate the calories based on the net weight. For actual calories, weigh the product and calculate the extra calories.

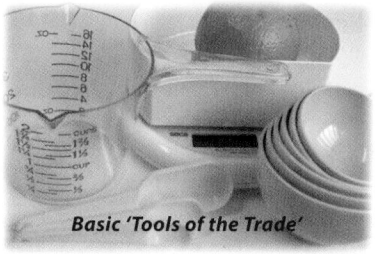

Basic 'Tools of the Trade'

CALORIEKING PORTION WATCH

Fries | Cal | Fat | Carb

Fries	Cal	Fat	Carb
Small	230	11	29
Medium	380	19	48
Large	500	25	63

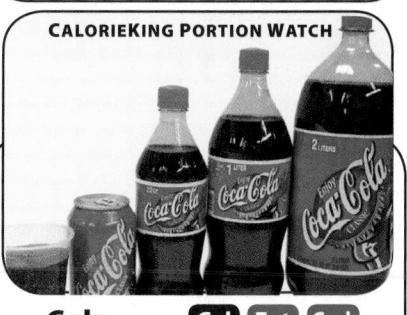

CALORIEKING PORTION WATCH

Cola | Cal | Fat | Carb

Cola	Cal	Fat	Carb
8 fl.oz Cup	100	0	25
12 fl.oz Can	150	0	37
20 fl.oz Bottle	250	0	63
1 Liter Bottle	400	0	100
2 Liter Bottle	800	0	200

Actual weight of this bun is 24% more than the stated net weight.

Recommended Fat Intake

► Fat in the Diet

Fats in the diet are essential for good health. However, too much fat can contribute to obesity and a higher risk of heart disease, high blood pressure, diabetes, gallstone and certain cancers.

Dietary fat and oils have over double the calories of carbohydrates and protein. (Example: Changing from whole-milk to non-fat milk halves the calories.)

MAXIMUM DESIRABLE FAT INTAKE (DAILY)	
Calories	**Fat**
1200 cals	30g fat
1500 cals	40g fat
1800 cals	50g fat
2000 cals	60g fat
2200 cals	70g fat
2500 cals	80g fat
3000 cals	110g fat

ZERO GRAMS TRANS FAT

*Don't be fooled by **Zero Grams Trans Fat** boldly displayed on some high-fat snacks. They are still high in fat and calories.*

Examples: Cheetos 99c pkg ~ 24g fat, 380 cals Lay's Chips (2¾ oz pkg) ~ 27g fat, 430 calories

0 grams Trans Fat

► Beware low-fat foods

It is a mistake to think that eating low-fat or fat-free foods allows you to eat double the quantity. You can end up with even more calories than eating smaller amounts of regular-fat products.

Food products which are fat-free but high in calories include soda drinks, fruit juices, beer, alcoholic spirits, sugar and candy. Bread, rice and pasta also have negligible fat but need to be eaten in controlled amounts.

Ultimately, **it is food portion size as well as total calories that count** whether from fat, carbohydrate or protein. Remember, cows get fat on grass!

Reduced fat and fat-free foods are not necessarily low calorie. Portion size is still important.

3 Cookies
140 Calories

6 oz Fat-Free Muffin:
450 calories

FOOD LABEL MEANINGS

FDA Nutrition Claim Definitions
(All are on a Per Serving Basis)

Low Calorie: 40 Calories or less

Light or Lite: One third fewer calories or, 50% or less fat than regular product

Fat-Free: Less than half a gram of fat

Low-Fat: 3 grams or less of fat

Reduced Fat: 25% less fat than regular product

Fewer or Less Calories: At least 25% fewer calories than regular product

▶ Meats, Poultry, Fish

- **Choose lean cuts** of meat with little marbling. **Trim all visible fat** from meat and remove the skin from poultry. Removal of fat after cooking, is okay (to prevent dryness). Choose 'extra lean' ground beef.
- **Avoid high-fat meat products** such as salami, bacon, sausage and franks.
- **Broil or bake. Avoid frying in oil.** Allow casseroles to cool and skim off surface fat.
- **Avoid fried fish**, frozen fish in batter and canned fish in oil.

▶ Fats & Oils

- **Use minimal amounts** of all types of fat and oil. All are high in calories.
- **Choose** 'light' and 'reduced fat' spreads but still use sparingly.
- Use minimal amounts of oil when stir-frying. Use no-stick sprays like Pam.

▶ Salad Dressings & Sauces

- **Avoid regular mayonnaise and oil dressings.** Choose 'light', 'reduced fat' or 'fat-free' brands.
- **Choose low-fat or fat-free sauces** (mainly tomato-based). Avoid 'pesto', 'alfredo', 'cheese' and 'creamy' sauces.

▶ Milk, Cheese

- **Choose low-fat or nonfat milks and yogurts.** Avoid full-cream milk, cream, Half & Half.
- **Cheese:** Choose fat-free, and low-fat cheese. Part-skim ricotta is still high in fat. Low-fat cottage cheese is a good choice. Cheese substitutes can still be high in fat.

▶ Snacks, Cookies, Candy

- **Avoid** high-fat snacks such as potato chips, corn/tortilla chips, cheese puffs, buttered popcorn, chocolate and carob bars.

▶ Desserts/Sweets

- **Avoid high-fat desserts**, such as cake, pie, pastries, cheesecake, full-fat puddings.
- **Choose** fresh fruits, fresh fruit salad, canned fruit in water pack, low-fat ice cream. Use low-fat yogurt in place of cream.

▶ Fast-Foods & Take-Out

Check the Fast-Foods Section of this book for actual fat and calorie counts.

- **Avoid deep-fried foods such as** chicken, french fries and onion rings.
- **Pizzas:** Avoid sausage/pepperoni. Choose vegetarian topping and modest quantity of cheese. Eat a moderate serving. Eat extra salad and fresh fruit.
- **Hamburgers:** Choose medium size, lower fat burgers. Avoid bacon. Have a side salad (with fat-free dressing).
- **Delis:** Choose sandwiches/bread rolls, pitas with low-fat fillings and plain salad. Limit meat/cheese to small portions.
- **Coffees:** Avoid large sizes of latte and frappuccino. Request nonfat milk and no whipped cream. Avoid cookies and pastries.

Extra Information: www.CalorieKing.com

FRYING ADDS FAT!

The greater the surface area of potato exposed to fat or oil, the higher the fat content and calories.

 Whole Potato (3 oz)
0g Fat 65 Cals

 Roasted Potato (3 oz)
5g Fat 155 Cals

 Fries (Large cut, 3 oz)
12g Fat 220 Cals

 Fries (Small, 3 oz)
15g Fat 265 Cals

 Potato Chips (3 oz)
30g Fat 450 Cals

Naturally-Friendly Carbs

- **Carbohydrate foods in their more natural forms** (not overly processed) are essential to good health. They are the main source of fuel for the body, and also provide important vitamins, minerals, antioxidants and fiber – all of which help protect against heart disease, diabetes, hypertension, constipation-related ailments and many other diseases.

Carbohydrate foods (minimally processed) are essential to good health.

Be sure to eat adequate fruit and vegetables (5 - 7 servings) every day.

- Carbohydrates even help the body produce serotonin, the 'feel good' brain chemical that helps control appetite and overeating. Too little serotonin can lead to mood swings and depression.

Carbohydrates are found in different forms in food as:

- Sugars in fruit, sugar cane, milk
- Starches in whole grains, legumes, nuts, seeds and vegetables
- Dietary fiber (See Fiber Guide ~ Page 264)

Glycemic Index & Diabetes ~ Page 21

RECOMMENDED CARBOHYDRATE INTAKE

Calories (Daily)	Carbohydrate (Grams)	Percent Carbohydrate Calories
1200 cals	100-120g	35-40%
1500 cals	140-170g	40-45%
1800 cals	180-200g	40-45%
2000 cals	200-250g	40-50%
2500 cals	310-350g	50-55%
3000 cals	410-450g	55-65%

How Much Do We Need?

- As shown in the chart, well-balanced diets above 2000 calories contain 50-60% of total calories from carbohydrates.
- At lower calorie levels used for weight control (1200-1500 calories), carbohydrates account for as little as 40% of total calories. This is because protein calories have nutritional priority.
- Carbohydrates & Diabetes ~ *See Page 21*

Low-Carbohydrate Diets

- Popular low-carbohydrate diets are extreme in their recommendations to initially cut carb intake to as little as 20 grams per day – the amount in 1 thick slice of bread, or 1 medium apple, or 1 small potato.

  This greatly increases the risk of nutritional deficiencies and compromises health, particularly if fat intake is excessive through fatty meats, high-fat dairy products, and fried foods.

- While overweight Americans do need to reduce carbohydrate intake, it should be done **sensibly as part of reducing portion size and total calories.**

- Simply eating 'low-carb' food products without regard to portion size, calories or fats, will do little to promote weight loss or good health.

- **Low-carb diets (and indeed any diet) only work if total calories are reduced.**

  FAT MATTERS CARBS COUNT BUT CALORIES ARE KING!

- Refined sugars should be one of the first targets in reducing carb intake.

Extra Info ~ www.CalorieKing.com

Sugar-free & lower carb products may still be high in calories and fat.

- **Excess Sugar:** Many overweight, inactive people consume over 500 calories of refined sugars per day, either self-added or as part of food products. This is equivalent to over 30 level teaspoons – a significant amount in weight control terms. Halving this amount would be reasonable and worthwhile.

Note: Naturally occurring sugars in fruits, vegetables and milk are fine when consumed in normal recommended amounts. These foods are also rich in other nutrients.

Refined sugar is referred to as having **'empty calories'**. Sugar supplies calories but negligible nutrients and no fiber.

- **Most sugar in our diet is 'hidden'** in processed foods such as soft drinks, fruit drinks, candy, cookies, cake, jam, sauces, ice cream, desserts, canned foods, and processed breakfast cereals.

For serious weight control, severely limit these foods and substitute healthier higher fiber wholefoods.

Note: Be careful not to substitute sugar-rich foods with high-fat foods which might boost calories even more!

- **Be aware that sugar comes in different forms** such as sucrose, glucose, fructose, malt, high-fructose corn syrup, molasses, honey and maple syrup. Check the label.

- **Sugar alcohols** such as sorbitol, mannitol and maltitol are carb-based and have ½ - ¾ the calories of regular sugar. While not counted as sugar on food labels, they do add to the carb count. Excess amounts can cause bloating, gas and diarrhea.

- **Sugar-free sweeteners** make it easy to reduce sugar in drinks and recipes. However, use minimally since research suggests possible ill-effects of some artificial sweeteners on friendly gut microbes. This may increase the risk of glucose intolerance and an increase in appetite.

Note: Most recipes can be adapted to contain less sugar with little effect on taste.

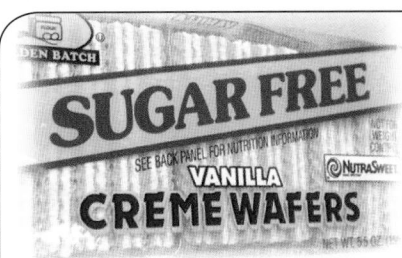

Sugar-free snacks and foods may be higher in fat and calories than the regular product.

Example	~ Creme Wafers (3):
Regular	~ 115 cals, 6g fat
Sugar-Free	~ 160 cals, 10g fat

SUGAR CONTENT OF SOME COMMON FOODS

Teaspoons of Sugar

Coca Cola or Pepsi, 12 fl.oz	10
20 fl.oz size	17
Iced Tea, sweetened, 12 fl.oz	8
Chocolate Milk, 12 fl.oz	6
Honey Smacks Cereal, ¾ cup, 1 oz	4
Popcorn, caramel, 1 cup	3.5
Chocolate Bar, 1.5 oz	6
M&M's 1.7 oz pkg	7
Muffin, large, 4 oz	6
Choc Chip Cookie, 1 oz	2
Donut, iced	6
Apple Pie, 1 piece	7
Jell-O, ½ cup	4.5
Jam, 1 Tbsp, ¾ oz	2.5
Syrup, maple, 1 Tbsp	3

Reach for fresh fruit when you want to snack instead of candy or snack products rich in sugar and fat.

Tips For Overweight Kids & Parents!

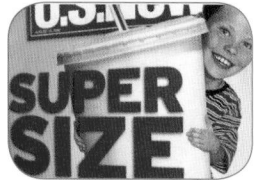

The XL Generation

Some 15% of American kids and adolescents are overweight; and childhood obesity has doubled over the last 20 years. Diabetes, high blood pressure and high cholesterol are major problem areas for overweight children and adolescents, as are depression, low self-esteem, sleep apnea and bone joint problems.

To address this problem, cooperation is required between kids, parents, schools and government. Weight control is a family and community affair.

Five Simple Tips To Get Started:

❶ Watch Soda Intake

Limit soda and sugary drinks to one serving on the weekends. Soda should not be an everyday beverage – water should be. When at restaurants or using a soda fountain, choose small servings with ice or choose diet soda instead. Schools should provide water and restrict access to soda as should parents when eating out or in the home!

❷ Cut back on Fast-Foods and Eating Out

Many more calories are consumed when you eat out. Healthy meals prepared at home are best for the whole family.

❸ Say "No" to Super-Sizing

When meals are upsized, loads more calories are consumed. Choose sensible portion sizes when eating out and at home. Use smaller plates and choose smaller packages.

❹ Limit Between-Meal Snacking

Watch out for high-fat and high-calorie snacks – they can have more calories than a meal! Keep your eye on portion sizes and limit salty snack foods and candy to parties and special occasions. Choose fresh fruit, vegetables, nuts and low-fat milk instead.

❺ Get Moving ~ Watch Less TV

Kids need at least 60 minutes of physical activity every day. It's critical for their fitness, and greatly lessens the risk of obesity.

Encourage kids to be active out of school hours. Wearing a pedometer can be highly motivational for kids to move more – as can playing dance video games such as *Dance Dance Revolution*. *Dance Central* (XBox360) and *Wii Fit (Nintendo)* are also excellent fitness motivators.

Limit TV and non-active computer games to just one hour per day. Also limit the accompanying snacks! Include exercise in family activities.

Extra information and tips ~ www.CalorieKing.com

Sample Meal Plan – 1400 Calories

For Healthy, Overweight Persons ~ Not for Persons With Any Medical Condition
~ Please Check With Your Doctor & Dietitian ~

Breakfast (approx. 300 cal)

	1 Small Fruit or ½ oz Dried Fruit
Plus	Cereal: 1½ oz Dry (high fiber)
	or 1 cup cooked Oatmeal
Plus	½ oz Almonds/Seeds
Plus	Milk (from daily allowance) or Yogurt (low-fat)

Daily Milk Allowance (approx.160 calories)
2 cups Non-Fat Milk or 1½ cups Low-fat (1%) Milk
or equivalent Soy Drink, Yogurt, Cheese, Tofu

Fat Allowance (140 calories; 15g Fat)
4 tsp Fat or 6-8 tsp Diet Margarine or 3 tsp Oil
or 1½ Tbsp Mayonnaise or ½ medium Avocado
or 1½ Tbsp Peanut Butter or 30g Nuts/Seeds

Breakfast ~ Choice 2

	1 Small Fruit
Plus	2 Eggs (no added fat)
	or 2 oz Cheese (low-fat)
	or 4 oz Cottage Cheese (low-fat)
	or 2 oz Lean/Canadian Bacon
Plus	1 Tomato
Plus	1 Slice Wholegrain Toast

Between Meals

Water, Coffee, Tea, Diet drinks,
Fruit from main meals; Raw vegetable
pieces, Milk from Daily Allowance

Lunch (approx. 440 calories)

	2 slices Wholegrain Bread (2 oz)
	or 4 Crispbreads/Crackers or 6" Pita
Plus	2 oz lean Meat, Chicken or Turkey
	or 3½ oz Tuna (in water) or 2½ oz Salmon
	or 1 oz Cheese or ½ cup (4 oz) Cottage Cheese
	or ½ cup (4 oz) Ricotta Cheese (low-fat)
	or ½ cup (4 oz) Fruit Yogurt (low-fat)
	or ½ cup (4 oz) Bean Salad
Plus	Large Salad (Oil-free dressing)
Plus	1 small Fruit or ½ oz Dried Fruit

Dinner (approx. 360 calories)

	Soup (fat-free)
Plus	3 oz lean Meat (cooked weight)
	or 4 oz Chicken Breast (no skin)
	or 3 oz Chicken Thigh/Leg (no skin)
	or 5 oz Fish (grilled, no fat)
	or ¾ cup (6 oz) Beans (Soy, Kidney, Pinto etc)/Lentils
	or Low-fat Entree (e.g. Lean Cuisine)
Plus	1 small Potato
	or ½ cup Rice/Pasta/Sweet Corn
	or 1 slice Wholegrain Bread
Plus	2-3 servings Vegetables/Salad
Plus	1 small Fruit + Diet Gelatin Dessert

- **Persons who exercise regularly lose more weight** and keep it off longer than non-exercisers. Blood glucose control also improves; as do beneficial gut microbes.
- **Exercise also improves general health and well-being.** Mood, confidence and self-esteem are also enhanced.
- **Exercise** is a good way to 'wake up' a sluggish metabolism and burn excess body fat.
- **Aerobic (huff and puff) exercise most days** is great for burning calories and for cardiovascular fitness. But, it is strength training that mainly builds the muscles that burn calories.
- **Strength training is the key to retaining or rebuilding muscles.** As we age, we lose some 6 pounds of muscle per decade. This results in a lower metabolism and fewer calories burnt.

  Muscles are the furnaces that burn calories. The more muscle you have, the more calories burnt – and as a bonus, the more food you can eat.
- **Regular strength training (2-3 times weekly)** can increase our metabolic rate for several days following exercise – with up to an extra 100 calories per day being burnt.

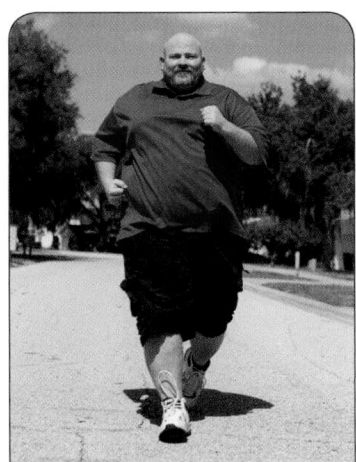

Brisk walking each day is a safe and effective way to burn calories and keep fit.
Try it – you'll like it!
Be sure to wear sun-protective clothing.

  While 2-3 pounds of muscle may be gained in the first 8-10 weeks, weight from exercised muscles is ok. It is excess fat (particularly abdominal fat) that is a potential health hazard.
- **Body reshaping** is enhanced by gaining muscle and losing fat - even if the scales don't show it.
- **Avoid injury** by beginning with walking, low impact aerobics, or weight-supported exercise (e.g. swimming, cycling). Avoid competitive sports. Allow 2-3 days of recovery between strength training sessions. Get professional advice.
- **How Much?** Start with 10-20 minutes per day and progress to 30-60 minutes per day. Also walk up stairs instead of using elevators. Take a brisk walk at lunch. Use an exercise bike, treadmill or stair machine while watching TV. Walk the dog.
- **How Often?** While aerobic fitness may require only 3-4 sessions weekly, **weight control is a daily event which requires daily exercise to burn calories.** Also add in strength training 2-3 times weekly.

Note: Persons on cholesterol-lowering statin drugs may experience muscle pains and weakness (as well as damage to muscle microfibrils). Supplementing with coenzyme Q10, magnesium, selenium, vitamins D and K2, may be beneficial. Check with your healthcare provider.

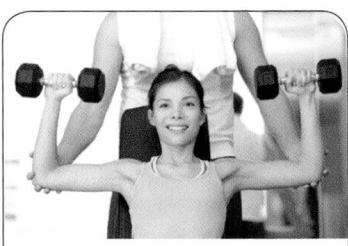

Strength training is the key to retain or rebuild muscles.
Exercized muscles burn extra calories even while you sleep.
For extra guidance and motivation, seek a qualified trainer or join a gym.

Calories Used in Exercise

LIGHT	MODERATE	HEAVY
130 lbs ~ 3 Cals/Min	130 lbs ~ 5 Cals/Min	130 lbs ~ 8 Cals/Min
170 lbs ~ 4 Cals/Min	170 lbs ~ 6 Cals/Min	170 lbs ~ 10 Cals/Min
220 lbs ~ 5 Cals/Min	220 lbs ~ 7 Cals/Min	220 lbs ~ 12 Cals/Min

LIGHT
- Walking, slow
- Cycling, light
- Frisbee playing
- Gardening, light
- Golf, social
- Tennis, doubles
- Housework, cleaning
- Calisthenics, light
- Bowling
- Ping-pong, social
- Ice Skating, light
- Aquarobics, light
- Skate Boarding
- Line/Square Dancing
- Tai Chi, Yoga
- Volleyball

MODERATE
- Walking, brisk
- Cycling, moderate
- Swimming, crawl
- Weight-training, light
- Tennis, moderate
- Racquetball, beginners
- Aerobics, light
- Football, touch
- Basketball, Baseball
- Walking Downstairs
- Snow Skiing (downhill)
- Shovelling snow
- Dancing (ballroom)
- Rowing, moderate
- Volleyball, competitive

HEAVY
- Walking (power), Jogging
- Cycling (vigorous)
- Swimming, strenuous
- Weight-training, heavy
- Wrestling/Judo, advanced
- Racquetball, advanced
- Tae Bo, Kick Boxing
- Football, training
- Basketball (Pro)
- Climbing Stairs
- Skipping Rope
- Skiing (cross country)
- Aquarobics, advanced
- Dancing (strenuous), Zumba
- Rowing, vigorous
- Martial Arts

Note: Only those sports or activities that are sustained over a period of time (e.g running) qualify for heavy exercise. Stop-start sports such as tennis are considered 'moderate'.

WALKING PROGRAM

USE DISTANCE, STEPS OR TIME

Weeks	Distance	Steps (Pedometer)	Time
1-2	1 mile	2000	20 mins
3-5	1.5 miles	3000	28 mins
6-8	2 miles	3500	35 mins
9-10	2.5 miles	4500	45 mins
11+	3.5 miles	6000	60 mins

10,000 STEPS PER DAY

A pedometer can motivate you to be more active. It clips to your belt or waist band and registers each step.

Alternatively, use a *Fitbit*, *Garmin* or *Striiv* activity tracker, or your smartphone inbuilt accelerometer.

Aim for 8,000 - 10,000 steps per day, insead of an average of only 3,000 - 4,000 steps.

- Eating is a behavior that is largely controlled by people with whom we live or socialize, places in which we carry out our lives, and our emotions. Become aware of those situations that commonly lead to extra food being eaten.

- We may also be unaware of 'bad' eating habits that can lead to excess calorie intake; e.g. eating quickly, large mouthfuls, eating when tense or bored, finishing a large serving of food when not hungry.

Tips to help uncover and correct those 'bad' or problem eating habits:

- **Don't eat while engaged in other activities;** for example, watching TV, reading. Eat only at the table, not at the fridge or while standing.

- **Don't eat quickly.** Chewing slowly allows time to register a feeling of fullness. Don't use fingers, only utensils. Cut food into smaller pieces. Don't load your fork until the previous mouthful is finished.

Practice saying 'NO' politely but assertively.

- **Don't purchase problem high calorie foods.** Shop from a set list to prevent impulse buying. Avoid shopping with children.

- **Buy snack foods** in the smallest package. The larger the serving size or package, the more you are likely to eat or drink.

- **Plan meals in advance. Stick to a set menu.**

- **Plan a strategy to avoid uncontrolled eating** and drinking at social events, or when your emotions urge you to binge.

  Rehearse repeatedly in your mind exactly what you will do in such situations. Remind yourself several times each day that you are in charge of your actions and that you can be strong-willed. Seek counseling or coaching on various strategies.

- **Distract yourself** when you feel the urge to snack impulsively. Engage in some activity that will distract you from thinking about food. Examples: go for a walk, brush your teeth, phone a friend.

  If you eat out of boredom, find some new hobby or interest that gets you out of the house. Even enrol in an adult education class.

Do you use food as an emotional crutch? If so, professional counseling may be helpful.

The food journal is the most powerful proven aid for dieters. Persons who keep a food and exercise journal not only lose more weight, they also keep it off. Here are some of the reasons:

- **Recording your eating and exercise habits** jolts you into realizing just what you do eat and drink each day; and also whether you exercise sufficiently.

- **Helps you identify problem foods** and drinks with excessive calories and fat.

- **Helps identify moods**, situations and events that lead to excessive eating of unwanted calories. You can then plan to overcome or avoid them.

- **Prevents 'calorie amnesia'**, the forgetfulness that leads to rebound weight gain after successful weight loss. Recording puts you back on the right track.

- **Helps you develop greater self-discipline.** You will think twice about overindulging if you have to record it - especially if someone checks your journal regularly. It certainly keeps you honest!

- **Motivates you** to carefully plan your meals and to exercise each day.

- **Serves as a check system** for your doctor, dietitian or counselor to assess your progress and make recommendations.

Write It Down!

"Keeping a journal gives me feedback on exactly what I eat and drink each day.

It helps prevent 'calorie amnesia' and reminds me to exercise each day.

It's a 'must' for successful weight control!"

3 Easy Ways to Track Your Food & Exercise Calories!

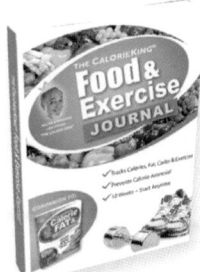

CalorieKing Online
Part of a comprehensive personalized program that includes tools, reports and a supportive community.

CalorieKing App
ControlMyWeight
Make smart food choices wherever you are!
Easy to use.

Book
A 10-week journal that fits in your pocket. Includes Weekly Summary page and Progress Checklist.

Extra Information ~ www.CalorieKing.com

Diabetes Guide

What is Diabetes?

Diabetes occurs when the body has difficulty processing glucose sugar in the blood.

- **After digestion**, sugar and starches are changed into **glucose** – the simplest form of sugar vital for body energy and growth.
- Insulin is the hormone which acts like a key that opens the door to body cells and allows glucose to enter.
- **Without enough insulin**, glucose builds up in the blood and passes into the urine. High blood glucose levels lead to frequent urination, extreme thirst, and tiredness.
- **Untreated diabetes increases the risk of damage to nerves and blood vessels.** This, in turn, increases the risk of heart disease, stroke, blindness, kidney damage, foot ulcers and gangrene (with amputation), impotence, Alzheimer's Disease and other prolems.

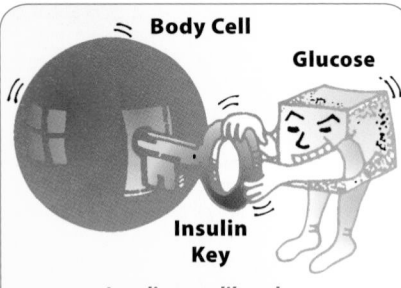

Insulin acts like a key.
It opens the door to body cells and allows glucose to enter.

People with type 1 diabetes and some with type 2 have too few or no keys and require insulin injections.

Others (primarily type 2) make enough insulin but the body doesn't use it as well as it should – particularly if obese and inactive.

SYMPTOMS OF DIABETES

- Frequent urination
- Extreme thirst
- Unusual hunger
- Rapid weight loss
- Extreme fatigue
- Blurred vision
- Skin infections that are slow to heal
- Tingling/numbness in feet

Note: Diabetes can be present even with no symptoms.

DON'T IGNORE DIABETES
IT'S A SERIOUS DISEASE!

TYPE 2 DIABETES

- Occurs in 90% of diabetes cases
- Occurs mainly in adults - particularly in overweight and inactive persons
- Insulin is produced but body cells resist its action and glucose   cannot enter cells
- Usually treated with meal planning and physical activity. Sometimes requires medication (pills or insulin)

TYPE 1 DIABETES

- Occurs in 10% of diabetes cases
- Usually in children and young adults
- Pancreas produces little or no insulin. Daily insulin injections (or use of an insulin pump) are necessary, as well as:
  - matching pre-meal insulin to the amount of carbohydrate eaten
  - weight control and regular physical activity

GESTATIONAL DIABETES

- Occurs in some women during pregnancy. It usually disappears after the baby's birth.
- Women who have had gestational diabetes still have a high risk of developing type 2 diabetes within 5 to 10 years. One in 3 do.
- Requires weight control, a healthy lifestyle and regular medical checks during and after pregnancy.

Are You At Risk for Diabetes?

Pre-Diabetes ~ An Early Warning!

Pre-diabetes means your blood glucose levels are higher than normal, but not high enough to be called diabetes.

If you have pre-diabetes, you have a higher risk for getting diabetes later on.

The good news is that you can start taking steps to prevent diabetes by making healthy lifestyle changes – such as losing weight if overweight, and being more physically active.

WHAT'S YOUR RISK?

Find out if you're at risk for diabetes by answering the following questions:

☐ I have been told I have pre-diabetes

☐ I have a family history of diabetes

☐ I am African American, Latino American, Asian American, Native American or a Pacific Islander

☐ I have had gestational diabetes (diabetes during pregnancy)

☐ I am over age 45

☐ I am overweight

☐ My waist is larger than: 35 inches (for a woman) or 40 inches (for a man)

☐ I get little or no physical activity

☐ My blood pressure is higher than 130 over 85

☐ My HDL (good cholesterol) is too low

☐ My triglycerides (blood fats) are too high

 CHECK YOUR RESULT

• If you've put a check mark in two or more of the boxes, you may be more likely to develop type 2 diabetes.

• Talk with your healthcare provider to see if you should have a blood test for diabetes.

BLOOD GLUCOSE CLASSIFICATION OF DIABETES

Normal:	**Below 100 mg/dl***
Pre-Diabetes:	**100-125 mg/dl***
Diabetes:	**Over 125 mg/dl***

(*Fasting Blood Glucose)

KNOW YOUR BGL

(Blood Glucose Level)
Everyone over the age of 45 should have a blood glucose test every three years.

Importance of Weight Control

• **Type 2 diabetes** is more common in people who are overweight.

• **Being overweight** means that your insulin doesn't work as well to control blood glucose levels.

• **Losing just 10 to 20 pounds** can help you better manage your diabetes and lower your risk for heart disease.

Keys to weight control include:

• Follow a healthy eating plan

• Control food portions.

• Be physically active every day. Track your daily activity.

• Keep food records ~ *See Page 15*

• Get the support of family and friends.

• **Work with a registered dietitian** who can help you reach a weight that's ideal for you.

KEEP MOVING!

Every day, do at least 30 minutes of moderate intensity exercise.
(even in 5-minute sets)

It's the key to improving insulin action.
Add muscle strength training 3-4 times a week to double the benefits.

Managing Diabetes

Don't battle diabetes alone. Establish a partnership with your doctor, dietitian, certified diabetes educator, and pharmacist.

Extra Support:
- American Association of Diabetes Educators
- American Diabetes Association
- BeyondType1.org
- Joslin Diabetes Center
- Juvenile Diabetes Research Foundation
- National Diabetes Education Program

Tips to keep blood glucose within safe limits:

- **Control your food intake.** Know what and when you will eat. Seek referral to a dietitian for expert advice.
- **Exercise regularly.** It assists weight control and can improve sensitivity of body cells to insulin. Plan physical activity into your daily routine.
- **Monitor your blood glucose** at home and work with a blood glucose meter. It will help you become familiar with your blood glucose patterns, and the effects of food, activity and medication.
- **Take insulin or oral medication as prescribed.** If on insulin, know what action to take if hypoglycemia (low blood glucose) occurs. Also educate your family and friends.

Be Heart Smart ~ Know Your ABCs

If you have diabetes, you are at a higher risk for heart attack and stroke than someone without diabetes. But you can fight back!

Be smart about your heart!

Take control of the ABCs of diabetes and live a long and healthy life. Talk to your healthcare provider about your ABC targets.

A is for A1C
The A1C (A-one-C) test – short for hemoglobin A1C. It reflects your average blood glucose (sugar) over the last 3 months.
Suggested Target: Below 7%

B is for Blood Pressure
High blood pressure makes your heart work too hard.
Suggested Target: Below 130/80

C is for Cholesterol
Bad cholesterol, or LDL, can build up and clog your arteries. **Suggested Target: Below 100**

Blood glucose meters and insulin pumps can greatly improve control of diabetes

BLOOD GLUCOSE METERS (EXAMPLES)

INSULIN PUMPS (EXAMPLES)

Roche
Accu-Chek

Medtronic
MiniMed

Be Smart About Your **Heart**
Control the ABCs of **Diabetes**
➤ A1C
➤ Blood Pressure
➤ Cholesterol

National Diabetes Education Program

Be smart about your heart!
Take control of the ABC's of diabetes and live a long and healthy life.

Talk to your healthcare provider about your ABC targets.

Take action now to lower your risk for heart attack, stroke and other diabetes problems.

◄ *Note: These targets are suggested by the National Institutes for Health and the American Diabetes Association*

Guidelines for choosing a healthy diet apply equally to people with or without diabetes. Eating a wide variety of foods that are mainly low in fat, low in refined sugars, and high in fiber, is recommended.

However, actual food quantities, as well as when you eat, will also influence control of b l o o d glucose. Your dietitian will individualize a meal plan to suit your food preferences, lifestyle and medical status.

Here are a few tips:

- **Maintain a healthy weight.** If overweight, even a modest weight loss plus daily physical activity can help manage blood glucose in type 2 diabetes.

- **Don't skip meals.** If you take insulin or an oral hypoglycemic agent, regular meals are important.

  If on insulin, eat meals at the same time each day. Eat a similar amount of food at each meal. Eating about the same amount of carbohydrate over the day will make best use of insulin and prevent wide variations in blood glucose levels.

- **Know which foods contain carbohydrate;** and learn how to check the *Nutrition Facts Label* on foods. Check the serving size, total fat and total carbohydrate – not just the sugar content. All carbohydrate breaks down to sugars after digestion.

- **Choose wholegrain breads, cereals and pasta.** Eat fresh fruits, vegetables and legumes. These foods contain more fiber and slow the release of glucose into your blood after a meal.

- **Limit foods high in saturated fat, trans fat and cholesterol.** Enjoy fish, soy foods, and other foods rich in omega-3 fats. *(Extra Notes: Page 259)*

- **Limit sugars and foods high in added sugar** particularly if overweight. Small amounts of sugar as part of a meal may occasionally be okay. Check with your dietitian. *(Extra Notes: Page 9)*

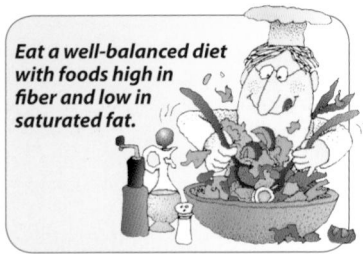

Eat a well-balanced diet with foods high in fiber and low in saturated fat.

A fiber-rich diet assists the growth of friendly gut microbes that can benefit our metabolism, weight and blood glucose levels – as well as hunger, mood and our immune system.
(Also see Fiber Guide ~ Page 264)

ALCOHOL TIPS

- **If you drink alcohol, have only moderate amounts:**
  Men ~ 1-2 drinks/day
  Women ~ 1 drink/day
  For some people, safe drinking will mean no alcoholic drinks at all.
  (Also see Alcohol Guide ~ Page 23)

- **Drink along with your food** – especially if you use insulin or diabetes pills.

- **Do not omit any carb food** in exchange for an alcoholic drink. However, non-alcoholic beers (12 fl oz) count as one carb exchange.

- **Alcohol increases the risk of hypoglycemia** (low blood sugar) and drug interactions if you take insulin and certain types of diabetes pills.

- **Check with your doctor and dietitian.**

The Plate Method – An Easy Way to Eat Healthfully

The plate method is a helpful tool to guide your food choices until you see a dietitian for your own meal plan.

For a healthy meal:

- Fill half of your plate with non-starchy vegetables (broccoli, green beans, carrots).
- Fill a quarter of your plate with carbohydrate (wholegrain bread, pasta, potato, brown rice).
- Fill the other quarter of your plate with 3-4 ounces of lean meat, poultry, or fish.
- Use 1-2 teaspoons of tub margarine or a heart-healthy vegetable oil.
- Add a small piece of fruit or 8 ounces of skim/low-fat milk or yogurt.

MAIN MEAL

Vegetables & Salad Greens

Bread • Starch • Grain

Meat • Protein

PLUS ONE CHOICE

Milk, Fruit, Dessert or other Carb Food

How Much Carbohydrate Should You Eat?

A dietitian can best determine how much carbohydrate you need at each of your meals, based on your lifestyle, food preferences, and overall diabetes control.

Until you see a dietitian, aim to keep the amount of carbohydrate you eat the same at each of your meals.

CARB CHOICES MEAL PLAN
One Carb Choice = 15 Grams of Carb

The amount in: 1 slice Bread
or ¾ cup Cereal (unsweetened)
or 1 small Potato **or** 1 small Fruit

Breakfast
- Eat 2-3 carb choices (30-45 grams)
- Include a low-fat protein source such as egg whites or skim milk.

Lunch and Dinner
- Eat 3-4 carb choices (45-60 grams carb)
- Include fruit and non-starchy vegetables. Choose small portions of low-fat protein foods.

Snacks: If needed, eat 1-2 carb choices (15-30 grams carb).

Note: Above plan is for adults. Carbohydrate amounts will vary with physical activity level.

Carb Type Affects Blood Glucose

The various forms of carbohydrate affect blood glucose levels in different ways. It is difficult to predict the effect of particular foods, sugars, or meals, simply by their carbohydrate content.

Thus the same amount of carbohydrate from different foods may affect blood sugar levels very differently. **Many factors affect the rate of digestion and absorption such as:**

- the type of sugar, starch, and fiber
- the degree of processing and cooking (which increases digestion rate)
- the amount of protein and fat (which slow stomach emptying and digestion).

Glycemic Index (GI)

The GI is a method of ranking carbohydrate foods on a scale (0-100) according to how they affect blood glucose levels. (See next column).

The higher the GI value, the greater the food's ability to rapidly raise blood glucose levels; and the more insulin that is needed by the body (not desirable).

Eating low-GI foods may lead to better control of blood glucose and insulin levels (which in turn lowers the risk of damage to blood vessels and nerves). The slower digestion of low-GI foods may also help to delay hunger pangs and benefit weight control.

Cautionary Notes on GI

Choosing low-GI foods is not a license to eat unlimited amounts. Calorie restriction and portion control for weight control is of prime importance.

Also remember, **low-GI foods are carbohydrate foods** and must still be counted as part of any dietetic carbohydrate plan.

GI is not meant to be used by itself without regard to portion size, and other dietary recommendations for healthy eating. Foods are not good or bad on the basis of their GI.

While GI may be a helpful tool for some people with diabetes, what is most important is to control the total amount of carbohydrate that you eat.

LOWER-GLYCEMIC FOODS

Slower-Acting Carbohydrates

These foods are more slowly digested and absorbed. They help maintain more even blood glucose levels, as long as excessive amounts are not eaten. Use these foods regularly but still limit portion size for weight control.

Examples:

- Dried beans, peas, lentils
- Nuts and seeds
- Wholegrain breads
- Bran cereals, oats
- Sweet corn, barley, quinoa buckwheat
- Wholegrain pasta, basmati rice
- Fresh fruit: apples, avocados, bananas (firm), berries, cherries, grapefruit, grapes, olives, oranges, pears, plums. Fresh juices.
- Vegetables: broccoli, yam, nopales, salad greens
- Milk, yogurt, soy drinks
- Dark chocolate, cacao
- Sugar alcohols (sorbitol, maltitol)

HIGHER-GLYCEMIC FOODS

Quicker-Acting Carbohydrates

These foods more rapidly raise blood glucose levels. Eat only in moderation.

- White bread, rice cakes, bagels, croissants, doughnuts
- Low-fiber cereals: Cornflakes, *Rice Krispies, Froot Loops*
- White potatoes, white rice
- Watermelon, ripe bananas, cantaloupe, pineapple
- Soda, sugar-sweetened sports and energy drinks
- Sugar, candy, popcorn (plain)
- Ice cream (low-fat), frozen yogurt

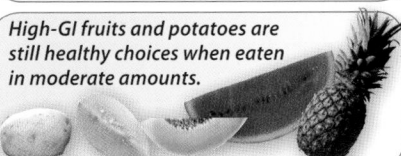

High-GI fruits and potatoes are still healthy choices when eaten in moderate amounts.

≫ **Calorie and fat values have been rounded off.**
Calories ~ to the nearest 5 or 10 calories.
Fat ~ to nearest half gram. **Note:** Trace amounts of fat (less than 0.3 grams) have been treated as zero.

≫ **Carbohydrate figures** in this book are for total carbohydrate, and not **Net Carbs** (which deducts fiber, polydextrose and sugar alcohols from total carbs).

≫ Because manufacturers' figures on labels are rounded off, figures in this book may differ slightly from the label. Serving sizes may also vary.

C ~ **Calories**
F ~ **Fat (grams)**
Cb ~ **Carbohydrate (grams)**

Abbreviations

tsp = teaspoon
Tbsp or T = Tablespoon
oz = ounce(s)
c = cup
fl.oz = fluid ounce(s)
g = gram(s)
avg = average
pkg = package

Volume Measures

(All measures are level)
3 tsp = 1 Tbsp
2 Tbsp = 1 fl.oz
½ cup = 4 fl.oz
1 cup = 8 fl.oz
2 cups = 1 Pint
2 Pints = 1 Quart
Note: 8 oz weight is not the same as 8 fl oz volume (space occupied). Dense foods weigh more per set volume. Examples:
1 cup popcorn weighs ½ oz
1 cup milk weighs 8½ oz
1 cup pudding weighs 10 oz

Metric Conversion

½ oz = 14 grams
1 oz = 28.4 grams
2 oz = 57 grams
3½ oz = 100 grams
1 fl.oz = 30 mls
1 cup (8 fl.oz) = 240 mls
33 fl.oz = 1 liter (volume)

IMPORTANT DISCLAIMER

* The authors and publishers of this book are not physicians and are not licensed to give medical advice. This book is not a substitute for professional advice. Users should consult their medical professional before making any health, medical or other decisions based on the material contained herein.

* This book is a compilation of original material from other sources intended for educational purposes only. Because food manufacturers constantly change their products, only they are the authoritative source for food's most current nutritional information.

* Persons using the information herein for any medical purposes, such as matching insulin dosage to carbohydrate intake, should not rely solely on the accuracy of figures herein and should independently check food labels or contact the food manufacturer for the latest data.

Canadian Readers:

Please note that figures in this book are based on U.S. food products and restaurants. Equivalent Canadian foods may vary and should be checked independently.

INFORMATION SOURCES
• U.S. Dept. of Agriculture
• U.S. Food Manufacturers
• Food Industry Boards & Councils
• Author extrapolations

FEEDBACK WELCOME!
Please contact the author with your queries and suggestions.
feedback@calorieking.com

- **Health Hazards: Excessive alcohol intake** contributes to obesity, high blood pressure, stroke, heart and liver disease, some cancers, and even impotence. **Concentration and short-term memory** are reduced as well as athletic performance.

  Other alcohol hazards include: Fetal Alcohol Syndrome, stomach upsets, gut dysbiosis, menstrual and menopausal problems, depression, snoring, sleep problems, work absenteeism, impaired judgement, risky behaviors and social/family problems.

- **Alcohol contributes to obesity** through its high calories and by lessening the body's ability to burn fat. Fat storage is promoted, particularly in the belly – a health danger zone. Alcohol can also stimulate the appetite; and weaken the dieter's resolve!

- **Alcohol is potentially more harmful while dieting:** Blood sugar levels may drop with resultant fatigue and further impairment of concentration, reflexes and driving skills.

Excess alcohol contributes to obesity, high blood pressure and many other health problems

LOWER RISK ALCOHOL LIMITS

WOMEN:
No more than
1 drink per day

MEN:
No more than
2 drinks per day
(1 drink if over 65 y.o.)

(At least 2 days a week should be alcohol-free)

1 DRINK CONTAINS 14 GRAMS ALCOHOL	12 fl.oz Regular Beer (5% Alc.)
	OR 14 fl.oz Light Beer (4.2% Alc.)
	OR 5 fl.oz Wine (12% Alc.)
	OR 1½ fl.oz Spirits (80 Proof)

Note: You cannot save daily drinks for one occasion. Binge drinking is particularly harmful: 4 drinks for males or 3 drinks for females (within 2 hours).

For some people, safe drinking means no alcohol at all. Even one drink may impair driving skills, particularly if tired. For women who drink frequently, breast cancer risk is increased by 9% for each drink after the first drink. In men, just 2 drinks a day doubles the risk of cancers of the mouth and throat.

It is advisable not to drink at all if you are:
- pregnant, trying to conceive or breastfeeding
- taking medication or have liver or heart disease (unless approved by your doctor or pharmacist)
- planning to drive, use machinery or play sports
- studying or needing to concentrate
- a child or adolescent

 Women and adolescents are more prone to alcohol's ill-effects due to their lower body weight, smaller livers and lesser capacity to metabolize alcohol. As we age, our ability to handle alcohol decreases.

HOW TO CALCULATE ALCOHOL CONTENT

Percent alcohol on label refers to alcohol volume (ml alcohol/100ml). **Note: 100ml = 3½ fl.oz**

To convert to grams (weight) of alcohol, multiply the alcohol volume by 0.8 – since 1 ml of alcohol weighs only 0.8 grams.

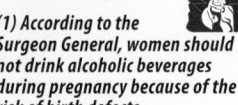

EXAMPLE:
12 fl.oz Can Beer (5% alcohol)
5% alc. volume
= 5% of 12 fl.oz = 0.6 fl.oz
= 18ml alcohol (Note: 1 fl.oz = 30ml)
Weight (18ml x 0.8) = 14.4g alcohol

GOVERNMENT WARNINGS!

(1) According to the Surgeon General, women should not drink alcoholic beverages during pregnancy because of the risk of birth defects.

(2) Consumption of alcoholic beverages impairs your ability to drive a car or operate machinery, and may cause health problems.

EXTRA INFORMATION
Alcohol & Diabetes ~ See Page 19
Alcohol & The Heart ~ See Page 18
Tips to Avoid Harmful Drinking ~ Page 19

Quick Guide   **Alc** ~ Alcohol (Grams)

Beer: **Cb** ~ Carbohydrate

Beer Contains Zero Fat: **C** **Alc** **Cb**

Regular Beer (5% Alc. Vol.):

	C	Alc	Cb
7 fl.oz Glass	80	8.5	4
12 fl.oz Bottle/Can/Glass	140	14	10
16 fl.oz/Pint	185	19	13
22 fl.oz Bottle	260	26	18
24 fl.oz Can	280	28	20
32 fl.oz/ ½ Yard	370	38	28
40 fl.oz Bottle	470	47	35
50 fl.oz Football	590	59	50

Light Beer (4.2% Alc. Vol.):

	C	Alc	Cb
7 fl.oz Glass	65	7	4
12 fl.oz Bottle/Can/Glass	110	12	7
16 fl.oz/Pint	145	16	9
22 fl.oz Bottle	200	22	13
24 fl.oz Can	220	24	14

Non-Alcoholic Brews:
(Less than 0.5% alcohol by volume)

	C	Alc	Cb
Average all Brands, 12 fl.oz	70	1	14

Beer ~ Brands

Note: Figure shown are for the United States except for the states of Utah, Colorado, Kansas and Oklahoma who have certain restrictions limiting the alcohol content to not more than 4% by volume (3.2% by weight).
Percentage alcohol listed is by volume - not by weight.
Per 12 fl.oz Serving

	C	Alc	Cb
Amstel, Light (3.5%)	95	10	5
Anchor: Porter (5.6%)	210	15	23
Steam (4.9%)	160	14	14
Asahi: Kuronama (5.3%)	165	14	14
Select (4.7%)	140	13	11
Super Dry (4.9%)	150	14	11
Bass, Pale Ale (5.1%)	155	14	12
Beck's: Original (5%)	145	14	11
Premier Light (2.3%)	65	7	4
Sapphire (6%)	160	17	9
Big Sky: Original IPA (6.2%)	195	18	17
Moose Drool (5.3%)	175	15	16
Scape Goat (4.7%)	155	14	14
Trout Slayer Ale (4.7%)	145	14	12
Blatz: Original (4.6%)	145	13	13
Light (3.9%)	110	11	8
Blue Moon:			
Belgian White (5.4%)	170	15	14
Cinnamon Horchata (5.5%)	175	15	16
Mango Wheat (5.4%)	175	15	16
Bohemia (4.73%)	140	14	12
Bud Ice (5.5%)	120	16	4

Brands (Cont)   **Alc** ~ Alcohol (Grams)

Per 12 fl.oz Serving

	C	Alc	Cb
Bud Light: Regular (4.2%)	110	12	7
& Clamato Chelada (4.2%)	150	12	16
Extra Lime (4.2%)	160	12	17
Coco-Nut-Rita Splash (4%)	205	12	32
Lime (4.2%)	115	12	8
Lime-A-Rita (8%), 8 oz	220	15	29
Lime Straw-Ber-Rita (8%), 8 oz	200	15	24
Budweiser: Lager (5%)	145	14	11
& Clamato Picante Chelada (5%)	200	14	23
Black Crown (6%)	165	17	10
Select (4.3%)	100	12	3
Select 55 (2.4%)	55	7	2
Busch: Original (4.3%)	115	12	7
Ice (5.9%)	135	17	4
Light (4.1%)	95	12	3
NA (0.4%)	60	1	13
Carlsberg, Pilsner (5%)	135	14	10
Carta Blanca (4.6%)	145	13	11
Castlemaine XXXX,			
Bitter (4.6%)	140	14	10
Cerveza, Aguila (4%)	125	11	11
Colt 45, Malt Liquor (5.6%)	155	16	11
Coors: Banquet (5%)	145	14	11
Extra Gold (5%)	150	14	12
Light (4.2%)	100	12	5
Corona: Extra (4.6%)	150	13	14
Light (4.1%)	100	12	5
Dos Equis XX: Ambar (4.7%)	145	14	12
Lager (4.5%)	140	13	11
Fosters: Lager (5%)	145	14	11
Premium Ale (5.5%)	160	16	13
Genesee: Lager (4.5%)	150	13	14
Genny Light Lager (4%)	100	10	4
George Killian's, Irish Red (5.4%)	170	16	15
Grolsch: Blonde (2.8%)	120	8	16
Light (3.6%)	95	11	6
Premium (5%)	145	14	10
Guinness: Draught (4%)	125	12	10
Extra Stout (6%)	175	17	14
Blonde American (5%)	150	14	11
Nitro IPA (5.8%), 11.2oz	155	19	5
Hamm's: Original (4.7%)	145	13	12
Special Light (3.9%)	110	12	8
Heineken: Lager (5%)	140	14	10
Special Dark (5%)	165	14	15
Premium Light (3.5%)	100	10	7
Hurricane: Malt Liquor (6%)	140	17	4
High Gravity (8.1%)	185	23	6
Icehouse: Original (5.5%)	150	16	10
Light (5%)	125	14	7
Keystone: Ice (5.9%)	145	17	6
Light (4.1%)	105	12	5

Brands (Cont)   Alc ~ Alcohol (Grams)

Cb ~ Carbohydrate   C   Alc   Cb

Beer Contains Zero Fat:
Per 12 fl.oz Serving

Per 12 fl.oz Serving Unless Indicated

	C	Alc	Cb
King Cobra (6%)	135	17	4
Kirin: Ichiban (5%)	145	14	11
Light (3.2%)	95	9	8
Kokanee Glacier (5%)	145	14	11
Labatt: Blue (5%)	135	14	10
Blue Light (4%)	110	11	8
Ultra Light, 52 Calories (2.2%)	52	6	2
Landshark, Lager (4.6%)	150	13	13
Leinenkugel's: Original (4.6%)	150	13	14
Summer Shandy (4.2%)	135	12	12
Lone Star: Pale Lager (4.65%)	135	13	11
Light (3.85%)	110	11	8
Lowenbrau, Original (5%)	140	14	12
Magic Hat, #9 (5.1% alc)	165	15	15
Magnum, Malt Liquor (5.6%)	155	16	11
Michelob: Amber Bock (5.1%)	150	14	12
Lager (4.8%)	160	14	14
Light (4.1%)	120	14	9
Golden Draft Light (4.1%)	110	12	7
Ultra Amber (4%)	95	11	3
Ultra Light (4.2%)	95	12	2.5
Ultra Lime Cactus (4%)	95	11	5.5
Mickey's, Malt Liquor (5.6%)	155	16	11
Miller: Chill, 100 Calorie (4.2%)	100	12	4
Genuine Draft /High Life (4.6%)	145	13	13
High Life Light (4.1%)	110	12	7
Lite (4.2%)	95	12	3
MGD 64 (2.8%)	65	8	2.5
Milwaukee's Best:			
Ice (5.9%)	145	17	7
Light (4.1%)	100	12	3.5
Premium (4.3%)	130	12	11
Minnesota's Best, Original (4.9%)	140	14	10
Modelo, Especial (4.4%)	145	13	14
Molson Canadian: Ice (5.6%)	170	16	14
Lager (5%)	150	14	11
Light (3.9%)	120	11	10
Moosehead, Lager (5%)	150	14	11
Natural: Ice (5.9%)	130	17	4
Light (4.2%)	95	12	3
Negra Modelo (5.4%)	175	15	14
Newcastle, Brown Ale (4.7%)	130	13	10
O'Douls: Amber (0.4%)	90	1	18
Original (0.4%)	65	1	13
Old Milwaukee:			
Lager (4.6%)	145	13	13
Light (3.8%)	110	11	8
Non-Alcoholic (0.4%)	60	1	12
Old Style: Lager (4.7%)	145	13	12
Light (4.2%)	115	12	7
Pabst: Blue Ribbon (4.7%)	145	13	12
Light (3.9%)	110	11	8

	C	Alc	Cb
Pacifico, Clara (4.4%)	145	13	13
Peroni, Nastro Azzurro	150	14	212
Piels, Lager (4.3%)	125	12	9
Pilsner Urquell, Lager (4.4%)	155	13	16
Point: Amber Classic (4.7%)	160	14	14
Special Lager (4.7%)	150	14	12
Redbridge, Lager (4%)	135	10	14
Red Dog, Lager (5%)	145	14	12
Red Hook: ESB (5.8%)	185	16	16
India Pale Ale (4.7%)	190	13	19
Red Stripe, Jamaican Ale (5%)	155	14	14
Redd's: Apple Ale (5%)	165	14	17
Wicked Hard Ale (8%), av.	275	22	30
Saint Archer: Blonde (4.8%)	150	14	13
Pale Ale (5.5%)	170	16	13
Samuel Adams:			
Boston Lager (4.9%)	175	14	17
Sam Adams, Light Lager (4%)	120	13	8
Sapporo, Prem. Lager (4.9%)	135	14	9
Schaefer: Lager (4.6%)	145	13	12
Light (3.9%)	110	11	8
Schell's: Deer (4.7%)	145	14	13
Light (3.5%)	100	10	7
Schlitz: Pale Lager (4.6%)	145	13	12
Light (3.8%)	110	11	8
Schmidt's: Pale Lager (4.6%)	145	13	13
Light (3.8%)	110	11	8
Sheaf, Stout (5.7%)	190	16	19
Shock Top: Belgian White (5.2%)	165	15	15
Lemon Shandy (4.2%)	145	12	15
Sierra Nevada: Bigfoot (9.6%)	330	28	32
Draft Pale Ale (5%)	155	14	13
Pale Ale (5.6%)	175	16	14
Sol (4.2%)	130	12	11
Sparks, Lager (6%)	250	17	34
Steel Reserve:			
High Gravity Malt Liquor (8.1%)	220	23	15
Steel 6 (6%)	160	17	11
Stella Artois, Pale Lager (5%)	155	14	13
Stroh's: Pale Lager (4.6%)	145	13	12
Light (3.9%)	115	11	7
Tecate: Pale Lager (4.6%)	140	13	11
Light (4%)	110	14	8
Third Shift, Amber Lager (5.3%)	185	15	18
Trader Jose: Premium, 11.2 fl.oz	145	14	14
Light (3.8%), 11.2 fl.oz	105	14	8
Victoria Lager (4%)	135	11	14
Widmer, Hefeweizen (4.9%)	155	14	13
Wild Blue, Lager (8%)	240	23	20
ZeigenBock, Amber (4.9%)	145	14	11

Alc ~ Alcohol (Grams)   **Cb** ~ Carbohydrate

Cider ~ Alcoholic/Hard

Per 12 fl.oz Unless Indicated

	C	Alc	Cb
Ace: Cider (5%), average all flavors	155	14	12
Joker (6.9%)	135	20	12
Angry Orchard: Crisp Apple (5%)	190	14	25
Easy Apple (4.2%)	150	12	19
Green Apple (5.5%)	210	14	31
Crispin: Original (5%), 12 fl.oz	150	14	15
Blackberry (5%), 12 fl.oz	160	14	16
Brut (5.5%), 12 fl.oz	165	16	14
Pacific Pear (4.5%), 12 fl.oz	160	13	17
Hornsby's: Amber (5.5%)	180	16	19
Crisp (5.5%), 12 fl.oz	190	16	26
Johnny Appleseed, (5.5%)	210	16	26
Magners, (4.5%)	125	13	9
Michelob, Ultra Light Cider (4%)	120	10	10
Saint Archer, Hard Cider (6.1%)	170	17	11
Smith & Forge, (6%)	220	17	26
Stella Artois Cidre, (4.5%)	170	13	21
Strongbow: *Per 11.2 fl oz*			
Cherry/Or. Blossom, (4.5%), av.	180	12	24
Gold Apple (5%)	170	13	20
Rose Apple (5%)	140	13	11
Woodchuck: Amber (5%)	200	14	21
Granny Smith (5%), 12 fl.oz	160	14	11
Pear (4%), 12 fl.oz	150	12	18
Raspberry (4%), 12 fl.oz	170	12	22
Semi-Dry (5.5%), 12 fl.oz	160	14	13
Wyder's: Dry Pear (4%)	140	12	22
Dry Raspberry (4%), 12 fl.oz	120	12	17
Prickly Pear (5%), 12 fl.oz	180	14	22
Reposado (6.9%), 12 fl.oz	250	19	30

Quick Guide

Table Wines:
Average all Varieties (11.5% Alc.)
(Wine Contains Zero Fat)

	C	Alc	Cb
4 fl.oz, 1 small wine glass			
OR ½ large wine glass	100	12	3
6 fl.oz, (¾ large wine glass)	145	18	5
8 fl.oz, (1 large wine glass)	195	25	7
½ Carafe/Bottle, 12 fl.oz	295	37	10
1 Bottle, 750ml, 25.4 fl.oz	620	78	21

Table Wines

	C	Alc	Cb
Red: *Per 4 fl.oz*			
Burgundy/Cabernet/Merlot, av.	100	11	4
White: *Per 4 fl.oz*			
Dry (Chenin; Fume Blanc; Chardonnay)	95	11	4
Sparkling, 4 fl.oz	95	11	4
Zinfandel Sweet,			
(Moselle/Sauterne), 4 fl.oz	85	11	2

Table Wines (Cont)

	C	Alc	Cb
Champagne: *Per 4 fl.oz*			
Average all types, 1 glass	85	11	2
with Orange Jce (3:1 orange)	75	8	4
with Orange Jce (1:1 orange)	65	5	7
Mulled Wine *(Gluhwein),* 4 fl.oz	180	14	20
Non-Alcoholic Wine: *Less than 0.5% Alcohol*			
Ariel: White varieties, average, 4 fl.oz	35	0.5	8
Red varieties, average, 4 fl.oz	25	0.5	5
Reduced Alcohol Wine:			
Average all types, (6%), 4 fl.oz	80	6	10
Skinnygirl, Red/White, (8.5%), 5 fl.oz	100	10	5
Sake *(Gekkeikan),* (16%), 4 fl.oz	120	15	5
Sangria *(Skinnygirl),* (4%), 5 fl.oz	130	5	23

Flavored Wines

Average All Brands (6% alcohol)
(Arbor Mist, Wild Vines, Boone's Farm):

	C	Alc	Cb
1 small wine glass, 4 fl.oz	80	6	10
1 large wine glass, 8 fl.oz	160	11	20
1 bottle, 750 ml (25.4 fl.oz)	510	35	64

Dessert Wines

	C	Alc	Cb
Madeira (18%), 2 oz	85	9	5
Marsala (18%), 2 oz	110	9	11
Port, Muscatel (18%), 2 oz	85	9	5
Sherry (15%), 2 oz:			
Dry, 1 Sherry glass	90	7	7
Sweet/Cream, average	90	7	8
Vermouth *(Martini & Rossi):*			
Extra Dry (18%), 2 oz	65	9	2
Martini Rosso (16%), 2 oz	90	8	8

Cooking Wines

	C	Alc	Cb
Holland House:			
Marsala, (14%), 2 T., 1 fl.oz	45	4	4
Red/White, (10%): 2 T., 1 fl.oz	20	2	1
1 cup, 8 fl.oz	160	24	8
Sherry (17%), 2 Tbsp, 1 fl.oz	45	5	2

Cooking with Wine:

For alcohol to evaporate, sufficient heat and cooking time (at least 30 minutes) is required.
Red and white table wines; Negligible residual calories.
Sweetened wines (Marsala/Sherry) Approx. 10 calories per 1 fl.oz.
Flambé Desserts: Only surface alcohol is burned off, so negligible reduction in alcohol or calories.

Quick Guide

Alc ~ Alcohol (Grams)

Spirits/Liquors:
Includess Bourbon, Brandy, Gin, Rum, Scotch, Tequila, Vodka, Whiskey.
Note: All spirits with same alcohol proof have similar calories and zero fat.

Average All Brands	C	Alc	Cb
80 Proof (40% Alcohol by Volume):			
1 fl.oz	65	9.5	0
1.5 fl.oz (1 shot)	100	14	0
3 fl.oz (Double shot)	195	28	0
1/2 Bottle, 350 ml (12 fl.oz)	770	113	0
1 Bottle, 700 ml (24 fl.oz)	1540	227	0
86 Proof (43% Alc):			
1 fl.oz	70	10	0
1.5 fl.oz (1 shot)	105	15	0
1 Bottle (24 fl.oz)	1670	247	0
100 Proof (50% Alc),			
1.5 fl.oz	125	18	0
Shochu (Soju),			
average all types (25% alc), 2 fl.oz	65	12	0

Flavored Spirits

	C	Alc	Cb
Captain Morgan: *Per 1.5 fl.oz*			
Original (35%)	85	12	0.5
Black Spiced (47.3%)	115	14	1
Parrot Bay (21%), average	90	7.5	10
Silver Spiced (35%)	95	12	2
Malibu Rum,			
Original/Fruit Flavors (21%), 1.5 fl.oz	80	8	8
Southern Comfort (35%), 1.5 fl.oz	100	13	3

Hard Lemonade, Sodas & Tea

	C	Alc	Cb
Margaritaville: *Per 12 fl.oz*			
Lime Margarita (8%)	310	23	30
Paradise Punch (8%)	340	23	46
Mike's:			
Lemonade:			
Hard (5%), 11.2 fl.oz	220	13	33
Harder (8%) average, 16 fl.oz	395	31	44
Margarita (5%), 11.2 fl.oz	220	14	34
Punch: Harder (8%), 12 fl.oz	300	23	36
Hard Mango (5.5%), 11.2 fl.oz	230	15	33
Sparks: *Per 16 fl.oz Can*			
Blackberry (8%)	385	31	44
Iced Tea (8%)	375	31	41
Lemonade (8%)	345	31	36
Original (6%)	335	23	45
Twisted Tea: Original (5%)	220	14	31
Half & Half (5%)	260	14	34
Zumbida Mango, (4.2%), 12 fl.oz	150	12	17

Coolers & Premix Cocktails

	C	Alc	Cb
Ready-To-Drink:			
Zero Fat Unless Indicated			
Bacardi: *Per 4 fl.oz*			
Party Drinks (Ready To Pour):			
Bahama Mama; Mai Tai (10%)	130	9	16
Mojito (15%)	160	14	16
Rum Island Ice Tea (12.5%)	150	12	16
Bacardi Silver: *Per 12 fl.oz*			
Lemonade/Sangria (6%), av.	270	17	41
Raz/Strawberry (5%)	240	14	36
Mojito (5%)	240	14	36
Bartles & Jaymes: *Per 11.2 fl.oz*			
Malt Based Coolers (3.2%):			
Exotic Berry	195	9	31
Margarita	245	9	43
Pina Colada	250	9	45
Sangria	240	9	40
Strawberry Daiquiri	205	9	34
Captain Morgan's,			
Parrot Bay (4.1%), all var. av., 11.2 fl.oz	210	10	35
Chi Chi's: Long Is. Iced Tea, 4 fl.oz	145	12	17
Mexican Mudslide, 4 fl.oz (8g fat)	240	1.5	42
Mojito, 4 fl.oz	160	11	21
Pina Colada, 4 fl.oz (6g fat)	240	4	42
White Russian, 4 fl.oz (7g fat)	245	1.5	43
Daily's, Frozen Pouches (5%),			
average all flavors, 10 fl.oz	285	12	47
Jack Daniels, Country Cocktails (4.8%),			
average all varieties, 10 fl.oz	200	9	30
Jose Cuervo:			
Margaritas:			
Classic Lime (10%), 6 fl.oz	210	14	29
Golden (12.7%), 4.7 fl.oz	170	14	19
Seagram's:			
Escapes Coolers (3.2%):			
Bahama Mama, 11.2 fl.oz	200	9	36
Strawb. Daiquiri, 11.2 fl.oz	225	9	41
Skinnygirl:			
Vodka with flavors (30%), 1.5 fl.oz	75	11	0
Cocktails (10%), av., 3 fl.oz	70	8	4
Smirnoff:			
Ice (4.5%): Original, 11.2 fl.oz	220	13	33
Mango; Pineapple, av., 11.2 fl.oz	230	13	35
Spiked Sparkling Seltzer,			
(4.5%), all flav., 12 fl.oz can	90	13	1
TGI Friday's:			
On The Rocks: *Per 6 fl.oz*			
Long Island Ice Tea (15%)	250	21	28
Margarita (7.5%)	185	11	29
Mudslide (10%)	365	14	31
Blenders (12.5%),			
Mudslide, 6 fl.oz	365	18	31

Coolers & Premix Cocktails (Cont)

Ready-To-Drink:

	C	**Alc**	**Cb**
The Club Premix Cocktails: *Per 3.4 oz Serving (½ can)*			
Censored on Beach; Margarita (7.5%)	105	6	17
Gin/Vodka Martini (21%), average	155	17	0.2
Ice Tea (15%)	145	12	17
Manhattan (17%)	115	13	5
Mudslide/Pina Colada (10%), average	200	8	16
Screwdriver (7.5%)	95	6	14
Whiskey Sour (10%)	95	8	11

Shooters — Alc ~ Alcohol (Grams)

Alabama Slammer	110	14	2
Amaretto Sour	120	6	19
B52	145	14	11
Beam Me Up Scotty	145	13	13
Blue Tequila	160	18	6
Jager Bomb	205	8	30
Jager Bomb, w/ Sugar-Free Red Bull	155	8	18
Jell-O Shot: 3 oz, with 1.5 oz Vodka	180	14	19
with Diet Jell-O	110	14	0
Kamikaze	75	8	3
Kool-Aid	160	15	14
Orgasm	100	12	6
Peppermint Patty	195	8	11
Stinger	170	18	12
Surfer on Acid	90	7	11

Cocktail Mixers ~ Non-Alcoholic

Bacardi: *Per 8 fl.oz, Prepared from 2 fl.oz Concentrate*			
Daiquiris; Rum Runner	120	0	32
Margarita	90	0	25
Mojito	110	0	30
Pina Colada	170	0	36
Baja Bob's: *Per 4 fl.oz*			
Cranberry Cosmo Martini	10	0	2
Pina Colada	30	0	4
Jose Cuervo:			
Margaritas: Av. all flav., 4 fl.oz	85	0	21
Light (Sugar Free), Lime, 4 fl.oz	5	0	1
Mr & Mrs T:			
Bloody Mary: Original, 5 oz	30	0	7
Bold & Spicy, 4 oz	35	0	7
Mai Tai	130	0	32
Margarita	100	0	26
Pina Colada	170	0	44
Strawberry Daiquiri	180	0	46
TGI Friday's:			
Mudslide, 2.3 fl.oz	110	0	23
Cosmo; Berrytini, 2 fl.oz	80	0	20
Strawb. Daiquiri; Marg., 4 fl.oz	190	0	46

Cocktails — Alc ~ Alcohol (Grams)

Made to Standard Recipes (Standard Size):
(Main Reference: The New American Bartender's Guide)
Zero Fat Unless Indicated

	C	**Alc**	**Cb**
Adios Mother F.	260	23	23
Bacardi & Coke (with 1.5 oz Bacardi)	160	14	17
Bellini, 4.5 fl.oz	95	11	7
Bloody Mary (with 1.5 oz Vodka)	125	10	7
Blushin' Russian (20g fat)	405	14	23
Bourbon & Soda (with 2 oz Bourbon)	130	19	0
Brandy Alexander (10g fat)	300	20	15
Chupa Naranjas (with 1.5 oz Tequila)	150	16	8
Cosmopolitan	215	24	12
Daiquiri (w/ 2 oz Rum), av. all types	140	19	4
Frozen Daiquiri (with 2 oz Rum):			
without fruit	155	19	6
with fruit (with 1.5 oz Rum)	145	14	11
Grasshopper	260	17	28
Harvey Wallbanger (2 oz)	200	19	17
Highball (1.5 oz Whiskey)	100	14	0
Irish Coffee (10g fat)	205	14	2
Kahlua Mudslide: with milk (3g fat)	145	11	12
with cream (12g fat)	230	11	10
Lemon Drop, 4 fl.oz	130	14	10
Long Island Iced Tea (with 3 oz Cola)	270	19	32
with 3 oz Diet Cola	235	19	22
Mai Tai (with 2 oz Rum)	290	24	33
Manhattan	130	17	5
Margarita	160	18	7
Martini: Dry, with 1.5 oz gin	100	14	0
Sour Apple, w/ 2 oz Vodka/1 oz Schnapps	250	31	10
Mint Julep (with 2½ oz Bourbon)	180	24	4
Mojito (with 2 oz rum)	170	19	9
Moscow Mule (with 1.5 oz Vodka)	180	14	20
Pina Colada (10g fat), 6 oz	250	15	18
Red Bull & Vodka (with 1.5 oz vodka)	210	14	28
with Sugar Free Red Bull	105	14	3
Rum & Coke (with 1.5 oz Rum)	160	14	17
Sake Bomb (1.5 oz Sake & 5 oz Beer)	105	12	7
Sangria: with 1 oz Fruit Juice, 5 oz	120	12	9
with 0.5 oz Brandy, 5.5 oz	150	17	9
Screwdriver	160	14	15
Sex On The Beach	235	19	25
Spritzer (with 3 oz Wine)	65	8	2
Tequila Sunrise	200	14	25
Tom Collins (with 2 oz Gin)	210	19	18
Vodka Soda (with 1.5 oz Vodka)	100	14	0
Vodka Tonic (with 1.5 oz Vodka)	165	14	18
Whiskey Sour (w/ 2 oz Whiskey)	155	19	7
White Russian (10g fat)	240	19	7
Non-Alcoholic:			
Cinderella	45	0	11
Shirley Temple (with 6 oz Ginger Ale)	140	0	34

Liqueurs/Cordials 🅒 🅐🅛🅒 🅒🅑

Per 1 fl.oz

	C	Alc	Cb
Advocaat (36 Proof; 2g fat)	85	4	9
Alizé: Cognac (80 Proof)	70	9	2
Gold/Red Passion (32 Proof)	105	4	11
Amaretto (56 Proof)	110	7	17
Baileys Irish Cream (34 Proof; 4g fat)	100	4	8
Benedictine (80 Proof)	90	9	5
Chambord (33 Proof)	105	4	11
Chartreuse (80 Proof)	100	9	9
Cherry Brandy (48 Proof)	80	6	9
Coffee Liqueur (53 Proof)	115	7	16
Cointreau (80 Proof)	95	9	7
Creme de Cacao (54 Proof)	100	6	15
Creme de Menthe (72 Proof)	125	9	14
Curacao (70 Proof)	95	8	6
Drambuie (80 Proof)	105	9	9
Frangelico (40 Proof)	65	5	12
Galliano (86 Proof)	100	10	8
Grand Marnier (80 Proof)	100	9	7
(40 Proof)	85	5	14
Kirsch (68 Proof)	80	8	6
Midori (42 Proof)	80	5	11
Ouzo (80 Proof)	105	9	11
Pernod (80 Proof)	75	9	11
Sambuca (84 Proof)	100	10	11
Schnapps (100 Proof)	115	12	9
Southern Comfort (70 Proof)	65	8	3
Tia Maria (40% Proof)	90	7	10

Liqueur Coffee & Hot Drinks

Per Standard Drink

	C	Alc	Cb
Liqueur Coffee: Av. all types	200	10	10
Irish, 1.5 oz Whiskey & 1 oz whip	205	9	4
Hot Toddy, with 1½ oz liquor, av. all	170	9	19
Mulled Wine (*Glühwein*), 4 fl.oz, av	195	14	25

"The doctor told him to cut down to just one glass a day."

TEN TIPS TO AVOID HARMFUL DRINKING

1. **Add up the alcohol** you typically drink each day and on social occasions. How does this compare with 'low risk' amounts? (*See page 23*)

2. **Compare the alcohol content** of different drinks and select the lowest. Request half shots of alcohol in cocktails and mixed drinks. Dilute them and keep topping off with non-alcoholic drinks.

3. **Go easy on 'Light' beers.** At 4% alcohol, on average, they are still high in alcohol compared to regular beer (5% alcohol).

4. **Try low alcohol or non-alcohol** alternatives such as fruit juices and mineral water. Take your own to parties.

5. **Before drinking alcohol,** quench your thirst with water and non-alcoholic drinks – particularly after vigorous exercise or sports.

6. **Slow the rate of drinking.** Chugging or drinking fast is the major cause of illness and death from alcohol poisoning.

7. **Avoid drinking in 'rounds'.**

8. **Have a non-alcoholic 'spacer'** between drinks (e.g. mineral water, orange juice).

9. **Don't drink on an empty stomach.** Food slows the rate of alcohol absorption.

10. **Keep track of the number of drinks** and know when to stop. Stick to a set limit.

Note: Alcohol can be very dangerous when taken with prescription or street drugs, or when you are very tired.

Extra Info: www.CalorieKing.com

Cocktail Mixers & Extracts

	C	Alc	Cb
Angostura Bitters, ¼ tsp	2	0	0.5
Grenadine, ½ tsp	6	0	2
Lime/Lemon Juice, 2 Tbsp, 1 oz	10	0	2
Maraschino Cherry, 1 small	8	0	2
Simple Syrup, 1 Tbsp, av.	50	0	14
Sweet & Sour Mix, 2 Tbsp, 1 oz	30	0	7
Tonic Water, 8 fl.oz	80	0	22
Flavor Extracts (*McCormick*):			
Pure Lemon (83%), 1 tsp	0	3.5	0
Pure Vanilla (35%), 1tsp	0	1.5	0

Baking Ingredients

Baking Ingredients	C	F	Cb
Almond Paste,			
(Marzipan), 2 Tbsp	170	7	24
Apple Pie Filling,			
Sweetened, 9.4 oz	290	0	69
(Bean Water), 1/4 c., 2 oz	10	0	2
Baking Powder: Regular, 1 tsp	5	0	1
Cream of Tartar, 1 tsp	10	0	2
Baking Mix (*Bisquick*):			
Original, 1/3 cup, 1.5 oz	160	5	26
Batter Mix (*Golden Dipt*),			
All Purpose, 1/4 cup	100	0	20
Butter/Margarine, 1/2 cup, 4 oz	800	88	1
Stick (*Land O' Lakes*), 0.5 oz	100	11	0
Cacao Butter, 2 Tbsp, 1 oz	240	28	0
Cacao Nibs, raw, 3 Tbsp, 1 oz	180	14	8
Cacao Powder, raw: 1 Tbsp, 0.3 oz	35	2	3
1/4 cup, 1 oz	150	9	11
Carob Flour, 1/2 cup	115	0.5	46
Chocolate Baking Bars: *Average all Brands*			
Sweet (*Baker's*):			
1 oz portion	120	7	16
4 oz bar	470	28	64
Semi-sweet, 1 oz	140	9	16
White Baking, 1 oz	160	9	16
Unsweetened: 1 oz	140	14	8
Grated, 1 cup, 4.5 oz	660	69	39
Chocolate Baking Chips: *Average all Brands*			
Milk Choc./Semi Sweet, 1 oz	140	8	18
1/2 cup, 3 oz	420	24	54
1 cup, 6 oz	840	48	108
Dark, 1 Tbsp, 0.5 oz	70	5	3
Mini Kisses (*Hershey*), 1 piece	5	0.5	1
Cocoa Powder, unsweetened:			
1 Tbsp, 0.2 oz	15	0.5	3
1/3 cup, 1 oz	60	4	17
Coconut, dried:			
Sweetened/Flaked:			
1 oz	130	8	15
1/2 cup, 1.3 oz	195	12	22
Toasted (*Baker's*), 1 oz	170	13	13
Unsweetened, 1 oz	190	18	7
Coconut Cream/Milk ~ *See Page 89*			
Coconut Manna (*Nutiva*), 1 Tbsp	100	9	3
Cornstarch, 1 Tbsp	30	0	7
Eggs: Large (1)	75	5	0
Jumbo (1)	90	6	0.5
Egg White: 1 Egg White	15	0	0
1/2 cup (4 egg whites), 4 oz	60	0	1
Flour: Whole Wheat, 1 cup, 4.2 oz	400	2	84
White: 1 Tbsp, 0.3 oz	25	0	5.5
1 cup, 4.2 oz	400	1	88

	C	F	Cb
Flavor Extracts: *Av. all Brands*			
Imitation, 1 tsp	10	0	2
Pure Extract, 1 tsp	10	0	0.5
Almond; Vanilla, 1 tsp	10	0	0.5
Fruit Pectin: Swtnd, 1/4 tsp	5	0	1
Unsweetened, 1/4 tsp	0	0	0
Gelatin, dry, unsweetened, 0.3 oz	20	0	0
Glaze (*Duncan Hines*): Choc., 2 T.	150	7	21
Vanilla, 2 Tbsp	140	6	22
Golden Dipt, Batter Mix			
1/4 cup, 1 oz	100	0	23
Honey, 1/2 cup, 6 oz	515	0	145
Lemon/Orange Peel, 1/4 cup	25	0	6
Lighter Bake (*Sunsweet*):			
(Butter & Oil replacement)			
1 Tbsp, 1/2 oz	35	0	9
1/4 Cup, 2.7 oz	140	0	36
Milk: Whole, 1 cup, 8 fl.oz	150	8	12
2%, 1 cup, 8 fl.oz	120	5	12
1%, 1 cup, 8 fl.oz	100	2.5	12
Fat-Free, 1 cup, 8 fl.oz	90	0.5	13
Pastry ~ *See Page 134*			
Pie Crusts ~ *See Page 134*			
Pie Fillings, Fruits ~ *See Page 134*			
Lemon Creme, 1/3 cup	130	1.5	28
Mincemeat, 3.5 oz	190	5	45
Pumpkin, 1 cup, 9.3 oz	270	1.5	60
Prune Puree, 1/4 cup, 3 oz	220	0	55
Raisins, 1/2 cup, 2.8 oz	240	0.5	63
Rennin, 0.4 oz pkt	10	0	2
Soy Milk ~ *See Pages 49-50*			
Sprinkles, all types, 1 tsp	20	1	3
Sugar: 1 Tbsp, 0.5 oz	55	0	14
1 oz	110	0	28
1 cup, 7 oz	775	0	195
16 oz (1 lb)	1760	0	454
Sweeteners & Sugar Substitutes ~ *See Page 156*			
Vinegar, average all types, 1 oz	5	0	1
Whey, sweet, dry, 1 oz	100	0.5	21
Yeast:			
Active, dry, 0.3 oz pkg	25	0.5	3
Bakers, compressed, 1 oz	30	0.5	5
Fleischmann's, 0.6 oz pkg	0	0	0

For Full Nutritional Data & Product Updates
~ *See Author's Website*
www.CalorieKing.com

Note: Actual weight of bars is usually 5-10% more than label Net Weight. Weigh bar and allow extra calories.

Bars ~ Brands   C F Cb

Per Bar

AdvantEdge ~ See EAS

Annie's Homegrown:

	C	F	Cb
Gluten Free, all varieties, 1 oz	110	3	20

Organic Chewy Granola Bars: *Per 0.9 oz Bar*

Chocolate Chip	100	2.5	18
Oatmeal Raisin	90	1.5	19
PB Chocolate Chip	100	3.5	16

Atkins:

Harvest Trail Bars: *Per 1.34 oz Bar*

Blueberry Vanilla & Almond	150	9	17
Coconut Almond	160	11	16
Dark Chocolate: Cherry & Nut	150	9	16
Peanut Butter	170	13	13
Sea Salt Caramel	180	14	13

Meal Bars: *Per 1.7 oz Unless Indicated*

Blueb. Greek Yog.; Cinn. Bun, av.	200	9	19
Choc. Chip Cookie Dough, 2 oz	220	10	32
Chocolate Chip Granola	210	9	17
Chocolate Peanut Butter, 2 oz	250	14	23
Choc. Peanut Butter Pretzel	210	10	19
Cookies 'n Crème, 1.76 oz	200	11	22
Raspberry Chia	180	7	19
Strawberry Almond	200	9	18

Snack Bars: *Per 1.55 oz Bar Unless Indicated*

Caramel Chocolate Nut Roll	190	13	19
Caramel Chocolate Peanut Nougat	170	11	20
Caramel Double Chocolate Crunch	160	9	22
Cashew Trail Mix, 1.4 oz	170	11	19
Choc. Chip Crisp, 1.23 oz	140	6	17
Classic Trail Mix, 1.34 oz	190	15	13
Coconut Almond Delight	200	15	18
Dark Chocolate Decadence	160	9	22
Lemon Bar, Triple Choc., av., 1.4 oz	160	8	16
Sweet & Salty Trail Mix, 1.34 oz	190	14	15

Note: Snack Bars Carb figures includes 4-15g sugar alcohol

Attune Bars:

Probiotic Bars: *Per 0.7 oz Bar*

Dark Chocolate	80	6	11
Milk Choc./Mint Crisp	90	6	12

Balance:

Original Bars:

Average, 1.8 oz	200	7	21
Dark Chocolate varieties, 1.6 oz	180	6	20

Duo-licious: *Per 2 Pieces*

Choc. C'rml P'nut Nougat, 1.55 oz	190	10	22
Choc. Pepeprmint Patty, 1.4 oz	160	4	27
Dulce de Leche & Caramel, 1.4 oz	150	5	24

Per Bar   C F Cb

Cascadian Farms *(General Mills):*

	C	F	Cb
Chewy Granola: Av. all var., 0.77 oz	85	2	16
1.23 oz Bars: Peanut varieties	160	7	22
Chocolate Chip	140	3	26
Crunchy Granola, av., 2 bars, 1.4 oz	185	8	27
Protein Granola Bars, av., 1.76 oz	250	15	20
Soft Baked Squares, av., 1.23 oz	150	5.5	23

Clif:

Energy: Av. all varieties., 2.4 oz	260	7	42
Mini size, average, 1.2 oz	100	2.5	17
Builder's, average, 2.4 oz	275	9	30
Crunch, average, 1.48 oz	200	9	24
Kid, ZBar, av. all varieties, 1.3 oz	135	3.5	23
Mojo, average, 1.6 oz	200	10	22
Nut Filled, av., 1.76 oz	230	11	26

Corazonas:

Heartbar Oatmeal Squares: *Per 1.8 oz Bar*

PB Oatmeal; White Choc. Macad.	200	7	29
Average other varieties	185	7	28

Detour:

Original, Caramel Peanut, 3 oz	350	11	32

Lean Muscle:

Cookie Dough Caramel Crisp, 3.2 oz	370	12	33
P'nut Butter Choc. Crunch, 3.2 oz	420	18	33

Lower Sugar, average all varieties:

1.4 oz Bar	170	6	16
2.8 oz Bar	340	13	33

Note: Low Sugar Bars Carb figures include 12-28g sugar alcohol

Simple:

Full size, 20g Protein, av., 2 oz	230	8	24
Snack size, 10g Protein, av., 1 oz	110	4	11
Smart: Coconut Almond, 1.3 oz	150	5	16
Fruit varieties, 1.3 oz	130	2.5	18
Peanut Butter Chocolate, 1.3 oz	160	6	16

dotFIT:

dotBAR:

Double Choc. Brownie, 3.3 oz	370	13	38
Peanut Butter Cup, 3.3 oz	370	13	38

Note: dotBARS Carb figures includes 21g sugar alcohol

dotSTICK, Iced, all varieties, 2 oz	190	6	26

Note: dotSTICK Bars Carb figures includes 8g sugar alcohol

EAS:

AdvantEDGE, Protein Bars,

average all varieties, 1.76 oz	190	7	20
Extend Bar: Yogurt, av., 1.4 oz	150	5.5	23
Anytime, av. all varieties, 1.4 oz	145	4	22

Note: Extend Bars Carb figure includes 3-9g sugar alcohol

B Bars ~ Granola ◆ Diet ◆ Sports

Bars ~ Brands (Cont)   C F Cb

Per Bar

Fiber One:

	C	F	Cb
90-Calorie Bar, av., 0.8 oz	90	2	17
Chewy: Layered, average, 1.27 oz	140	4	25
Oat varieties, average, 1.4 oz	140	4	29
Protein: Av. all varieties: 1.2 oz	140	6	18
Nut, Chocolate Pretzel, 1.4 oz	180	11	15

General Mills: *Per 1.6 oz Bar*

	C	F	Cb
Milk'n Cereal Bar, Honey Nut Cheerios	160	4	28

Glucerna:

	C	F	Cb
Crispy Delights, Peanut/Choc. Chip, av., 1.4 oz	155	5.5	20

Note: Carbohydrate figure includes 7g sugar alcohol

	C	F	Cb
Mini Snack Bar, average, 0.7 oz	80	3.5	11

Note: Carbohydrate figure includes 3g sugar alcohol

Great Value (Walmart):

	C	F	Cb
Chewy Granola: 90 calorie, 0.8 oz	90	1.5	18
Other varieties, 0.8 oz	100	2.5	18
Dipped, Choc. Chip, 1.1 oz	140	5	22
Protein, average, 1.4 oz	190	12	14
Sweet & Salty, Peanut, 1.2 oz	180	9	19
Crunchy Granola, Oats & Honey, 2 bars, 1.48 oz	200	7	29
Fiber, Oats & Chocolate, 1.4 oz	140	4	30
Fruit & Grains, Cereal, av., 1.3 oz	130	3	25

Health Valley,

	C	F	Cb
Multigrn, Cobbler Cereal Bars, .3 oz	130	2.5	27
HMR, Benefit Bars, av. all, 1.4 oz	160	5	22

Init: *Per 1.4 oz Bar*

	C	F	Cb
Dark Choc., average	180	10	23
Mixed Nut & Sweet Berries	180	9	24
Roasted Nuts & Honey Chipotle	190	13	18
Jenny Craig, all var., 1.2 oz	110	3	14

Kashi:

	C	F	Cb
Cereal Bars, 1.3 oz	120	3	23
GoLean, Plant Based Bars, av., 1.6 oz	195	10	21
Granola Bars: Chewy, average all varieties, 1.3 oz	135	5	23
Chewy Nut Butter, av., 1.23 oz	150	7	21
Crunchy, all varieties, 2 bars, 1.4 oz	175	6	26
Layered, av. all, 1.1 oz	125	4	21

Kellogg's:

Fiber Plus Antioxidants,

	C	F	Cb
Protein Chewy Bars, Peanut, 1.4 oz	170	8	18

Nutrigrain ~ *See page 33*
Special K ~ *See page 34*

Per Bar

Kind:

	C	F	Cb
Breakfast: Peanut Butter (2), 1.76 oz	230	11	28
Blueb. Alm; Honey Oat (2), 1.76 oz	220	8	33
Other varieties (2),1.76 oz	215	10	26

Fruit & Nut: *Per 1.4 oz*

	C	F	Cb
Almond & Coconut	190	12	21
Caramel Almond & Sea Salt	200	16	15
Dark Choc. Almond & Coconut	190	12	22
Healthy Grains, av. all varieties, 1.2 oz	145	5	24

Plus: *Per 1.4 oz Bar*

	C	F	Cb
Dark Chocolate Cherry Cashew	170	9	24
Average other varieties	185	12	20
Protein, average, 1.76 oz	250	17	18
Sweeet & Spicy, average, 1.58 oz	230	16	16
Kudos, av. all varieties, 0.9 oz	100	3	17

Labrada:

	C	F	Cb
Cookie Roll, average, 2.8 oz	315	10	34

Lean Body Protein Bar: *Per 2.54 oz*

	C	F	Cb
Cookie Dough; PB Choc Chip, av.	270	6	33
Fudge Brownie	260	6	31
Lean Body Gold, all var., 2.96 oz	330	9	32
Rockin' Roll, 2.47 oz	290	16	25

Larabar:

	C	F	Cb
Apple Pie, 1.6 oz	190	10	24
Cherry Pie, 1.7 oz	200	8	30
Chocolate Chip Brownie, 1.6 oz	200	9	31
Peanut Butter & Jelly, 1.7 oz	210	10	27
Snickerdoodle, 1.6 oz	190	9	25
Lindora: Chewy Choc. Chip, 1.6 oz	160	6	19
Peanut Butter Crunch, 1.48 oz	150	4.5	18
Salted Caramel Pretzel, 1.55 oz	160	6	18
Zesty Lemon Crisp, 1.55 oz	160	7	16

Luna:

	C	F	Cb
Regular, av., 1.7 oz	195	7	26
Rica, av., 1.4 oz	165	9	22
5G Sugar, average, 1.48 oz	175	9	20
Protein, av. all varieties, 1.6 oz	175	5	21

Marathon (Snickers):

	C	F	Cb
Energy: Chewy, av. all var., 2 oz	210	8	26
Crunchy, Dark Chocolate, 1.6 oz	150	4.5	22
Protein, average all var., 2.8 oz	285	9	40

Mariani: *Per 1.4 oz Bar*

	C	F	Cb
Honey Bars: Granola	160	6	25
Sweet & Salty	200	14	15

Market Pantry (Target):

Chewy Granola Bars:

	C	F	Cb
Choc. Chip; Monster, av., 0.8 oz	100	2	18
Dipped, Chocolate Chip, 1.1 oz	140	5	22

Bars ~ Brands (Cont)	C	F	Cb

Per Bar

Mars, Protein Bar, 2 oz | **200** | 4.5 | 22

Medifast:

	C	F	Cb
Chewy, all varieties, 1.3 oz	**110**	3	15
Crunch, av. all varieties, 1.2 oz	**110**	3	13

Note: Crunch Bars Carb figure includes 2-3g sugar alcohol

	C	F	Cb
Maintenance, Cararmel Nut, 1.5 oz	**170**	5	22

Met-Rx:

	C	F	Cb
Big 100, av. all varieties, 3.5 oz	**375**	6	49
Big 100 Colossal: Sweet & Salty	**430**	15	44
Other varieties, 3.5 oz	**410**	13	45
Protein Plus: Choc. Choc. Chunk, 3 oz	**310**	10	29
Choc. Roasted Peanut w/ Crml, 3oz	**320**	10	33
Peanut Butter Crisp, 3 oz	**310**	10	33

Mojo Bars ~ *See Clif*

Muscle Milk *(Cytosport):*

Protein Bars:

	C	F	Cb
Almond Cookie Flav.; Choc PB, 2.25 oz	**250**	9	28
B'Day Cake; Cookies 'N Crm, 1.76 oz	**185**	6	23
Blueberry Waffle, 2.18 oz	**230**	6	27
Doube Fudge; Salted C'rml, 2.22 oz	**240**	7	28

Note: Protein Bars Carb figures include 6-14g sugar alcohol

Nature's Path:

	C	F	Cb
Chewy Breakfast, aveage, 1.2 oz	**140**	4	25
Love Crunch, average, 1.1 oz	**150**	7	19
Superfood Snack, average, 1.34 oz	**185**	10	20

Nature Valley:

	C	F	Cb
Chewy Trail Mix, av. all, 1.3 oz	**135**	3	24
Crunchy Granola,			
average all var., 0.75 oz	**100**	4	15
Nut Crisp, average, 0.9 oz	**135**	9	11
Protein, all varieties, 1.4 oz	**190**	12	14
Sweet & Salty, average, 1.3 oz	**165**	7	22

NuGo:

	C	F	Cb
Dark, average all varieties, 1.76 oz	**200**	6	28
Family:			
Choc. Banana, 1.76 oz	**190**	3.5	25
Av. other var., 1.76 oz	**170**	3	26
Fiber d'Lish: Orange Cranb., 1.58 oz	**130**	3	32
Coc. Macaroon; P'nut Choc. Chip, 1.58 oz	**160**	6	28
Average other varieties, 1.58 oz	**140**	4	31
Gluten Free, av. all varieties, 1.58 oz	**180**	4	28
Organic, all varieties, 1.58 oz	**190**	5	26
Slim: Espresso, 1.58 oz	**170**	5	20
Average other varieties	**185**	5	19

Per Bar

NuGo (Cont):

	C	F	Cb
Smarte Carb: Choc. Black Berry, 1.76 oz	**150**	3	22
Peanut Butter Crunch, 1.76 oz	**160**	4	19

Note: Smarte Carb Carb figures include 12-14 g sugar alcohol

Stronger: *Per 2.8 oz Bar*

	C	F	Cb
Cookies 'N Crm; Caramel Pretzel, av.	**290**	10	37
Dark Choc C'rml.; Peanut Cluster, av.	**315**	13	35

Nutri-Grain *(Kellogg's):*

Bakery Delights,

	C	F	Cb
average, 1.4 oz	**160**	5	27

Soft Baked B'fast Cereal Bars,

	C	F	Cb
all varieties, 1.3 oz	**120**	3	24

NutriSystem:

	C	F	Cb
Breakfast: Cinnamon Bun	**150**	3.5	26
Harvest Nut	**160**	6	22
Lunch: Choc. P'nut Butter; Trail Mix	**200**	8	24
Double Chocolate Caramel	**180**	6	28
Snacks: Dark Chocolate & Sea Salt Nut	**200**	13	16
Average other varieties	**150**	4	23

Oh Yeah! *(ISS):*

Original:

	C	F	Cb
Chocolate Caramel Candies, 3 oz	**350**	17	36
Cookie Caramel Crunch, 3 oz	**340**	13	32
Peanut Butter & Caramel, 3 oz	**360**	19	36
Good Grab, average, 1.6 oz	**190**	10	19
Victory Bar, P'B Cup, 2.3 oz	**200**	6	27

Optifast:

800 Bars:

	C	F	Cb
Apple Cinnamon, 1.52 oz	**160**	4	18
Chocolate, 1.65 oz	**160**	4.5	18
Peanut Butter Chocolate, 1.52 oz	**160**	5	18

Note: 800 Bars Carb figures include 1-4g sugar alcohol

PowerBar:

	C	F	Cb
Performance Energy, average	**230**	4	45
Protein: Clean Way, average, 2.1 oz	**190**	5	25

Note: Protein Bars Carb figures include 8g sugar alcohol

	C	F	Cb
Protein Plus, average, 2.1 oz	**205**	7	25

Note: Protein Plus Bars Carb figures include 16-18g sugar alcohol

Power Crunch *(BNRG):*

	C	F	Cb
Orig. Protein Bar, av. all var., 1.4 oz	**205**	12	10
Power Crunch, Choklat, av., 0.75 oz	**105**	6	8

PR:

	C	F	Cb
Protein: Chocolate Mint, 2.1 oz	**200**	6	22
Chocolate Peanut, 1.8 oz	**200**	7	21
Oatmeal Raisin Granola, 1.8 oz	**210**	7	22

Premier Protein *(Premier Nutrition):*

	C	F	Cb
Chocolate Peanut Butter, 2.54 oz	**290**	8	25
Dark Chocolate Crunch, 2.54 oz	**270**	6	25
Yogurt Peanut Crunch, 2.54 oz	**290**	8	25

Note: Actual weight of bars is usually 5-10% more than label Net Weight. Weigh bar and allow extra calories.

Bars ~ Brands (Cont)

Per Bar

C F Cb

Promax:

Original, av. all varieties, 2.6 oz	**290**	8	37
Lower Sugar, av. all varieties, 2.4 oz	**230**	7	33
Pro Series, av. all varieties, 3.17 oz	**340**	12	39
Proti Bars *(Bariatrix),* av. all var.	**160**	5.5	16
PureFit, av. all varieties, 2 oz	**220**	7	25

Pure Protein:

Hi Protein, average all varieties:

1.76 oz bar	**190**	5	18
2.1 oz	**195**	7	24
2.75 oz bar	**300**	8	27

Note: Carbohydrate figures include 5-8g Sugar Alcohol

Quaker:

B'fast Squares: P'nut Butter, 2.1 oz	**250**	10	35
Other flavors, 2.1 oz	**210**	4.5	41

Note: Carbohydrate figures include 2-6g Sugar Alcohol

B'fast Flats: Banana Honey Nut (3)	**180**	7	27
Av. other varieties (3)	**175**	6.5	28

Granola Bars:

Chewy: 25% Less Sugar, average, 0.8 oz	**95**	3	17
Big, average all varieties, 1.9 oz	**175**	6	30
Bites, average, 8 pieces	**135**	5	21
Dipps, average, 1.2 oz	**140**	6	22
Snackwich, av., 1.4 oz	**165**	6	29
Yogurt, all varieties, 1.2 oz	**150**	4.5	25

Quest Bar:

Beyond Cereal Protein, 1.34 oz	**110**	4.5	17
Hero: Choc. Caramel Pecan, 2.1 oz	**200**	11	27
Average other varieties, 2.1 oz	**175**	8	30

Note: Carbohydrate figure include 1-4g Sugar Alcohol

Protein,, av., 2.1 oz	**195**	9	22

Note: Carbohydrate figures includs 1-6g Sugar Alcohol

Revival Soy *(Direct):*

Chocolate Temptation	**270**	7	32
Marshmallow Krunch	**220**	2.5	30
Peanut Chocolate	**260**	7	30
Peanut Pal	**240**	6	28
Low Carb, average all varieties	**235**	8	31

Note: Low Carb Bars Carb figure includes 20-22g Sugar Alcohol

Skratch Bars:

Anytime Energy: *Per 1.76 oz Bar*

Cherries & Pistachios; Ginger & Miso	**210**	10	27
Chocolate Chips & Almonds	**200**	8	30
Energy Chews, all flavors, 0.78 oz	**80**	0	20

Per Bar

C F Cb

Slim-Fast:

Bake Shop Bars, average all, 1.6 oz	**180**	6.5	17

Note: Carbohydrate figures include 12-13g Sugar Alcohol

Snickers, Protein Bar, 1.8 oz	**200**	7	18
Solo, Gi, average all varieties 1.8 oz	**200**	7	26

Special K:

Chewy Snack Bars,

av. all varieties, 0.88 oz	**100**	2	19

Nourish: *Per 1.16 oz*

Bites, 6 pieces	**180**	9	20
Chewy Nut Bars: Cranberry Amond	**150**	6	20
Average other varieties	**170**	10	16

Protein Meal Bars,

average all varieties, 1.58 oz	**175**	5	25
Protein Snack, av. all var., 1.23 oz	**155**	7	17

Supreme Protein:

High Protein:

Caramel Nut Chocolate, 3.4 oz	**390**	15	26
PB Crunch, 3 oz	**390**	18	26
PB Jelly, 3.4 oz	**390**	15	35

Note: Carbohydrate figures include 14-15g sugar alcohol

thinkThin,

High Protein, Choc. Strawb., 2oz	**250**	9	24

Note: Carbohydrate figure includes 12g sugar alcohol

Protein Nut, average all var., 1.4 oz	**190**	12	16

Tiger's Milk:

Protein Rich, 1.2 oz	**140**	5	19
Peanut Butter Crunch, 1.2 oz	**150**	6	18
King Size, average all varieties, 2 oz	**225**	9	28

Toaster Strudel ~ *see page 64*

Toaster Strudel ~ *see page 64*

Trader Joe's:

Chewy Coated Granola Bars, 6-Packs:

Chocolate Chip, 1.3 oz	**150**	4	26
Peanut Butter & Oats, 1.2 oz	**130**	4	25
Raises the Bar, av., 1.2 oz	**140**	4	23

Fruit Bars: Fig 1.5 oz	**120**	2	24
Average other varieties, 1.5 oz	**140**	2.5	27

Granola Bars, 6-packs:

Fiberful, average,1.2 oz	**125**	5	21
Trail Mix, 1.3 oz	**150**	5	23

Tri-O-Plex *(Chef Jay's):*

High Protein,

Ban. Walnut, 4.2 oz	**405**	14	40
Duo, Bursting Peanut Butter	**395**	17	35

Zone Perfect:

Choc. Chip Cookie Dough, 1.58 oz	**180**	5	24
Chocolate Peanut Butter, 1.76 oz	**210**	7	24
Dark Choc. Almond, 1.58 oz	**190**	6	22
Fudge Graham, 1.76 oz	**210**	7	23
Salted Caramel Brownie, 1.58 oz	**200**	9	19

Cocoa & Hot Chocolate 🅒 🅕 🅒ᵇ

Cocoa:

	C	F	Cb
Small (8 fl.oz):			
with Whole Milk	205	8.5	22
with Nonfat Milk	145	1	23
Tall (12 fl.oz): with Whole Milk	280	12	26
with Nonfat Milk	185	1	28
Hot Chocolate:			
Small (8 fl.oz): with Whole Milk	180	7	26
with Nonfat Milk	140	2	27
Tall (12 fl.oz): with Whole Milk	260	10	36
with Nonfat Milk	190	2	37
Cinnabon, Mochalatta Chill, 16 oz	420	17	63
Swiss Miss, Mixes, av., 1 packet	120	2.5	22

Cocoa - Chocolate Mixes

Add extra cals/fat/carbohydrate for milk
Carnation Breakfast Drinks ~ *See Page 38*

	C	F	Cb
Carnation: *Per 3 Tbsp*			
Malted Milk: Original	90	2	15
Chocolate	90	1	18
Ghirardelli:			
Premium Hot Cocoa: Caramel, 0.8 oz	90	1	20
Chocolate Mocha, 3 Tbsp	120	1.5	29
Double Chocolate, 3 Tbsp	120	1.5	30
Hershey's, Cocoa,			
Natural, unsweetened,			
1 Tbsp, 0.2 oz	10	0.5	3
Land O Lakes:			
Arctic White Coccoa, 1.3 oz	160	6	26
Other varieties, 1.3 oz	140	3.5	26
Nestle: *Per Per Single Serve Envelope*			
Chocolate Caramel	100	3	19
Dark Chocolate	100	3	19
Rich Milk Chocolate:			
Regular	80	3	14
Fat Free	20	0	4
No Sugar Added Fat Free	20	0	5
Nesquik Powder: *Per 2 Tbsp*			
Chocolate; Strawberry	50	0.5	12
Chocolate No Added Sugar	35	1	7
Ovaltine, All Natural Cocoa Mixes,			
average all varieties, 2 Tbsp	40	0	10
Swiss Miss: *Per Single Serve Envelope*			
Breakfast Blends: Great Start	60	1	11
Pick Me Up	110	2	23
Classics, Milk Chocolate:			
Hot Cocoa Mix	90	2	16
No Added Sugar	60	1	11
with Marshmallow	90	2	16
Rich Chocolate	120	2	23

Instant Coffee 🅒 🅕 🅒ᵇ

	C	F	Cb
Powder/Granules: *Regular or Decaffeinated,*			
1 level tsp	2	0	0.5
1 rounded tsp	4	0	1
Ground, 3 tsp	7	0	2
Brewed/Percolated, 1 cup, 8 fl.oz	4	0	1
Coffee with Milk/Cream/Creamers: *Per 8 oz Cup*			
Black:	4	0	1
with Whole Milk: Dash, 1 Tbsp	15	0.5	2
2 Tbsp, 1 fl.oz	25	1	2.5
with 2% Milk, 2 Tbsp	20	0.5	2.5
with 1% Milk, 2 Tbsp	20	0.5	2.5
with Fat Free Milk, 2 Tbsp	15	0	2.5
with Soy Milk: 1 Tbsp	10	0	1.5
2 Tbsp, 1 oz	15	0.5	2
with Half & Half: 2 Tbsp	50	3	3
¼ cup, 2 fl.oz	90	6	4
with Cream (light coffee), 2 Tbsp	65	6	2
with Coffee Mate: Liquid, reg., 1 T.	20	1	3
Liquid Fat Free, 1 Tbsp	25	0	2
Powder, 1 heaping tsp	15	1	2
Sugar ~ Add Extra: 1 heaping tsp	25	0	6
Single portion, 1 package	25	0	6
Sweeteners, *(Equal/Splenda/Sweet N Low),*			
Powder, 1 package	0	0	0

Flavored Coffee Mixes

	C	F	Cb
Chicory:			
Instant Coffee, 1 tsp	5	0	1
Coffee Essence, 1 tsp	15	0	4
Caffé D'Vita:			
Hot Cocoa, 1 oz	110	1.5	24
Hot Cocoa, Sugar Free, 0.5 oz	70	4.5	7
General Foods International:			
Average all varieties, 0.5 oz	60	3	10
Sugar-free, av. all varieties, 1 tsp	30	2.5	2
Cappuccino Coolers, all varieties, 0.5 oz	60	0	15
Hills Bros: *Per 3 Tbsp, 1 oz*			
Cappuccino: French Vanilla	120	4.5	19
Chocolate Hazelnut	110	3.5	19
Classic Cappuccino	120	5	17
Dark Chocolate	110	4	19
Mocha Mint	120	4	20
Nescafe, Memento, 1 stick,			
average all varieties	100	2.5	19
Starbucks, VIA, Iced Coffee,			
all varieties, 1 stick/packet	100	0	24

Coffee Shops/Restaurants

Per 8 fl.oz Cup (Unless Indicated)

	C	F	Cb
Coffee, Regular/Percolated/Filtered	5	0	0
Americano Drip Coffee, 1 cup	7.5	0	1
Cafe Au Lait: 1 cup, 8 fl.oz	60	3.5	5
Nonfat Milk, 1 cup, 8 fl.oz	35	0	5
Caffe Latté:			
8 fl.oz cup: with Whole Milk	110	6	9
with 2% Milk	100	3.5	9
with Nonfat Milk	70	0	10
12 fl.oz: with Whole Milk	180	9	14
with Nonfat Milk	100	0	15
16 fl.oz: with Whole Milk	220	11	18
with Nonfat Milk	130	0	19
Cafe Mocha (Mochaccino): 8 fl.oz	150	6	20
12 fl.oz	230	9	31
16 fl.oz	290	12	41
Cappuccino:			
8 fl.oz cup: with Whole Milk	90	3.5	7
with 2% Milk	80	3	8
with Nonfat Milk	50	0	8
12 fl.oz: with Whole Milk	110	6	9
with 2% Milk	90	3.5	9
with Nonfat Milk	60	0	9
16 fl.oz: with Whole Milk	140	7	11
with 2% Milk	120	3.5	11
with Nonfat Milk	80	0	12
Mocha: *With Cream*			
8 fl.oz: with Whole Milk	200	11	22
with Nonfat Milk	160	6	22
12 fl.oz: Whole Milk	290	15	33
with Nonfat Milk	230	8	34
Iced Mocha: *Without Cream*			
12 fl.oz: with Whole Milk	170	6	26
with Nonfat Milk	130	2	27
Espresso: Single (Solo), 1 fl.oz	5	0	1
Double (Doppio), 2 fl.oz	10	0	2
Espresso con Panna,			
(w/ dollop wh. cream), solo, 1 fl.oz	30	2.5	2
Espresso Macchiato, solo, 1 fl.oz	5	0	1
Frappuccino: Tall, 12 fl.oz	180	2.5	37
Grande, 16 fl.oz	240	3	48
Frappuccino Mocha:			
(with Cream): Tall, 12 fl.oz	280	11	43
Grande, 16 fl.oz	380	15	57
Iced Latte, Similar to Caffe Latte			

McCafe (McDonald's) ~ See Fast Food, Page 216
Starbucks ~ See Fast-Foods Section , Page 243

Coffee Substitute Mixes

	C	F	Cb
Roasted Cereal Beverages ~ *(No Caffeine)*			
Cafix, Instant Beverage, 1 tsp	5	0	1
Kaffree Roma, Instant Beverage, 1 tsp	10	0	2
Teeccino, Herbal Coffees, 1 tsp	10	0	2

Irish & Liqueur Coffees

	C	F	Cb
Irish Coffee, without sugar	175	10	0
Liqueur Coffee, with cream,			
all varieties, av., 1 fl.oz	100	5	7

Coffee Extras

	C	F	Cb
Chocolate (Cocoa) Topping, $\frac{1}{2}$ tsp	5	0	1
Flavored Syrups: Regular, 2 Tbsp	80	0	20
Sugar-free, 2 Tbsp	0	0	0
Half & Half Cream: 2 Tbsp	40	3.5	1
Single serve pkg, $\frac{3}{8}$ fl.oz	15	1.5	0.5
Light whipped cream, 2 Tbsp	15	1.5	1
Marshmallows, miniature (2)	5	0	1
Sugar:			
1 single portion package	20	0	5
1 level tsp	15	0	4
1 heaping tsp	25	0	6
Equal/Splenda/Sweet 'N Low	0	0	0

Coffee Shop ~ Cakes, Cookies

	C	F	Cb
Cookies:			
Biscotti, 1 oz	140	6.5	18
Chocolate Chip, 3 oz	350	15	54
Oatmeal Raisin, 3 oz	350	12	56
Peanut Butter, 3 oz	410	25	39
White Choc. Macadamia, 3.33 oz	420	20	55
Cakes/Pastries:			
Almond Croissant, 5 oz	620	35	67
Apple Danish, 5 oz	450	18	67
Banana Walnut, 4.5 oz	410	17	60
Brownie, 3 oz	390	24	42
Bundt, Chocolate, 4 oz	440	21	61
Carrot Cake, 4 oz	400	22	45
Chocolate Cake, 5 oz	530	28	65
Crumble Coffee Cake, 4.5 oz	500	25	65
Cupcake, 3 oz	330	16	43
Pound Cake, av., 3 oz	330	17	40
Cinnamon Roll, 6 oz	500	15	83
Donuts:			
Sugared, 1.8 oz	220	11	27
Glazed, 2 oz	250	12	34
Pretzel, large, 4 oz	290	5	52

Starbucks Bakery Items ~ See Page 244

READY TO DRINK COFFEE C F Cb

Bottled & Chilled:

Califia Farms: *With Almond Milk*

	C	F	Cb
Cold Brew Coffee, av., 10.5 fl.oz	115	4.5	18
Dunkin Donuts,			
Iced Coffee, av., 13.7 fl.oz	290	6	47
International Delight:			
Iced, all flavors, 8 fl.oz	150	2.5	29
Light varieties, 8 fl.oz	90	2.5	14
Java Monster Energy ~ *See Page 39*			
Kahlua, Cappuccino Shake, 10.5 fl.oz	130	2	24
Starbucks:			
Doubleshot Energy: *Per 15 fl.oz Can*			
Coffee Drink	210	2.5	36
Hazelnut Drink	210	3	31
Mocha/Vanilla Drink	205	2.5	34
White Chocolate Drink	210	3	31
Doubleshot Espresso: *Per 6.5 fl.oz Can*			
Espresso & Cream	140	6	18
Espresso & Cream Light	70	4	5
Frappuccino Coffee Drink: *Per 9.5 fl.oz Bottle*			
Mocha	180	3	33
Light Mocha	100	3	12
Vanilla	200	3	37
Iced Coffee: *Per 11 fl.oz Bottle*			
Coffee: with Milk, sweetened	110	0.5	23
Light. sweetened	50	0	11
Caramel; Vanilla, swtnd, av.	110	0.5	23
Vanilla	120	0.5	22
Iced Espresso Classics (Chilled): *Per 8 fl.oz Bottle*			
Caffe Mocha	140	2.5	23
Caramel Macchiato; Van. Latte	130	2.5	21
Skinny, Caramel Macchiato, Van. Latte	70	0	10
Starbucks Refreshers ~ *See Page 40*			
TruMoo:			
Coffee Milk:			
Low-Fat (1%), 8 fl.oz	130	2.5	20
Fat-Free, 8 fl.oz	110	0	20

Tips to Reduce the Calories in Your Coffee Drinks:

- Request non-fat milk in place of whole or 2% milk
- Downsize to 8 fl.oz or 12 fl.oz
- Avoid cream on frappuccinos
- Replace sugar with *Equal, Splenda, Stevia* or *Sweet 'N Low*
- Avoid syrup add-ons

CAFFEINE COUNTER

Moderate caffeine intake is not harmful to healthy adults. However, frequent large amounts (over 350mg/day) may cause dependency ('caffeinism') and adversely affect health. **To be safe, limit caffeine to 200mg/day.** Avoid if pregnant, breast feeding, a child under 8, have sleep problems, an overactive bladder or heart arrhythmia.

	Caffeine (mg)
Coffee: Instant: Weak, 1 level teaspoon	30
Medium, 1 rounded teaspoon	60
Strong, 1 heaping teaspoon	100
Decaffeinated, 1 rounded teaspoon	2
Bags (Folgers), 1 bag (6-8 fl.oz)	115
Ground, 1 Tbsp, 0.2 oz	60
Bottled (Ready-To-Drink), 9.5 fl.oz	70
Coffee Shop: Brewed, 8 fl.oz	110 -150
Cappuccino/Latte: 1 cup, 8 fl.oz	75
Tall, 12 fl.oz	110
Large, 16 fl.oz	150
Decappuccino, decaffeinated	5
Espresso: Regular/Single/Solo	75
Double/Doppio	150
Iced Coffee w/o Milk, 12 fl.oz	140
Latte, 1 cup, 8 fl.oz	75
Mocha, 1 cup, 8 fl.oz	90
Hot Chocolate, 8 fl.oz	15
Black Tea: Weak, 1 cup	20
Medium Strength, 1 cup	40
Strong, 1 cup	70
Decaffeinated Tea, 1 cup	0-5
Herbal Tea, 1 cup	0
Green Tea, 1 cup	20
Iced Tea, tall glass/can, 12 fl.oz	20-30
Soft Drinks: *Per 12 fl.oz Can*	
Coca-Cola; Pepsi (Regular/Diet)	35
Diet Coke; TAB; RC Cola (Regular)	45
Dr. Pepper; Sunkist Orange	40
Pepsi One; Mountain Dew; Mellow Yellow; Surge	55
Pepsi Max (Regular/Diet) Sun Drop (Reg/Diet)	70
7-Up, Fanta, Sprite, Fresca, Diet Rite Cola	0
Energy Drinks (with added caffeine):	
(AMP, Adrenaline Rush, Full Throttle Monster, No Fear, Red Bull, Rockstar)	
Average all brands: 8 fl.oz	80
16 fl.oz	160
NOS Energy, 16 fl.oz	260
Chocolate Bars: Milk Chocolate, 2 oz	20
Dark Chocolate, 2 oz	30
Choc Chip Cookies, 2 medium, 2 oz	6
Chocolate Syrup, 2 Tbsp, 1.4 oz	5
Guarana, GNC, 1 tablet	90
Medicinals: *Excedrin Extra/Migraine*, 1 tab.	65
Jet Alert/NoDoz, 1 tablet	200
Stay Awake (Walgreens), Vivarin, 1 tab.	200

Energy/Protein Drinks

	C	F	Cb
5-hour Energy, 2 fl.oz	4	0	1
A.B.B:			
Energy: Speed Shot, 8.5 fl.oz	0	0	0
Ripped Force, 18 fl.oz	90	0	23
Pure-Pro:			
Pure Pro 35 Shake, all flav., 12 fl.oz	160	0.5	5
Pure Pro 50, all flavors, 14.5 fl.oz	240	1.5	7
Maxx Recovery, all flavors, 18 fl.oz	400	0.5	60
AdvantEDGE *(EAS)*,			
RTD Shakes, av., 11 fl.oz	100	2.5	5
AllSport Hydration:			
Regular, all flavors, 20 fl.oz	150	0	40
Zero, 20 fl.oz	0	0	0
AMP Energy: *Per 16 fl.oz Can*			
Orig.; Strawb. Limeade; P'Fruit	220	0	58
Cherry Blast	120	0	31
Tropical Punch	100	0	26
Boosted, Wild Berry Cherry	100	0	26
Arizona: *Per 11.5 fl.oz Can*			
Nat. Energy: Arnold Palmer	70	0	20
Other Fruit Flavors	100	0	26
Atkins, Shakes, av., 11 fl.oz	155	9	4
Bariatrix, Proti-Max,			
Anytime Shakes, av., 11 fl.oz	160	9	3
Bawls Guarana: *Per 10 fl.oz Bottle*			
Original; Cherry, average	120	0	31
Ginger; Orange; Root Beer	135	0	33
Blue Sky,			
Blue Energy Drink, 8 fl.oz	120	0	29
BodyArmor, SuperDrinks,			
all flavors, 16 fl.oz	140	0	36
Bolthouse: *Per 8 fl.oz*			
Breakfast Smoothies,			
Peach/Strawberry Parfait, av., 8 fl.oz	190	2.5	35
Protein Plus: Chocolate, 8 fl.oz	210	3	29
Mango, 8 fl.oz	200	0.5	33
Vanilla Bean, 8 fl.oz	170	3	21
Boost *(Nestle Health Care): Per 8 fl.oz*			
Original, all flavors	240	4	41
Glucose Control, all flavors	190	7	16
High Protein, all flavors	240	6	33
Plus, all flavors	360	14	45
Carnation:			
B'Fast Essentials, Powder:			
Av. all flav., 1 env., 1.3 oz	130	0	27
Light Start, av., 0.7 oz	60	0	12
Ready To Drink: Reg., all flav., 8 fl.oz	240	4	41
High Protein, average, 8 fl.oz	220	6	28
Celestial Seasoning,			
Kombucha, all flavors, 2 oz shot	30	0	8
CeraSport, EX1, Lime Flavor, 8.5 fl.oz	20	0	1
Champion Lyte,			
Sports Drink, 8 fl.oz	0	0	0
Champion Performance:			
Heavywt Gainer 900,			
average all flavors, 4 scps, 5.4 oz	600	7	102
Metabolol II, 2 scoops, 2.3 oz	260	3	40
Pure Whey Plus, av., 1 scoop, 1.2 oz	130	2	5
UltraMet, 2.7 oz pkt	280	4	20
Clif: Protein Mix, Chocolate, 1.6 oz	160	0	31
Shot, Energy Gel, av., 1.2 oz pkt	100	0	24
Cocaine, Energy, 8.4 fl.oz can	70	0	18
Core Power:			
26g, av. all flavors, 11.5 fl.oz	240	3.5	27
Elite, 42g, av. all flav., 14 fl.oz	240	3.5	12
Light, 20g, av. all flavors, 11.5 fl.oz	150	3.5	12
Curves, Protein Drink,			
Choc.; Vanilla, 2 scoops, 1 oz	120	1	12
EAS ~ *See AdvantEdge & Myoplex*			
Ensure: *Per Bottle*			
Original, all flavors, 8 fl.oz	220	6	33
Clear, all flavors, 10 fl.oz	180	0	37
Enlive, av. all flavors, 8 fl.oz	350	11	44
High Protein , all flav., 8 fl.oz	160	2	19
Plus, all flavors, 8 fl.oz	350	11	50
Enterex, Diabetic, all flavors, 8 fl.oz	240	9	27
Enu, Nutritional Shakes, av., 11 fl.oz	450	17	53
FRS, Energy & Endurance, all flav., 11.5 fl oz	80	0	22
Fruit₂O (Veryfine): Classic 20 fl.oz	0	0	0
Sparkling, 20 fl.oz	0	0	1
Full Throttle: *Per 16 fl.oz*			
Energy: Citrus; Blue Agave	220	0	58
Orange	220	0	52
Fuze:			
Blends, average, 16.9 fl.oz	185	0.5	43
Juice: Berry Punch, 8 fl.oz	80	0	21
Strawb. Lemonade, 8 fl.oz	100	0	26
Gatorade:			
G Series: *Ready To Drink*			
Endurance: Carb Energy Drink, f fl.oz	120	0	0
Thirst Quencher: 12 fl oz	80	0	21
32 fl oz bottle	215	0	56
Recover,			
Protein Shake, av., 11.2 fl.oz	270	1	46
Genisoy, Prot. Pdr, Choc.; Van., 1.3 oz	125	0	18

	C	F	Cb
Glaceau:			
Smartwater, 8 fl.oz	0	0	0
Vitaminwater, av. all flav., 20 fl.oz	120	0	33
Glucerna: Shakes, all flavors, 8 fl.oz	180	9	16
Advance Shakes, average., 8 fl.oz	200	7	27
Hunger Shakes, average, 8 fl.oz	180	8	15
GNC:			
Pro Performance:			
Amplified: Mass XXX,			
all flavors, 4 scoops	750	6	124
RTD, Wheybolic, Vanilla, 14 fl.oz	190	1	2
Total Lean:			
Adv., Lean Shake Burn, all flav., 14 fl.oz	170	6	8
Lean Shake, all flavors, 2 scoops	180	2	30
Lean Shake 25, all flavors, 2 scoops	195	3	17
Guru:			
Org. Energy Drink: Regular, 8 oz can	80	0	21
Lite,12 oz can	10	0	3
Hammer, Gel, av., 1.2 oz	90	0	21
Hansen's: Energy Pro, 8 fl.oz	130	0	34
Energy Diet Red, 8 fl.oz	20	0	6
Herbalife: Nutr. Shake, 0.9 oz	90	1	13
with 8 fl.oz non-fat milk	170	1	26
Hormel: Protein Powder, 1.2 oz pkt	130	1.5	3
Mighty Shakes, all flav., 8.45 fl.oz	500	22	54
Vital Quisine, all flavors, 14. fl.oz	210	9	8
Hype:			
Enlite, 8.5 fl.oz	25	0	4
Energy: After Dark, Hype, 8.5 fl.oz	130	0	30
MFP, 8.5 fl.oz	110	0	25
Up, Ice Berry Max, 8.5 fl.oz	120	0	28
Shot, 3.5 fl.oz	35	0	8.5
Jarrow:			
Whey Protein: Unflavored, 0.8 oz	95	2	2
Chocolate; Vanilla, 1 oz	105	1	6
Kellogg's:			
To Go, Breakfast Shakes:			
RTD, all flavors, av., 10 fl.oz bottle	185	5	29
Shake Mix, all flavors, av., 1 pkt	130	0.5	27
Knudsen: Recharge, average, 8 fl.oz	75	0	18
Simply Nutritious, av. all, 8 fl.oz	120	0	30
Kombucha,			
Wonder Drink, all flavors, 7 fl.oz	50	0	13
Kroger: *Per 8 fl.oz Bottle*			
Nutrutional Shake, all flavors	190	7	23
Nutrition Shake, Fortify Plus, av.,	350	11	50
La Brada:			
Lean Body, Meal Repl., 2.8 oz scoop	330	8	34
RTD, Lean Body, 17 fl.oz	260	9	9
Liquid Ice: Black, 8.3 fl.oz	110	0	26
Other Flavors, 8.3 fl oz	120	0	28
Liquid Lightning, Reg., 8.5 fl.oz	90	0	22

	C	F	Cb
Max Velocity:			
Energy, 16 fl.oz can	240	0	62
Sugar Free, 16 fl.oz can	15	0	1
MLO,			
Mus-L Blast, Chocolate, 4 scoops	570	3	114
Monster:			
Energy: 16 fl.oz can	210	0	54
Lo-Carb, 16 fl.oz	20	0	6
M-80, 16 fl.oz	180	0	46
Mixxd (with Juice), 16 fl.oz	220	0	54
Java Monster: All flavors, 15 fl.oz	190	3	33
Light, Vanilla, 15 fl.oz	95	3	13
Shakes, 16 fl.oz can	220	4	20
MRM: All Natural Whey, 1 scoop, 0.9 oz	90	1	2
Low Carb Protein, 1 scoop, 1.1 oz	120	2.5	2
Muscle Milk *(Cytosport)*:			
Gainer, powder, av. all flav., 2.85 oz	315	4.5	55
Non Dairy Ready To Drink:			
Chocolate, 11 fl.oz	130	4	7
Vanilla Creme, 11 fl.oz	100	1.5	5
100 Calorie Shakes, av., 11 fl.oz	100	1	6
Pro Series, av. all flavors, 14 fl.oz	200	2.5	9
Yogurt Protein Shakes, 16 fl.oz	260	4.5	28
Muscle Tech:			
Mass-Tech Advantage:			
Milk Choc., 5 scoops, 9 oz	840	8	131
Nitro Tech Ripped, all flavors, 1.5 oz	170	4	3
Myoplex *(EAS)*:			
Ready To Drink Shakes:			
Original, av. all flavors, 17 fl.oz	300	7	19
Shred, Muscle Mocha, 16 fl.oz	210	2	8
Powder: Original Choc. 1 pkt, 2.8 oz	300	6	21
Lite, Choc.Cream, 1 pkt, 1.9 oz	180	2	24
Nature's Best:			
Carb Up, all flavors, 16 fl.oz	400	0	100
Isopure: Alpine Punch, 20 fl.oz	260	0	25
Mass, all flavors, 20 fl.oz	350	0	53
Zero Carb, all flavors, 20 fl.oz	160	0	0
JavaPro Ready To Drink + Coffee,			
Whey Prot. Complex, all flav, 8 fl.oz	110	1.5	3
Nestle Health Science,			
Diabetishield, Mixed Berry, 8 fl.oz	150	0	30
No-Fear: Regular, 16 fl.oz	260	0	72
Sugar Free, 16 fl.oz	20	0	4
NOS, High Performance Energy,			
Grape, 16 fl.oz can	210	0	54
Av. other flavors, 16 fl.oz	200	0	55
Zero, 16 fl.oz	0	0	0
Nutrament *(Nestle)*, 12 fl.oz	360	10	52
Nutrilite *(Amway)*:			
BodyKey Meal Replacement Shakes:			
Powder, av. all flavors, 1.2 oz scoop	110	3	8
Ready To Drink, av. all flav., 11 fl.oz	140	3	15

Energy/Protein Drinks (Cont)

	C	F	Cb
Optifast: (Nestle):			
800: Shake Mix, 1 pkg	160	3.5	18
Ready To Drink Shakes, 8 fl.oz	160	3.5	18
HP Shake Mix, 1 pkg	200	6	10
Optimum Nutrition:			
Gold Standard:			
100% Whey, av. all flavors, 1 oz scp	120	1	4
Gainer, av. all flav., 7.9 oz scoop	770	10	113
Hydro Whey, average. 1.4 oz scoop	140	1	3
Oats & Whey, average, 1.9 oz scoop	205	1.5	23
Optisource (Nestle),			
Very High Prot. Drink, Strawb., 8 fl.oz	200	6	12
OrGain: Per			
Nutr. Prot. Shake, Choc Fudge, 14 fl.oz	150	4	11
Prot. Shake, Iced Cafe Mocha, 11 fl.oz	255	7	32
Powerade,			
ION4, av. all flavors, 20 fl.oz bottle	150	0	35
PowerBar: Protein Shakes, 14 fl.oz	160	3	5
Perfect Energy Blends, av., 1 pouch	80	0	21
Power Gel, average, 1.5 oz pkg	110	0	27
Simple Fruits, av. all flav., 1 pouch	100	0	25
Premier Protein (Premier Nutrition):			
Powder, Choc./Vanilla, average, 1.65 oz	180	3.5	8
Shakes, average, 11 fl.oz bottle	160	3	5
Propel, Purified Water, 12 fl.oz	0	0	0
Protein2O, av. all flavors, 16.9 fl oz	60	0	2
Pure Protein: Per 11 fl.oz Bottle or Can			
23 Gram Shakes, average	115	0.5	8
35 Gram Shakes: Banana	150	1	1
Average other flavors	165	1.5	2
Powder, av., 1 scoop, 1.16 oz	130	2	6
Radioactive:			
Regular: 10.5 oz	150	0	37
16 oz	220	0	56
Sugar Free, all sizes	0	0	0
Red Bull:			
Energy Drink: Average, 8.3 fl.oz	110	0	28
12 fl.oz can	160	0	40
Sugar-Free, 8.4 fl.oz	10	0	3
Zero Calories, 8.4 fl.oz	0	0	0
Revival:			
Soy Mix, unsweetened:			
Plain, 2 scoops, 0.95 oz	105	1	4
Average all flavors, 2 scoops	115	2.5	5
Rhino's, Energy Drink, all flav., 100ml	50	0	11
Rip It, Energy Fuel, Citrus X, 16 fl.oz	200	0	52
Rockstar: Per 16 fl.oz Can			
Energy Drink: Punched, av.	270	0	62
Sugar Free	20	0	0
Rumble, Supershake, 12 fl.oz	250	8	28
Rush: Per 8.4 fl.oz			
Energy Drink: Regular	120	0	32
with Maca, 8 fl.oz	130	0	30

	C	F	Cb
Skratch Labs:			
Hydration Drink Mix: 16 fl. oz Prepared			
Anytime Mix, all flav., 1 scoop, 0.46 oz	50	0	12
Hyper, Mango, 0.9 oz	70	0	16
Rescue, Lemons & Limes, 0.76 oz	70	0	17
Sport Mix, average, 1 scoop, 0.78 oz	80	0	20
Sport Recovery Mix, all flav., 1.76 oz	200	3.5	35
Slim-Fast:			
Original, Protein Shakes, av., 11 fl.oz	185	6	24
Advanced Nutrition:			
Meal Replacement Shakes, av., 11 fl.oz	180	8	6
Smoothies, Powder, av., 1 scoop, 0.9 oz	105	3.5	8
SoBe: Per 20 fl.oz Can/Bottle			
Citrus Energy Fruit Drink	250	0	64
Lifewater: Strawberry Kiwi	100	0	26
Coconut Water	80	0	21
O-Cal, all flavors	0	0	9
Note: Carb figure inlude 7-10g sugar alcohol			
Solixir, Energy Drink, av. all, 12 fl.oz	55	0	13
Special K,			
Protein Shakes, av. all flav.	185	5	23
Spiru-Tein:			
Energy Meal Shake Powder:			
Chai Latte, 1.2 oz scoop	130	0	16
Choc. Chip Cookie Dough, 1.2 oz	130	1.5	14
Gold: Strawberry,1.3 oz scoop	130	0	20
Average other flavors, 1.2 oz	100	0	21
PureTrition, av., 1.3 oz scoop	115	0.5	10
Sport, average, 2.25 oz scoop	260	9	26
Whey, Cookies & Cream, 1.2 oz scp	125	2	15
Starbucks:			
Refreshers, av. all flav.,12 fl.oz	65	0	19
Doubleshot Energy ~ See page 37			
Steaz: Energy, all flav., 12 fl.oz	135	0	35
Zero Calorie, Berry, 12 fl.oz	0	0	0
The Sports Club/LA:			
Beachbody Whey Prot. Powder,			
Chocolate; Vanilla, av., 1 scoop, 1 oz	110	2	4.5
Twin Lab, MVP Fuel, av.,1 sc., 0.5 oz	25	0	6
Vemma: Bod-e Burn, 8 fl.oz can	110	0	12
Energy Drinks, 8.3 fl.oz can	80	0	21
Vemma, 8.3 fl.oz can	50	0	14
Venom: Mojave Rattler, 16 fl.oz	50	0	8
Av. other varieties, 16 fl.oz	235	0	57
Vital Whey, 100% Whey, 0.7 oz	85	1	2
Weider: 100% Whey, av., 1.4 oz sc.	155	3	11
Creatine ATP, ½ cup, 1.7 oz	210	0	37
Dynamic Wt Gainer, av., 4.5 oz	460	2	96
Mega Mass 2000, av., 3.5 oz	400	7	61
Pro Carb, Ult. Mass Gainer,			
6 scoops, average, 7 oz	770	6	161
Worx, Energy, all varieties, 2 fl.oz	0	0	0
XS (Quixtar), Energy Drink, 8.4 oz	10	0	0
Zola Acai: Original Juice, 8 fl.oz	125	2	25
Pomegranate, Blueberry, 8 fl.oz	120	2	25

Quick Guide C F Cb

Orange Juice
Average ~ Fresh

	C	F	Cb
½ Cup, 4 fl.oz	55	0	13
Small Glass, 6 fl.oz	85	0	19
Regular Cup 8 fl.oz	110	0.5	26
Regular Glass, 12 fl.oz	160	0.5	39
10 fl.oz Bottle	140	0.5	32
11.5 fl.oz Can	160	0.5	37
16 fl.oz Bottle	225	1	52
20 fl.oz Bottle	280	1	64

Juices ~ Generic
Average All Brands:

	C	F	Cb
Aloe Vera Juice, unsweetened, 2 oz	10	0	0
Apple Juice: 8 fl.oz	120	0	29
10 fl.oz Bottle	145	0.5	36
16 fl.oz	235	0.5	58
Cactus Water, 1 Cup, 8 oz	25	0	6
Carrot Juice: Fresh, 6 fl.oz	35	0	8
Sweetened, 6 fl.oz	75	0	17
Coconut Water, 8 fl.oz	50	0.5	9
Cranberry Juice, Cocktail/Blend	140	0	34
Fruit Blends, average all, 8 fl.oz	110	0	27
Fruit Nectars, average all, 8 fl.oz	140	0	36
Grape Juice, 8 fl.oz	155	0	38
Grapefruit Juice, 8 fl.oz	95	0	22
Lemon/Lime Juice: 1 Tbsp	5	0	1
1 cup, 8 fl.oz	50	0.5	16
Concentrate, 1 tsp	0	0	0
Noni Juice:			
Tahitian, 2 Tbsp, 1 fl.oz	15	0	3
Tahiti Traders, 1 fl.oz	20	0	5
Papaya/Peach Nectar, av., 8 fl.oz	140	0	36
Passion Fruit Juice, Fresh:			
Purple, 1 cup, 8 fl.oz	125	0	34
Yellow, 1 cup, 8 fl.oz	80	1.5	14
Pear Nectar, 8 fl.oz	150	0	40
Pineapple Juice, 8 fl.oz	130	0	32
Pomegranate Juice, 8 fl.oz	160	0	40
Prune Juice, 8 fl.oz	180	0	45
Strawberry/Raspberry Juice, 8 fl.oz	100	0	23
Tangerine Juice, 8 fl.oz	105	0.5	25
Tomato Juice, 8 fl.oz	40	0	10
Vegetable Juice, 8 fl.oz	45	0	11
Wheat Grass Juice:			
1 fl.oz 'Shot'	10	0	1.5
2 fl.oz 'Shot'	20	0	3

Quick Guide C F Cb

Fruit Smoothies (Jamba Juice; Smoothie King)
Average All Brands

	C	F	Cb
Fruit Only: 8 fl.oz	115	0.5	29
12 fl.oz	175	1	43
16 fl.oz	230	1	58
24 fl.oz	350	1	78
Fruit + Non-Fat Milk/Soy:			
12 fl.oz	135	0	29
16 fl.oz	155	0	37
24 fl.oz	265	1	59
Fruit + Non-Fat Frozen Yogurt/Sherbet:			
12 fl.oz	200	0.5	47
16 fl.oz	265	1	63
24 fl.oz	395	1.5	95

Juice ~ Brands

Per 8 fl.oz Unless Indicated

Apple & Eve:

100% Juice, No Sugar Added:

	C	F	Cb
Cherries & Berries; Cranb. Raspb., av.	120	0	29
Cranberry Apple	130	0	33
Cranberry Pomegranate	140	0	34
Fruitables, av. all flav., 6.75 fl.oz	60	0	14
Organic Quenchers, all flav., 6.75 fl.oz	40	0	10
Bolthouse Farms: *Per 8 fl.oz*			
Juice: 100% Carrot	70	0	15
100% Pomegranate	150	0	38
Acai + 10 Superblend	120	0	31
Mango Ginger + Carrot	110	0.5	27
Orange + Carrot	100	0	22
Fruit Smoothies: Amazing Mango	130	0	31
Berry Boost	120	0	27
Blue Goodness	170	1.5	41
C-Boost	110	0	27
Green Goodness	130	0	30
Strawberry Banana	130	0	32
Bright & Early *(Minute Maid)*,			
Orange Flavored Drink, 8 fl.oz	110	0	30
Cactus Cooler, Orange Pineapple Blast,			
12 fl oz can	150	0	40
Campbell's:			
Tomato Juice: 5.5 fl.oz can	30	0	7
8 fl.oz	50	0	10

Juice Brands (Cont)

	C	F	Cb

Per 8 fl.oz Unless Indicated

Califia Farms: *Per 8 fl.oz Unless Indicated*

Agua Fresca:

	C	F	Cb
Strawberry Basil	80	0	20
Watermelon Ginger Lime	60	0	14
Ginger Limeade	90	0	21
Meyer Lemonade	80	0	21
Orange Juice, 10.5 fl.oz	140	0.5	32
Tangerine	100	0	24

Capri Sun: *Per 6 fl.oz*

	C	F	Cb
100% Juice, average,	85	0	21
Juice Drinks,			
(25% Less Sugar), all flavors	50	0	14
Roarin' Waters, all flav., 6 fl.oz	30	0	8

Clamato: *Per 8 fl.oz*

	C	F	Cb
Original Tomato Cocktail	60	0	12
Picante	60	0	13
Coco Joy, Coconut Water, 8.4 fl.oz	30	0	7
Coco Libre, Coconut Water, 11 fl.oz pkg	60	0	14

CocoZia, Coconut Water:

	C	F	Cb
100% Organic, 11.1 fl.oz pkg	70	0	16
Original, 8 fl.oz	40	0	10
Chocolate, 8 fl.oz	60	0.5	13

Dole: *Per 8 fl.oz*

	C	F	Cb
100% Pure, Chilled or Frozen, av.	120	0	28
Blended Juices, average all flavors	120	0	30

Florida's Natural: *Per 8 fl.oz*

	C	F	Cb
Apple Juice	120	0	29
Cranberry Ruby Red Cocktail	130	0	32
Orange, No Pulp	110	0	26
100% Blends: Orange Mango	110	0	27
Orange Pineapple	130	0	31
Orange Strawberry	110	0	26
Ruby Red Grapefruit, Original	90	0	22

Goya: *Per 12 fl.oz Can*

	C	F	Cb
Nectar: Guava; Tamarind	240	0	59
Mango	230	0	56
Papaya; Peach, average	220	0	55
Average other varieties	220	0	55

Per 8 fl.oz Unless Indicated

Great Value *(Walmart):*

100% Juice: *Per 8 fl.oz*

	C	F	Cb
Apple	110	0	28
Cranberry Pomegranate	140	0	35
Grape	160	0	40
Orange, all varieties	110	0	26
White Grape	150	0	38

Hansen's:

Juice Box: *Per 6.75 fl.oz Box*

	C	F	Cb
Awesome Apple; Loud Lemonade, av.	90	0	23
Burstin Berry; Totally Tropical	100	0	24
Strawberry Banana	110	0	27

Junior Juice,

	C	F	Cb
100% Juice, av. of flavors, 4.23 oz box	60	0	16

Natural, (64 fl.oz Bottles): *Per 8 fl.oz*

	C	F	Cb
Apple	120	0	28
Apple Strawberry	110	0	27
Cranberry Apple	110	0	27
Cranberry Grape	140	0	35
Grape	120	0	33
White Grape	140	0	36

Hawaii's Own, Frozen Concentrate,

	C	F	Cb
10% Juice, average all flavors, 8 fl.oz prepared	105	0	27

Hi-C Juice Drinks: *Per 6.75 fl.oz Box*

	C	F	Cb
Flashin' Fruit Punch	90	0	25
Orange Lavaburst	90	0	25
Poppin' Lemonade	100	0	27

Hood: *Per 8 fl.oz*

	C	F	Cb
Apple	120	0	31
Lemonade	110	0	29
Orange	120	0	30

Jamba Juice ~ *See Fast-Foods Section*

Juicy Juice *(Nestle):*

Average all flavors:

	C	F	Cb
4.23 fl.oz box	60	0	15
6.75 fl.oz box	100	0	24

Kerns:

Nectars: *Per 11.5 fl.oz Can*

	C	F	Cb
Guava; Strawberry	210	0	53
Pear; Strawb. Banana, av.	220	0	53
Pineapple Coconut	280	8	53

Kool Aid, Jammers,

	C	F	Cb
Scary Blackberry; Trop. Punch, 6 fl.oz	80	0	20

L & A: *Per 8 fl.oz*

	C	F	Cb
All Cherry	180	0	45
All Cranberry	60	0	14
Papaya Delight	130	0	32
Pineapple Coconut	140	3	28

Juice Brands (Cont) — C F Cb

Per 8 fl.oz Unless Indicated

Lakewood Organic: *Per 8 fl.oz*

	C	F	Cb
Blends: Acai Amazon Berry	130	1.5	29
Blueberry Blend	120	0	31
Cranberry Lemonade	100	0	24
Lemonade	100	0	25
Pineapple Coconut	190	8	29
Pomegranate Lemonade	100	0	26
Super Kale	100	0	24
Super Tomato	70	0	15
Super Veggie	60	0	13
Pure: Apple	120	0	30
Beet	100	0	23
Blueberry	110	0	26
Carrot	90	0	21
Cranberry	80	0	19
Noni	5	0	1
Orange	120	0	28
Pineapple	130	0	31
Pink Grapefruit	100	0	24
Prune	180	0	42

Langers: *Per 8 fl.oz*

	C	F	Cb
100% Juice: Apple Cider	120	0	28
Apple Juice	120	0	28
Red/White Grape Juice	160	0	40
Juice Cocktails (27% Juice):			
Blueberry Cranberry	135	0	34
Cranberry	140	0	35
Cranberry Grape	165	0	41
Cranberry Raspberry	140	0	35
20% Juice, all flavors	120	0	30

Martinellli's: *Per 8 fl.oz*

	C	F	Cb
Juice, 100% Apple, all varieties	140	0	35
Sparkling: Apple Cider	140	0	35
Apple-Cranberry	110	0	27
Apple Grape	120	0	31
Apple-Mango/Pomegranate	140	0	34
Apple-Pear/Marionberry, av.	125	0	31

Minute Maid:

15.2 fl.oz Bottles: *Per Bottle*

	C	F	Cb
Apple Juice	210	0	52
Cranb. Apple Raspberry	230	0	61
Cranberry Grape	270	0	74
Pineapple Orange	220	0	55

Per 8 fl.oz Unless Indicated

Minute Maid (Cont): — C F Cb

	C	F	Cb
Orange Juice,			
Pure, No Pulp, 8 fl.oz	110	0	26
Coolers, average all flavors, 6.75 fl.oz	100	0	26
Kid's Juice Boxes, 100% Juice,			
Apple White Grape, 6.75 fl.oz	90	0	22
Light Juices: Orange, 8 fl.oz	50	0	13
With Tea; Light Lemonade, 8 fl.oz	15	0	3
Soft Frozen Concentrate,			
Limeade, 3 fl.oz tube	70	0	19

Mott's:

100% Juice:

	C	F	Cb
Original Apple, 8 fl.oz	120	0	29
Apple White Grape, 6.75 fl.oz	130	0	31
Fruit Punch, 4.23 fl.oz	60	0	15
Light, Apple, 8 fl.oz	50	0	12
Juice Drink:			
Fruit Punch Rush, 8 fl.oz	60	0	16
Strawberry Boom, 8 fl.oz	60	0	15
Wild Grape Surge, 8 fl.oz	60	0	16
Medleys:			
Apple, 8 fl.oz	110	0	25
Grape, 8 fl.oz	140	0	33
Mott's For Tots (47-54% Juice):			
40% Less Sugar:			
Apple Wh. Grape; Fruit Punch, 8 fl.oz	70	0	17
Average other flavors, 8 fl.oz	60	0	16

Naked Juice: *Per 15.2 fl.oz*

	C	F	Cb
100% Juice, No Sugar Added:			
O-J	210	0	51
Orange Mango	250	0	59
Pomegranate Blueberry	290	0	68
100% Juice Smoothie, No Sugar Added:			
Berry Blast; Strawb. Banana	250	0	55
Mighty Mango	290	0	68
Boosted: Acai Machine	300	6	59
Blue Machine	170	0	40
Green Machine	270	0	63
Power-C Machine	230	0	55
Red Machine	320	9	59
Coconut Water: Pure, 16.9 fl.oz	80	0	21
Kale Coconut, 16.9 fl.oz	120	0	30
Pineapple Coconut, 8 fl.oz	50	0	13

Juice Brands (Cont)

Per 8 fl.oz Unless Indicated

	C	**F**	**Cb**
Nantucket Nectars:			
100% Juice: *Per 16 fl.oz*			
Peach Orange	270	0	64
Pineapple Orange Banana	290	0	69
Pomegranate Cherry	230	0	57
Premium Orange Juice	220	0	51
Pressed Apple	240	0	59
Juice Cocktail, Cranberry	240	0	59
Juice Drinks: *Per 16 fl.oz*			
Orange Mango	220	0	59
Pineapple Orange Guava	210	0	52
Pomegranate Pear	230	0	57
Red Plum	220	0	53
Watermelon Strawberry	220	0	55
Lemonade, Squeezed	180	0	47
Newman's Own: *Per 8 fl.oz*			
Lemonade, Regular; Pink	110	0	27
Limeade	140	0	34
Fruit Juice Cocktail:			
Gorilla Grape	110	0	29
Orange Mango Tango	130	0	33
Northland: *Per 8 fl.oz*			
100% Juice:			
Blueberry Blackberry Acaí	110	0	25
Cranb. Blackberry/Raspberry, av.	110	0	25
Cranberry Cherry	140	0	35
Cranberry Grape	100	0	25
Cranberry Mango	120	0	29
Superfruits, Raspb. Pomegr. Goji	130	0	32
Ocean Spray: *Per 8 fl.oz*			
Juice Cocktails:			
Blueberry; Cranberry	110	0	28
100% Juice Blends:			
Citrus Tangerine Orange	110	0	28
Cranberry Concord Grape	130	0	33
Cranberry Mango	120	0	30
Cranberry Raspberry	120	0	30
Juice Drinks:			
Cran-Apple	120	0	31
Cran-Grape	120	0	31
Cran-Tangerine	110	0	28
Diet Juice Drinks, all flavors	5	0	2
Light Juice Drinks, av. all flavors	50	0	13
Sparkling, av. all flavors, 8.4 fl.oz	85	0	22
Wave, average all flavors, 8 fl.oz	80	0	20

Per 8 fl.oz Unless Indicated

	C	**F**	**Cb**
Odwalla:			
100% Juice: *Per 15.2 fl.oz Bottle*			
Berry Greens	160	0	39
Groovin' Greens	150	0	37
Orange	210	0	47
Smoothies: *Per 15.2 fl.oz Bottle*			
Citrus C Monster	240	0	58
Mango Tango	260	0	65
Mo' Beta	250	0	59
Original Superfood	240	0	58
Red Rhapsody	210	0	52
Strawberry C Monster	240	0	58
Orange Julius:			
Originals: *Per Medium*			
Mango P'apple, 22.2 oz	450	0	114
Orange, 18.2 oz	270	0	68
Pina Colada, 21.6 oz	470	7	99
Strawberry Banana, 20.9 oz	530	8	114
Smoothies ~ *See Fast-Foods Section*			
Orangina, 10 fl.oz bottle	130	0	32
Pom Wonderful,			
100% Juice (8 fl.oz Bottle),			
Pom Blueberry/Cherry/Pomegranate	150	0	37
R.W. Knudsen: *Per 8 fl.oz*			
Organic, 100% Juice: Apple	110	0	28
Concord Grape	150	0	39
Cranberry Blueberry	120	0	31
Natural, 100% Juice:			
Mango Peach	120	0	30
Papaya Nectar	130	0	32
Razzleberry	110	0	28
Rio Red Grapefruit	140	0	34
Just Juice:			
Just Blueberry	100	0	24
Just Black Cherry	150	0	36
Just Black Currant	110	0	25
Simply Nutritious: Mega C	120	0	30
Average other flavors	125	0	31
Sparkling: Blueberry; Cranberry, av.	110	0	28
Cherry; Pomegranate	130	0	32
Organic Pear	120	0	31

Juice Brands (Cont)   C   F   Cb

Per 8 fl.oz Unless Indicated
R.W. Knudsen (Cont):
Sensible Sippers: *Per 4.23 fl oz*

	C	F	Cb
Organic Apple; Fruit Punch	30	0	7
Organic Berry	35	0	9
Very Veggie, Original, 8 fl.oz	60	0	12

ReaLemon – ReaLime:
Lemon/Lime Juice (from concentrate):

	C	F	Cb
1 teaspoon	0	0	0
2Tbsp, 1 fl.oz	10	0	2.5

Santa Cruz: *Per 8 fl.oz*
Organic, 100% Juice:

	C	F	Cb
Apple; Red Tart Cherry	120	0	30
Concord/White Grape	160	0	39
Orange Mango	120	0	29
Pear Nectar	130	0	33

Carbonated Beverages,

	C	F	Cb
Lemonade, 10.5 fl.oz can	130	0	32
Lemonade: Regular; Peach; Mango	90	0	22
Cherry	100	0	26
Raspberry; Strawberry, average	90	0	24

Simply Orange Juice Company:

	C	F	Cb
Lemonade; Limeade, average	120	0	31
Mixed Berry; Fruit Punch; Tropical	100	0	26
Orange Juice, with or without pulp	110	0	26

Snap·E· Tom,

	C	F	Cb
Tomato & Chili Cocktail, 11.5 fl.oz can	70	0	15

Snapple: *Per 16 fl.oz Bottle*
Juice Drink Blends:

	C	F	Cb
Go Bananas; Rasp. Peach, av.	225	0	55
Grapeade; Lemonade; Orangeade	190	0	46
Fruit Punch	200	0	48
Diet, Cranberry Raspberry	20	0	5

Ssips, Juice Boxes,

	C	F	Cb
av. all flavors, 6 fl.oz box	80	0	21

Stonyfield Farm: *Per 10 fl.oz Bottle*

	C	F	Cb
Smoothies: Strawb.; Wild Berry	230	3	39
Peach	230	3	42
6 oz Bottle, Strawb. Banana	140	2	25

Per 8 fl.oz Unless Indicated   C   F   Cb
SunnyD:
Original: *Per 64 fl.oz Ctn*

	C	F	Cb
Orange, all var., 8 fl.oz	50	0	15

Blends, 64 fl.oz Containers,

	C	F	Cb
average all flavors, 8 fl.oz	60	0	15

Baja Juice: *Per 12 fl.oz Bottles*

	C	F	Cb
Red Punch	170	0	43
Other flavors	190	0	46

Chillers: *Pe 16 fl.oz*

	C	F	Cb
Blue Raspberry	110	0.5	28
Grape	120	0	30

Sunsweet: *Per 8 fl.oz*

	C	F	Cb
Plum Smart: Original	160	0	36
Light	60	0	15
Prune Juice: Original	180	0	42
Light	100	0	26

Trader Joe's:
All Natural Pasteurized, 32/64 fl.oz Bottle: *Per 8 fl.oz*

	C	F	Cb
100% Cranberry	70	0	16
Blueberry Pomegranate	140	0	34
Just Blueberry	100	0	24
Just Pomegranate	150	0	37
Mango PassionFruit	130	0	32
Omega Orange Carrot	110	0	26

Organic, 32/64 fl.oz Bottle: *Per 8 fl.oz*

	C	F	Cb
100% Pomegranate	140	0	35
Apple Juice	120	0	30
Concord Grape Juice	160	0	39
Cranberry	70	0	18
Grapefruit Sunset; Lemonade	120	0	30
Mango Nectar	130	0	32
Pink Lemonade	130	0	32
Strawberry Lemonade	120	0	29
White Grape Juice	160	0	40

Joe's Kids: *Per 6.75 oz Box*

	C	F	Cb
From Concentrate: Apple	90	0	23
Apple Grape	100	0	24
White Grape	120	0	30
10% Juice, Lemonade	90	0	22

Sparkling Juices, 25.4 fl.oz Botle:

	C	F	Cb
Blueberry, 8 fl.oz	120	0	30
Cranberry, 8 fl.oz	140	0	35
Pomegranate, 8 fl.oz	130	0	31

Juice Brands (Cont)   **C** **F** **Cb**

Per 8 fl.oz Unless Indicated

Tree Top:
100% Juice Concentrates:
64 fl.oz Bottle: *Per 8 fl.oz*

	C	F	Cb
Apple Berry/Grape, average	125	0	32
Apple Cranb.; Or. Passionfruit, av.	115	0	28
11.5 fl.oz Can: *Per Can*			
Apple Berry/Grape, av.	180	0	46
6.75 fl.oz Box, average	105	0	26
Smoothie, Ban. Strawb., 4.5 fl.oz	100	0	23

Tropicana:
20% Juice, 15.2 fl.oz Bottle,

	C	F	Cb
Cranberry	270	0	66
Farmstand, 32 fl.oz bottle,			
average all flavors, 8 fl.oz	120	0	27
100% Juice Pure Premium:			
Grapefruit, 15.2 fl.oz	170	0	42
Ruby Red Grapefruit, 15.2 fl.oz	250	0	59
Strawberry Kiwi, 15.2 fl.oz	230	0	58
Trop50, 50% less sugar, 59 fl.oz bottle,			
average all flavors, 8 fl.oz	50	0	13
Trop Twisters, 20 fl.oz bottle:			
Or. Strawb. Banana Burst	330	0	80
Tropicana Twister , 20 fl.oz	340	0	85
Tropics, 59 fl.oz container,			
average all flavors, 8 fl.oz	125	0	30

Tru Nopal:

	C	F	Cb
Cactus Water: 1 Cup, 8 fl.oz	25	0	6
16.9 fl.oz carton	50	0	12

Turkey Hill: *Per 8 fl.oz*

	C	F	Cb
All Natural Lemonade: Classic	100	0	26
Blackberry	110	0	27
Regular Lemonade flavors	120	0	29
Fruit Punch	100	0	26
Orangeade	110	0	26

V8 Juices & Drinks (Campbell's):
Original/Spicy 100% Vegetable Juice:

	C	F	Cb
5.5 fl.oz can	35	0	7
8 fl.oz cup	50	0	10
11.5 fl.oz can	70	0	14
12 fl.oz bottle	75	0	15
Blends: Pineapple Passion, 8 fl.oz	70	0	17
Red Radiance, 8 fl.oz	70	0	17
Healthy Greens; Carrot Mango, 8 fl.oz	60	0	14
V-Fusion: Average all flavors	115	0	28
Light Varieties, av. all flavors	50	0	13

Veryfine:

	C	F	Cb
100%: Apple, 8 fl.oz	120	0	29
Apple Strawb., Krazy Kiwi, 11.5 fl.oz	170	0	43
Orange, 8 fl.oz	120	0	30

Per 8 fl.oz Unless Indicated   **C** **F** **Cb**

Vita Coco:

	C	F	Cb
Coconut Water: 8 fl.oz	45	0	11
with Pineapple, 8 fl.oz	60	0	15
Chocolate, 11 fl.oz	90	3	16

Walnut Acres: *Per 8 fl.oz*

	C	F	Cb
Organic: Apple; Cranberry, av.	110	0	28
Apricot; Raspberry	130	0	32
Cherry	140	0	34
Incredible Vegetable	50	0	12
Mango Nectar	120	0	29

Welch's: *Per 8 fl.oz Unless Indicated*

	C	F	Cb
100% Juice: Concord Grape	140	0	36
Red Grape juice	160	0	41
White Grape	140	0	38
White Grape Cherry/Peach	140	0	34
Fruit Shots, all flavors, 5.5 fl.oz can	90	0	22
Frozen Concentrates,			
100% Juice, Grape; all var., 2 fl oz	140	0	39
Light Juice, 52 fl.oz Bottle			
Concord/White Grape, 8 fl.oz	45	0	12
Sparkling Juice Cocktail:			
Blueberry Grape, 8 fl.oz	150	0	38
Other flavors, 8 fl.oz	160	0	40

Zola:
Acai: *Per 12 fl.oz Bottle*

	C	F	Cb
Original	185	3	38
with Blueberry/Pomegranate	180	3	38
Coconut Water, 17.5 oz Can:			
Original,	50	0	13
Chocolate, 8 fl.oz	50	0	12
Espresso, 8 fl.oz	60	0	13

CALORIEKING PORTION WATCH

ORANGE JUICE	C	Cb
8 fl.oz	110	26
16 fl.oz	220	52
24 fl.oz	330	78
32 fl.oz	440	104

Quick Guide   C   F   Cb

Cow's Milk ~ Average All Brands
Whole (3.25% fat):

	C	F	Cb
2 Tbsp, 1 fl.oz	20	1	1.5
1 Cup, 8 fl.oz	150	8	12
1 Large Glass, 12 fl.oz	220	12	17
1 Pint, 16 fl.oz	295	16	22
1 Quart, 946 ml	590	32	44

Reduced-Fat (2% fat):

2 Tbsp, 1 fl.oz	15	0.5	1.5
1 Cup, 8 fl.oz	120	5	12
1 Large Glass, 12 fl.oz	180	7.5	18
1 Pint, 16 fl.oz	245	10	23
1 Quart, 946 ml	490	20	46

Light/Low-Fat (1% fat):

2 Tbsp, 1 fl.oz	13	0.3	1.5
1 Cup, 8 fl.oz	100	2.5	12
1 Large Glass, 12 fl.oz	150	4	18
1 Pint, 16 fl.oz	205	5	25
1 Quart, 946 ml	410	10	49

Fat Free/Skim (0% fat):

2 Tbsp, 1 fl.oz	10	0	1.5
1 Cup, 8 fl.oz	90	0.5	13
1 Large Glass, 12 fl.oz	135	0.5	19
1 Pint, 16 fl.oz	180	1	26

Half & Half ~ *See Page* [89]

Other Milks   C   F   Cb

Buttermilk: *Average All Brands*

	C	F	Cb
Reduced-Fat (2%), 1 cup, 8 fl.oz	120	5	10
Low-Fat (1%), 1 cup, 8 fl.oz	100	2.5	12

Lactose Free:

Lactaid 100: Whole	160	8	13
2% Reduced-Fat	130	5	12
1% Low-Fat	110	2.5	13
Fat Free; Calcium Enriched	90	0	13
Smart Balance,			
FF + Omega-3s & Vit. E	100	0	14

Lower Calorie/Carb Dairy Drinks: *Per 8 fl.oz Cup*

Calorie Countdown (*Hood*):			
2% Reduced-Fat: Plain	70	4.5	3
Chocolate	80	4.5	6
Fat-Free	35	0	4

Goat/Sheep Milk, Kefir

Goat's Milk (*Meyenberg*):

Whole, 1 cup, 8 fl.oz	140	7	11
Low-Fat (1%), 8 fl.oz	100	2.5	11
Evaporated, reconst., 8 fl.oz	140	8	12

Kefir: *Per 8 fl.oz*

Lifeway: Original, Plain	150	8	12
Greek, Plain, whole milk	210	14	12
Lowfat, average all flavors	140	1.5	20
Nancy's: Plain, low fat	140	3	17
Fruit flavors, average	205	2.5	38
Trader Joe's: Plain, 1%	110	2.5	8
Strawberry	160	2	21
Sheep's Milk, Whole, 1 cup	265	17	13

Canned & Dried Milk

Condensed: Sweetened, 2 T., 1 fl.oz	130	3	22
Low Fat, 2 Tbsp	120	1.5	23
Fat-Free, 2 Tbsp	110	0	24
Evaporated: Whole, 2 Tbsp	40	3	3
Whole, 1/2 cup, 4 fl.oz	170	10	13
Carnation: Low Fat, 2 Tbsp, 1 oz	25	0.5	3
1/2 cup, 4 fl.oz	115	2.5	14
Fat-Free, 2 Tbsp, 1 oz	25	0	4
Dried: Whole, 1/4 cup, 1 oz	160	9	12
Skim/Non-Fat, 1/3 cup	80	0	12
Made-up, 1 cup, 8 fl.oz	80	0	12
Buttermilk (sweet cream): 1 oz	110	2	14
Non-Fat, 1 Tbsp	25	0	3
Carnation, Malted, dry, 3 Tbsp, 0.7 oz	90	2	15
Horlick's, Malt Powder, dry, 1 oz	180	4	27

Soy/Non-Dairy Drinks ~ See Page 49

SWITCH & SAVE

Switch from whole milk to either 2%, 1% or 0% milk and save significant calories.

Per 8 oz Cup/Glass

WHOLE MILK 3.3% Fat 150 Cals

2% MILK 120 Cals	SAVE 30 Cals
1% MILK 100 Cals	SAVE 50 Cals
0% FAT-FREE 90 Cals	SAVE 60 Cals

Switching to low-fat or fat-free milk also greatly reduces saturated fat.

Quick Guide   C   F   Cb

Chocolate Milk:
Average All Brands:

	C	F	Cb
Whole Milk, (3.3%):			
8 fl.oz cup	220	8	29
1 Pint, 16 fl.oz	440	16	58
Reduced-Fat, (2%):			
8 fl.oz cup	190	5	30
1 Pint, 16 fl.oz	380	10	60
Low-Fat, (1%):			
8 fl.oz cup	160	3	26
1 Pint, 16 fl.oz	315	5	52

Flavored Milk ~ Brands   C   F   Cb

	C	F	Cb
Ready-To-Drink: *Per 8 fl.oz Cup Unless Indicated*			
Albertson's, Choc Milk	180	2.5	29
Great Value *(Walmart),*			
Low Fat Choc. Milk, 8 oz	160	2.5	26
Hood: Chocolate	220	8	30
Low-Fat (1%), Chocolate	160	2.5	28
Horizon Organic:			
Low-Fat:			
Chocolate with Omega 3	150	2.5	23
Vanilla with Omega 3	150	2.5	22
Kellogg's:			
To Go, Breakfast Shakes: *Per 10 fl.oz*			
Chocolate; Strawberry, av.	180	5	29
Mixes, average all flavors,			
1 packet	130	0	26
Kroger, Simple Truth,			
Choc Milk, Low-Fat, 1%	150	2.5	22
Land O Lakes: *Per 8 fl.oz*			
Grip 'n Go:			
Swiss Chocolate (2% red-fat)	190	5	26
Strawberry (whole milk)	190	8	22
Muscle Milk ~ *See Energy Protein Drinks*			
Nesquik: *Per 8 fl.oz*			
Low Fat, average all flavors	150	2.5	24
Chocolate: Fat Free, 8 fl.oz	95	0	24
No Sugar Added	100	2	13
Prairie Farms: *Per 8 fl.oz*			
Chocolate, 2% Reduced Fat	180	5	26
Strawberry, 1% Low Fat	160	2.5	28
Ralphs,			
Choc., Low-Fat, 8 fl.oz	210	2.5	36
Starbucks *~See Page 37*			

Flavored Milk ~ Brands (Cont)

	C	F	Cb
Ready-To-Drink:			
TruMoo:			
Chocolate/Strawberry*:*			
Whole, 8 fl.oz	220	8	29
1% Low-Fat: 8 fl.oz	140	2.5	20
14 fl.oz Bottle	250	5	35
Fat-free, 8 fl.oz	120	0	20
High Protein 1% (25g),			
average all flavors, 8 fl.oz	205	2.5	31
Yoo-Hoo, Chocolate,15.5 fl.oz bottle	230	2	51
Bottled Coffee Drinks ~ *See Page 37*			

Shakes

	C	F	Cb
Arby's: *Per Small Size*			
Jamocha, Ultimate Choc.,	545	18	88
Burger King: *Per Medium 16 oz*			
Hand Spun Shakes: Chocolate	760	21	131
Strawberry	640	15	113
Vanilla	580	15	98
Other flavors ~ *See Fast Food Section*			
Denny's: Cake Batter, 21 oz	1310	69	160
Chocolate, 16 oz	860	44	104
Oreo, 16 oz	1180	61	174
Strawberry, 15 oz	730	33	95
Vanilla, 16 oz	870	44	107
Hardees, all flavors, av., 14 oz	710	33	87
McDonalds, McCafe Shakes:			
Chocolate/Strawberry, average:			
12 fl.oz cup	530	16	86
16 fl.oz cup	635	18	104
22 fl.oz cup	850	24	141
Other Restaurants ~ *See Fast-Foods Section*			

Smoothies

	C	F	Cb
Made Up Ready-To-Drink:			
8 fl. oz Milk/Soy + Fruit: *Per 12 fl.oz*			
Average all flavors:			
with Whole Milk	300	8	50
+ Ice Cream, 1 scoop	400	13	62
with Non-Fat Milk	240	0	50
Kroger/Ralph's Smoothies: *Per 8 fl.oz*			
Mixed Berry	210	2.5	40
Strawberry Banana	200	2.5	37
Freshens; Jamba Juice; TCBY ~ *See Fast-Foods*			

Nut, Rice & Cereal Drinks

Per 8 fl.oz Cup Unless Indicated **C F Cb**

Almond Breeze *(Blue Diamond):*

	C	F	Cb
Original: Regular	60	2.5	8
Reduced Sugar	40	2.5	4
Chocolate	120	3	22
Vanilla	80	2.5	14
Unsweetened: Original; Vanilla	30	2.5	2
Chocolate	40	3.5	2

Almond Dream: *Per 8 fl.oz*

	C	F	Cb
Almond Drink: Pumpkin Spice	50	1.5	9
Orig, Enriched Unswtn'd	50	3.5	3
Amazake, Oh So Original, Rice Shake	150	0	31

Better Than Milk:

	C	F	Cb
Rice Vegan Powder Mix, Orig.; Van., 2 Tbsp, 0.7 oz	70	0	17
Cacique, Horchata Rice Drink	160	3.5	31

Califia Farms: *Per 8 fl.oz Cup*

	C	F	Cb
Almond Milk: Original	60	4	6
Unsweetened	35	3	1
Vanilla	50	3	4
Toasted Coconut Almond	45	4	1

Don Jose: *Per 8 fl.oz Cup*

	C	F	Cb
Cereal Match	100	3	17
Horchata Rice Drink	140	4	25

Dream: *Per 8 fl.oz Cup*

	C	F	Cb
Boosted: Original Almond	120	7	6
Coconut	130	8	5
Enriched, unsweetened	50	3.5	3
Ultimate: Original Almond	150	11	9
Unsweetened	130	11	4

Milkadamia: *Per 8 fl.oz Cup*

	C	F	Cb
Macadamia Nut Milk: Original	70	5	7
Original; Vanilla, unsweetened	50	5	1
Latte da	70	4.5	8

Pacific Foods: *Per 8 fl.oz Cup*

	C	F	Cb
Hazelnut: Original	110	3.5	19
Chocolate	120	5	19
Organic Almond:			
Original; Vanilla, av.	65	3	10
Chocolate, single serve container	100	3	19
Organic Oat, Original/Vanilla, av.	130	2.5	25

Rice Dream: *Per 8 fl.oz Cup*

	C	F	Cb
Organic Original Rice: Classic	120	2.5	23
Vanilla	130	2.5	26
Enriched: Unsweetened	70	2.5	11
Chocolate	160	3	34
Horchata, 8 fl.oz cup	160	2.5	33

Note: Rice/Oat/Nut drinks are very low in protein. Unless enriched with protein (and calcium), they are not suitable for infants as a substitute for milk or calcium-enriched soy drinks.

Nut & Rice Drinks (Cont)

Per 8 fl.oz Cup Unless Indicated **C F Cb**

Silk: *Per 8 fl.oz Cup*

	C	F	Cb
Almond: Original	60	2.5	8
Dark Chocolate	100	2.5	19
Unswt'nd, Orig.; Vanilla	30	2.5	0.5
Cashew:			
Original	60	2.5	9
Unsweetened/ Vanilla	25	2	1
Chocolate	90	2	18

Trader Joe's: *Per 8 fl.oz Cup*

	C	F	Cb
Rice Drinks:			
Unsweetened:			
Original, Organic	120	2.5	23
Vanilla	130	2.5	26
WestSoy, Rice, Plain; Vanilla	110	2.5	20

Soy Milk ~ Ready-To-Drink

365 Organic *(Whole Foods): Per 8 fl.oz Cup*

	C	F	Cb
Original, unsweetened	70	4	4
Chocolate	140	3.5	22
Vanilla	90	3.5	10
Light: Original	70	1.5	9
Vanilla	70	1.5	10

8th Continent: *Per 8 fl.oz Cup*

	C	F	Cb
Original	80	2.5	7
Complete Vanilla	80	2.5	8
Vanilla	100	2.5	11
Light: Original	50	2	2
Chocolate	90	1.5	12
Vanilla	60	2	5
Better Than Milk, Orig., 8 fl.oz cup	90	1.5	18

Edensoy: *Per 8 fl.oz Cup*

	C	F	Cb
Organic: Original	140	5	14
Carob	170	4	28
Unsweetened	120	6	5
Vanilla	150	3	24
Extra: Original	130	4	13
Vanilla	150	3	23

	C	F	Cb
Great Value *(Walmart),* **Vanilla Soy Milk,** 8 fl.oz	100	3.5	10

Kikkoman ~ See Pearl *(next page)*

Odwalla: *Per 15.2 fl.oz Bottle*

Soy & Dairy Protein Shakes:

	C	F	Cb
Chocolate	410	8	53
Strawberry	300	6	36
Vanilla	370	6	46

Soy Milk ~ Ready-To-Drink (Cont)

Per 8 fl.oz Unless Indicated

	C	F	Cb
Pacific: *Per 8 fl.oz Cup*			
Organic, Original, unsweetened	90	4.5	4
Select Soy: Original	70	2.5	9
Vanilla	80	2.5	11
Ultra: Original	140	5	12
Vanilla	140	5	14
Pearl *(Kikkoman): Per 8 fl.oz Cup*			
Chocolate	150	4.5	21
Coffee Flavor	150	4	24
Creamy Vanilla	110	3.5	11
Original	110	3.5	12
Unsweetened	80	2.5	6
Silk *(Whitewave): Per 8 fl.oz Cup*			
Original	110	4.5	9
Chocolate	120	3	21
Vanilla	100	3.5	12
Very Vanilla	130	3.5	18
Light: Original	60	2	5
Chocolate	90	1.5	16
Vanilla	70	2	7
Organic: Orig., unsweet'nd	80	4	4
Vanilla	100	3.5	10
Slim-Fast ~ *See Page 40*			
Soy Dream: *Per 8 fl.oz Cup*			
Enriched: Original	100	4	8
Vanilla	120	4	14
Organic: Original	130	4	16
Vanilla	140	4	18
Trader Joe's: *Per 8 fl.oz Cup*			
Soy Milk: Original	110	2	13
Chocolate	130	2.5	23
Vanilla	100	2	16
Organic: Original	130	3	17
Chocolate	120	3	17
Vanilla	130	3	19
WestSoy: *Per 8 fl.oz Cup*			
Organic Plus, (25% Less Sugar):			
Plain	110	4.5	11
Vanilla	110	4.5	11
Low-Fat: Plain	90	2	15
Vanilla	120	2	23
Non-Fat: Plain	70	0	10
Vanilla	80	0	12
Unsweetened: Plain	100	5	4
Vanilla	100	4.5	5

Soy Powder Mix

1 oz (¼ cup) mix makes 8 fl.oz Cup

	C	F	Cb
Soy Protein Isolate, dry, 1 oz	95	1	2
Better Than Milk:			
Original, 2 Tbsp	90	1.5	18
Vanilla, 2 Tbsp	90	1.5	18
Genisoy: *Per Scoop*			
Protein Shake Powder:			
Natural, 1 oz	100	0	0
Chocolate, 1.2 oz	120	0	17
Vanilla, 1.2 oz	130	0	18
Now:			
Soy Protein Isolate:			
Plain, ⅓ cup, 0.8 oz	90	0.5	0.5
Natural:			
Chocolate, 1 level scoop, 1.6 oz	160	1.5	9
Vanilla, 1 level scoop, 1.6 oz	180	2.5	13
Revival: *Per Packet*			
Unsweetened Shakes: Plain	105	1	4
Chocolate	120	2.5	7
Strawberry Banana	115	2	4
Strawberry Smile	115	2	4
Vanilla Pleasure	120	2	6
Average other flavors	115	2	4
Whole Foods:			
Chocolate, with Spirulina, 1 oz	100	1	10
Vanilla, with Spirulina, 1 oz	100	0	11

Coconut Milk Drinks

	C	F	Cb
Silk: *Per 8 fl.oz Cup*			
Original	80	5	7
Unsweetened	45	4	0.5
Vanilla	90	5	10
Blends, Almond Coconut:			
Original	50	3	5
Unsweetned	35	3	0.5
So Delicious: *Per 8 fl.oz cup*			
Original	70	4.5	8
Chocolate	90	5	13
Vanilla	80	4.5	9
Unweetened, Original	45	4.5	1
Trader Joes: *Per 8 fl.oz cup*			
Unsweetened	60	5	1
Vanilla	90	5	9
(Enriched with calcium + vitamins D & B12)			

Quick Guide

C **F** **Cb**

Cola:
Drinks: *Average all Brands*

	C	F	Cb
8 fl.oz Cup/Can	100	0	26
12 fl.oz Can	150	0	39
16 fl.oz Bottle	200	0	52
20 fl.oz Bottle	250	0	65
24 fl.oz (Pepsi)	300	0	84
1-Liter Bottle (34 fl.oz)	400	0	100
2-Liter Bottle (68 fl.oz)	800	0	200

Other Soda Drinks: *Per 12 fl.oz, average all brands*

	C	F	Cb
Club Soda	0	0	0
Cream Soda	190	0	48
Ginger Ale	125	0	31
Lemonade, Regular/Pink	180	0	45
Orange	180	0	45
Root Beer	150	0	39
Tonic Water	125	0	32
Mineral Water: Plain	0	0	0
Sweetened/flavored	150	0	37
with Fruit Juice	120	0	30
Soda Water/Seltzer: Plain/Diet	0	0	0
Sweetened/flavored	155	0	39
with Fruit Juice	160	0	40

Fountain, Movie Theater & Take-Out

Average All Flavors

	C	F	Cb
Small Cup, 12 fl.oz: No Ice	160	0	40
with 1/3 Ice	120	0	30
Regular, 16 fl.oz: No Ice	215	0	53
with 1/3 Ice	160	0	40
Medium, 22 fl.oz: No Ice	295	0	73
with 1/3 Ice	220	0	55
Large, 32 fl.oz: No Ice	430	0	105
with 1/3 Ice	320	0	80

Note: 1/3 Cup of Ice = 1/4 Cup Liquid

Soft Drink ~ Brands

Per 12 fl.oz Unless Indicated

	C	F	Cb
365 Organic *(Whole Foods)*, Spritzers, all flavors	110	0	28
A&W: Root Beer, 20 fl.oz	290	0	78
Ten, 20 fl.oz	10	0	3
Albertson's:			
Super Chill: Cola	160	0	43
Root Beer	180	0	48
Barq's, Root Beer	170	0	47
Big Red, Soda, 12fl.oz	150	0	38
Blue Sky, Natural Soda, Cola	170	0	43

Soft Drink Brands (Cont)

Per 12 fl.oz Unless Indicated

C **F** **Cb**

	C	F	Cb
Bubble Up, Lemon-Lime Soda, 8 fl.oz	110	0	28
Cactus Cooler	150	0	40
Canada Dry:			
Club Soda; Diet Ginger Ale	0	0	0
Ginger Ale; Tonic Water, average	140	0	36
Cheerwine	150	0	42
Coca-Cola:			
Classic; Caffeine Free	140	0	39
Diet Coke, all varieties	0	0	0
Cherry Coke; Vanilla Coke	150	0	42
Crush:			
Grape; Orange	160	0	43
Peach; Pineapple, average	190	0	51
Strawberry	170	0	46
Dad's: Cream Soda	200	0	51
Root Beer	165	0	42
Diet Rite, Pure Zero	0	0	0
Dr Pepper: *Per 12 fl.oz Can*			
Regular	150	0	40
Cherry	160	0	43
Ten	10	0	3
Fanta: Orange	160	0	45
Other flavors	180	0	48
Fresca, all flavors	0	0	0
GuS, average all flavors	95	0	23
Hansen's: *Per 12 fl.oz*			
Natural Cane Sugar:			
Creamy Root Beer	170	0	45
Original Cola	160	0	41
Pomegranate	130	0	35
Diet, all flavors	0	0	0
Hawaiian Punch:			
Aloha Morning, 40% less sugar, Orange/Strawb./Mixed Berry Citrus	60	0	13
Average other flavors	60	0	14
Henry Weinhard's: Root Beer	170	0	43
Orange/Vanilla Cream, av.	180	0	44
Hires, Root Beer	170	0	45
IBC: Cream Soda; Black Cherry	175	0	44
Root Beer	160	0	40
Icee: Cola; Orange, 6 fl.oz	80	0	20
Lemon Lime	80	0	20
Raspberry Lemonade	80	0	21
Watermelon	80	0	20
Jarritos, all flavors, 8 fl.oz	110	0	28
Jelly Belly, all flavors	180	0	42
Jolt, Cola	150	0	41

Soft Drink Brands (Cont)

Per 12 fl.oz Unless Indicated

	C	F	Cb
Jones Soda:			
Regular, all flavors, 12 fl.oz	170	0	42
Stripped, all flavors, 12 fl.oz	30	0	8
Zilch, sugar free, 12 fl.oz	0	0	0
Kool Aid, Bursts, av., 6.75 fl.oz	35	0	9
Mello Yello, Regular	170	0	47
Mountain Dew: All flavors	170	0	46
Diet varieties	0	0	0
Dewshine	160	0	42
Black Label, 16 fl.oz	210	0	54
Mug, Root Beer	160	0	43
Natural Brew: Chai Cola	170	0	41
Draft Root Beer	170	0	43
Outrageous Ginger Ale	180	0	44
Vanilla Cream Soda	160	0	39
Nehi, Peach	190	0	51
Pepsi: *Per 12 fl.oz*			
Regular; Caffeine Free	150	0	41
Diet Pepsi; Jazz; Pepsi One	0	0	0
Pepsi Next	60	0	16
Pepsi True: 7.5 fl.oz can	60	0	17
12 fl.oz can	100	0	27
Perrier, Carbonated Water	0	0	0
Pibb, Xtra	155	0	39
RC Cola: Regular	160	0	43
Ten	10	0	3
Reed's, Ginger Brew,			
all varieties	145	0	38
7•UP: Lemon Lime; Cherry	140	0	39
Diet flavors	0	0	0
Ten, Lemon Lime	10	0	3
Safeway: *Per 8 fl.oz*			
Refreshe: Cola; Lem. Lime, av.	110	0	28
Grape	140	0	36
Mtn Breeze; Strawberry	120	0	30
Refreshe Ice, all flavors, 17 fl.oz	0	0	0
Santa Cruz, Lemonade, 12 fl.oz	130	0	32
Schweppes: Ginger Ale	120	0	33
Tonic Water	130	0	33
Shasta: Cream Soda	190	0	47
Cherry Cola	180	0	45
Club Soda; Diet, all flavors	0	0	0
Dr. Shasta	150	0	38
Ginger Ale	130	0	33
Tiki Punch; Pineapple; Orange	200	0	50
Average other flavors	170	0	41
Sierra Mist, Lemon Lime	120	0	30
Sprite: Regular, 12 fl.oz	140	0	38
Zero	0	0	0

Per 12 fl.oz Unless Indicated

	C	F	Cb
Squirt, Ruby Red	170	0	45
Stewarts: Root Beer	150	0	38
Grape; Orange 'n Cream	180	0	45
Sun Drop: Citrus Soda, 20 fl.oz	290	0	76
Diet Citrus Soda	10	0	1
Sunkist: Orange, with sugar, 20 fl.oz	170	0	44
Pineapple, 20 fl.oz	320	0	85
Surge, 16 fl.oz	230	0	62
TAB	0	0	0
Tampico: *Per 12 fl.oz*			
Punch: Blue Raspberry	90	0	21
Pineapple Coconut	105	0	26
Average other flavors	90	0	21
Soda, all flavors, 12 fl.oz	180	0	42
Thomas Kemper: *Per 12 fl.oz*			
Black Cherry	170	0	44
Ginger Ale; Vanilla Cream	150	0	36
Root Beer	160	0	41
Trader Joe's:			
Sparkling:			
French Berry Lemonade:			
1 cup, 8 fl.oz	130	0	31
1 bottle, 33.8 fl.oz	520	0	124
Lime Ade: 1 cup, 8 fl.oz	110	0	28
1 bottle, 33.8 fl.oz	440	0	108
Pink Lemonade: 1 cup, 8 fl.oz	130	0	31
1 Bottle, 33.8 fl.oz	520	0	124
Vernors, Ginger Soda, 20 fl.oz	240	0	65
Virgil's, Root Beer	160	0	42
Walgreens: *Per 20 fl.oz*			
Orchard Grape Soda	300	0	84
Cola; Zesty Lemon Lime, av.	225	0	65
Root Beer	225	0	75
Zevia, all flavors	0	0	4
(Contains between 4-7g Erythritol)			

Powdered Soft Drink Mixes

Per 8 fl.oz Prepared, Unless Indicated

	C	F	Cb
Country Time:			
Lemonade; Pink Lemonade	60	0	16
Strawberry Lemonade	80	0	19
Crystal Light *(Kraft):*			
Fruit Drinks, all flavors, ½ tsp	5	0	0
Pure Fitness, average all flavors, 1 pkt	15	0	4
Flavor Aid, ⅛ package	0	0	0
Kool-Aid, sweetened, 0.6 oz	60	0	16
Tang, Regular, 2 Tbsp, 1 oz	90	0	24

Quick Guide   C   F   Cb

Teas

	C	F	Cb
Regular: Bag, Loose or Instant			
Brewed, 1 cup, 8 fl.oz	2	0	0.5
(Add extra for sugar/milk)			
Herbal: All flav., av., 1 cup	2	0	0.5
Bigelow, all flavors	0	0	0
Celestial Seasonings, all flavors	0	0	0
Bubble Milk Tea, w/ Pearls, 8 fl.oz	175	0	41
Chai Tea, 2 Tbsp	120	3.5	21
Starbucks ~ *See Fast-Foods Section*			

Iced Tea

Average All Brands

Sweetened: 8 fl.oz cup	90	0	22
12 fl.oz glass/can	140	0	35
16 fl.oz bottle	180	0	45
20 fl.oz bottle	225	0	55
Unsweetened, 8 fl.oz	0	0	0

Iced Tea Mixes

Per 8 fl.oz Made-Up

4C Iced Tea:			
Average all flavors, 0.67 oz	70	0	18
Totally Light, all flavors	0	0	0
Crystal Light, sugar free	5	0	0
Lipton:			
Sweetened: Lemon	70	0	18
Mango; Peach	80	0	19
Unsweetened	0	0	0
Diet, all varieties	5	0	1

Bottled & Canned Teas

Arizona: *Per 8 fl.oz*			
Black: Cranberry	80	0	22
Sweet	90	0	23
with Ginseng	60	0	15
Green Tea, average all flavors	70	0	18
Bigelow: *Per 8 fl.oz*			
Green Tea, average all flavors	60	0	15
Half & Half Tea, Lemonade	70	0	16
Unsweetened Tea	0	0	0
Fuze, Iced Lemon	70	0	19
Gold Peak, Lemon, 12 fl.oz	120	0	30
Health-Ade, Kombucha Tea, 8 fl.oz	30	0	7
Honest Tea: *Per 16 fl.oz Bottle*			
Assam Black	35	0	9
Just Black/Green	0	0	0

Bottled & Canned Teas (Cont)

	C	F	Cb
Lipton:			
Iced Tea: *Per 20 fl.oz Unless Indicated*			
Citrus Green Tea, 8 fl.oz	70	0	19
Diet, all flavors	0	0	0
Half & Half	120	0	31
Lemon	120	0	32
Peach	120	0	30
Sparkling: Peach	70	0	18
Diet	0	0	0
Sweet Iced Tea, 12 fl.oz	130	0	35
White Tea, with Raspberry, 16.9 fl.oz	110	0	29
Nestea:			
Iced Tea, with Lemon:			
8 fl.oz	50	0	13
20 fl.oz bottle	125	0	33
Diet, Green/Lemon	0	0	0
POM:			
Antioxidant Super Tea: *Per 12 fl.oz*			
Pomegranate:			
Honey Green Tea	130	0	35
Lemonade Tea	140	0	35
Peach Passion White Tea	130	0	32
Sweet Tea	120	0	30
Snapple: *Per 16 fl.oz*			
Green Tea	120	0	31
Diet Green Tea	0	0	0
Lemon/ Raspberry Tea	150	0	37
Diet Lemon/Raspberry Tea	10	0	0
Straight Up Tea: *Per 18.5 fl.oz Bottle*			
Honey Green; Sorta Sweet	90	0	22
Rooibos	90	0	23
Sweet	180	0	45
SoBe, Elixir, Green Tea, 20 fl.oz	200	0	52
Ssips, Lemon Iced Tea, 6 fl.oz	70	0	17
Steaz, Iced Green Tea,			
lightly sweetened, av., 16 fl.oz	80	0	20
Tampico, Iced Tea,			
average all flavors, 12 fl.oz	135	0	35
Tazo, Org. Iced Black Tea, 13.8 fl oz	60	0	15
TeaZazz, all flavors, 12.8 fl.oz	70	0	20
Trader Joe's: *Per 8 fl.oz*			
Organic Tea & Lemonade	100	0	25
Pomegranate Green Tea	60	0	15
Turkey Hill, Iced Tea, 16 fl.oz	180	0	42
Peach Tea, 16 fl.oz	200	0	46
Green Tea, Mango, 16 fl.oz	180	0	42
365 Organic *(Whole Foods):*			
Unsweetened: Black Tea	0	0	0
Green Tea	0	0	0

Note: Most breads have similar calories on a weight basis. However, volume may vary.

For example, 1 oz of bread may equal 1 slice regular bread or 2 slices of a lighter bread. It is best to weigh bread used and calculate using: 1 oz bread = 70 calories, 14g carb.

Quick Guide

C   F   Cb

Bread

White or Wheat: *Average Per Slice*

		C	F	Cb
Thin or Light, 0.75 oz		50	0.5	9
Sandwich slice, 1 oz		70	1	14
Thick or Large, 1.5 oz		105	1.5	18
Thick, 2 oz		140	2	23
Extra Thick, 3 oz		210	3	35
Whole Loaf: 16 oz		1120	15	185
24 oz Loaf		1680	24	280

Multi Grain/Whole Grain: *Per Slice*

	C	F	Cb
Sandwich Slice, 1 oz	75	1.5	12
Thick Slice, 2 oz	150	2.5	25

Toast: *Based on same counts as White/Wheat as above*

1 Slice (1 oz fresh):

	C	F	Cb
with 1 tsp butter/margarine	105	5	12
with 1 tsp "light" butter/marg.	90	3.5	12
with 2 tsp butter/margarine	140	9	12
with 2 tsp "light" butter/marg.	110	6	12

Breads

Per Slice Unless Indicated

	C	F	Cb
12-Grain, 1.5 oz	110	1.5	22
Bran style/Dark, 1 oz	70	1	14
Buttermilk, average, 1.5 oz	110	1	22
Challah, 0.75 oz	85	1.5	17
Chapati, 1 oz	110	3	18
Ciabatta, 2 oz	130	1	26
Cornbread, average, 3 oz	220	6	37
Cracked Wheat Sourdough, 1.5 oz	130	0.5	27
Croissants ~ See Page 134			
Crustless Bread, regular, slice, 0.75 oz	40	0.5	8.5
Crusts Only, regular slice, 0.25 oz	30	0	7
English Toasting, 2 oz	140	1.5	27
Flax & Grain, 1.5 oz	120	3	19
Foccacia: Plain, 2 oz serve	150	2.5	28
Cheese & Garlic; Pesto, 2 oz serve	160	6	21
Tomato & Olive, 2 oz serve	150	5	21

Breads (Cont)

C   F   Cb

Per Slice Unless Indicated

	C	F	Cb
French Stick/Baguette, 1 oz	70	1	15
French Toast: Slices, 1.5oz	140	2	26
Aunt Jemima, Sticks, av., 2 oz	110	2	18
Garlic Bread/Toast:			
Small slice + 1 tsp spread, 0.75 oz	80	5	7
Medium slice + 2 tsp spread, 1.5 oz	160	10	14
Thick slice + 3 tsp spread, 1.8 fl.oz	220	14	20
Pepperidge Farm, 1 slice, 1.4 oz	160	10	15
Hawaiian Sweet Bread, 1.5 oz	110	2	19
Hemp Bread, 1.2 oz	95	2	12
Italian Bread, 2 oz	140	1	28
Lower Carb, (higher protein/fiber),			
average all brands, 1 oz	60	1.5	9
MultiGrain, 1.5 oz	100	2	21
Naan Flatbread, 2 oz	160	3.5	29
Nut/Health Nut, 1.35 oz	90	1.5	18
Oatmeal/Oatbran Bread, 1.5 oz	90	0.5	19
Pita, average all types:			
Small (4" diam), 1 oz	90	0	18
Large (6½" diam), 2 oz	140	1.5	27
Extra Large (9" diam), 4 oz	300	1.5	60
Popovers, (1), without butter	130	2	18
Pumpernickel:			
Cocktail/Party size	30	0.5	6
Large slice, 1.35 oz	80	0	15
Raisin Bread, 1 oz	80	1	15
Rye: 1 thin slice, av., 1 oz	80	1	14
1 thick slice, 2 oz	150	2	25
Cocktail size, 0.4 oz	25	0.5	4
Sandwich Pockets, 2 oz	140	1.5	27
Sourdough: Regular, 1.5oz	120	1	25
French Style,1 oz	75	0	14
Spelt, 1.6 oz	130	1	26
Sprouted 7-Grain, 1.5 oz	110	0.5	18
Squaw, 1.1 oz	85	0.5	13
Tacos/Tortillas ~ See Page 172			
Turkish/Middle Eastern, 1 oz	80	1.5	16
Wheat-Free Breads: Spelt, 1.6 oz	130	1	26
Rice, with Fruit Juice, 1.5 oz	110	2	21
Healthseed Rye, 1.6 oz	90	1	20
Millet, 1.5 oz	100	1	20

Bread ~ Brands

	C	F	Cb
Per Slice Unless Indicated			
Ener-G, Gluten-Free Breads:			
Brown Rice Loaf,			
Regular, 1.3 oz	100	3	16
High Fiber Loaf, 1.4oz	90	4.5	16
Seattle Brown Loaf, 1.3 oz	90	3	15
Tapioca, regular, sliced, 1 oz	80	3	11
Ezekiel:			
Sprouted: 7 Sprouted Grains, 1.2 oz	80	0.5	15
Sesame, 1.2 oz	80	0.5	14
Whole Grain, 1.3 oz	80	0.5	15
Francisco International:			
Extra Sourdough Loaf,			
1 slice, 1.7 oz	130	1	24
French, 2 slices, 1.6 oz	120	1	22
Sourdough Sliced Bread, 2 sl., 1.4 oz	110	1	22
Oroweat:			
3 Seed Oatnut, 1.34 oz	120	3	18
100% Whole Wheat, 1.34 oz	90	1	16
Dill Rye, 1.2 oz	80	0	16
Extra Grainy, 17 Grains & Seeds, 1.2 oz	110	2.5	18
Pepperidge Farm:			
100% Whole Wheat	110	2	20
15 Grain	110	2	20
Family, White Sandwich	150	3	20
Italian, with Sesame Seeds	90	1.5	20
Light Style, av. all varieties	135	1	20
Frozen Breads:			
Garlic Bread:			
Original	180	8	20
Five Cheese	200	10	20
Texas Toast, Cheddar	160	9	20
Roman Meal: Orig. Multigr., 2 slices	110	1.5	21
Honey Oat Bran, 1.5 oz	110	1.5	20
Sara Lee: Honey Wheat, 1 oz	70	0.5	13
100% Whole Wheat, 1 oz	60	1	12
Cracked Wheat, 1 oz	80	0.5	15
Schwan's, Frozen:			
Cheese Stuffed Breadsticks, 1.7 oz	130	5	15
French Baguette, 1/4 loaf, 1.7 oz	120	0	25
Trader Joe's: Gourmet White, 1.5 oz	120	3.5	19
Soft 10 Grain, 1.5 oz	90	1.5	16
Sprouted Rye, 1.2 oz	90	1	15

Biscuits, Bread Rolls & Buns

	C	F	Cb
Biscuits: *Average, 2½" diameter*			
Plain/Butter Milk:			
Prepared from Recipe	210	10	27
Refrig. Dough, Baked	95	4	13
Brown 'n Serve, av., 1 oz	70	1	13
Refrigerated Dough:			
Pillsbury, Buttermilk Biscuit,			
(3), 2.25 oz	150	2	30
Buns:			
Frankfurter/Hot Dog: 1.25 oz	110	1.5	21
1.5 oz	130	2	25
Hamburger: Regular, 1.5 oz	110	1.5	22
Large, 3 oz	210	3	40
Hoagie/Submarine, Plain, 2.3 oz	200	1	38
Rolls:			
Ciabatta Roll, 3.5 oz	230	4	41
Crescent Roll, Original, 1 oz	100	6	11
Dinner:			
1 small, 1 oz	90	1.5	17
1 medium (3" diam),1.5 oz	110	1	23
French: 1 med, 1.3 oz	110	1.5	22
1 large, 3 oz	230	2.5	42
Kaiser:			
Small, 2 oz	200	2.5	35
Large, 3.5 oz	350	4	61
Plain, 6", average all, 2.5 oz	200	1	38
Sourdough, 1.3 oz	110	1	21
Wheat Rolls: Small, 1.2 oz	100	1	17
Medium, 1.8 fl.oz	130	1.5	23
Large, 3.5 oz	260	3	46

Breadsticks, Croutons

	C	F	Cb
Breadsticks:			
Salt Sticks, plain, 1 oz	110	1	20
Fresh baked (1), 2 oz	180	2.5	34
Stella D'oro: Original (1)	45	1	7
Sesame (1)	50	2	7
Croutons: Seasoned, 2 Tbsp, 0.3 oz	35	1.5	4
Pepp. Farm, Zesty Italian, 6 croutons	30	1	5

Bread Products

	C	F	Cb
Bread Crumbs, dry:			
Plain or seasoned: 1 oz	110	1.5	20
1 cup, 3.5 oz	385	5	70
Corn Flake Crumbs, 1 oz	120	0	29
Graham Cracker Crumbs *(Keebler),* 1 oz	110	2.5	20
Bread Dough, average:			
Frozen, 1 slice, 2 oz	140	2	26
Refrigerated: French, 1" sl.	60	1	13
Wheat; White, 1" slice	80	2	14
Coating Mixes, av., 2 Tbsp., 1 oz	100	0.5	20
Stuffing: Dry mix, average all,1 oz	110	1	10
Prepared, ½ cup, 4 oz	180	9	22

Quick Guide | C | F | Cb

Bagels
Average All Brands
Plain/Onion:

	C	F	Cb
1 mini/bagelette, 1 oz	65	0.5	13
1 small bagel, 2 oz	145	1	29
1 medium bagel, 3 oz	220	1.5	43
1 large bagel, 4 oz	290	2	57
Bagel Chips, 1 oz	130	4.5	19
Pizza Bagel Bites (Bagel Bites),			
average all varieties., 4 pieces, 3 oz	190	5.5	27
Bagel Crisps (New York Style),			
average all varieties, 6 crisps, 1 oz	130	5	17
Bagel Thins (Thomas'), 1, 1.5 oz	110	1	25

Bagel ~ Brands

Per Bagel

	C	F	Cb
Bubba's: Plain	220	1.5	45
Blueberry	150	0.5	32
Cinnamon Raisin	250	1.5	51
Costco Bakery: Plain	330	1.5	70
Cinnamon Raisin	340	1.5	73
Whole Grain	300	5	56
Lender's, Fresh, NY Style:			
Plain, 3.3 oz	240	2	46
Blueberry, 3.3 oz	240	2	46
Cinnamon, 3.3 oz	240	2	46
Whole Wheat, 3.3 oz	240	2	46
Panera Bread: Plain	290	1.5	58
Cinnamon & Raisin Swirl, 3.8 fl.oz	320	2	66
Everything, 4 oz	300	2	58
Whole Grain, 4.3 oz	330	2.5	67
Sara Lee: Mini, average, 1.3 oz	100	0.5	20
Plain, 3.4 oz	260	1	52
Blueberry, 3.4 oz	260	1	54
Cinnamon Raisin, 3.7 oz	260	0.5	54
Everything, 3.4 oz	270	3	50
Onion, 3.4 oz	260	1	53
Western, The Alternatives, av., 2 oz	120	0.5	29

Bagel Spreads

Cream Cheese:	C	F	Cb
Plain: 2 Tbsp, 1 oz	100	9	1
2 oz mini-tub	200	18	2
Reduced Fat: 2 Tbsp, 1 oz	60	5	2
2 oz mini-tub	120	10	4
Flavors: Lox, 1 oz	90	8	2
Honey Nut, 1 oz	80	7	4
Strawberry, 1 oz	90	7	5
Sundried Tomato, 1 oz	80	7	2
Vegetable, 1 oz	90	8	2

English Muffins | C | F | Cb

Average All Brands

	C	F	Cb
Plain/Whole Wheat: Regular, 2 oz	135	1.5	26
Heavier, 2.5 oz	155	2	31
Super Size, 3.2 oz	190	2	38
Raisin-Cinnamon, 2.2 oz	150	1	30

Note: Actual weight of packaged muffins can be 10-15% heavier than stated net weight.

Rice Cakes

	C	F	Cb
Regular size (1), average, 0.3 oz	35	0.5	7.5
Hain, Mini, White Cheddar (10), 1.2 oz	70	2.5	11
Lundberg: Brown Rice (1), 0.7 oz	60	0.5	14
Caramel Corn (1)	80	0.5	17
Cinnamon Toast (1), 0.8 oz	80	0	20
Quaker, Apple Cinn., 0.5 oz	50	0	11

Tortillas & Shells

Tortillas: *Per Tortilla*

Corn Flour:	C	F	Cb
White/Yellow: 6", 1 oz	55	1	11
7", 1.2 oz	75	1	14
Wheat Flour:			
6", 1.2 oz	100	3	16
8", 1.4 oz	130	4	20
10", 2.3 oz	200	6	31

Shells: *Per Shell, without Fillings*

Corn Taco Shells:	C	F	Cb
Mini, 3", 0.2 oz	25	1	3
Medium, 5", 0.5 oz	60	2.5	8
Large, 6½", 0.7 oz	100	4.5	13
Salad Shell, 10"	310	17	34
Tostada Shells, fried:			
White Corn, 5½" diam., 0.4 oz	55	2.5	8
Yellow Corn, 5½" diam., 0.5 oz	80	3.5	11
Sopes, 1 shell, 4" 2 oz	110	1.5	23

La Tortilla Factory:

	C	F	Cb
100 Calorie, Whole Wheat, 2 oz	100	1.5	24
Hand Made Style,			
White Corn & Wheat, 1.45 oz	90	1	15
Low Carb, Flour, 1 oz	45	1.5	10
Traditional, Flour,			
Soft Taco Size, 1.2 oz	130	3.5	18

Mission Foods:

	C	F	Cb
Corn, Yellow/White, Super Soft:			
Regular size, 2 Tortillas, 1.7 oz	100	1.5	20
Super size (1), 1.1 oz	70	1	13
Flour: Homestyle, 1 Tortilla, 2.2 oz	190	6	29
Super Soft, 1 Tortilla, 1.7 fl.oz	140	3.5	24

Quick Guide	**C**	**F**	**Cb**
Cooked Cereals			
Barley, pearled, cooked, 1 cup	195	0.5	44
Buckwheat Groats, roasted:			
Dry, ¹/₂ cup, 3 oz	285	2	61
Cooked, 1 cup, 6 oz	155	1	34
Bulgur: Dry, ¹/₂ cup, 2.5 oz	240	1	53
Cooked, 1 cup, 6.5 oz	150	0.5	34
Corn/Hominy Grits:			
Dry: Regular, ¹/₄ cup, 1.4 oz	140	0.5	32
Instant: 0.8 fl.oz packet	75	0	18
w/ Imitation Bacon Bits, 1 oz	100	0.5	22
Cooked, ³/₄ cup, 6.5 oz	110	0.5	23
Cream of Rice, cooked, ³/₄ cup, 6.5 oz	95	0	21
Cream of Wheat:			
Cooked: Regular, ³/₄ cup, 6.5 oz	95	0.5	20
Instant, ³/₄ cup, 6.5 oz	105	0.5	21
Quick, ³/₄ cup, 6.5 oz	100	0.5	22
Farina, cooked, ³/₄ cup, 6 oz	95	0.5	19
Millet, dry, ¹/₂ cup, 1.8 fl.oz	190	2	36
Oat Bran: Raw, ¹/₃ cup, 1 oz	70	2	19
Cooked, ¹/₂ cup, 3.8 fl.oz	45	1	13
Oatmeal:			
Dry: Regular, ¹/₃ cup, 1 oz	100	1.5	18
Instant: Regular, average, 1 oz	105	1.5	18
Flavored, average, 1.5 oz	165	2	34
Cooked: Regular, ³/₄ cup, 6 oz	125	2.5	21
1 cup, 8 fl.oz	165	3.5	28
Whole Wheat, cooked, ³/₄ cup, 6.5 oz	115	0.5	25

Brans, Wheat Germ, Add-Ons			
Bee Pollen Granules, 1 Tbsp, 0.3 oz	25	1	2
Bran:			
Oat Bran: Raw, 1 Tbsp, 0.2 oz	20	0.5	3
¹/₃ cup, 1 oz	100	2	17
Rice Bran: Raw, 1 Tbsp, 0.2 oz	15	1	2.5
¹/₄ cup, 1 oz	95	6	15
Fruit: Dried, average, 1 oz	70	0	18
Banana, ¹/₂ medium	55	0	14
Prunes in Syrup (5), 3 oz	90	0	23
Honey, 1 Tbsp, 0.75 oz	65	0	17
Lecithin Granules, 1 Tbsp, 0.4 oz	55	4	0.5
Nuts, Almonds (6), 0.3 oz	40	4	1.5
Psyllium Husks, 1 Tbsp, 0.2 oz	10	0	4
Wheat, unprocessed, 1 Tbsp	5	0	2
Wheat Germ: Raw, 1 Tbsp, 0.3 oz	25	0.5	4
¹/₄ cup, 1 oz	105	3	15

Hot/Cooked Cereals ~ Brands			
Per Serving, Dry Mix only	**C**	**F**	**Cb**
Albers,			
Quick Grits, ¹/₄ cup, 1.4 oz	140	0.5	31
B&G:			
Cream of Wheat Instant:			
Original, 1 oz	100	0	19
Cinn. Swirl; Maple Br. Sugar, 1.3 oz	130	0	29
Bobs Red Mill:			
Organic Kasha, ¹/₄ cup, 1.45 oz	160	1	33
Rolled Spelt Flakes, ¹/₂ cup, 1.4 oz	130	1.5	28
Whole Oat Groats, ¹/₄ cup, 1.6 oz	170	3	31
Dr. McDougall's: *Without Sugar*			
Mighty Omega Superfood, 2.6 oz	240	7	38
Milled Flax Oatmeal, 1.2 oz pkt	120	3	21
Superfood Chia Crunch, 1.3 oz pkt	140	3	24
Great Value *(Walmart):*			
Instant Oatmeal:			
Apple Cinnamon, 1.5 oz pkt	130	1.5	27
Maple & Brown Sugar, 1.5 oz pkt	160	2	33
McCann's:			
Instant Irish Oatmeal:			
Regular, 1 oz package	100	2	19
Apple & Cinn., 1.3 oz	130	1.5	28
Maple & Brown Sugar, 1.5 oz	160	2	32
Malt-O-Meal: Original; Choc., 1.2 oz	130	0.5	27
Maple Brown Sugar, ¹/₄ cup	170	0	37
Natures Path:			
Oatmeal: Flax Plus, 1 oz	110	1.5	23
Apple Cinnamon, 1.7 oz	210	2.5	40
Maple Nut, 1.7 oz	210	4	38
NutriSystem,			
Oatmeal, Apple Cinnamon, 1 pkt	130	1.5	26
Quaker:			
Instant Grits, av. all flavors, 1 oz	100	1	22
Quick Grits, Original, ¹/₄ cup, 1.3 oz	130	0.5	29
Instant Oatmeal:			
Maple & Brown Sugar,	160	2	32
Organic, Regular, 1 oz	100	2	19
Peaches & Cream, 1.3 oz	130	2	27
Old Fash'nd/Quick Oats, ¹/₂ c., 1.4 oz	150	3	27
Real Medleys:			
Apple, Pear, Pecan, 2.1 oz	250	8	41
Blueb. Hazelnut, 2.47 oz	270	7	49
Summer Berry, 2.47 oz	250	3	51
Super Grains: Ban. Walnut, 2.47 oz	280	8	49
Maple Pecan Raisin, 2.47 oz	270	7	49
Wegmans:			
Instant Oatmeal: Orig., 1.4 oz pkt	150	2.5	27
Maple & Spice, 1.4 oz pkt	150	2	28

Quick Guide	**C**	**F**	**Cb**
Cold Cereals			
Average All Brands			
Bran Flakes, ³/₄ cup, 1 oz	95	0.5	24
Corn Flakes, 1 cup, 1 oz	100	0	22
Frosted Flakes, ³/₄ cup, 1 oz	110	0	27
Granola, 100% Nat., ¹/₂ cup, 1.7 oz	205	6	35
Oat Bran Cereal, ¹/₂ cup, 1.5 oz	145	3	25
Puffed Rice, 1 cup. 0.5 oz	55	0	13
Puffed Wheat, 1 cup, 0.5 oz	45	0	10
Raisin Bran, ¹/₂ cup, 1 oz	90	0.5	22
Rice Crisps, 1 cup, 1 oz	105	0.5	24
Shredded Wheat, 1 biscuit, 1 oz	85	0.5	20
Wheat Flakes, ³/₄ cup, 1 oz	105	1	24

Breakfast/Cereal Bars ~ *See Page 31*

Ready-To-Eat Cereal ~ Brands

	C	**F**	**Cb**
Arrowhead Mills:			
Flakes: Amaranth, 1.2 oz	140	2	26
Kamut, 1 oz	120	1	25
Oat Bran, 1.2 oz	140	2.5	24
Spelt, 1 oz	120	1	24
Sprouted Wheat Berry & Quinoa, 1.5 oz	100	1	22
Breadshop Granola,			
Blueberry 'n Cream, ½ cup, 1.8 fl.oz	210	6	36
Puffed: Corn, 0.5 oz	60	1	12
Kamut, 0.5 oz	50	0	11
Millet, 0.5 oz	60	0.5	11
Rice, 0.5 oz	60	0	14
Wheat, 0.5 oz	60	0	12
Shredded Wheat:			
Bite Size:			
Regular, 1.7 oz	190	1	38
Sweetened, 1.8 fl.oz	200	1	42
Back to Nature: *Per ¹/₂ Cup*			
Granola: Apple Blueberry, 1.8 fl.oz	190	2.5	37
Chocolate Delight, 1.8 fl.oz	200	5	36
Classic, 1.8 fl.oz	200	2.5	38
Cranberry Pecan, 1.6 oz	180	5	34
Dark Chocolate Coconut, 1.76 oz	230	11	31
Sunflower & Pumpkin Seed, 1.8 fl.oz	210	7	31
Vanilla Almond Agave, 1.8 fl.oz	200	6	34
Granola Clusters:			
Peanut Butter, 1.8 oz	220	9	27
Av. other varieties, 1.8 oz	200	4.5	36

	C	**F**	**Cb**
Barbara's Bakery:			
Classics, Organic & Sweetened:			
Brown Rice Crisps, 1.4 oz	150	1	33
Corn Flakes, 1.4 oz	150	0	35
Honest O's, Original, 1 oz	120	2	24
High Fiber Medley:			
Original, 2 oz	180	1.5	42
Cranberry, 2 oz	190	1.5	42
Morning Oat Crunch:			
Original, 2 oz	210	2	44
Cinnamon, 2 oz	230	3	43
Vanilla Almond, 2 oz	220	3	42
Puffins:			
Original; Cinnamon, 1 oz	90	1	24
Honey Rice, 1 oz	110	0.5	25
Multigrain; Pumpkin, 1 oz	110	0	25
PB/PB & Choc., av.,1 oz	115	1.5	24
Snackanimals, all varieties, 1 oz	110	0.5	26
Shredded Wheat, 2 biscuits, 1.4 oz	140	1	32
Spoonfuls, Multigrain, 1.1 oz	120	1.5	29
Squarefuls, Multigrain, 1.95 oz	200	1	47
Bear Naked, Granola:			
Fruit & Nutty, 1 oz	140	6	20
Original Cinnamon, 1 oz	140	6	15
Triple Berry, 1 oz	120	2	23
Vanilla Almond, 1 oz	120	2.5	22
Bob's Red Mill,			
Muesli, Old Country, ¹/₄ cup, 1 oz	110	3	21
Cascadian Farm:			
Buzz Crunch, 2.1 oz	230	3	47
Cinnamon Crunch, 1 oz	110	2.5	22
Graham Crunch, 1 oz	110	2	23
Granola: Ancient Grains, 2 oz	240	6	41
French Vanilla Almond, 2 oz	250	7	42
Oats & Honey, 2.2 oz	260	7	46
Honey Nut O's, 1 oz	110	1	25
Multi Grain Squares,			
1 cup, 1.9 oz	210	1	44
Raisin Bran, 1.8 fl.oz	180	1	41
EnviroKidz: *Per 1 oz*			
Amazon Frosted Flakes, 1 oz	120	0	26
Gorilla Munch, 1 oz	120	1	26
Leapin' Lemurs, 1 oz	120	1.5	25
Panda Puffs, 1 oz	130	3.5	23
Erewhon:			
Corn Flakes, 1.2 oz	130	0	30
Crispy Brown Rice,			
Original/Cinn. av. 1 oz	110	0.5	24
Harvest Medley, 1 oz	110	1	24
Honey Rice Twice, 1 oz	120	0	26
Simply Vanilla Granola, 2 oz	240	6	41

Ready-To-Eat Cereal (Cont)

Ezekiel 4.9:

	C	F	Cb
Sprouted Whole Grain Cereals:			
Original, ¹/₂ cup, 2 oz	190	1	40
Almond, ¹/₂ cup, 2 oz	200	3	38
Cinnamon Raisin, 2 oz	190	1	41
Golden Flax, ¹/₂ cup, 2 oz	180	2.5	37

General Mills:

Cheerios: *Per ³/₄ Cup Unless Indicated*

Original, 1 cup, 1 oz	100	2	20
Ancient Grains, ³/₄ c., 1 oz	110	2	22
Apple Cinn., ³/₄ cup, 1 oz	120	1.5	24
Chocolate, av., ³/₄ cup, 1 oz	100	1.5	21
Frosted, ³/₄ cup, 1 oz	100	1.5	22
Fruity, Nat Flav., ³/₄ c., 1 oz	100	1.5	21
Honey Nut, ³/₄ cup, 1 oz	110	1.5	22
Multi Grain, Regular, 1 c., 1oz	110	1.5	24
Protein: Cinn. Almond, 1¹/₄ c., 2 oz	220	4.5	40
Oats & Honey, 1¹/₄ cups, 2 oz	210	2.5	41
Chex: Choc., ³/₄ cup, 1 oz	130	2.5	26
Cinnamon, ³/₄ cup, 1 oz	120	2	25
Corn, 1 cup, 1 oz	120	0.5	26
Honey Nut, ³/₄ cup, 1 oz	120	0.5	28
Rice, 1 cup, 1 oz	100	0.5	23
Vanilla, ³/₄ cup, 1 oz	120	2	25
Wheat, ³/₄ cup, 1.7 oz	160	1	39
Cinn. Toast Crunch, ³/₄ cup, 1 oz	130	3	25
Fiber One: Original, ¹/₂ cup, 1 oz	60	1	25
Honey Clusters, 1 cup, 1.8 fl.oz	170	1.5	44
French Toast Crunch, ³/₄ cup, 1 oz	110	1	24
Kix: Original, 1¹/₄ cups, 1 oz	110	1	25
Berry Berry; Honey,			
1¹/₄ cups, 1.2 oz	120	1.5	28
Lucky Charms,			
Original; Chocolate, ³/₄ cup, 1 oz	110	1.5	23
Monsters: Count Chocula, ³/₄ c., 1 oz	100	1.5	23
Other varieties, 1.2 oz	130	1.5	28
Total, Whole Grain, 1 oz	110	0.5	25
Trix, 1 cup, 1.1 oz	130	1.5	27
Wheaties, 1 oz	100	0.5	23

Great Value *(Walmart):*

Apple Blasts, 1.2 oz	120	0	29
Cinnamon Crunch, ¾ cup	130	3	23
Cocoa Crunch, ³/₄ cup, 1 oz	120	1.5	26
Corn Flakes, 1 cup	110	0	26
Crunchy Raisin Bran, 1.87 oz	190	1	20

Great Value Cont. *(Walmart):*

	C	F	Cb
Extra Raisin Raisin Bran, 1 cup	200	1	43
Frosted Shredded Wheat, 1.9 oz	180	1	42
Fruit Spins, 1 cup	150	0	26
O's Oat, 1 oz	120	1	23
Sugar Frosted Flakes, 1 oz	120	0	28
Toasted Multi-Grain Spins, 1 cup	110	1.5	24

Health Valley:

Crunch-Ems!, Rice, 1¹/₄ cups, 1 oz	110	0	26

Organic Flakes:

Oat Bran, 1 cup, 1.8 fl.oz	190	1.5	39
Sprouted Amaranth,			
1¹/₄ cups, 2 oz	210	2	43

Heartland:

Granola: Original, ¹/₂ cup, 2 oz	240	6	41
Fruit & Nut, ¹/₂ cup, 1.8 fl.oz	210	6	34
Harvest Spice, ¹/₂ cup, 1.8 fl.oz	210	5	37
Low-Fat var., ¹/₂ cup, 1.8 fl.oz	200	3	40
Oat Bran, ¹/₂ cup, 1.4 oz	160	3	23
Raisin, ¹/₂ cup, 2 oz	240	6	40

Kashi:

7 Whole Grain: Flakes, 1 c., 1.8 fl.oz	170	0.5	41
Honey Puffs, 1½ cups, 1.4 oz	150	1	34
Nuggets, ¹/₂ cup, 2 oz	200	1.5	46
Whole Grain Puffs,			
1½ cups, 1.4 oz	150	1.5	32
GoLEAN: Original, 1¹/₄ cups, 2 oz	180	2	40
Crunch: Original, ³/₄ cup, 2 oz	190	3	38
Chocolate, ³/₄ cup, 1.83 oz	220	7	32
Cinnamon Crisp, ³/₄ cup, 1.8 oz	180	4	32
Honey Almond Flax, ²/₃ cup, 2 oz	200	5	35

Heart to Heart:

Oat Flakes & Blueb. Clusters, 1 c., 2 oz	200	2.5	42
Other varieties, ³/₄ cup, 1.2 oz	120	1.5	26

Organic Corn:

Indigo Morning, 1.37 oz	140	1.5	32
Simply Maize, 1.37 oz	140	1.5	32

Organic Promise:

Sprouted Grains, 1¹/₄ cups, 2 oz	190	1	45
Sweet Potato Sunshine, 1 c., 1.8 fl.oz	180	1	43

Whole Wheat Biscuit,

Island Vanilla, 27 biscuits	190	1	44

Kellogg's:

All-Bran: Original, ½ cup, 1 oz	80	1	23
Bran Buds, ¹/₃ cup, 1 oz	80	1	24
Compl. Wheat Flakes, 1 oz	90	0.5	24
Apple Jacks, 1 cup, 1 oz	110	1	25
Cinnabon, 1 cup, 1 oz	120	2	25

continued next page...

Ready-To-Eat Cereal (Cont)

Kellogg's (Cont):

	C	F	Cb
Corn Flakes, Orig., 1 c., 1 oz	100	0	24
Cracklin' Oat Bran,			
³/₄ cup, 1.8 fl.oz	200	7	34
Crispix, Original, 1 cup, 1 oz	110	0	25
Despicable Me 3 Minion, 1 c., 1.2 oz	120	1	27
Disney Princess, Strawb., 1.2 oz	120	1	27
Froot Loops: Orig., 1 c., 1 oz	110	1	25
Marshmallow, 1 c., 1 oz	110	1	26
Frosted Flakes: *Per 1 oz*			
Chocolate, ³/₄ cup	120	1	26
w/ Marshmallows, ³/₄ cup	120	1	26
Cinnamon, ³/₄ cup,	110	0	26
Original Flakes, ³/₄ cup	110	0	26
w/ Marshmallows, ³/₄ c.,	110	0	26
Honey Smacks, 1 oz	100	0.5	24
Krave, Double Choc., 1.1 oz	120	3.5	23
MarioKart, 1 pouch, 0.78 oz	70	0	17
Mini-Wheats, Frosted:			
Bite Size, Orig. (21), 1.8 oz	190	1	46
Little Bites: Orig., 1 c., 2 oz	200	1	47
Chocolate, 1 cup, 2 oz	200	2	46
Touch of Fruit In Middle,			
Raspberry (24), 2 oz	190	1	45
Mini Wheats, unfrosted:			
Bite Size (30), 1.8 oz	190	1	46
Little Bites, 1 cup, 2 oz	200	1	47
Mueslix, ²/₃ cup, 2 oz	200	3	41
Raisin Bran: Reg., 1 c., 2 oz	190	1	46
Crunch, 1 cup, 2 oz	190	1	45
Rice Krispies: Orig., 1.2 oz	130	0	29
Frosted, ³/₄ cup, 1 oz	120	0	27
Treats, ³/₄ cup, 1 oz	120	1	26
Smart Start, Orig. Antioxidants,			
1 cup, 1.8 fl.oz	190	1	43
Special K:			
Apple Cinn. Crunch, 1.1 oz	120	1.5	27
Chocolate Almond, 1 oz	110	1.5	23
Cinn. Brown Sugar Crunch, 1.1 oz	110	1	22
Nourish, C'nut Cranb. Alm., 1.8 oz	200	4	40
Oats & Honey, ²/₃ cup, 1 oz	100	0.5	25
Protein, average, ³/₄ cup, 1.1 oz	115	1	21
Red Berries, 1 cup, 1.1 oz	110	0	27
Vanilla Almond, 1.1 oz	110	1.5	25
Super Mario, 1 cup, 1.2 oz	120	1	27
Kind: *Per ¹/₂ Cup, 1.8 oz*			
Clusters: Banana Nut; Raspb. Chia	190	3	36
Cinnamon Oat, with Flax	190	5	34
Dark Chocolate	190	4.5	30
Maple Quinoa, with Chia	200	4.5	34
Peanut Butter Whole Grain	210	6	28

Malt-O-Meal:

	C	F	Cb
Apple Zings, 1 cup, 1.2 oz	130	1	29
Cocoa Dyno-Bites, ³/₄ c.	120	1	26
Coco Roos, ³/₄ cup, 1 oz	120	1.5	26
Frosted Flakes, ³/₄ cup, 1 oz	120	0	28
Frosted Mini Spooners,			
Blueberry, 1 cup, 1.95 oz	190	1	45
Golden Puffs, ³/₄ cup, 1 oz	100	0	24
Honey Nut Scooters,			
1 cup, 1 oz	120	1.5	24
Raisin Bran, 1 cup, 2 oz	200	1	47

Nature's Path:

	C	F	Cb
Flax Plus: Flakes, 1 oz	110	1.5	23
Mesa Sunrise Flakes, 1 oz	120	1	24
Multibran Flakes, 1 oz	110	1.5	23
Pumpkin Raisin Crunch, 1.95 oz	210	4.5	40
Heritage Flakes, 1 oz	120	1	24
Honey'd Corn Flakes,			
³/₄ cup, 1 oz	120	1	25
Kamut Puffs, 1 cup, 0.5 oz	50	0	11
Love Crunch, Dble Choc Chunk, 1 oz	135	4.5	21
Multigrain Oatbran Flakes,			
³/₄ cup, 1 oz	110	1	24
Optimum Power,			
Blueb. Cinnamon Flax, 1 oz	120	1.5	25
Qi'a, Superfod, Original, 1 oz	140	7	13

New England Natural Bakers:

Organic Granola:

	C	F	Cb
Berry Coconut, unswteetened,			
¹/₂ cup, 1.5 oz	250	12	31
Blueberry Harvest, ²/₃ cup, 2 oz	260	10	35
Cranberry Almond, ²/₃ cup, 2 oz	240	9	36
Pumpkin Spice, ¹/₂ cup, 2 oz	240	7	40

NutriSystem,

	C	F	Cb
Granola Cereal, 1 pkg	150	3	28

Peace:

Clusters & Flakes:

	C	F	Cb
Blueberry Pomegranate, 2 oz	240	6	41
Blueberry Walnut, 1 oz	220	3	43
Coconut Chia Almond, 2 oz	220	3.5	42
Maple Pecan, 2 oz	240	6	42
Vanilla Almond, 2 oz	240	6	42
Granola: Coconut Craze, 2 oz	270	12	37
French Vanilla, 2 oz	240	6	41
Maple Pecan, 2 oz	250	8	40
Purple Corn Flakes, 1 oz	90	1	23
Raisin Bran, 1 oz	170	0.5	42

= B

Breakfast Cereals

Ready-To-Eat Cereal ~ Brands (Cont)

	C	F	Cb
Post:			
Alpha Bits, 1 cup, 1 oz	120	1.5	24
Bran Flakes, ³/₄ cup, 1 oz	100	0.5	24
CoCo Wheats, 1.1 oz	120	0	24
Good Mornings, 1 oz	120	1.5	25
Grape-Nuts: Original, 2 oz	210	1	47
Flakes, ³/₄ cup, 1 oz	110	1	24
Great Grains:			
Banana Nut Crunch, 1 cup, 2 oz	230	5	43
Cranb. Alm. Crunch, 1cup, 2 oz	210	3.5	41
Crunchy Pecan, ³/₄ cup, 2 oz	210	6	38
Honey Bunches of Oats:			
Chocolate,1.2 oz	130	1.5	27
Honey Roasted, 1 oz	120	1.5	25
Pecan & Maple Brown Sugar	120	2.5	23
With Almonds, 1 oz	130	2.5	26
With Cinnamon, 1 oz	120	1.5	25
Honey-Comb, 1.1 oz	130	1	28
Malt O Meal ~ see Page 60			
Oreo O's, 2 cup, 1 oz	120	1.5	25
Pebbles, av. all varieties, ³/₄ cup, 1 oz	115	1	24
Raisin Bran, 1 cup, 2 oz	190	1	47
Shredded Wheat, Spoon Size:			
Original, 1.7 oz	170	1	40
Honey Nut, 2.1 oz	220	2	49
Waffle Crisp, 1 cup, 1 oz	120	1.5	25
Quaker			
King Vitaman, 1¹/₂ cups, 1 oz	120	1	26
Life, all types, ³/₄ cup, 1 oz	120	1.5	25
Oatmeal Squares,			
all varieties, 2 oz	210	2.5	44
Quisps, 1 cup 1 oz	100	1.5	23
Simply Granola:			
Apple Cranberry Almond, 1.7 oz	200	5	37
Oats, Honey, & Almonds,1.7 oz	200	6	35
Stop & Shop:			
Fiber Select, ¹/₂ cup, 1 oz	50	0.5	23
Granola,			
Oats & Honey, ¹/₂ c., 1.8 oz	230	9	31
Oats & O's, 1 cup, 1.1 oz	110	1.5	22
Raisin Bran, 1 cup, 2 oz	190	1	46
Shredded Wheat, Bite Size, 1 c., 1.5 oz	140	1	33
Sweet Home Farm:			
Blueberry, w/Flax, ³/₄ cup, 2 oz	250	8	40
Cinnamon, w/Raisins, ¹/₂ c., 1.8 oz	200	3	43
French Vanilla, w/Alm., ²/₃ c., 2 oz	250	8	40
Honey Nut, w/Alm., ¹/₂ c., 2 oz	260	10	37
Maple Pecan, w/Syrup, ¹/₂ c., 2 oz	250	8	40
Pumpkin Flax, ²/₃ cup, 2 oz	240	9	37

	C	F	Cb
Trader Joe's:			
Bran Flakes, ³/₄ cup, 1 oz	100	0.5	24
Cinnamon Squares, 1 cup, 1.5 oz	170	3	31
Clusters: Raisin Bran, 1 cup, 1 oz	190	3	41
Super Nutty Toffee, ³/₄ cup, 2 oz	250	9	38
Vanilla Almond, ²/₃ cup, 2 oz	220	8	34
Av. other Flavors, 1 c., 2 oz	230	8	40
Cornflakes, 1 cup, 1 oz	110	0	26
Frosted Flakes, ³/₄ c., 1 oz	110	0	24
High Fiber Cereal: Reg., ²/₃ cup, 1 oz	80	0.5	23
Fruit & Nut, Multigrain, ²/₃ cup, 1 oz	90	1.5	25
Granola: Gluten Free, ³/₄ cup, 2 oz	60	12	35
Low Fat, av., ³/₄ cup, 2 oz	210	3	44
Org., Apple/Mango, av., ²/₃ cup, 2 oz	240	8	37
Joe's O's, 1 cup, 1 oz	110	2	20
Just The Clusters, av., ²/₃ cup, 2 oz	240	9	36
O's, av. all flavours, ³/₄ - 1 cup, 1 oz	120	2	24
Oatmeal (Instant): *Per 1.4 oz Pkt*			
Ancient Grains	160	6	24
Mango; Maple & Brown Sugar, av.	160	2	32
Unsweetened	160	3.5	24
Oatmeal Complete: Plain, 1.4 oz pkt	170	3	29
Maple Brown Sugar, 1.4 oz pkt	210	3	38
Raisin Bran: Regular, 1 cup, 1 oz	170	1	41
Clusters, 1 cup, 2 oz	190	3	41
w/ Pomegr. Blue. Flakes/Clusters, 1 c.	210	2	44
Shredded Wheat, 1 cup, 1.7 oz	180	1	38
Toasted Oatmeal Flakes, ³/₄ c.,1 oz	110	1	23
Udi's:			
Granola: Orig.; Cranb., ¹/₄ c., 1 oz	140	6	21
All Naturel; Vanilla, av., ¹/₄ cup, 1 oz	120	4	19
Uncle Sam:			
Original, Wheat Berry,			
³/₄ cup, 1 oz	210	6	37
Skinner's Raisin Bran, 1 cup, 2 oz	200	1	45
Weetabix, 2 bisc., 1.3 oz	130	1	29
Wegmans:			
Chocolaty Rice Crisps, 1 oz	120	1	26
Crunchy Raisin Bran, 1 cup, 1.8 oz	190	1	44
Granola, Vanilla & Almonds, 1 oz	140	4	22
Peanut Butter Corn Crunch, 1 oz	110	2.5	20
Shredded Wheat,			
Bite Size, 1 cup, 2 oz	200	1	44
Whole Foods 365:			
Corn Flakes, 1 oz	110	0	26
Frosted Flakes, 1 oz	110	0	27
Honey Flakes & Oat Clusters,			
³/₄ cup, 1 oz	120	1	25
Protein & Fiber Crunch, 1.8 oz	190	1	33
Raisin Bran, 1 cup, 2 oz	180	1	44
Wheat Squares:			
Bite Sized, 1.7 oz	180	1	38
Frosted, 1 cup, 1.9 oz	210	1	45

Ready-to-Eat

	C	F	Cb
Per Piece/Slice			
Angel Food, Plain: without oil, 2 oz	145	0	33
with oil, 2 oz	145	1	27
with Cream Frosting	255	7	45
Almond Croissant, 5 oz	620	35	67
Apple Danish, 5 oz	450	18	67
Apple Pie ~ *See Pies/Tarts Page 134*			
Baklava, 1½" square, 1.75 oz	200	10	27
Banana Cake, with Butter Cream, 2 oz	230	9	37
Banana Walnut Cake, 3 oz	270	11	40
Bear Claw, 4.5 oz	540	24	71
Black Forest, 3 oz	345	11	59
Brownie: Small, 2" Square, 1 oz	130	8	14
Large, 3 oz	390	24	42
Bundt Cakes, average all types:			
3 oz slice	300	13	42
Mini-Bundt, 5 oz	500	22	70
Cannoli's: Mini, 1 oz	85	3	11
Regular, 2.5 oz	215	8	28
Carrot Cake: Plain, 3 oz	300	16	37
with Cream Cheese Frosting	400	22	48
Cheesecake:			
Small serving, 3 oz	240	13	26
Large serving, 5 oz	400	21	44
with Low-Fat Cheese/Fruit, 3 oz	170	4	28
Denny's, NY Style, 5oz	510	34	43
Chocolate Cake:			
with Chocolate Frosting, 4 oz	415	18	62
without Frosting, 1/12 of 9", 3.5 oz	340	14	51
Chocolate Croissant, 4.25 oz	470	26	54
Chocolate Eclair, w/ custard, 3.5 oz	260	16	24
Chocolate Fudge Cake, 3 oz	270	12	40
Chocolate Meringue, 2.5 oz	320	13	48
Churros, 1 stick, 1.5 oz	165	8	21
Cinnamon Crumb Cake, 2.5 oz	260	9	40
Cinnamon Rolls: Small, 2 oz	220	8	34
Regular, 4 oz	440	16	68
Large, 6 oz	660	24	102
Brands ~ *See Page 67*			
Coffee Cake, 2 oz	180	6	30
Concha: Small, 2 oz	240	9	33
Large (5" diameter), 5.5 oz	615	23	85
Cream Puff, custard filled, 4.6 oz	335	20	30
Cream Horn, 3 oz	210	5	36
Crumble Coffee Cake, 4.5 oz	500	25	65
Danish Pastries:			
Small, 2.5 oz	250	14	25
Large, 5 oz	500	28	50
Donuts ~ *See Page 66*			
Eclair, Chocolate, custard filled, 3.5 oz	260	16	24
Fig Bars, average	160	3	31

Ready-to-Eat (Cont)

	C	F	Cb
Per Piece/Slice			
Fruit Cake, Dark/Light, 2 oz	185	5	34
Fudge Nut Brownie, 3.5 oz	380	18	54
Gingerbread, from mix, 3" square	210	4	41
Honey Bun, 2.7 oz	310	15	39
Jelly Roll, 1/12 roll, 1.8 oz	150	2	32
Key Lime Pie, 4.3 oz	400	25	41
Kringles: Almond; Pecan, average	205	12	24
Blueberry: Cherry; Raspberry, av.	165	8	24
Lady Finger, 3 oz	310	4.5	59
Lemon Cake, 4 oz	440	24	49
Lemon Poppy Seed Creme, 1.6 oz	180	9	23
Marble Cake, 4 oz	430	23	50
Mississippi Mud Pie, 4 oz	480	22	67
Mud Cake, 4.5 oz	380	20	44
Muffins ~ *See Page 67*			
Palmier Cookie, large, 4.5 oz	490	25	62
Pineapple Upside Down Cake,			
2.5 oz	230	9	36
Peach Melba, 3.5 oz	300	8	52
Pecan Sticky Roll, 6.5 oz	690	22	91
Pecan Twirls, 1.3 oz	170	7	26
Pies & Tarts ~ *See Page 134*			
Pound Cakes: Iced Lemon, 3.5 oz	360	17	50
Marble, 3.75 oz	350	13	53
Raspberry Rugulah,			
1.2 oz	110	9	7
Scone, fruit, 2 oz	200	9	30
Sponge Cake: Plain, 2.5 oz	220	10	33
with Chocolate Frosting	290	12	45
with Cream & Strawberry Jam	390	12	69
Starbucks Cakes ~ *Page 244*			
Strawberry Cream Cake, 4.7 oz	400	27	33
Strudel Bites, 0.75 oz	60	2.5	9
Strudel, fruit, av., 4.5 oz	300	17	32
Swiss Rolls, 1 oz	135	6	19
Tiramisu, 4.5 oz	440	22	34
Turnovers, fruit, average, 3 oz	290	15	35

Cupcakes

	C	F	Cb
Average all Varieties			
Regular:			
Cake only, 1.5 oz	140	5.5	20
Cake + Icing, 2.5 oz	260	13	34
Large, (Muffin Size):			
Cake only, 2.5 oz	235	9	34
Cake + Icing, 5 oz	520	27	67
Mini, (2-Bite):			
Cake only, 0.4 oz	40	1.5	5.5
Cake + Icing, 1 oz	110	5.5	13
Icing Only: Per 1 oz	115	7	13
Thick/Tall amount, 2.5 oz	290	17	32

Cakes ~ Brands	**C**	**F**	**Cb**
Albertson's Bakery:			
Ring Cakes: *Per ⅛ Cake*			
Angel Food, 2 oz	160	0	36
Butter; Chocolate, av., 3 oz	305	15	39
Cake Slices: *Per Slice Unless Indicated*			
Banana Nut Loaf	330	17	39
Butter Creme	110	6	20
Creme Cake (2), 3.2 oz	300	12	43
Cinnamon Streusel (2), 3.2 oz	350	18	43
Bimbo Bakery:			
Concha, Vanilla, 2 oz	260	11	35
Pound Cakes: *Per Slice*			
Panquecitos, 1.8 oz	170	4.5	29
Pecan, 2.3 oz	260	11	36
Raisin, 2.3 oz	240	9	38
Bon Appetit Bakery:			
Banana Bread, 4 oz	440	25	49
Cream Cheese Cake,			
4 oz slice	430	24	49
Danish: Apple (1), 5 oz	210	11	25
Bear Claw (1), 5 oz	240	13	27
Cheese & Berries (1), 5 oz	250	14	26
Vienna Cream (1), 5 oz	240	14	27
Slices: Cheesecake, 4 oz	430	24	49
Lemon Cake, 4 oz	430	24	49
Marble Cake, 4 oz	430	24	50
Walnut Brownie, 3.5 oz	380	18	54
Cheesecake Factory ~ *See Fast-Foods Section*			
Entenmann's: *Per Slice*			
Crumb Cakes: All Butter French, 1.8 oz	210	10	29
Cheese-Filled, 2 oz	200	10	25
NY Style, ⅛ cake	270	12	39
Danish: Pecan Twist, ⅙ cake	260	16	27
Raspberry Twist, 2 oz	220	11	29
Walnut Twist, ⅙ cake	260	15	26
Dessert Cakes:			
Chocolate Fudge, 2.3 oz	240	10	37
Lemon/Louisiana Crunch, 3 oz	330	14	49
Strawberry Iced Cake, ⅙ cake	350	17	47
Loaf Cakes: Chocolate, ⅙ loaf	190	8	29
Cinnamon Crunch, ⅙ loaf	270	14	33
Glenny's:			
100 Calorie:			
Blondie, Choc. Chip, 1.5 oz	100	4	15
Brownies: Chocolate Chip, 1.5 oz	100	4	12
Peanut Butter, 1.5 oz	100	4	15
Muffins/Sweet Rolls ~ See Page 67			

Great American Cookies:	**C**	**F**	**Cb**
Cookie Cakes: *Per Slice*			
By the Slice, 4.5 oz	580	27	83
Heart Shaped, 3.5 oz	440	21	64
M&M, 4 oz	500	24	73
Great Value *(Walmart)*:			
Chocolate Cup Cake, (1), 1.8 oz	170	5	31
Devil's Food Cake, (1), 1.4 oz	160	7	23
Snack Cakes: Fudge Swirl, (1), 1.3oz	165	8	23
Choc./Lemon Snack Cake, 1 oz	120	6	18
Swiss Roll Snack Cake (1), 1 oz	120	5	17
Hostess:			
Cup Cakes:			
100 Calorie Packs, av.,			
3 minicakes	100	2.5	21
8 Pack, Chocolate, 1 cake, 1.5 oz	160	6	26
Ding Dongs, (1)	165	9	22
Ho Hos, (1)	120	5	18
Twinkies:			
Original; Banana, av., (1)	140	5	24
Deep Fried: Original (1)	220	9	32
Chocolate (1)	220	8	36
Zingers, (2)	250	9	41
Donettes ~ *Page 66*			
Little Debbie:			
Boxed: Boston Creme Roll, (1)	270	12	40
Choc. Chip Cake, 2 oz	300	14	42
Choc. Cup Cake, Crm Filled (1), 1.9 oz	210	8	33
Cocoa Cremes, (1), 1.5 oz	170	8	24
Devil Cremes ,(1), 1.66 oz	200	9	29
Devil Squares, (2), 2.2 oz	260	11	38
Fancy Cakes, (2), 2.4 oz	310	15	43
Frosted Fudge Cake, (1), 1.5 oz	190	9	27
Fudge Brownie (1)	280	12	40
S'mores Cake Rolls, (1), 2.2 oz	260	11	40
Zebra Cake, (1), 2.6 oz	320	14	48
Ne-Mo's:			
Breads: Banana, 4 oz	460	23	57
Carrot, 4 oz	450	22	56
Cheese Coffee Cake, 4 oz	460	21	62
Wild Blueberry Bread, 4 oz	430	20	58
Brookie, (1), 1.5 oz	160	7	26
Bundt: Chocolate, 4 oz	380	14	62
Coconut Pineapple, 4 oz	410	18	60
Key Lime, 4 oz	440	18	67
Orange Dreamswirl	440	18	67
Cake Squares: Carrot, 3.6 oz	390	21	47
Banana; Chocolate, av, 3 oz	300	12	45
Crumble Cake: Blueberry (1), 4 oz	390	17	54
Cinnamon Streusel (1), 4 oz	420	18	59
Lemon Rasp. (1), 4 oz	400	19	55

Cakes ~ Brands (Cont)	C	F	Cb

Pepperidge Farm:
3-Layer Cakes: Per 1/8 Cake

	C	F	Cb
Chocolate Fudge	240	13	32
Coconut	250	12	34
Key Lime; Vanilla	240	12	34
Average other varieties	240	11	33
Turnovers (Frozen):			
Apple; Cherry (1)	260	13	31
Chocolate (1)	350	22	35
Peach; Raspberry (1)	270	13	34
Pop Tarts (Kellogg's):			
Chocolate Chip	210	6	36
Fruit/Frosted/Unfrosted, av.	200	5	36
Wholegrain, Strawberry	180	2.5	38
Safeway Select,			
Molten Chocolate Lava Cake, 4.5 oz	440	26	50
Sara Lee:			
Carrot Cake, 1/6 cake	340	18	41
Cheesecakes:			
Classic: French, 4.7 oz sl.	410	26	38
Strawberry, 4.3 oz sl.	320	18	37
New York Style, 5 oz sl.	480	29	48
Limited Edition,			
NY Style, Chocolate, 5 oz slice	500	29	55
Original Cream:			
Cherry, 4.8 oz slice	320	11	50
Classic, 4.3 oz slice	340	18	38
Strawberry, 4.7 oz slice	330	12	51
Coffee Cake, Butter Streusel, 1/6 cake	190	9	24
Pound Cakes:			
All Butter, 1.9 oz slice	260	9	42
Lemon, 2.7 oz slice	270	9	42
Individual Slices:			
All Butter, 1 oz	100	3	15
Double Choc., 1.8 oz	180	7	28
Lemon, 1 oz	100	3.5	15
Original, 1.6 oz	160	5	25
Special K,			
Pastry Crisps, all varieties, (2), 1 oz	100	2	20
Tastykake:			
Choc Cupkakes:			
Chocolate Koffee Kake, 2.1 oz	240	9	37
Cream Filled, 2.1 oz	220	8	34
Banana Pudding, 2 oz	180	6	31

Tastykake (Cont):	C	F	Cb
Kandy Kake:			
Lemon Flavored, 2 oz	290	16	34
Peanut Butter, 1.4 oz	190	11	19
Krimpets, Spice Kake Cake, (2)	220	7	37
Mini Cupcakes, Koffee Kake (3)	180	8	25
Toaster Strudel (Pillsbury): Per 2 oz			
Boston Cream Pie	180	7	26
Cream Cheese,			
average all varieties	180	9	26
Fruit flavors, all var.	180	7	27
Trader Joe's:			
Bakery Fresh:			
Apricot Almond Tart,			
4 oz slice	450	24	56
Cheesecake Brownie Bites (1)	110	7	9
Chocolate Ganache Cake, 3 oz slice	390	22	44
Flourless Chocolate Cake,			
1 slice, 2 oz	260	17	23
Lemon Cake, 3.3 oz slice	350	19	43
Mini Carrot Cake, 5 oz	450	19	68
Whoopie Pie (1), 2.5 oz	350	14	54
Bread Cake:			
Banana Bonanza, 2.6 oz slice	250	9	39
Pumpkin Nut, 2.6 oz slice	270	10	43
Walnut Streusel Coffee, 2 oz slice	180	8	25
Zucchini Carrot, 2 oz slice	200	7	32
Loaf Cake:			
Cranberry Pumpkin, 2 oz slice	140	2	30
Pumpkin Nut, 2.6 oz slice	270	10	43
Frozen:			
Apple Raspberry Turnover, 3.2 oz	280	14	34
Chocolate Dilemma Cheesecake:			
Plain, 3.5 oz	320	19	30
Choc. Chip; Triple Choc., av., 3.5 oz	345	20	35
Tuxedo, 3.5 oz	320	17	34
Choc Lava Cake, 4 oz	360	23	40
Karat Cake, 3 oz slice	320	19	37
N.Y. Style Cheesecake, 4.5 oz slice	400	28	32
Tiramisu Torte, 3.2 oz slice	230	12	24
Tarts			
Pear, 3.5 oz slice	250	9	39
Raspberry, 5 oz slice	290	10	51
Wild Blueberry, 3.5 oz slice	260	6	52

Cakes ~ Mixes

	C	F	Cb

Prepared as Directed
Arrowhead Mills:
Brownie Mix:

	C	F	Cb
Regular, $^1/_{20}$ package, 1 oz	150	7	21
Gluten Free,			
Fudge Brownie, $^1/_{20}$ pkg., 1 oz	160	8	21
Cake Mix:			
Chocolate, organic, $^1/_{12}$ pkg., 1.75 oz	280	11	42
Vanilla, $^1/_{12}$ package, 1.7 oz	270	10	39

Betty Crocker: *Prepared as Directed*
Brownie Mix:

Dark Choc. Fudge, $^1/_{20}$ pkg	160	6.5	24
Fudge, $^1/_{20}$ package	160	7	22
Low-Fat Fudge, $^1/_{18}$ pkg	140	2.5	28
Gluten Free, Chocolate, $^1/_{16}$ pkg	150	5	24
Premium:			
Chocolate Chunk, $^1/_{16}$ pkg	170	7	26
Original Supreme, $^1/_{16}$ package	190	8	27
P'nut Butter; Walnut, av., $^1/_{16}$ pkg	170	7	24
Triple Chunk, $^1/_{20}$ package	180	8	25
Ultimate Fudge, $^1/_{16}$ package	170	6.5	26

Gluten Free Cake Mix:

Devils Food, $^1/_{10}$ Pkg	260	12	36
Yellow, $^1/_{10}$ Pkg	260	11	37

SuperMoiste Cake Mixes: *Per $^1/_{10}$ Package*

Butter Recipe Yellow	240	9	36
Carrot	310	18	35
Cherry Chip	280	14	36
Devil's Food; French Vanilla	280	14	35
Lemon	280	14	36
Milk Chocolate	250	10	35
Triple Chocolate Fudge	280	14	34

If using No-Cholesterol Recipe, deduct 40 cals and 4g fat.

Dessert Bars: Reeses, 1 oz mix

Reeses, 1 oz mix	180	12	20
Sunkist Lemon, 1 oz mix	140	4.5	24

Duncan Hines: *Prepared as Directed*
Brownie Mix:

Chewy Fudge Brownie, $^1/_{20}$ pkg	150	7	22
Decadent, Caramel Turtle, $^1/_{15}$ pkg	170	7	25
Double Fudge, $^1/_{16}$ pkg	170	8	25
Cake Mix,			
Classic, Dark Choc. Fudge, $^1/_{10}$ pkg	260	13	33
Decadent: *Per $^1/_{12}$ Pkg*			
Classic Carrot	260	10	39
German Chocolate	290	14	37

Prepared as Directed

	C	F	Cb

Duncan Hines (Cont):
Signature: *Per $^1/_{12}$ Pkg*

Banana Supreme	270	12	36
French Vanilla; German Choc., av.	270	12	34
Red Velvet	250	12	33

Jell-O:
No Bake Cheesecake:

Cherry, $^1/_8$ pkg, 2.2 oz	360	20	41
Real Cheesecake, $^1/_8$ pkg, 2.2 oz	350	16	49

Krusteaz:

Cinn. Swirl Crumb Cake, $2^1/_2$x2" pce	210	5	39
Lemon; Key Lime Bar, 2" bar	140	3	26

Pillsbury:
Brownies, Premium Mix: *Dry Mix Only*

Caramel Swirl, $^1/_{12}$ pkg, 1.2 oz	120	1	28
Cheesecake Swirl, $^1/_{15}$ pkg, 1 oz	110	1.5	25
Chocolate Extreme, $^1/_{15}$ pkg, 1 oz	120	2	24
Double Chocolate, $^1/_{16}$ pkg, 1 oz	100	0.5	24

Cakes:

Funfetti: Bold Purple $^1/_6$ pkg, 1.4 oz	140	1.5	21
Neon Yellow, $^1/_6$ pkg, 1.4 oz	140	1.5	21
Moist Supreme: *Per $^1/_{10}$ Pkg, Dry Mix Only*			
Devils Food, 1.5 oz	150	2	34
White/Yellow, 1.5 oz	160	1.5	35

Cake Frostings

Betty Crocker:
Rich & Creamy,

average all flavors, 2 Tbsp, 1.2 oz	135	5	22
Whipped, av. all flavors.,2 T., 0.9 oz	100	4.5	15
Cool Whip, Original, 2 Tbsp, 0.3 oz	25	1.5	2

Duncan Hines:

Creamy Homestyle, av. all flav., 2T.	140	6	23
Whipped, av. all flavors, 3 Tbsp	150	7	21

Pillsbury: *Per 2 Tbsp*
Creamy Supreme:

Choc Fudge; Milk Choc., 1.2 oz	130	6	21
Classic White; Vanilla, 1.2 oz	140	5	22
Fluffy, av. all flavors, 2 Tbsp, 0.8 oz	100	5	14
Funfetti, av. all flavors, 2 Tbsp,1.2 oz	140	5	23
Sugar Free, average, 2 Tbsp, 1.1 oz	100	6	16

Quick Guide

	C	F	Cb
Donuts			
Average All Brands			
Cake: Plain, 1.8 oz	205	12	23
Chocolate Iced, 2 oz	255	14	29
Sugared, 0.8 oz	205	10	29
Non-Cake, Glazed, 2 oz	225	11	29
Croissant-Donuts			
(Includes Cronuts/Frissants)			
Average all Brands			
Cream-filled, 3.5 oz	430	26	45
Custard-filled, 3.5 oz	360	19	45

Extra Listings ~ *See CalorieKing.com*
(Cronut is a trademark of Dominique Ansel Bakery, New York)

Donuts ~ Brands

	C	F	Cb
Albertson's:			
Donut Holes:			
Glazed Old Fashioned (4)	240	12	31
Powdered Sugar (4)	210	12	24
Gem Donuts: Plain Cake (3)	190	12	20
Cinnamon Sugar (3)	240	15	23
Glazed (1)	140	6	21
Bon Appetit:			
Mini Donuts:			
Chocolate (4)	270	16	29
Crumb (4)	240	12	32
Powdered (4)	250	12	34
Dunkin' Donuts:			
Apple Crumb	320	15	42
Apple N' Spice	260	14	29
Barvarian Kreme	270	15	31
Blueberry Butternut	420	17	60
Blueberry Crumb Cake	380	18	50
Boston Kreme	300	16	37
Chocolate Frosted Cake	350	19	40
Chocolate Headlight	330	18	39
Choc. Peanut Butter Flav. Cream	360	19	44
Glazed Chocolate	340	19	38
Jelly Filled	270	14	32
Powdered	320	19	33
Vanilla Creme	330	20	35

Extra Listings ~ *See Fast Food Section*

Donuts ~ Brands (Cont)

	C	F	Cb
Entenmann's:			
8 Pack: *Per Donut*			
Plain	220	13	24
Crumb Topped	250	12	36
Glazed	260	13	34
Rich Frosted	290	19	30
Pop'ems:			
Pumpkin (4)	230	13	29
Rich Frosted (4)	320	23	28
Hostess:			
Mini Donettes: Crumb, 6-pack, 4 oz	430	18	63
Frosted, 6-pack, 3 oz	360	22	38
Powdered, 6-pack, 3 oz	340	17	43
Krispy Kreme:			
Apple Fritter, 3.5 oz	350	19	42
Chocolate: Iced Cake, 2.5 oz	280	13	37
Iced Custard Filled, 3 oz	300	15	37
Iced Glazed Cruller, 2.5 oz	260	10	40
Iced Glazed, 2.2	240	11	33
Iced Kreme Filled, 3 oz	350	19	41
Iced Glazed w/ Sprinkles, 2.3 oz	250	11	36
Cinnamon Twist, 1.9oz	210	11	26
Glazed Cruller, 1.9 oz	210	10	29
Glazed Doughnut Holes:			
Original (5)	220	11	25
Blueberry (4)	190	7	28
Cake (4)	190	8	28
Chocolate Cake (4)	180	7	27
Glazed Kreme Filled, 3 oz	340	19	40
Maple Iced Glazed, 2.2 oz	240	11	34
New York Cheesecake, 3.3 oz	310	17	35
Original Glazed, 1.7 oz	190	11	22
Powdered Cake, 2.3 oz	240	11	29
Traditional Cake, 2 oz	230	12	26
Little Debbie,			
Donut Sticks, 1.9 oz	270	16	29
Tastykake:			
Cinnamon, (3), 2 oz	230	11	31
Mini: Crunch, 3 oz pkg	330	13	50
Powdered Sugar, 2.5 oz pkg	300	14	41

Quick Guide   C F Cb

Muffins: Ready-To-Eat
Average All Brands

	C	F	Cb
Small, 1 oz	90	3.5	14
Medium, 2 oz	185	6.5	28
Large, 3 oz	275	10	42
Extra Large, 4 oz	365	13	57
Giant, 6 oz	550	20	84
Super Size, 8 oz	730	27	112

Muffins Ready-To-Eat ~ Brands

Albertsons:
	C	F	Cb
Minis: Banana Nut (2)	200	12	20
Blueberry (2)	180	10	21
Honey Raisin Bran (2)	170	7	24

Entenmann's,
	C	F	Cb
Blueberry; Choc. Chip; Corn (1), av.	190	9	25
Garden Lites: Chocolate (1), 2 oz	120	4	21
Banana Choc. Chip (1), 2 oz	120	3	23
Blueberry Oat (1), 2 oz	120	2	25
Av. other flavors (1), 1 oz	70	2	13

Great Value *(Walmart):*
	C	F	Cb
Double Banana Filled, (1), 4 oz	360	16	52
Double Blueberry Filled, (1), 4 oz	430	16	65
Triple Chocolate Filled, (1), 4 oz	420	18	61
Little Debbie: Banana Nut (1), 1.9 oz	210	9	30
Blueberry (1), 1.9 oz	190	8	27
Chocolate Chip (1), 1.9 oz	210	9	28

My Favorite Muffin: *Per Large*
	C	F	Cb
Banana Nut	650	38	71
Blueberry	590	28	78
Boston Cream Pie	740	33	105
Chocolate Chip	790	39	100
Lemon Poppyseed	670	32	90

Otis Spunkmeyer:
	C	F	Cb
Banana, 2 oz	220	10	30
Blueberry, 2 oz	210	9	29
Choc. Chip Minis (3), 2.25 oz	270	14	32

Starbucks ~ *See Fast-Foods Section*

Trader Joe's: *Per Muffin*
	C	F	Cb
Apple Cranberry, 4.8 oz	220	5	38
Banana Chocolate Chip, 4 oz	400	18	57
Carrot, 4 oz	320	11	52
Triple Berry, 4 oz	310	11	49

Vitalicious:
	C	F	Cb
VitaTops: Deep Choc./Choc Mint, 2 oz	100	1.5	26
Wild Blueberry, 2 oz	120	2	25
Protein, hoc. P'nut Butter, 2 oz	150	4	23
Sugar free, Velvety Choc., 2 oz	90	2	24

Weight Watchers,
	C	F	Cb
Blueb.; Double Choc, av., 2.5 oz	185	2.5	42

Muffin Mixes   C F Cb

Per Muffin, Prepared
	C	F	Cb
Betty Crocker: Banana Nut	170	8	22
Cinnamon Streusel	190	8	27
Wild Blueberry	160	6.5	24
Pouch Mix, with Milk:			
Banana Nut	130	4	24
Blueberry	130	3	23
Chocolate Chip	130	3	23
Krusteaz:			
Choc Chunk	260	12	33
Lemon Poppyseed	170	4	31
Oat Bran	180	4.5	32
Trader Joe's, Triple Berry	150	2	28

Sweet Rolls & Buns

Note: It is best to weigh for accuracy as actual weight can be 10-50% higher than label weight·

Per Sweet Roll or Bun Unless Indicated
	C	F	Cb
Bimbo, Bimbolete, 2.2 oz	250	10	36
Bon Appetit,			
Cinnamon Roll, 2.5 oz	230	8	34
Cinnabon: Classic	880	37	127
Caramel Pecanbon	1080	51	146
Cloverhill Bakery,			
Jumbo Glazed Honey Bun, 4.75 oz	600	35	64
Entenmann's, Cinn. Swirl Bun, 3 oz	320	14	44
Little Debbie:			
Honey Bun: 2.3 oz	280	16	32
Individual: 3 oz Bun	360	20	41
4 oz Bun	480	26	56
with White Icing, 4 oz	490	25	60
Pecan Spinwheels: Single, 1 oz	100	3.5	17
2 Pack, 2.1 oz	210	7	32
O&H Danish: *Per 1.95 oz*			
Kringles: Apple	180	7	26
Almond; Turtle, average	215	10	30
Cinn. Roll; Cream Cheese, average	205	11	26
Wisconsin,	170	5.5	28
Pillsbury:			
Sweet Rolls, Refrigerated: *Per Roll Unless Indicated*			
Cinnamon, w/ Crm Cheese Icing	140	4.5	23
Cinn., Flaky w/ Butter Cream Icing	160	7	23
Twists, Flaky Cinnamon, with Icing	160	7	23
Grands, Refrigerated: *Per Roll*			
Cinnabon: Cinnamon Roll,			
with Cream Cheese Icing	300	7	54
Caramel Rolls, with Icing, 3.5 oz	300	8	53
Flaky Supreme Cinnamon Roll,			
with Icing, 3.5 oz	360	17	47
7-Eleven: Iced Honey Bun, 6 oz	820	58	68
Glazed Honey Bun, 5 oz	620	35	70
Sara Lee, Cinnamon Roll, 2.4 oz	260	12	33

Quick Guide

	C	F	Cb
Chocolate:			
Average All Brands			
Milk Chocolate: regular:			
Plain/Nuts/Fruit, average, 1 oz	150	9	17
1.5oz Bar	230	13	25
2 oz Bar	305	17	34
4 oz Block	610	34	68
8 oz Block	1220	68	136
1 Pound, 16 oz	2440	136	272
Dark/White Chocolate: 1 oz	155	9	17
Hershey's, Sugar Free, 5 pieces	110	13	24
Milk Chocolate-Coated:			
Almonds, 5-6, 1 oz	150	10	15
Cherry Cordial Centers, 2 pcs, 1 oz	145	6	21
Clusters, Nut, 3 pieces, 1.2 oz	210	14	20
Coffee Beans, 1.4 oz	220	13	22
Macadamias, 10 pieces, 1.4 oz	220	16	21
Mints, 1 medium, 0.5 oz	55	1	11
Nougat & Caramel, 1 oz	150	9	15
Peanuts, 12 medium, 1 oz	145	10	14
Raisins, 28 medium, 1 oz	110	4	19
Baking Chocolate:			
Baker's: Bittersweet, 1 oz	140	12	14
Semi-sweet, 1 oz	140	9	16
Nestle, Chips: Dark, 1 Tbsp. 0.5 oz	70	5	3
Semi-Sweet, 1 Tbsp. 0.5oz	70	4	9
Unsweetened, 1 oz	140	14	8
Carob, Plain, 1 oz	155	9	16

Candy ~ Brands & Generic

Per Piece/Serving

	C	F	Cb
3 Musketeers: Orig., 1 bar, 1.9 oz	240	7	42
2 To Go, 1.7 oz Bar	200	6	36
Fun Size, 3 bars, 1.6 oz	190	6	34
Minis, 7 pieces, 1.4 oz	170	5	32
100 Grand: 1.5 oz bar	190	8	30
Snack Size (1), 0.8 oz	95	4	15
Super Size, 2.8 oz	360	14	58
Abba Zabba, 2 oz bar	250	5	48
After Dinner Mints, 1 small	25	1.5	3
After Eight Mint, each	35	1.5	4
Airhead, 1 bar, 0.5 oz	60	1	14
Almond Joy: 2 bars, 1.6 oz	220	13	26
King Size, 4 bars, 3.2 oz	440	26	53
Snack Size, 0.6 oz bar	80	4.5	10
Pieces (46), 1.4 oz	200	10	27

Per Piece/Serving

	C	F	Cb
Almond Roca, 3 pieces, 1.3 oz	200	15	17
Almond: Sugar-coated (15), 1.4 oz	190	7	27
Jordan, 15 pieces, 1.4 oz	180	8	28
Almond Clusters:			
True North, 1 oz	170	12	9
Trader Joe's, 1.2 oz	190	14	13
Altoids, 3 pieces	10	0	2
Andes, Thins (8), av. all var., 1.4 oz	205	13	22
Anthon Berg:			
Creamy Mint (4), 1.4 oz	180	6	31
Marzipan with Plum, in Madeira	120	6	14
Atomic Fireball, 1 piece, 0.3 oz	35	0	9
Baby Ruth: King Size, 3.5 oz bar	500	24	66
2 oz bar	280	14	39
Fun size, 2 bars	170	8	24
Minis, 4 bars	210	11	28
Baci *(Perugina),*			
1 piece, 0.5 oz	75	6	7
Bark Thins, Snacking Chocolate,			
Dark Choc. Mint/Pretzel, av., 1 oz	140	6	20
Baskin-Robbins: Sugar Candy, 3 pcs	60	1	12
Sugar Free, 4 pieces, average, 0.6 oz	40	1	16
Note: Carb figure includes 16g sugar alcohol			
Big Hunk, 2 oz Bar	230	3	47
Bit-O-Honey: 1.7 oz bar	180	3.5	39
Chews, 6 pcs, 1.4 oz	150	3	32
Bliss *(Hershey's):*			
Milk/Dark Choc./Caramel, 6 pieces	120	14	25
Meltaway Centers,			
Milk Chocolate/Raspberry, 6 pcs	220	15	24
Blow Pops, each, 0.6 oz	60	0	17
Bon Bons, 3 pieces	65	0	15
Boston Baked Beans, (11)	70	2	11
Brach's: Almond Supremes (10)	200	14	20
Bridge Mix (15)	190	10	26
Double Dippers (15)	210	14	22
Gummi Bears (14)	130	0	30
Lemon Drops, Sugar Free, 4 pieces	35	0	17
Note: Carb figures include 17g Sugar Alcohol			
Mandarin/Orange Slices (3), 1.6 oz	150	0	37
Maple Nut Goodies (8)	190	9	27
Milk Maid Crmls (4)	150	4	25
Peanut Cluster (3)	210	15	20
Breath Savers, (1),all var.	5	0	2
Bubble Gum – *See Page 75*			
Bulls Eyes, 3 pieces, 1.2 oz	130	3	23
Buncha Crunch: 1.4 oz	180	9	25
Movie Box, 3.2 oz	450	20	65
Burnt Peanuts, 1.4 oz	170	6	29

Candy ~ Brands & Generic (Cont)

Per Piece/Serving	C	F	Cb
Butterfinger: 2 oz bar	270	11	43
King Size (3 bars), 3.5 oz	480	18	75
Fun Size, (1), 0.8 oz	100	4	15
Giant, (Pieces in Choc.),		
$^{1}/_{4}$ bar, 1 oz	150	8	21
Miniatures:		
1 piece, 0.4 oz	45	2	8
4 pieces, 1.4 oz	180	8	32
Crisp Bar: Original, 2 oz bar	270	11	43
King Size, 3 pieces, 2 oz	310	17	38
Minis, 2 bars, 1.4 oz	210	11	25
Snackerz:		
Single, 1.3 oz	170	8	23
Fun Size, 2 pcs, 1.2 oz	150	7	21
King Size, 10 pcs, 1.4 oz	190	8	25
Butter Mints, 7 pieces, 0.5 oz	50	0	12
Butterscotch: 3 pieces	60	0	15
Discs (*Walgreens*), 3 pieces, 0.6 oz	70	0	17
Cadbury: Caramello Bar, 1.6 oz	220	10	29
Caramel Egg, 1.2 oz	170	8	22
Dairy Milk Bar, 7 pcs, 1.4 oz	200	11	23
Mini Eggs (Candy), 12 pcs, 1.4 oz	190	8	28
Candy Apple, medium, 6.5 oz	280	0	60
Candy Cane, medium, 5", 0.5 oz	40	0	14
Candy Corn, 20 pieces, 1.4 oz	150	0	38
Candy Jar Mix (*Jewel*), 3 pcs, 0.6 oz	60	0	14
Candy Necklace (*Smarties*), (1), 0.8 oz	90	0.5	20
Caramels: Each, 0.4 oz	40	1	8
Chocolate, each, 0.3 oz	25	0.3	6
Creams (3), 1.3 oz	130	3	23
Caramel Popcorn, $^{2}/_{3}$ cup	150	6	23
Cella's,		
Milk Choc. Cherries, 3 pieces, 1.5 oz	160	6	27
Certs, Breath Mints, 1 piece	5	0	2
Charleston Chew:		
Chocolate Bar (1), 1.4 oz	160	4.5	30
Mini Bars, 13 pieces	190	6	34
Charms: Blow Pop	60	0	17
Flat Pop, 0.5 oz	50	0	14
Chew-ets, Peanut Chews,		
Original (4), 1.6 oz	230	12	29
Chewz, 1 roll, 1 oz	120	1	28
Chick O Stick, 2 oz	240	9	42

Per Piece/Serving	C	F	Cb
Chunky Bar (*Nestlé*),		
King Size, 2.5 oz	340	19	44
Chupa Chups, 1 Pop	50	0	12
Cinn. Buttons (*Walgreens*), 3 pieces	60	0	16
Cinnamon Disks (*Walmart*), 3 pieces	70	0	18
Circus Peanuts (*Spangler*),		
6 pieces, 1.3 oz	165	0	41
CocoaVia, Orig., 0.8 oz	100	6	12
Coconut Stacks, (8)	320	16	46
Coffee Go, Candy, (4)	60	1	12
Conversation Hearts (*Necco*):		
Small (40), 1.4 oz	160	0	39
1 large	10	0	3
Cookie Dough Bites, 1.4 oz	200	10	27
Cote d'Or: Dark 86% Coca, 4 pcs	270	22	14
Dark, 70%, Orange, 3.5 oz	575	46	34
Dark, Raspberry, 3.5 oz	580	46	34
Milk, Intense, 3.5 oz	575	40	45
Cotton Candy, 1 oz	110	0	28
Cough Drops ~ *See Page 75*		
Cracker Jack, $^{1}/_{2}$ cup, 1 oz	120	2	23
Creme Savers:		
3 pieces, 0.5 oz	60	1	11
Sugar-Free, 3 pieces	30	1	8
Crisped Rice, Choc Chip, 1 bar, 1 oz	115	4	20
Crows, 11 pieces, 1.4 oz	130	0	33
Crunch Bar ~ *See Nestle*		
Dots, 11 dots, 1.4 oz	130	0	33
Double Dip Stick, 1 stick	15	0.5	3
Dove:		
Milk Choc: Singles Bar, 1.4 oz	220	13	24
Large Tablet Bar, 9 pcs, 1.5 oz	230	13	25
Choc. Cov. Almonds, 13 pcs, 1.4 oz	220	15	19
Promises: Milk Choc., 1 pce, 0.3 oz	45	2.5	5
w/ Caramel, 1 piece, 0.3 oz	40	2	5
w/ Peanut Butter, 1 pce, 0.3 oz	45	3	4
Swirls, all var., 9 pieces 1.5 oz	230	14	25
Dark Choc: Singles Bar, 1.3 oz	220	13	24
Large Tablet Bar, 9 pcs, 1.5 oz	220	14	25
Choc. Cov. Almds, 13 pcs, 1.4 oz	210	15	19
Promises, Almond, 1 piece, 0.3 oz	40	3	4
Swirls, Raspberry, 9 pcs, 1.4 oz	220	14	24
Sugar Free, all flav., 5 pcs, 1.4 oz	195	15	21
Dum Dum Pops (*Spangler*), 1 pop	25	0	7
Drops (*Hershey's*):		
Cookies 'n' Creme, 14 pieces, 1.5 oz	210	11	26
Milk Chocolate, 15 pieces, 1.4 oz	200	12	25

Candy ~ Brands & Generic (Cont)

Per Piece/Serving	C	F	Cb
English Toffee, 1 piece, 0.4 oz	70	4	6
5th Avenue: 2 oz bar	260	12	38
King Size, 3.5 oz	440	20	64
Fannie May:			
Mint Meltaway (1)	230	15	24
Pixie (1), 1.5 oz	210	12	24
Trinidad (1), 1.5 oz	200	12	23
Fast Break (Reese's): 2 oz bar	260	12	35
3.5 oz bar	460	22	62
Ferrero Rocher: 1 piece	75	5	5
3 pieces, 1.3 oz	220	16	16
Rondnoir, 3 pieces, 1 oz	180	13	14
Fifty 50 Snack Bars:			
Milk Chocolate:			
5 pieces, 1 oz	135	11	14
Almond, 5 pieces, 1 oz	135	12	14
Crunch Bar, 7 pcs, 1 oz	140	12	16
Dark Chocolate, 5 pieces, 1 oz	120	11	15
Note: Carb figures include 9-12g Sugar Alcohol			
Fluffy Stuff *(Charms),*			
Cotton Candy, 1.4 oz	150	0	40
Fondant: Choc-coated, 1.2 oz	125	3	27
Mint, 1 oz	105	0	25
Fran's: Gold Bar, Macadamia (1)	250	14	27
GoldBite, Almond (1)	120	7	13
Fruit Drops, (1), ¼ oz	20	0	4
Fruit Gems *(Sunkist),* (4), 1.4 oz	130	0	33
Fruit Leathers, average, 0.5 oz	50	0.5	12
Fruit Pastilles *(Rowntree),* 1 roll	185	0	45
Fruit Roll-Ups *(Betty Crocker/Sunkist),*			
1 roll, 0.5 oz	50	1	12
Fruit Runts *(Walgreens),*			
12 pieces	60	0	14
Fruit Flavored Shapes *(Betty Crocker),*			
all varieties, 0.8 oz	80	0	19
Fudge:			
Chocolate; Mint, 1 oz	130	8	14
P'nut Butter & Choc., 1 oz	130	8	13
Brevin's: Cashew, 1 oz	195	9	28
Triple Decker, 1 oz	165	7	25
Ghirardelli:			
3 oz Bars: Dark Choc., 4 squares	220	17	23
Filled, P'nut Butter, 4 squares	250	17	22
Intense Dark Bars,			
Ev'ng Dream, 3 pcs	190	15	20
Squares:			
Dark Choc., (4), 1.5 oz	210	16	23
Milk & Caramel (3), 1.5 oz	220	12	27
Sea Salt Escape (4), 1.5 oz	210	15	24

Per Piece/Serving	C	F	Cb
Godiva:			
Bars: Milk/Dark, av., 1.5 oz	230	14	26
Extra Dark: 75%, 1.5 oz	230	17	18
85%, 1.4 oz	260	21	14
Chocoiste: Dk Choc. Cherries (12)	190	7	30
Milk Chocolate Cashews (14)	230	15	19
Hearts: Dark Ganache (4)	200	12	23
Milk Praline (4)	220	13	23
Go Lightly:			
Assorted Toffee, 5 pieces, 1 oz	85	2	24
Fruit Chews, 5 pieces, 1 oz	95	2	26
Hard Candy, Assorted (4), 0.5 oz	45	0	15
Note: Carb figures include 15-25g sugar alcohol			
Goobers Peanuts, 1 package, 1.4 oz	200	13	21
Good & Plenty *(Hershey's),* (33), 1.4 oz	140	0	35
GooGoo Clusters, 1 piece, 1.8 oz	240	12	30
Gum ~ *See Page 75*			
Gum Drops: 1 small, 0.1 oz	15	0	3
5 pieces, 0.5 oz	75	0	15
Gummi *(Shur Fine):*			
Bears (15), 1.4 oz	130	0	29
Chewy Sweet Tarts (4)	160	0	36
Worms (9), 1.5 oz	140	0	31
Guylian:			
Bars: Dark Chocolate (3), 1 oz	150	12	11
Milk Choc. w/ Hazelnuts (3),1 oz	170	11	11
No Sugar Added Bars:			
Milk Chocolate, 3 squares	150	11	16
54% Cocoa, Dark Choc., 3 sqrs.	140	11	16
Seashells:			
Bar, 1.4 oz	210	13	21
Boxed, Originals (1), 0.4 oz	60	4	6
Truffles, (1), 0.4 oz	70	5.5	5
Heath: Original (1), 1.4 oz	210	13	24
King Size, 2.8 oz	410	22	49
Snack Size, 3 pieces, 1.5 oz	230	14	27
Hershey's:			
Cookie Layer Crunch, av., 1.4 oz	300	17	36
Cookies 'n' Creme, 1.55 oz Bar	230	12	26
Milk Chocolate:			
Bars: 1.55 oz	220	13	26
with Almonds, 1 bar, 1.4 oz	210	14	21
King Size, 1 Bar, 2.5 oz	370	22	44
Kisses, 9 pieces, av., 1.4 oz	200	12	25
Nuggets: 4 pieces, 1.4 oz	200	13	20
w/ Toffee & Alm., 4 pcs, 1.3 oz	200	13	21
Extra Dark Choc., 4 pcs, 1.4 oz	180	14	21
Simple Pleasures, 6 pcs, av.	180	8	29
Special Dark Choc., 1.5 oz bar	190	12	23
Sugar Free Choc., 5 pieces, 1.4 oz	160	13	24

Candy ~ Brands & Generic (Cont)

Per Piece/Serving

	C	**F**	**Cb**
Hershey's, (Cont):			
Pot of Gold Chocolate Asstd:			
Carmel, 4 pieces, 1.4 oz	**190**	10	26
Av. other var., 4 pieces, 1.4 oz	**210**	12	24
Candy-Coated Eggs:			
Milk Chocolate: (8) 1.2 oz	**170**	8	27
w/ Almonds (8) 1.2 oz	**200**	12	18
Honeycomb: Plain, 1 oz	**115**	0	27
Choc-coated, 2 pieces	**180**	7	31
Hot Tamales,			
20 pieces, 1.4 oz	**150**	0	36
Hugs ~ *See Kisses*			
Jawbreakers *(Sathers)*, (15), 0.6 oz	**60**	0	16
Jells *(Joyva)*, Raspb., 3 pieces, 1.6 oz	**160**	0	38
Jelly Beans, average all brands:			
Small Size (Jelly Belly): 1 bean	**5**	0	1
12 beans, 0.5 oz	**50**	0	13
Regular Size: 1 bean	**10**	0	2
10 beans, 1 oz	**105**	0	26
Large Size: 1 bean	**15**	0	38
10 beans, 1.5 oz	**150**	0	38
Sugar Free,			
average all brands, 25 beans, 1 oz	**60**	0	26
Note: Carb figure include 26g sugar alcohol			
Jelly Belly: 25 beans, 1 oz	**105**	0	26
3.5 oz package	**360**	0	90
Sugar Free,			
25 beans, 1 oz	**60**	0	26
Note: Carb figure include 26g sugar alcohol			
Chocolate Dips:			
All flavors: 1 bean	**4**	0	1
10 beans	**40**	1	8
2.8 oz bag	**300**	8	62
Jelly Rings *(Jewel)*, 5 pieces, 1.4 oz	**110**	0	26
Jolly Rancher:			
Bites: Soft, 15 pieces	**150**	1.5	32
Sours, 16 pieces	**130**	0	34
Crunch 'N Chew, 1 oz pkg	**160**	0.5	40
Filled Fruity Bites, 22 pieces	**140**	1	31
Gummies, 9 pieces	**120**	0	28
Hard Candy, 3 pieces	**70**	0	17
Jelly Beans/Sours, 1.4 oz	**140**	0	36
Lollipops (1), 0.55 oz	**60**	0	15
Jujubes, all varieties (52), 1.4 oz	**110**	0	28
Juju Bears, 5 pieces	**130**	0	34
Juju Mix (Sathers), 11 pieces, 1.5 oz	**150**	0	36
Jujyfruits, 16 pieces, 1.4 oz	**120**	0	32
Junior Caramels: 13 pieces, 1.5 oz	**190**	6	33
Mini, 2 boxes, 1 oz	**130**	4	23

Per Piece/Serving

	C	**F**	**Cb**
Junior Mints: 1.8 oz	**220**	4	45
16 pieces, 1.4 oz	**170**	3	35
Justin's, Peanut Butter Cups,			
Milk Choc, 2 cups, 1.4 oz pkg	**200**	14	18
Kinder Joy, 1 egg, 0.7 oz	**110**	6	12
Kisses *(Hershey's):*			
Milk Chocolate: (1), 0.16 oz	**25**	1.5	3
(9), 1.4oz	**200**	12	25
with Almonds (9), 1.4 oz	**200**	13	22
Caramel Filled (9), 1.5 oz	**190**	9	27
Air Delights (11), 1.4 oz	**200**	12	24
Cookies 'n' Creme (9), 1.5 oz	**220**	12	26
Hugs (9), 1.4 oz	**210**	12	24
Special Dark, (9), 1.4 oz	**180**	12	25
Kit Kat *(Nestle):*			
Halloween:			
Miniatures, 1.34 oz bar	**190**	12	22
Snack Size: Triple Choc. 1.48 oz	**200**	11	27
White Choc., 1.48 oz	**220**	11	27
Milk Chocolate: 4 pce bar, 1.5 oz	**210**	11	28
Extra Crispy, 1.6 oz bar	**220**	12	29
King Size, 8 pcs, 3 oz bar	**420**	22	56
Minis, 5 pieces	**210**	11	28
Snack Size, 6 pcs, 1.5 oz	**210**	11	27
White Chocolate, 4 pcs, 1.5 oz	**220**	12	26
Lemon Drops: (4), 0.6 oz	**60**	0	16
Walgreens, Sugar Free (3), 0.6 oz	**50**	0	17
Lemonhead, (26), 1.4 oz	**140**	0	36
Lance, Peanut Bar, 2.2 oz	**340**	19	29
Licorice:			
Average all varieties, 1oz	**100**	0	25
Chews *(Panda)*, (1)	**10**	0	3
Tid Bits (1)	**10**	0	2
Twists: Black/Red, av., 1 pc	**35**	0	8
Sugar Free, 1 piece	**15**	0	2.5
American Licorice Co.:			
Natural Vines: Black (9), 1.4 oz	**140**	1	33
Strawberry (9), 1.4 oz	**150**	1	34
Red Vines (4), 1.4 oz	**140**	0	34
Sip-n-Chew, 1 oz package	**100**	1	23
Snaps (31), 1.4 oz	**140**	0.5	33
Sour Punch (6), 1.4 oz	**150**	0.5	34
Super Ropes (1), 2 oz	**200**	0	46
Lifesavers: Large size, 1 candy	**15**	0	3
Regular: All flavors, 1 candy	**10**	0	3
1 Roll (14 candies), 1.2 oz	**140**	0	35
Creme Savers, 3 pcs, 0.5 oz	**60**	1	11
Pep-o-mint (3), 0.2 oz	**20**	0	5
Fruit Splosion (10), 1.4 oz	**130**	0	31
Sugar-Free, Pep-O-Mint (4), 0.5 oz	**35**	0	14
Note: Carb figure includes 14g sugar alcohol			

Candy ~ Brands & Generic (Cont)

Per Piece/Serving	C	F	Cb
Lik-m-aid *(Nestle)*, Fun Dip, 1 package	50	0	13
Lindt: Lindor Truffles (1), average	75	6	5
Swiss Milk Chocolate Bars:			
70% Cocoa, 4 pieces	220	17	13
Classic, with Hazelnuts, 10 pieces	230	16	20
Raspberry filled, 7 pieces	200	10	25
Dark Choc. Truffles,			
with filling, 7 pieces	240	18	18
Lollipops: Mini, 0.3 oz	25	0	6
Small, 0.5 oz	50	0	12
Medium, 1 oz	100	0	25
Giant (4" diam), 7 oz	790	0	198
M & M's:			
Dark Chocolate: 1.5 oz package	210	10	29
Peanuts, 1.5 oz	220	12	25
Halloween:	210	10	29
Mini, Whitet Candy Corn Choc., 1.5 oz	220	11	29
White Pumpkin Pie Candy, 1.5 oz	210	11	29
Milk Chocolate: 28 piece, 1 oz	145	6.5	21
1.5 oz package	210	9	30
1.7 oz package	240	10	34
Almond Choc., 1.5 oz	220	12	25
Minis, 1 tube, 1 oz	150	7	21
Peanut: 28 pieces, 1 oz	155	8	17
1.75 oz pkg	250	13	30
Peanut Butter, 1.6 oz pkg	240	14	26
Premiums: Chocolate Trio, 1.5 oz	230	14	25
Mint Thrills, 1.5 oz	240	14	25
Pretzels, 1/2 pkg, 1.4 oz	180	6	29
Snack Mix, av. 1/3 cup, 1.5 oz	200	9	25
Mamba Sours, Fruit Chews,			
6 pieces, 1 oz	100	1	22
Marshmallow Egg, 1 egg, 1 oz	120	3	22
Mary Jane *(Necco)*, 5 pieces, 1.4 oz	160	3.5	32
Marshmallows: Firm/Soft, 1 oz	90	0	23
Regular size, 4 pieces, 1 oz	100	0	24
Mini-Marshmallow, 2/3 cup, 1 oz	95	0	24
Joyva, Choc-coated Twists	95	2	10
Fluff, 2 Tbsp, 0.6 oz	60	0	15
Kraft: Creme, 0.5 oz	45	0	11
Funmallows, 2/3 cup, 1 oz	100	0	24
Jet-Puffed, 5 pieces, 1 oz	100	0	24
Mini, 1 oz	90	0	23
Marzipan, 2 Tbsp, 1.4 oz	160	4	29
Mauna Loa, Mountains, 4 pcs	230	17	21
Mexican Hats, (7), 1.4 oz	120	0	30
Mentos: Regular	10	0	3
Sugar Free	5	0	2
Mike & Ike:			
Original: 2.1 oz package	220	0	55
23 pieces, 1.4 oz	140	0	36
Milk Duds, 1 box, 1.8 oz	230	8	38

Per Piece/Serving	C	F	Cb
Milky Way *(Mars):*			
Bars: Single, 2 oz	240	9	37
Fun Size, 2 bars, 1.2 oz	160	6	24
To Go, 1.8 oz	230	9	36
Minis, 5 pieces, 1.5 oz	190	7	30
Midnight Bars: 1.8 oz	230	8	36
Minis, 5 pieces, 1.4 oz	190	7	30
Simply Caramel, 1.9 oz	250	11	37
Mints: Uncoated, 3 pieces	70	0	17
1 mint, medium	7	0	1
1 large mint	15	0	3
Mon Cheri *(Ferrero)*, 4 pieces, 2 oz	260	18	20
Mounds: 1.75 oz bar	240	13	28
King Size, 4 pieces, 3.5 oz	480	26	56
Snack Size, 1 piece, 0.6 oz	80	4.5	10
Mr Goodbar: 1.8 oz bar	250	17	26
King Size, 2.6 oz bar	380	26	38
Munch Bar, 1.4 oz	220	15	18
Necco, Candy Wafers (40), 2 oz	220	0	56
Nestle: Original, 1.6 oz bar	220	11	30
Fun Size, 3 bars, 1.4 oz	180	9	26
Miniatures, 4 bars, 1.4 oz	200	10	27
Buncha Crunch, 1/3 cup, 1.2 oz	180	9	25
Crunch Crisp, 1.8 oz	240	13	32
Newman's Own:			
Milk Choc.: Caramel Cups (3)	160	8	21
Peanut Butter Cups (3)	180	12	17
Dark Choc.: Caramel Cups (3)	160	9	20
Peanut Butter Cups (3)	180	13	16
Nips, all varieties, 2 pieces, 0.5 oz	60	2	11
Nougat: 3 pieces, 1.5 oz	170	1	39
Chocolate Covered, 1 oz	125	4	22
Nuggets ~ *See Hershey's*			
Nutrageous Bar *(Reese's)*, 1.8 oz	260	16	28
Oh Henry!: Fun Size, 0.9 oz	120	5	16
1.8 oz bar	230	11	33
Orange Slices:			
Jewel, 3 pieces, 1.5 oz	140	0	35
Walgreens, 4 pieces, 1.6 oz	160	0	39
Pastel Mints *(Walgreens)*, 20 pieces	60	0	14
PayDay Bar: 1.8 oz bar	240	13	27
King Size, 3.5 oz bar	440	24	50
Snack Size, 0.7 oz	90	5	10
Avalanche, 1.8 oz bar	250	13	29
Peanut Bar *(Planter's)*, 1.6 oz	240	14	21
Peanut Butter Cups ~ *See Reese's; Newman's Own*			
Peanut Brittle: 1 piece, 1.5 oz	190	5	32
Sugar Free *(Russell Stover)*,			
4 pieces, 1.3 oz	140	10	24

Candy ~ Brands & Generic (Cont)

Per Piece/Serving

	C	F	Cb
Peanuts, choc-covered, 14 pieces	230	14	23
Pearson's, Mint Patties, (5), 1.3 oz	150	2.5	31
Peppermints: 7 small, 0.5 oz	60	0	15
Brach's, Star Brites (3)	60	0	16
Pez, 1 roll	35	0	9
Planters,			
Double Peanut Bar, 1.6 oz	240	14	21
Pop Rocks, 0.4 oz package	35	0	9
Pot of Gold *(Hershey's):*			
Assortment: Caramel, 4 pieces	190	10	25
Nut, 4 pieces	210	13	23
Pretzels: Choc-covered, Mini (6)	200	9	25
White Chocolate Bites (23), 1.4 oz	200	9	25
Pretzel Flipz *(Nestlé)*, 8 pcs, 1 oz	130	5	20
Raisinets:			
Milk Choc: 1.58 oz pkg	190	8	32
Movie Pack, 3.5 oz	380	16	64
Dark Chocolate, 1/4 cup, 1.6 oz	180	8	32
Reese's:			
Clusters, 3 pieces, 1.5 oz	220	12	24
Crispy Crunchy Bar: 1.7 oz	260	18	22
2 pieces, 1.2 oz	170	10	19
King Size, 3 oz	480	32	40
Fast Break, 2 oz bar	260	12	35
P'nut Butter Chips, 0.5 oz	80	4	8
P'nut Butter Cups:			
Milk Choc: (2), 1.5 oz	210	13	24
Miniatures (5), 1.5 oz	220	13	26
Minis (11)	200	12	23
Big Cup (1), 1.4 oz	200	12	22
Sugar Free, Minis (5), 1.4 oz	180	13	27
Dark Chocolate (2), 1.5 oz	210	14	23
Pieces, Peanut Butter (51)	200	9	25
Sticks: 1.5 oz pkg	220	13	23
King Size, 3 oz pkg	440	26	46
Snack Size (1), 0.6 oz	90	5	9
Snacksters, 1 package, 0.8 oz	100	4	14
Whipps, 1.5 oz	230	9	37
Rice Krispies Treats *(Kellogg's)*,			
1 bar, average all varieties, 0.8 oz	95	2.5	17
Riesen, Choc. Chew, 4 pcs, 1.3 oz	170	6	28
Rocky Road, Milk/Dark, 1.8 oz bar	240	11	34
Roca Thins, 3 pieces, av. all var.	210	14	24
Rolo: Regular, all var., 1.7 oz roll	220	10	33
Mini Chews, Caramel in milk choc. (11)	190	9	26
Root Beer Barrels, (3), 0.6 oz	60	0	17

Per Piece/Serving

	C	F	Cb
Russell Stover Candy:			
Boxed Chocolates Choc. Coated:			
Assorted (2), 1.2 oz	150	7	22
Cherry Cordials (3), 0.4 oz	150	5	25
Dairy Crm Caramels (2), 1.2 oz	160	7	22
Elegant Collection (3), 1.6 oz	210	10	25
French Choc. Mints (4), 1.4 oz	220	13	22
Nut, Chewy & Crisp Centers (2)	160	8	21
Sugar Free:			
Ass'td Hard Candies (3), 1.6 oz	210	16	24
Bags: Caramel (3), 1.3 oz	180	8	25
Coconut (3), 1.5 oz	160	10	28
Mint Patty (3), 1.5 oz	180	12	26
Peanut Butter Cups (2), 1.2 oz	160	12	17
Pecan Delight (2), 1.2 oz	160	12	19
Note: Carbohydrate figures include sugar alcohol			
Salt Water Taffy *(Brach's)*, (5)	170	2.5	36
Seashells *(Guylian)*, (4), 1.6 oz	260	17	24
See's Candies:			
Almond Royal (5)	190	13	18
Butterscotch Chews (5)	210	12	27
Krispy's: Caffe Latte (5)	180	8	27
Mint (5)	170	8	27
Little Pops:			
Butterscotch (4), 0.5 oz	60	2	12
Av. other flavors (4)	55	3	10
Lollypops, average, 0.7 oz	90	3	17
Milk Molasses Chips (6), 1.4 oz	180	8	27
Milk Peppermints, 2 pieces, 1.3 oz	150	4	28
Peanut Brittle Bar, 1 oz	150	10	15
Peanut Butter Patties (2), 1.2 oz	170	16	16
Peppermint Twists (3)	60	0	15
Toffee-ettes, 3 pieces	270	21	18
Sugar Free:			
Dark Bar, 1.5 oz	180	16	24
Dark Walnut Clusters (4), 1.5 oz	230	21	17
Peanut Brittle, 1.5 oz	170	14	17
Note: Carbohydrate figures include 12-18 g sugar alcohol			
Skinny Cow:			
Dreamy Clusters, all var., 1 pouch	120	6	20
Heavenly Crips, all varieties, 1 bar	110	6	14
Skittles: Original, 2 oz	230	2.5	52
Sour, 1.8 oz	200	2	44
Tropical; Wild Berry, 2.2 oz	250	2.5	56
Fun Size, 1 bag, 0.5 oz	60	1	14
Tear & Share, 4 oz bag	420	4.5	93
Skor, Toffee Bar (1), 1.4 oz	200	12	25
Smarties: Candy Rolls (1), 0.3 oz	25	0	6
Giant, 1 roll, 1 oz	100	0	25

Candy ~ Brands & Generic (Cont)

Per Piece/Serving

	C	F	Cb
Snickers:			
Milk Chocolate:			
1.9 oz bar	250	12	33
Fun Size, 2 bars, 1.2 oz	160	8	21
To Go Bar, 1.6 oz	220	10	29
Almond Bar, 1.8 oz	230	11	32
P'nut Butter Squared, 2 bars, 1.8 oz	250	13	30
Miniatures: (4)	170	8	22
Sugar Free, 5 pcs	180	13	27
Dark Chocolate Bar, 1.8 oz	250	12	31
Sno Caps, 1/4 cup, 1.4 oz	180	8	30
Soft 'N Chewy, Butter Toffee, 1 piece	30	0.5	5
Sorbee, Crystal Light Hard Candy, 4 pieces	25	0	13
Note: Carb figure includes Isomalt which has fewer calories than sugar.			
Sour Patch: Kids, average, 2 oz	210	0	52
Extreme, 1.8 oz	190	0	47
Spearmint Leaves:			
Jewel, 5 pieces, 1.4 oz	140	0	35
Walgreens, 4 pieces, 1.6 oz	160	0	39
Spree Candies: Original, 15 pieces	50	0	13
Chewy, 8 pieces	60	0	13
Starburst:			
Candy Canes, 0.5 oz	70	0	18
Fruit Chews: Original (1)	20	0.5	4
8 pieces, 1.4 oz	160	3.5	33
Gummibursts, 9 pieces, 1.4 oz	130	0	31
Jellybeans, 1.4 oz	150	0	37
Starlight Mints, 3 pieces, 0.5 oz	60	0	15
Suckers *(Walgreens)*, 1 piece, 0.4 oz	45	0	11
Sugar Babies, Original, 1.4 oz	160	1.5	37
Sugar Coated Peanuts, 1 oz	120	8	10
Sunbursts Sunflowers *(Kimmie)*:			
ChocoRocks Milk, 3.5 oz	525	25	67
Habanero Corn, 3.5 oz	500	23	70
Sunburst Mix, Milk, 3.5 oz	500	28	55
Swedish Fish, 7 pieces, 1.5 oz	150	0	38
SweeTARTS:			
Orig., 8 pieces, 0.5 oz	50	0	13
Mini Chewy, 23 pieces, 0.5 oz	50	0.5	12
Symphony *(Hershey's)*:			
Milk Choc: 1.5 oz bar	220	14	23
Large Block: 5 pieces, 1.4 oz	200	12	22
w/ Alm. & Toffee, 5 pcs, 1.3 oz	200	13	21

Per Piece/Serving

	C	F	Cb
Taffy,			
Fruit Chews, 1 piece	20	0.5	4
Take 5 *(Hershey's)*: Orig., 1.5oz	200	11	25
King Size, 2.3 oz	300	16	37
Snack Size, 2 pcs, 1 oz	150	8	19
3 Musketeers:			
Original, 1.9 oz	240	7	42
2 To Go, 1 bar, 1.6 oz	200	6	35
Fun Size, 3 bars, 1.6 oz	190	6	34
Minis, 7 pieces, 1.4 oz	170	5	32
Tang-a-Roos, 1 roll	25	0	6
Terry's: Chocolate Orange (5), 1.5 oz	230	12	27
Dark Chocolate Orange (5), 1.5 oz	240	13	28
Tic Tac, all flavors, 1 piece	2	0	0
Toblerone: 1.3 oz bar	190	10	22
1.8 oz bar	270	15	31
3.5 oz bar	540	30	63
5.3 oz Package, 5 pieces, 1.5 oz	230	13	27
Toffees, Regular, 1 oz	160	9	18
Tootsie Pops, (1), 0.6 oz	60	0	15
Tootsie Roll: 2.3 oz roll	245	2	55
Midgees, 1.4 oz	140	3	28
Truffles: Reg., 1 piece, 0.4 oz	60	4	6
Large *(Godiva)*, 0.8 oz	110	6.5	12
Extra Large *(J.Schmidt)*, 1.5 oz	220	13	24
Turtles: Original, 1 piece, 0.6 oz	85	5	10
Sugar Free, 1 piece, 0.4 oz	50	3.5	7
Twists, Licorice; Strawb., sugar free, 7 pieces, 1.4 oz	90	0	25
Twix:			
Caramel: 2 cookies, 1.8 oz	250	12	34
Fun Size, 2 cookies, 1.7 oz	250	14	27
4 To Go, 1 cookie, 0.8 oz	110	5	15
6 To Go, 1 cookie, 0.5 oz	80	4	11
Minis, 3 pieces, 1 oz	150	7	20
Peanut Butter:			
Single, 2 cookies, 1.7 oz	250	14	27
4 to Go, 1 cookie, 0.8 oz	250	12	34
Twizzlers: Cherry Bites (17), 1.4 oz	140	0.5	32
Cherry Nibs, 29 pieces, 1.4 oz	140	1	32
Pull 'n' Peel, Cherry, 1 piece, 1.2 oz	110	0.5	26
Twists, Strawb., 1.3 oz	120	0.5	29
U-No Bar, 1.5 oz	250	17	22
Weight Watchers *(Whitman's)*:			
Caramel Medallions (3)	160	9	24
Coconut (3)	150	9	23
English Toffee Squares (3)	150	9	21
Mint Patties (3)	150	9	23
Peanut Butter Cups (4)	180	8	31
Pecan Crowns (3)	160	10	24

Candy ~ Brands & Generic (Cont)

Per Piece/Serving	C	F	Cb
Werther's:			
Hard Candy: Original (3), 0.5 oz	70	1.5	14
Sugar-Free Original (5)	40	1.5	15
Note: Carb figure includes 14g sugar alcohol			
Soft, Chocolate Caramel (4), 1.4 oz	190	8	28
Whatchamacallit: 1.5 oz Bar	230	12	28
King Size Bar, 2.5 oz	370	20	45
Whitman's, Boxed Chocolates:			
Sampler (4), 1.6 oz	220	12	27
12 oz Box, 3 pieces, 1.2 oz	170	9	21
Reserve, 7 oz Box, 2 pieces, 1.2 oz	160	9	21
Sugar Free, 10 oz Box, 3 pcs, 1.5 oz	190	13	25
Whoppers, av. all varieties, 18 pcs	190	7	31
Wonka:			
Bar (1), 2.5 oz	360	19	49
Exceptional Bars, average, 4 pieces	200	13	23
Gobstopper, 9 pieces, 0.5 oz	60	0	14
Laffy Taffy: Ropes, all var., 0.8 oz	80	1.5	18
Stretchy & Tangy, all var., 1.5 oz	150	3.5	29
Nerds, Giant, Chewy, 1.8 oz package	180	0	42
Yogurt Candy,			
Coated Raisins, 27 pieces, 1.4 oz	180	8	28
York: Mints, (3)	10	0	3
Peppermint Pattie, reg, 1.4 oz	140	2.5	31
Pieces (50)	170	8	28
Zagnut, 1.75 oz bar	220	9	35
Zero Bar: 1.8 oz bar	230	8	37
King Size, 3.5 oz	400	14	68

Gum

Per Piece	C	F	Cb
Bazooka	15	0	4
Beechies	6	0	2
Big League Chews	10	0	2
Bubble Yum: Original	25	0	6
Sugarless	10	0	3
Candilicious	30	0	2
Carefree, Sugarless/Regular	5	0	2
Chiclet	5	0	1
Dentyne	5	0	0.5
Double Bubble Ball	20	0	5
Estee, Bubble/Regular	5	0	2
Extra (Wrigley's), Sugar-Free	5	0	2
Freshen-Up	10	0	3
Hubba Bubba: Regular	25	0	6
Sugar-free, average	14	0	0.5
Ice Breakers	5	0	2
Jolt Gum	5	0	2
Super Bubble	15	0	4
Trident, Orig.; White	5	0	1
Wrigley's, all flavors	10	0	2

Carob Candy

	C	F	Cb

Per Piece/Serving	C	F	Cb
Carob, Plain/Natural, 1 oz	155	9	15
Carob Coated: Raisins, 1 oz	130	8	15
Almonds/Peanuts, 1 oz	150	10	14
Caramels, 1 oz	110	4	18
Dates, 1 oz	125	5	20
Malt Balls, 1 oz	135	8	15
Soybeans	145	9	16
Trail/Party Mix, 1 oz	150	9	15

Cough Drops

	C	F	Cb

Per Drop/Piece	C	F	Cb
Beech Nut, 1 drop	10	0	2
CVS, Honey Lemon Cough Drops	15	0	4
Diabetic Tussin	0	0	0
Halls, Defense Vitamin C: Regular	15	0	4
Sugar Free	5	0	3
Fruit Breezers	15	0	4
Menthol Drops: Regular	15	0	4
Sugar Free	5	0	2
Plus	20	0	5
Listerine (Amer. Chicle), Lozenge	10	0	2
Luden's, Throat Drops: Reg., all var.	10	0	2
Sugar Free	0	0	0
Pine Bros, Cough Drops	10	0	2
Ricola, Cough Drops:			
Natural Herbs	10	0	3
Sugar-Free Lemon Mint	0	0	1
Rolaids, Sodium Free	5	0	1
Sathers, Peppermint Lozenges	15	0	3
Sucrets (Beecham), Lozenges	10	0	2.5
Wintergreen, Lozenges	15	0	3

Eat at least 5 servings of fruit and vegetables every day . . . and Enjoy Better Health!

C Cheese

Quick Guide   C   F   Cb

Firm/Hard Cheeses
American, Cheddar, Jack, Swiss:
Average All Brands
Regular Cheese:

	C	F	Cb
Thin Deli slice, 0.8 oz	80	6	0.5
1 oz slice/piece	110	9	0.5
8 oz package	880	72	3
Cubes: 1" cube, 0.6 oz	70	5.5	0.5
1¼" cube, 1 oz	115	9	0.5
Diced, 1 cup, 4.5 oz	510	41	3
Melted, ¼ cup, 2 oz	245	20	1
Shredded: ¼ cup, 1 oz	110	9	0.5
1 cup, 4 oz	440	36	2

Cheese & Cheese Products

Per 1 oz Unless Indicated

	C	F	Cb
Almond *(Lisanatti)*, Chunks, average	50	1	3
American:			
Regular: 1 slice, 1 oz	105	9	0.5
Kraft, Regular, 0.67 oz slice	60	4	1
Land O'Lakes, 0.67 oz slice	70	4	2
Reduced Fat:			
Alpine Lace, Yellow/White, 1 oz	90	6	2
Borden 2%, 1 slice, 0.8 oz	50	3	2
Kraft, 2% Milk, 0.67 oz	45	2.5	1
Land O Lakes,			
2% Milk, 1 oz	90	6	2
Babybel *(Laughing Cow)*, Mini:			
Original (1), 0.75 oz	70	6	0
Light (1), 0.75 oz	50	3	0
Light Original (1), 0.75 oz	50	3	0
Gouda (1), 0.75 oz	70	6	0
Mozzarella (1), 0.75 oz	50	3.5	0
Blue/Bleu: *Average all Brands*			
Crumbled, ¼ cup, 1 oz	100	8	0
Light, 0.8 oz	35	1.5	2
Brie: Average, 1 oz	95	8	0
Alouette, 1 oz	100	9	1
Camembert, 1 oz	85	7	0
Caraway, 1 oz	105	8	1
Castello, 1 oz	120	12	0
Cheddar:			
Regular: Medium/Sharp, av., 1 oz	110	9	1
Shredded, ¼ cup, 1 oz	110	9	1
Cracker Barrel: Extra Sharp, 1 oz	110	10	0
Vermont Sharp White, 1 oz	110	10	0

Cheese & Cheese Products (Cont)

Per 1 oz Unless Indicated   C   F   Cb

	C	F	Cb
Cheddar (Cont):			
Reduced Fat, 2% Milk,			
Kraft, Shredded, 1 oz	90	6	1
Curds, Cheddar Cheese,			
Cheese Curds ~ *See Cottage Cheese*			
Cheese Logs *(Kaukauna)*, average	100	7	4
Cheez Whiz ~ *See Dips*			
Cheshire, 1 oz	110	9	1.5
Colby, Regular, 1 oz	110	8	0
Colby-Jack:			
Big Slice, 0.8 oz	90	7	0
Cottage Cheese (Curds): *Average All Brands*			
Creamed (4% milk fat):			
2 Tbsp, 1 oz	30	1	1.5
½ cup, 4 oz	110	5	4
with fruit, ½ cup, 4 oz	115	4	5
Reduced-Fat (2%): 2 Tbsp, 1 oz	25	0.5	1
½ cup, 4 oz	100	3	4
Low-Fat (1%): 2 Tbsp, 1 oz	20	0.5	1
½ cup, 4 oz	80	1	3
Fat-Free/Non-Fat: 2 T., 1 oz	20	0	1
½ cup, 4 oz	80	0	5
Cottage Cheese (Curds): *Brands*			
Fiber One, 1% Fat, ½ c., 4 oz	80	2	8
Friendship:			
1% Low-Fat with Pineapple, 5 oz	150	1.5	22
Nonfat with Pineapple, ½ cup, 4 oz	110	0	18
Pot Style, 2%, ½ cup, 4 oz	100	2.5	4
Hood, Low Fat, 4 oz	90	1.5	5
Knudsen/Breakstone's:			
Free, Non-Fat, ½ cup, 4.25 oz	80	0	7
2% Milk Fat, ½ cup, 4 oz	90	2.5	6
On the Go!,			
Low-Fat, 4 oz carton	90	2.5	7
Lactaid, 1% Low-Fat, ½ cup, 4 oz	80	1	7
Light n' Lively:			
Fat-Free, ½ cup, 4.4 oz	80	0	8
Low-Fat, ½ cup, 4.4 oz	80	1.5	6
Breaded & Fried:			
A&W, 5 oz	570	40	27
Culver's, Wisconsin, 5.3 oz	510	25	51

Cheese & Cheese Products (Cont)

Per 1 oz Unless Indicated — **C** **F** **Cb**

	C	F	Cb
Cream Cheese: *Average All Brands*			
Regular/Soft:			
2 Tbsp, 1 oz	95	10	1
3 oz package	290	29	3.5
8 oz package	780	78	9
Light, Plain, 1 oz	60	4.5	2.5
Fat-Free, Plain, 1 oz	30	0	2
Better Than Cream Cheese (Tofutti),			
all varieties, 1 oz	85	5	9
Easy Cheese (Kraft),			
American, 2 Tbsp, 1.2 oz	80	6	1
Edam, 1 oz	100	8	0.5
Farmer, Low-Fat, 1 oz	40	2.5	0
Feta: Regular, 1 oz	75	6	1
Crumbled, ¹/₂ cup, 2.5 oz	190	15	3
Athenos, Reduced-Fat,			
1 oz	50	3	1
Fontina, 2 Tbsp, 1 oz	110	9	0.5
Galaxy, Cheese Substitute:			
Grated Parmesan Flavor, 2 tsp, 0.2 oz	15	0.5	0
Slices: Mozzarella, 1 slice, 0.6 oz	40	3	0.5
Cheddar, 1 slice, 0.67 oz	35	2	5
Goat's Milk Cheese:			
Chevre: Original, 2 Tbsp	75	6	0.5
Semi-Soft, 1 oz	100	8.5	1
Hard, 1 oz	130	10	0.5
Chavrie, Logs:			
Original, 2 Tbsp, 1 oz	80	7	1
Sundried Tomato & Garlic, 1 oz	80	6	2
Pyramid, Original, 1 oz	50	3.5	1
Gjetost, fresh, 1 oz	130	8	12
Myzithra, grated, 1 oz	80	4	2
Gorgonzola, 1 oz	100	8	0.5
Galbani, Dolcelatte, 1 oz	95	8	1
Gouda, 1 oz slice	100	8	0.5
Gruyere, 1 oz	115	9	1
Handi-Snacks *(Kraft):*			
Breadsticks 'n Cheez Single, 1 oz	110	4.5	14
Ritz Crackers 'n Cheez Dip, 1 oz	100	6	11
Havarti *(Land O'Lakes),* 0.7 oz	80	6	1
Jarlsberg: Average, 1 oz	100	8	0
Reduced Fat, shredded, 1 oz	70	3.5	0
Labneh, (Lebanese Cream Chse), 1.8 oz	70	4	4

Cheese & Cheese Products (Cont)

Per 1 oz Unless Indicated — **C** **F** **Cb**

	C	F	Cb
Laughing Cow, Wedges:			
Creamy Asiago (1)	35	1.5	1
Swiss: Original Creamy (1)	50	4	1
Light Swiss (1)	35	1.5	1
Lifetime, Cholesterol Reducing,			
Low Fat, all varieties, 1 Slice, 1 oz	45	1.5	1
Limburger, 1 oz	95	8	0
Mascarpone, av., 1 oz	125	13	0.5
Mexican:			
Cacique: Asadero, sliced	70	5	1
Cotija	100	8	0
Enchilado; Manchego	90	7	0
Panela	80	7	0
Queso Fresco	80	6	0
Queso Quesadilla	90	7	0
Ranchero	80	6	0
Chi-Chi's, Salsa Con Quéso, Mild	45	3	4
El Mexicano: Asadero, Regular	90	7	0
Cotija, grated, 2 Tbsp	40	3	0
Kraft, Mexican Four Cheese; Taco,			
Shredded,	100	8	0
Sargento, 4 Cheese Mexican	110	9	2
Supremo, Quéso Chihuahua, 1 oz	100	8	0
Verole, Quéso Oaxaca, 1 oz	70	8	0
Monterey Jack:			
Regular, shredded, 1 oz	100	8	1
Land O Lakes, Co-Jack, 1 oz	110	9	0
Kraft, 1" cube, 1 oz	100	9	0
Mozzarella:			
Whole Milk: Average 1 oz	85	6.5	0.5
Land O'Lakes/Polly-O:			
Slice, average, 1 oz	80	6	1
String, 1 oz	90	6	1
Fat-Free,			
Kraft, Shredded, 1 oz	45	0	2
Reduced Fat,			
Kraft, 2% Milk Fat	70	5	1
Part Skim:			
Borden/Kraft, Shredded	80	5	2
Kraft, String	80	6	0
Polly-O, Shredded, 1 oz	80	5	0
Muenster:			
Regular, 1 oz	105	9	0.5
Low-Fat, 1 oz	85	5	1

Cheese & Cheese Products (Cont)

Per 1 oz Unless Indicated

	C	F	Cb
Parmesan:			
Fresh/Block, Dry, 1 oz	110	7.5	1
Grated (Packaged): 2 tsp	20	1.5	0
1 oz	120	8	1
1/2 cup, 1.8 oz	215	14	2
Kraft, Reduced-Fat Topping, 1 Tbsp	20	1	2
Philadelphia:			
Cream Cheese: Original, 2 T. 1 oz	80	7	2
3 oz package	240	21	6
Flavored:			
Blueberry, 1.16 oz	80	4.5	7
Chive & Onion, 1.1 oz	80	7	2
Pinapple, 1 oz	70	4.5	5
Salmon, 1.1 oz	70	5	2
Strawberry, 1.1 oz	80	6	5
1/3 Less Fat: Plain, 2 T., 1 oz	70	5	3
Neufchatel, 2 T., 1 oz	70	6	1
Fat-Free, Plain, 1 oz	30	0	3
Cheesecake Filling, 3 oz	240	17	6
Milk/White Chocolate:			
2 Tbsp, 1.27 oz	110	6	12
Dark Chocolate, 2 T., 1.23 oz	100	5	12
Whipped:			
Original, 0.8 oz	50	4.5	2
Mixed Berry, 0.7 oz	50	3.5	5
Pizza Four Cheese, shredded,			
Kraft/Sargento, Regular, av., 1 oz	90	7	1
Port de Salut, 1 oz	100	8	0
Port Wine *(Kaukauna/WisPride):*			
10 oz Ball, 1 oz	100	6	4
10 oz Log, 2 Tbsp, 1 oz	100	7	4
11.3 oz Tub, 0.85 oz	80	6	3
Provolone: Regular, 1 oz	100	7.5	0.5
Alpine Lace, Reduced-Fat, 1 oz	80	6	1
Sargento, 1 slice, 0.67 oz	70	5	0
Pub *(President)*, average all varieties	75	7	1
Quark: 40% fat	45	3	1
20% fat	30	1.5	1
Skim/Non-Fat	20	0	1.5
Rice Cheese Chunks *(Lisanatti),*			
average, 1 oz	60	3	2

Cheese & Cheese Products (Cont)

Per 1 oz Unless Indicated

	C	F	Cb
Ricotta Cheese:			
Whole Milk: 1 oz	50	3.5	1
1/2 cup, 4.5 oz	215	16	4
Part Skim: 1 oz	40	2	1.5
1/2 cup, 4.5 oz	170	10	6
Light/Low-Fat: 1 oz	25	1	1.5
1/2 cup, 4.5 oz	125	5	6
Fat-Free, 1/2 cup, 4.5 oz	100	0	10
Baked Ricotta, 2 oz	130	9	3
Romano: Block/Loaf	110	8	1
Grated: 1 oz	120	9	1
1 Tbsp, 0.2 oz	20	1.5	0
Roquefort, 1 oz	105	9	0.5
Sheep's Milk, (Manchego),			
Trader Joes/Wegman's, 1 oz	120	10	1
Soy Cheese:			
Trader Joe's, Cheddar flavor, 0.7 oz	45	2	3
Soy Kaas: Cheddar, 1 oz	50	2	8
Monterey Jack, 1 oz	60	4	0
Soy Sation, Chunks,			
all varieties, 1 oz	60	3	2
Smoked Cheddar, average, 1 oz	110	10	0
Stilton, average, 1 oz	110	10	0
String:			
Regular, average all brands	80	6	0.5
Kraft, Twist-Ums & String-ums,			
Super Long, 1 stick, 1.1 oz	90	6	1
Light/Lite:			
Frigo, String (1), 0.85 oz	50	2.5	0.5
Polly-O, String,			
2% Red-Fat, 1 oz	70	4.5	0
Sargento: 1 piece, 1 oz	80	6	1
Light, , 0.75 oz	50	2.5	1
Swiss: Regular, 1 oz	110	8	1.5
Alpine Lace, Reduced-Fat, 1 oz	90	6	1
Kraft Singles, 2% Milk, 0.75 oz	60	4.5	1
Tilsit, 1 oz	100	7.5	0.5
Tofutti, Better Than Cream Cheese,			
all flavors, 2 Tbsp	60	5	2
Tybo, 1 oz	100	7	0.5
Velveeta *(Kraft):*			
Original, 1 oz	80	5	3
Reduced Fat, 2% Milk, 1 oz	60	3	4
Mexican, 1 oz	60	4	3
Queso Blanco, Mild, 1 oz	70	4	3

Dips/Spreads | C | F | Cb

Per 2 Tbsp, 1 oz, Unless Indicated

Average All Brands

	C	F	Cb
Avocado/Guacamole	45	4	2
Baba Ghanoush (Eggplant/Sesame)	70	6	2
Cheese Fondue, 1/2 cup, 4 oz	260	15	4
French Onion Dip	60	4.5	3
Hummus: 2 Tbsp	50	1	5
1/2 cup, 4.5 oz	220	4.5	23
Tzatziki (Cucumber/Yogurt)	30	2.5	2
Clearman's, Original Spread	150	16	0
De La Casa, 5 Layer Party Dip	45	2.5	4
Fritolay, French Onion Dip, 2 Tbsp	60	5	3

Fritos: *Per 2 Tbsp*

Dips:

	C	F	Cb
Bean; Hot Bean w/ Jalapeno	35	1	5
Jalapeno Cheddar Cheese	40	2.5	3
Mild Cheddar	40	3	3

Guiltless Gourmet,

	C	F	Cb
Black Bean/Spicy Black Bean Dip	40	0	7

Heluva Good Cheese,

	C	F	Cb
French Onion Dip, 2 Tbsp	50	4.5	2

Kaukauna *(Wisconsin)*:

Spreadable Cheddar,

	C	F	Cb
Sharp/Smokey Cheddar	80	6	3

Kemps: *Per 2 Tbsp*

	C	F	Cb
Dips: French Onion	60	5	2
Ranch Style	60	5	2

Top The Tater,

	C	F	Cb
Taco Fiesta; Veggie Ranch, av.	60	5	3
Kroger, Dips, all varieties	60	5	2

Kraft: *Per 2 Tbsp*

	C	F	Cb
Dips: Average all varieties	60	5	3
Cheez Whiz: Orig., 1.2 oz	90	7	4
Light	80	3.5	6

Salsa Con Queso ~ See Velveeeta

	C	F	Cb
Spreads: Olive & Pimento, 1.1 oz	80	6	3
Old English Sharp; Roka Blue, av	88	7	3

Marzetti: *Per 2 Tbsp*

	C	F	Cb
Dips: Chocolate Fruit, 2 Tbsp	110	1	25
Old Fashioned Caramel, 1.25 oz	130	4	22
Veggie: Dill, Light, 1.1 oz	60	5	4
Ranch, 1 oz	110	12	2
Light Ranch, 1.1 oz	60	5	4

Dips/Spreads (Cont) | C | F | Cb

Per 2 Tbsp, 1 oz, Unless Indicated

Marie's:

	C	F	Cb
Dips: Buttermilk Ranch; Crmy Dill. av.	100	10	2
Guacamole	40	3	3

Naturally Fresh: *Per 2 Tbsp*

	C	F	Cb
Dips: Chocolate, 1.3 oz	90	0	23
Crm Cheese Strawb., 1 oz	90	3	15
Caramel, 1 oz	100	4	16

Old Dutch:

	C	F	Cb
Dips: French Onion, 1 oz	50	3	5
Mild Cheddar, 1 oz	40	3	2
Nacho Cheese, 1 oz	35	2.5	2

Old El Paso: *Per 2 Tbsp*

	C	F	Cb
Dips: Cheese & Salsa, 1.2 oz	40	3	3
Thick N' Chunky Salsa	10	0	2

Price's: *Per 2 Tbsp*

	C	F	Cb
Dips: Pimiento Cheese	90	7	4
Light Pimiento	50	3	3

Stop & Shop: *Per 2 Tbsp*

	C	F	Cb
Dips: Veggie	100	10	3
Sour Cream French Onion	60	4.5	2

TGI Fridays,

	C	F	Cb
Spinach, Cheese & Artichoke Dip, 1 oz	30	2	2
Toby's, Original Tofu Spread, 2 Tbsp	80	8	2

Tostitos:

	C	F	Cb
Dips: Chunky Salsa, 2 Tbsp	10	0	2
Creamy Spinach, 2 Tbsp	50	4	2
Salsa Con Queso, 2 Tbsp	40	2.5	5

Wise: *Per 2 Tbsp*

	C	F	Cb
Dips: French Onion	60	5	3
Salsa con Queso	45	3	3

*New Diet Aid
- The Refrigerator Air Bag!*

POOF!

Condiments, Sauces C F Cb

Average of Brands & Homemade

Apple Sauce:

	C	F	Cb
Sweetened, ¼ cup, 2.5 oz	55	0	13
Unsweetened, ¼ cup, 2 oz	25	0	7
Barbecue Sauce:			
Regular, av. all flavors, 2 Tbsp, 1 oz	40	0	10
Bull's Eye, Original, 1 oz	60	0	14
Bearnaise Sauce, ¼ cup, 2.5 oz	190	19	5
Buffalo Wing Sce: Hon. Mustard, 1 T.	40	3	3
Average other varieties, 1 Tbsp	25	2	2
Cheese, h/made, ¼ cup, 2.5 oz	150	10	12
Chef-Mate, Hot Dog, ¼ cup	70	2.5	9
Chili Sauce *(Heinz),* 1 Tbsp	20	0	5
Cocktail Sauce: ¼ cup	110	0	15
Walden Farms, Fat-Free, 1 Tbsp	0	0	0
Cranberry Sauce, av. all varieties: 2 T.	45	0	11
¼ cup, 2.5 oz	110	0	27
Demi Glaze Gold, 2 tsp	30	0.5	3
Honey Mustard *(French's),* 2 Tbsp	60	0.5	12
Horseradish: 1 tsp	2	0	0
Kraft, 1 tsp	15	1.5	1
Ketchup: Regular, 1 Tbsp	15	0	4
Heinz: Reduced Sugar, 1 Tbsp	5	0	1
Simply Heinz, 1 Tbsp	15	0	4
Mole:			
Dona Maria, av. all varieties., 2 T.	150	10	10
Rogelio Bueno, 2 Tbsp, 1 oz	160	11	12
Mushroom Sce, ½ cup, 2 oz	50	2	5
Mustard, average, 1 tsp	5	0	0.5
Pesto Sauce, ¼ cup, 2 oz	270	28	2
Pizza Sauce, ¼ cup, 2 oz	30	0	6
Seafood Cocktail Sce, ¼ cup	60	0	15
Soy Sauce: Average all, 1 Tbsp	10	0	1
Kikkoman, Lite Soy, 1 Tbsp	10	0	1
Spaghetti Sce, ½ cup, 4.5 oz	135	6	19
Steak Sauce:			
Kraft, A1, 1 Tbsp, 0.5 oz	15	0	3
Lea & Perrins, 1 Tbsp, 0.5 oz	20	0	5
Strawb. Puree Sauce, Unsweet., 2 T.	10	0	2
Sweet & Sour Sauce:			
Contadina, 1.2 oz	40	1	8
Kraft, 1 Tbsp	60	0	13
Tabasco Sauce, 1 tsp	2	0	0
Taco Sauce, average all, 2 Tbsp, 1 oz	10	0	1
Tartar Sauce: *(Heinz),* 2 Tbsp, 1 oz	120	11	4
Hellmann's, Regular, 2 Tbsp, 1 oz	80	7	4
McCormick, Fat-Free, 2 Tbsp, 1 oz	30	0	7
Teriyaki Sauce *(Kikkoman),* 1 T., 0.5 oz	15	0	2
Vinegar, White or Wine, 2 T.	4	0	1
White Sauce, ½ cup, 5 oz	130	7	10
Worcestershire Sauce, 1 tsp	5	0	1

Pickles & Relish C F Cb

Average All Brands

	C	F	Cb
Bread & Butter Pickles, 4 sl.,1 oz	25	0	6
Chutney, 2 Tbsp, 1.25 oz	50	0.5	11
Dill Pickles:			
Slices, 4 slices, 1 oz	4	0	1
1 large, (3¾"x 1¼" diam.), 2.25 oz	12	0	3
Extra large (4"x 1¾" diam.), 5 oz	30	0	6
Halves: Small, 1 oz	3	0	0.5
Large, 2.5 oz	8	0	2
Gherkins, sweet, 1 medium, 1 oz	30	0	7
Green Chiles, chopped, 2 Tbsp	5	0	1
Horseradish, 1 Tbsp	10	0	2
Jalapenos, pickled (2), 2 oz	10	0.5	2
Jalapeno Relish, 1 Tbsp, 0.5 oz	5	0	1
Mustard, av. all brands, 1 tsp	5	0	0.5
Peppers, Hot/Mild (1), 1.5 oz	20	0	4
Pickled: Beets, ½ cup, 4 oz	75	0	19
Cocktail Onion, 1 onion	2	0	0
Red Cabbage, ½ cup, 3 oz	65	0	15
Pickles: Sweet, 2 Tbsp, 1 oz	35	0	8
Large (3"x ¾ diam.),1.25 oz	40	0	10
Pickle in a Pouch, 1 large	12	0	3
Relishes:			
Cranberry-Orange, 1 Tbsp	30	0	7
Hot Dog *(Heinz),* 1 T., 0.5 oz	17	0	3
S'wich Spread, 1 tsp	20	1	5
Sweet Pickle, 1 Tbsp, 0.5 oz	20	0	5
Sweet Cauliflower, 1 oz	35	0	8
Sugar Free Relish, 1 tsp	5	0	1
Sweet Gherkins (2), 1 oz	5	0	1
Sauerkraut,			
Drained, 1 cup, 5 oz	25	0	6

Salsa

Average all Types:

	C	F	Cb
Regular, w/out oil, 2 T., 1 oz	15	0	3.5
Made with oil, 2 Tbsp, 1 oz	40	3	8
La Victoria, 2 Tbsp, 1 oz	10	0	2
Old El Paso, 1 Tbsp, 1 oz	10	0	3
TGI Friday's, 1.2 oz	15	0	4

Quick Guide

Cookies:

Average All Brands: *Per Cookie*

	C	F	Cb
Biscotti: Small, 0.5 oz	70	3	10
Regular, 1 oz	140	6.5	18
Chocolate Chip:			
Small/Thin, 0.5 oz	70	3.5	9
Regular, 1 oz	140	7	18
Large (*Mrs Fields*), 3 oz	350	17	45
Extra Large, 4 oz	555	28	73
Oatmeal/Oatmeal Raisin:			
Small/Thin, 0.5 oz	65	2.5	10
Regular, 1 oz	130	5	20
Large (*Mrs Fields*), 2.5 oz	330	14	44
Extra Large, 4 oz	510	20	78
Peanut Butter:			
Small/Thin, 0.5 oz	70	3.5	9
Regular, 1 oz	135	7	17
Large (*Mrs Fields*), 2.5 oz	330	17	41
Extra Large, 4 oz	540	27	67
Low-Fat Cookies:			
Choc Chip (Low-Fat), (1), 0.5 oz	65	2	10
Oatmeal Raisin (Fat-Free), (1), 1 oz	95	0.5	22
Peanut Butter (Low-Fat), (1), 1 oz	105	5	15

Quick Guide

Crackers

Average All Brands: *Per Cracker Unless Indicated*

	C	F	Cb
Cheese Crackers:			
Plain: 1" square	5	0	0.5
Bag, single serving, 1 oz	140	7	16
Cheese/P'nut Butter filled	30	1.5	4
Crispbread, Rye	35	0	8
Grahams, 2¹⁄₂" square	30	0.5	5
Melba Toast, Plain, 1 piece	20	0	4
Matzo, Plain, 1 oz	110	0.5	23
Oyster/Soup, ¹⁄₂ cup	95	2	17
Rice: 1 crackers	70	1.5	11
Oriental Style, 1 oz	130	3.5	23
Saltines, 5 crackers	65	2	11
Snack-type, 1 round cracker	15	1	2
Soda Crackers (*Saltine*), 2	25	1	4.5
Water Cracker (*Carr's*), Original	15	0.5	2.5
Wheat:			
Wheat Thins	10	0.5	1.5
Cheese/Peanut Butter filled	35	2	4

Cookies & Crackers ~ Brands

Per Cookie/Cracker, Unless indicated

	C	F	Cb
Albertsons:			
Animal Crackers (6), 1 oz	130	3.5	22
Chocolate Chip:			
Original (3), 1 oz	150	7	20
Chewy (2), 1 oz	130	6	18
Chunky (1), 0.5 oz	80	3.5	10
Chocolate S'wich Cremes: (3) 1 oz	150	6	25
Double Filled (2), 1 oz	140	6	22
Fudge Graham (3), 1 oz	140	7	18
Fudge Wafer (3), 1 oz	140	8	18
Fudge Marshmallow Ring	120	5	19
Pinwheels, Chocolate Marshmallow	120	5	20
Vanilla Wafers (9), 1 oz	140	4	25
Graham: Cinnamon (2)	150	3	28
Honey (2), 1 oz	140	2	28
Annie's:			
Bunny Grahams:			
Chocolate; Choc Chip, 1 oz	130	4.5	22
Cinnamon; Honey, 1 oz	130	4.5	22
Friends, 1 oz	130	4.5	22
Gluten Free: Cocoa & Vanilla, 1 oz	120	3.5	22
SnickerDoodles, 1 oz	130	4	21
Cheddar Bunnies:			
Regular, 1 oz Snack Pack	140	6	19
Extra Cheesy, 1 oz	150	7	18
White Cheddar; Whole Wheat, 1 oz	145	7	19
Arnott's: Original Tim Tams (2)	190	10	24
Caramel (2)	190	9	26
Austin:			
Sandwich Crackers: *Per Package*			
Cheese: with Cheddar Cheese	190	10	23
with Peanut Butter	190	10	23
Grilled Cheese, 1.4 oz	190	9	24
Pepperjack 1.4 oz	190	9	24
Sour Cream & Chives, 1.4 oz	200	10	27
Toasty, with Peanut Butter	190	9	23
Zoo Animals (16), 1 oz	130	2	25
Barbara's Bakery:			
Fig Bars: Raspberry, 1.4 oz	120	0	27
Wheat/Multigrain	110	0.5	26
Snackimals:			
Choc Chip, 1 oz	120	4	19
Double Chocolate, 1 oz	140	4.5	23
Oatmeal, 1 oz	120	5	17
Bear Naked:			
Soft-Baked Granola Cookies,			
Double Choc.; Fruit & Nut, av.	130	6	19

Cookies & Crackers ~ Brands (Cont)

Per Cookie/Cracker, Unless Indicated **C** **F** **Cb**

BelVita *(Nabisco):*
Breakfast Biscuits:

	C	F	Cb
Crunchy, 1 pack (4 biscuits), average	230	8	36
Soft Baked, 1 biscuit, average	190	7	32
Bites, (46), av., 1.8 oz	230	8	37

Blue Diamond:
Nut Thins:

	C	F	Cb
Almond,(19),1 oz	130	2.5	24
Pecan (16), 1 oz	130	3.5	23

Brent & Sam's:
Natural: *Per 2 Cookies*

	C	F	Cb
Chocolate Chip Pecan	120	7	15
Key Lime White Choc.	120	6	16
White Choc. Macadamia	130	7	14

Soft Baked: *Per 1 Cookie*

	C	F	Cb
Chocolate Chunk	130	5	20
Oatmeal Raisin	140	6	20
Snickerdoodle	130	4	21

Carr's:
Crackers:

	C	F	Cb
Original (4)	60	1	10
Roastd Garlic & Herbs (4)	50	1	10
Rosemary (4)	70	2.5	11
Whole Wheat (2)	80	3.5	11

Cheez•It ~ *See Sunshine, Page 87*
Chips Ahoy! ~ *See Nabisco, Page 85*

Country Choice:
Sandwich Cremes,

	C	F	Cb
all varieties, 2 pieces	130	5	19

Snacking:

	C	F	Cb
Ginger Snaps (5); Vanilla Wafers (7)	140	5	22
Iced Oatmeal (4)	120	4	21

Dr. Kracker:
Crispbread:

	C	F	Cb
Klassic 3 Seed (1)	100	4	15
Pumpkin Seed Cheddar (1)	110	5	15
Snackers, Pumpkin Seed Cheddar (8)	125	5	13

Erin Baker's:
Original Breakfast: *Per 3 oz*

	C	F	Cb
Banana Walnut	300	8	53
Peanut Butter	320	11	48

Minis: *Per 1 oz Cookie*

	C	F	Cb
Peanut Butter	100	3.5	16
Dble Chocolate; Oatmeal Raisin, av.	100	2.5	18

Famous Amos:
Bite Size: Choc. Chip,

	C	F	Cb
4 Cookies, 1 oz	150	7	20
Choc. Chip & Pecans (4)	150	8	18
Sandwich, Creme Filled,			
Choc.; Vanilla, 3 cookies, 1 oz	170	7	25

Per Cookie/Cracker, Unless Indicated **C** **F** **Cb**

Fig Newtons ~ *See Nabisco, Page 85*

Fifty50:

	C	F	Cb
Chocolate Chip (4)	170	9	22
Hearty Oatmeal (4)	160	7	24
Wafers, average all varieties, (6)	150	9	17

Gamesa:

	C	F	Cb
Animalitos, 14 cookies, 1 oz	110	1	25
Arcoiris Marshmallow,			
2 oz pkg, 6 cookies	220	5	38
Chocolatines Marshmallow,			
2 cookies, 1 oz	130	5	18
Chokis, Chocolate Chip, 1.4 oz pkg	190	9	27
Emperador: Cream Cookie Sandwich			
Lemon Creme, 1 pkg, 6 cookies	270	8	45
Av. other flavors, 1 pkg, 6 cookies	360	12	57
Fruitbars, average, 1 cookie, 1 oz	110	4.5	18
Giro, 3 cookies, 1 oz	140	6	20
Mamut, Choc Marshmallow,			
1 cookie, 1 oz	130	5	19
Marias, 8 cookies, 1 oz	120	2	24
Sugar Wafers, (3), average, 1.2 oz	160	7	25

Girl Scouts Cookies:

	C	F	Cb
Caramel DeLites/Samoas, (2)	130	6	19
Girl Scout S'Mores (2)	180	9	25
Peanut Butter S'wich, (3)	170	9	19
Shortbread (4)	120	4.5	19
Thin Mints (4)	160	7	22

Goya:

	C	F	Cb
Lady Fingers , 1 oz	130	1	25
Maria, 5 cookies, 1 oz	130	3	24
Wafers, average all flavors,			
4 wafers, 1 oz	150	7	20

Grandma's:
Homestyle: *Per Cookie*

	C	F	Cb
Chocolate Brownie	190	8	27
Chocolate Chip	200	10	25
Minis, 1 pkg	210	8	31
Oatmeal Raisin	180	7	26
Peanut Butter	190	10	22

Sandwich Cremes:

	C	F	Cb
Peanut Butter (5)	200	9	25
Strawberry (5)	190	9	27
Vanilla (5)	190	9	27
Minis (9)	150	7	22

Cookies & Crackers ~ Brands (Cont)

Per Cookie/Cracker, Unless Indicated **C** **F** **Cb**

Great American Cookies:

	C	F	Cb
Chewy Choc. Supreme	200	9	29
Chewy Pecan Supreme	230	12	31
Double Fudge with Reese's	230	11	33
Original, w/ Reese's or M&M's	240	12	31
Peanut Butter w/ M&M's	250	14	29
White Chunk Macadamia	250	14	30
Double Doozies:			
Original, 5.3 oz	690	34	94
M&M Big Bite, 2.5 oz	340	17	46
Cookie Cakes:			
16", 3.5 oz	460	22	67
16" M&M, 4 oz	500	24	73
Heart Shaped, 3.5 oz	440	21	64

Great Value *(Walmart): Per Cookie Unless Indicated*

	C	F	Cb
Caramel Coconut Fudge	130	6	18
Chocolate Chip: Chewy	120	5	17
Chunky	160	7	21
Classic	160	7	23
Double Filled Twist & Shout			
Chocolate Sandwich	140	6	20
Fudge Marshmallow	120	5	19
Pecan Shortbread, 2 cookies	150	8	17
Soft Cookies, Fudge & Cream	150	6	22
Twist & Shout, Chocolate; Vanilla	160	6	25
Crackers:			
Buttery, Baked, 0.5 oz	70	4	8
Cheddar Cheese, Baked, 1 oz	150	8	18

Joseph's:

Sugar Free: *Per 4 Cookies*

	C	F	Cb
Almond (4)	95	5	13
Chocolate Chip; Coconut, aerage	95	5	14
Average other varieties	95	4	15

Note: Carb figures include 6 grams Maltitol

Kashi: *Per Cookie*

	C	F	Cb
Chocolate Almond Butter	130	5	19
Oatmeal: Dark Chocolate	130	5	20
Raisin Flax	120	4.5	20
Crackers:			
Original 7 Grain, (15)	120	3.5	20
Fire Roasted Veggie, (15)	120	3.5	20
Pita Crisps:			
Original 7 Grain with Salt (11), 1 oz	120	3	23
Garlic Pesto (11), 1 oz	120	3	23

Per Cookie/Cracker, Unless Indicated **C** **F** **Cb**

Keebler:

Animals:

	C	F	Cb
Crackers: 8 Crackers, 1 oz	130	4	22
Variety Pak, 1.4 oz	180	6	30
Frosted Cookies: 8 pieces	160	7	22
Variety Pak, 1.4 oz	200	10	28
Iced Cookies: 6 pcs, 1 oz	140	4.5	20
Variety Pak, 1.4 oz	180	6	30
Chips Deluxe: Original (2)	160	8	19
Chocolate Lovers (2)	170	9	20
Coconut (2)	160	9	18
Peanut Butter Cups (2)	170	9	19
Soft 'n Chewy (2)	140	6	21
Rainbow:			
Triple Choc. Chip wih M&M's (2)	150	8	19
Choc Chip Minis, with M&M's, 5 cookies, 1 oz	140	7	19
Cinnamon Roll, Original (2)	150	6	23
Danish Wedding, (4)	140	7	19
E.L. Fudge: Original (2)	180	7	25
Double Stuffed (2)	180	9	24
Fudge Shoppe:			
Coconut Dreams (2)	160	9	20
Deluxe Grahams (3)	140	7	18
Fudge Sticks:			
Original (3)	150	8	20
Fudge Stripes:			
Original (2)	140	6	19
Mini, Original, 1.4 oz pkg	200	9	27
Grasshopper (4)	140	7	20
Gripz, Chips Deluxe, 0.9 oz pouch	120	5	18
Oatmeal, with Raisins (2)	140	6	19
Pitter Patter, P'nt Butter Creme (2)	140	6	19
Sandies Cookies:			
Dark Choc. Almond; Pecan Shtbrd, av.	170	10	19
Toffee Shortbread (2)	160	9	20
Vienna Fingers:			
Creme Filled (2)	150	6	23
Reduced Fat (2)	140	4.5	24
Wafers: Vanilla (8)	140	5	22
Mini Vanilla (18)	140	5	22

continued next page...

Cookies & Crackers ~ Brands (Cont)

Per Cookie/Cracker, Unless Indicated **C** **F** **Cb**

Keebler (Cont):
Crackers:

	C	F	Cb
Club: Original (4)	70	3	9
Reduced Fat (5)	70	2	12
Grahams: Original (8)	120	3.5	22
Honey (8)	140	4.5	23
Town House: Original (5)	90	5	9
Reduced Fat (6)	60	1.5	12
Pita: Cinnamon Sugar; Sea Salt (6)	70	2.5	11
Mediterranean Herb (6)	70	2.5	12
Kraft, Macaroni & Cheese Crackers, av. all varieties, 1. oz	150	7	18

Kroger:

	C	F	Cb
Chip Mates: Orig. (3), 1.5 oz	150	7	22
Chunky (2), 1 oz	120	6	17
Peanut Butter (2), 1 oz	120	7	15
White Chip (2), 1 oz	120	6	16
Chocolate Sandwich:			
Original (3), 1.2 oz	150	6	24
Double Filled (2), 1 oz	140	6	22
Olde Southern Pecan Shortbread (2)	150	9	16
Vanilla Wafers (7)	130	3.5	23
Crackers:			
Grahams, Orig.; Honey, (4)	120	3	20
Saltines, Original (5), 0.5oz	60	1.5	10

Lance:
6 Pack: *Per Pack of 4 Cookies*

	C	F	Cb
Choc-O-Lunch/Van-O-Lunch, av.	150	6	22
Crackers:			
Cracker Sandwiches: *Per 6 Crackers*			
Malt, with Peanut Butter Filling	180	8	21
Nekot, Peanut Butter	240	11	33
Nip Chee, Cheddar Cheese	200	9	24
Toastchee, Peanut Butter	210	10	25
Toasty, Peanut Butter	180	9	21
Wholegrain, Cheddar Cheese	200	10	26

Little Debbie:

	C	F	Cb
Caramel Apple Oatmeal Pies (1)	140	4.5	24
Chocolate Chip Cream Pie (1), 3 oz	380	16	58
Cookie Wreaths (1)	100	5	12
Marshmallow Puffs	150	5	25
Oatmeal Creme Pie (1)	170	7	26
Star Crunch(1)	150	6	22

Lu:

	C	F	Cb
Petit Beurre Milk Chocolate (2)	130	6	7
Petit Ecolier Extra Dark Chocolate(2)	130	7	15
Petit Ecolier, Milk Chocolate (2)	130	6	17
Pim's, Orange(2), 0.9 oz	100	3	17

Manischewitz:
Crackers:

	C	F	Cb
Tam Tams: Original (10)	110	4	16
Everything; Garlic (10)	140	5	19

Mary's Gone Crackers:

	C	F	Cb
Chocolate Chip (2)	130	6	19
Crackers:			
Original (13)	140	5	21
Super Seed, Classic (12)	160	8	19
Other varieties, (13)	140	5	21

Miss Meringue:
Meringue Classiques:

	C	F	Cb
Cappuccino (4), 1 oz	110	0	26
Mint Choc. Chip (4), 1 oz	120	1.5	25
Triple Chocolate (4), 1 oz	120	1.5	25
Vanilla Rainbow/Van. (4), 1 oz	110	0	27

Meringue Minis, Low Fat:

	C	F	Cb
Mini: Chocolate Chip (12), 1 oz	130	1.5	27
Mint Chocolate Chip (12), 1 oz	120	1.5	26

Meringue Minis, Fat Free:

	C	F	Cb
Peppermint Crush (9), 1 oz	110	0	25
Rainbw Vanilla; Vanilla (13), 1 oz	110	0	27

Meringue Petites: Cafe au Lait (7) 100 | 0 | 25

	C	F	Cb
Toasted Coconut (6)	120	2.5	23

Mother's:

	C	F	Cb
Circus Animal, (7), 1 oz	150	7	21
Coconut Cocadas, (5), 1.2 oz	160	8	21
Double Chocolate Chips, (4)	150	8	19
Double Fudge, (2), 1.3 oz	190	8	27
Iced Oatmeal, (4), 1.2 oz	150	6	23
Peanut Butter Gauchos, (2), 1.3 oz	190	9	26
Taffy; Vanilla Cream, (2), av., 1.3 oz	190	8	28

Mrs Fields Cookies ~ *See Page 219*

Cookies & Crackers ~ Brands (Cont)

Per Cookie/Cracker, Unless Indicated **C** **F** **Cb**

Nabisco Cookies:

Chips Ahoy!, Chocolate Chip:

Original:

	C	F	Cb
3 cookies, 1.2 oz	160	8	22
Single Serve, 1.4 oz	190	9	27
Reduced Fat (2), 1.2 oz	150	6	24
Mini Choc. Chips: 1.1 oz	150	7	21
3 oz Package	450	21	63
Go-Pak, 3.5 oz	525	25	74

Chewy:

Regular (2), 1.1 oz	140	6	21
Chewy, Fudge Filled (2), 1.1 oz	150	7	21
Chunky, Choc. Chunk (2), 1.2 oz	160	8	20
Made with Reeses PB Cups, 1.1 oz	160	9	18
S'Mores Filled Soft (2), 1.1 oz	150	7	21
White Fudge Chunky Chocolate (1)	80	4	11

Lorna Doone:

100 Calorie Pack, Shortbread Cookie Crisps (6), 0.7 oz	100	3	16
Shorbreads: 1 oz cookie	140	6	19
1.5 oz cookie	210	10	28
Mallomars (1), 1 oz	120	5	18

Newtons:

100% Whole Grain:

Blueberry (2), 1 oz	100	1.5	22
Original Fig: 2 cookies, 1.1 oz	110	2	22
Fat-Free, 2 cookies, 1 oz	100	0	24
Fruit Thins, Crispy (3), all var., 1 oz	140	5	22

Nilla Wafers:

8 wafers, 1 oz	140	6	21
Reduced-Fat (8), 1 oz	120	1	24

Nutter Butter, Peanut Butter Sandwich:

16 oz package, 1 cookie 1 oz	130	5	20
4.8 oz package, 2 cookies, 0.9 oz	120	5	17
1.9 oz package, 4 cookies	250	10	37
Bites, Go-Paks!, 3.5 oz pkg	460	20	69

Oreo, Chocolate/Golden: *Average All fillings*

100 Calorie Pack, Thin Crisps (6)	100	2	19
Original: 1 cookie	55	2.5	8
3 cookies, 1.2 oz	160	7	25
Single Serve pkg (6), 2 oz	270	11	41

Per Cookie/Cracker, Unless Indicated **C** **F** **Cb**

Nabisco (Cont):

Oreo, Choc./Golden (Cont): *Average All Fillings*

Original Continued:

	C	F	Cb
Reduced Fat (3), 1.2 oz	150	5	27
Mini Bite: Bite Size (9), 1 oz	130	6	21
Go-Paks, average, 3.5 oz	490	22	70
Chewy, 1.2 oz	150	7	21

Double Stuf:

2 cookies, 1 oz	140	7	20
Single Serve, 1.5 oz	210	10	30
Fudge Cremes: 1 cookie	60	3	8
3 cookies	180	9	24
Thins, all flavors, 1 oz	140	6	21
Triple Double Chcolate (1), 0.75 oz	100	5	15

Teddy Grahams, 10 oz Box:

Snacks: Honey (24), 1 oz	120	4	21
Chocolate; Cinnamon (24), 1 oz	130	4	22

Nabisco Crackers:

Barnum's Animals:

8 crackers, 1 oz Pack	120	3.5	22
Snack Saks, 1.2 oz Pack	140	4	24

Cheese Nips:

Cheddar: 19 pieces, 1 oz	140	6	19
Mini, Despicable Me, 1 oz Pack	130	4	19

Honey Maid:

Grahamfuls,

S'Mores; PB & Choc. 0.9 oz pkg, av.	115	4	18
Grahams (8) average all varieties,	130	3	24

Premium:

Saltine: Original, 5 crackers, 0.5 oz	70	1.5	12
Unsalted Tops (5), 0.5 oz	70	1.5	13
Rounds: Original (6), 0.5 oz	60	1.5	12
Wholegrain (6), 0.5 oz	60	1.5	11

Triscuit:

Original (6), 1 oz	120	4	20
Reduced Fat (7), 1.1 oz	110	2.5	21
Brown Rice & Wheat (6), average all varieties	130	3	22

Wheat Thins: *Per 9 oz Box*

Original (16), 1.1 oz	140	5	22
Reduced Fat (16), 1 oz	130	3	22
Av. other flav. (14), 1.1 oz	140	5	21
Multigrain (14), 1.1 oz	130	4	22
Popped, av. all flavors, 24 pcs	125	3	23

Per Cookie/Cracker, Unless Indicated **C** **F** **Cb**

Nana's: *Per Cookie*

	C	F	Cb
Choc. Chip; Oatmeal Raisin, av.	410	17	59
Coconut Chip; Peanut Butter, av.	370	18	50
Double Chocolate	420	20	58
Gluten Free: Choc. Crunch	360	12	62
Ginger	360	10	64
Lemon	360	14	60
Cookie Bars, average	150	6	23
Bites, P'Nut Butter (1), 1 oz	130	6	17

Newman's Own Organics:

	C	F	Cb
Alphabet: Chocolate (10)	110	3	21
Other varieties (10)	120	3	21
Double Choc Chip, (5)	150	8	22

Fig Newman's:

	C	F	Cb
Fat-Free (2)	100	0	24
Low-Fat (2)	110	1.5	23
Wheat/Dairy-Free (2)	110	1.5	23
Ginger Snaps, (5)	130	3.5	24
Hermits, all varieities, 0.75 oz	80	1.5	16
Newman-O's: Original (2)	130	5	20
Choc.; Hint O Mint Creme, (2), av.	130	5	20
Peanut Butter (2)	120	5	18
Oatmeal Chocolate Chip, (2)	140	6	23
Orange Chocolate Chip, (2)	160	7	22

Nonni's:

Biscotti:

	C	F	Cb
Original, 1 piece, 0.8 oz	90	3	14
Av. other varieties, 1 piece, 0.8 oz	110	4	17
THINAddictives: Cranb. Alm., 1 oz	130	4.5	20
Chocolate varieties, average, 0.5 oz	75	3	10
Pistachio/Mango Coconut Alm., 1 oz	145	6	18

Oreo Cookies ~ *See Nabisco, Page 85*

Payaso:

	C	F	Cb
Animalitos, 19 pieces	120	1.5	23
Marias, (8)	120	2.5	22
Orejitas Finas, (4)	100	5	13

Pepperidge Farm:

Cookies:

Chunk:: *Per Cookie*

	C	F	Cb
Chesapeake, Dark Chocolate Pecan	140	8	20
Lexington, Milk Chocolate, Toffee Almond	130	6	17
Monauk, Milk Chocolate	140	6	20
Nantucket, Dark Chocolate	130	6	18
Sausalito, Milk Choc. Macadamia	130	7	17
Tahoe, White Chocolate Macadamia	130	7	17

Per Cookie/Cracker, Unless Indicated **C** **F** **Cb**

Pepperidge Farm (Cont):

	C	F	Cb
Brown Butter Rum, (3)	130	6	20
Brussels (3)	150	7	20
Geneva (3)	160	9	19
Milano: Milk Chocolate (3)	170	9	21
Double Dark Chocolate (2)	140	7	20
Mint; Orange; Raspb. (2)	130	7	16
Melts, Boston Cream Pie (2)	150	8	20
Slices (3), av. all varieties	145	7	20
Pirouettes, (2), average all varieties	120	5	19
Tahiti, Coconut (2)	170	10	20

Crackers:

	C	F	Cb
Cracker Trio, (3)	60	2	9
Flavor Blasted, av, ½ cup, 1.1 oz			
Golden Butter, (4)	70	2	10

Goldfish:

	C	F	Cb
Cheddar: ½ cup, 1.1 oz	140	5	20
Carton, small, 2 oz	280	10	40
Lunch Pack, 0.9 oz pouch	120	4.5	17
Grahams, av., ½ cup, 1.1 oz	140	5	22
Parmesan, ½ cup, 1.1 oz	140	5	20
Pretzel, ½ cup, 1.1 oz	130	2.5	20
Saltine, ½ cup, 1.1 oz	150	6	20

Ritz:

	C	F	Cb
Originals: Original (5)	80	4.5	10
Bacon; Roasted Veg. (5)	80	4	10
Whole Wheat (5)	70	2.5	10
Crisp & Thins, all varieties (21)	130	4.5	21

Toasted Chips:

	C	F	Cb
Original (14)	130	4.5	20
Cheddar (5)	80	4.5	10
Sour Cream & Onion (12)	130	6	19

Safeway Select:

	C	F	Cb
Homestyle, Oatmeal Raisin, 1 oz	130	6	18
Indulgent: Double Choc Chunk, 1 oz	130	7	18
Milk Chocolate Macadamia Nut, 1 oz	140	8	17

Gourmet Sandwich Cremes:

	C	F	Cb
Maple Creme (2)	170	7	25
Raspberry Swirl (2)	130	5	20
Strawberry Swirl (2)	130	6	19

Sedano's:

	C	F	Cb
Cinnamon, (5)	160	6	24
Maria, (5)	120	3	22

Shar Gluten Free ~ *See CalorieKing.com*

Cookies & Crackers ~ Brands (Cont)

Per Cookie/Cracker, Unless Indicated	C	F	Cb
Special K: *Per 1 oz Serving*			
Crackers, Parm. Sesame Quinoa (14)	130	4.5	21
Cracker Chips, all varieties, (25)	120	4	22
Stella D'Oro:			
Breakfast Treats (1), av. all var.	90	3	15
Margherite: Chocolate (2)	130	6	19
Vanilla (2)	120	4	20
Roman Egg Biscuits, 1 oz	130	4.5	19
Swiss Fudge (3)	180	9	22
Toast & Sponge:			
Almond Toast (2)	100	2	20
Anisette Sponge (3)	90	1	18
Anisette Toast (3)	130	1	27
Streit's:			
Flavored Wafers:			
Chocolate (3)	170	11	18
Vanilla (3)	170	11	18
Sunshine:			
Cheez-It:			
Crackers, average, 1 oz	150	8	17
1.25 oz bag	180	9	20
Big, 1 oz	150	8	17
Grooves, Sharp White Chedd., 1 oz	140	6	19
Sandwich Crackers, av.,	210	10	24
Snack Mix, 1 oz	140	4.5	20
Zings, (18), average, 1 oz	150	7	18
Trader Joe's:			
100 Calorie Packs, average	100	2.5	18
Almond Windmill (2)	140	6	18
Charmingly Chewy Choc Chip (2)	130	5	20
Cherry Granola (2)	110	4	18
Chocolate Chip: Small (4)	140	7	18
Large, singles, 1.7 oz	280	14	35
Deep Dish: $^1/_{10}$ cookie, 1.6 oz	200	9	28
$^1/_4$ Cookie, 4 oz	500	23	70
Vegan (1)	130	6	18
Caramel Cashew (3)	140	7	16
Crispy Crunchy Choc. Chip (12)	150	9	19
Crispy Oatmeal Choc. Chip (12)	150	7	19
Dark Choc Chunks with almonds (3)	140	7	17
Dunkers: Chocolate Chip (2)	160	7	21
Choc. Coated Choc. Chip (2)	190	9	25

Per Cookie/Cracker, Unless Indicated	C	F	Cb
Trader Joe's (Cont):			
Ginger Snaps, Gluten Free (5)	140	6	21
Highbrow Chocolate (2)	140	7	17
Joe Joe's Sandwich Cremes,			
Chocolate/ Vanilla (2)	130	6	19
Macarons A La Parisienne (2)	90	3	10
Meringues, Vanilla (4)	110	0	27
Oatmeal Raisin, 1.8 oz	270	12	35
Pecan Southern Style (4)	150	9	15
Thins: Meyer Lemon (9)	130	4.5	22
Toasted Coconut (8)	130	4.5	22
Triple Choc Chunk, 1 oz	140	7	20
Ultimate Vanilla Wafers (5)	120	6	15
Way More Chocolate Chip (3)	160	11	14
Crackers:			
Multigrain (14)	150	6	22
Savory Thin Edaname (38)	120	2	21
Water (4)	60	1	12
Triscuits ~ *See Page 85*			
Voortman: *Per Cookie Unless Indicated*			
Almond Delight	120	6	16
Chocolate Chip	90	4	13
Coconut	100	5	9
Coconut Dark Chocolate	90	5	10
Fudge Striped Almonette	110	6	13
Iced Almonettes	100	4.5	11
Oatmeal Choc Chip	90	4	12
Sugar Free: Choc Chip	80	5	13
Fudge Striped Shortbread	130	8	17
Oatmeal	80	4	13
Wafers (3), average all flavors	130	7	19
Whole Foods (365 Organic):			
Chocolate Chip (2)	150	7	21
Classic Fig Bars (2)	140	2.5	27
Lemon Wafers (7)	110	3	19
Oatmeal (2)	130	4.5	20
Sandwich Cremes; Sugar, (2), average	130	5	20

Cookie ~ Mixes

Prepared as Directed	C	F	Cb
Betty Crocker:			
Pouch Mix: *Per 2 Cookies*			
Double Choc. Chunk; P'nut Butter, av.	140	6	21
Walnut Chocolate Chip	170	9	20
Average other varieties	145	6	22

Thaw, Bake & Serve   C   F   Cb

Per Cookie/Cracker Unless Indicated

Pillsbury Cookies:

Refrigerated Cookie Dough: *Per Cookie*

	C	F	Cb
Chocolate Chip Cookie, 1.1 oz	140	7	20
P'nut Butter, 1 oz	120	5	17
Sugar, 1 oz	120	5	18

Ready To Bake:

Big Deluxe Classics:

	C	F	Cb
Chocolate Chip (1)	160	7	23
Oatmeal Raisin (1)	150	5	24
White Chunk Macadamia (1)	170	8	22
Simply Cookies, Choc. Chip (1)	150	7	20
Choc. Chunk & Chip (2)	160	7	24
Holiday Cookies, Sugar, average all shapes, (2)	120	6	15
Melts: Caramel Brownie (1)	140	5	22
S'mores Sensation (1)	150	6	23
Sugar Shapes, (2), av. all var.,1 oz	120	6	15

Refrigerated Sweet Buns/Rolls~ *See Page 67*

Toll House (Nestle):

Refrigerated Doughs: *Per Cookie*

	C	F	Cb
Bars: Chocolate Chip	90	4	11
P'B Chocolate Chip	80	4.5	10
Sugar Bar	80	3.5	11
Walnut Chocolate Chip	90	4.5	11
Blueberry Lemon (1)	80	3	4
Peanut Butter (1)	130	7	15
Pecan Turtle Delight (1)	160	7	24
Triple Chip (1)	90	4.5	4

Ultimates Refrigerated Dough: *Per Cookie*

	C	F	Cb
Chocolate Chip Lovers	180	9	23
Chocolate Pecan Deluxe	190	10	22
Choc. P'nut Butter Deluxe	180	9	23
Dark Chocolate Delight	160	8	21
Pecan Turtle Delight	160	7	23

Crispbreads   C   F   Cb

Per Crispbread Unless Indicated

Finn Crisp:

	C	F	Cb
Classic: Caraway	20	0	4
High Fibre	40	0.5	7
Sourdough	20	0.5	4
Traditional	40	0.5	7
Round: Multigrain	50	0	7.5
Original	45	0.5	8

New York Flatbread Crisps,

	C	F	Cb
Sesame, 0.4 oz	50	1.5	8
Ry-Krisp: Natural (2)	50	0	11
Seasoned (2)	50	0	11
Sesame (2)	50	0	9

Ryvita:

	C	F	Cb
Crackerbreads, Original; Ched. Chse	20	0	4
Crispbreads, Original; Dark	35	0	6.5

WASA:

Crisp'n Light Thins:

	C	F	Cb
Fiber (2), 0.7 oz	60	1	14
Hearty (1), 0.5 oz	50	0	12
Light Rye (2), 0.5 oz	60	0	15
Whole Grain (1), 0.5 oz	40	0	10

Matzos

Manischewitz:

	C	F	Cb
Matzos: Egg & Onion, 1 oz	80	0.5	17
Thin Salted/Tea, average, 0.9 oz	95	0	20
Whole Wheat, 1 oz	110	1	21
Yolk Free, 1.2 oz	100	0	20

Crackers:

	C	F	Cb
Tam Tam Snack:: Original (10), 1 oz	110	4	16
Everything; Onion (10), 1 oz	140	5	19
Rye (10), 1 oz	110	4	16

Streit's:

	C	F	Cb
Lightly Salted, (1)	110	0.5	23
Unsalted Matzos, (1)	100	0	23

Quick Guide C F Cb

Cream
Average All Brands

Half & Half Cream:

	C	F	Cb
1 Tbsp, 0.5 oz	20	1.5	0.5
2 Tbsp, 1 oz	40	3	1
$^1/_4$ cup, 2 oz	80	6	2
Light: Coffee/table (20% fat): 1 Tbsp	30	3	0.5
2 Tbsp, 1 oz	60	6	0.5

Sour Cream:

Regular: 1 Tbsp, 0.5 oz	25	2.5	1
1 cup, 8 oz	445	45	7
Low-Fat/Light: 1 Tbsp, 0.5 oz	20	1.5	1
2 Tbsp, 1 oz	40	3	2
Fat-Free: Av., 2 Tbsp, 1 oz	20	0	3
Knudsen, 2 Tbsp, 1 oz	30	0	2
Kroger, 2 Tbsp, 1 oz	20	0	3

Sour Cream Substitute:

Albertson's, 2 Tbsp, 1 oz	60	5	4
Tofutti, Sour Supreme, 2 Tbsp, 1 oz	85	5	9

Whipping Cream:
Heavy, (37% fat):

1 Tbsp fluid/2 Tbsp whipped	50	5.5	0.5
½ cup whipped	105	11	1
1 cup whipped	410	44	3.5
Light, (30% fat):			
1 Tbsp fluid/2 Tbsp whipped	45	4.5	0.5
½ cup fluid/1 cup whipped	350	37	3.5

Coconut Cream/Milk

Coconut Cream, (Canned):

Plain/unsweetened: 2 Tbsp, 1 oz	75	6.5	3
½ cup, 4 oz	285	26	12
Sweetened:			
Coco Lopez: 1 oz	130	5	21
½ cup, 4 oz	520	20	84

Coconut Milk: (Canned):

Thai Kitchen: Lite, $^1/_3$ cup, 2 fl.oz	50	4.5	1
Premium/Organic, 2 fl.oz	115	10	4
Unsweetened, $^1/_3$ cup	140	14	3
Coconut Water, (Center), 1 cup	45	0.5	9

Whipped Toppings

Average All Brands

Cream (Pressurized): 2 Tbsp	20	1.5	1
$^1/_4$ cup	40	3.5	2
Cream Topping, Lite, 2 Tbsp	20	1	3

Whipped Toppings (Cont)

Kraft:

	C	F	Cb
Cool Whip: Regular, Original, $^1/_3$ oz	25	1.5	2
Extra Creamy, 2 Tbsp	25	2	2
Lite, Sugar Free, $^1/_4$ oz	20	1	3
Free, 2 Tbsp, 0.3 oz	20	0	3
Seasons Delight, Fr. Vanilla, 0.3 oz	25	1.5	2
Dream Whip Mix, $^1/_{16}$ envolope	10	0	1

Reddi-wip:

Original, 2 Tbsp, 0.3 oz	15	1	1
Extra Creamy, 2 Tbsp, 0.3 oz	15	1	1
Fat-Free, 2 Tbsp, 0.3 oz	5	0	1
Chocolate, 2 Tbsp, 0.3 oz	15	1	1

Creamers (Non-Dairy)

Powder:
Coffee-Mate/Cremora/N-Rich:

Original: 1 tsp	10	0.5	1
Lite, 1 tsp	10	0	2
Flavors: Av., 0.4 oz	60	3	9
Fat-Free, average, 4 tsp	50	0	11
Sugar Free, Chocolate, 0.2 oz	30	0.5	2

Liquid/Refrigerated:
Per Tablespoon

Baileys, Coffee Creamer,			
all flavors, 1 Tbsp, 15ml	25	0.5	5
Califia Farms, all flavors, 1 Tbsp	15	0	4
Coffee-Mate: *Per Tbsp, 15 ml Unless Indicated*			
Flavors: Average all flavors	35	1.5	5
Fat-Free, all flavors	25	0	5
Sugar free, all flavors	15	1	2
Shelf Stable, Ital. Swt Creme	35	1.5	5
Unflavored: Original	20	1	2
Fat-Free	10	0	1
2Go, all flavors, 5 ml	25	1.5	3
Natural Bliss, all flavors	35	1.5	5
Hood, Country Creamer, 1 Tbsp	20	1.5	2
International Delight: *Per Tbsp*			
American/Classic/Coffee House:			
Regular, all flavors	35	1.5	6
Fat-Free, all flavors	30	0	7
Sugar-Free, all flav.	20	2	1
Simply Pure, all flavors	30	1	5
Kroger: *Per Tbsp*			
Coffee Creamers: Original	20	1	3
Caramel Vanilla; Hazelnut	35	1.5	6
Fat-free, Hazelnut	30	0	6
Silk: Almond, Vanilla	20	1	3
Soy: Original	20	1.5	2
Hazelnut	30	1.5	4

Ready-To-Serve

	C	F	Cb
Hunt's:			
Snack Pack Puddings:			
3.3 oz Container:			
Butterscotch	100	2.5	20
Choc./Fudge; Tapioca, av.	110	3	20
Vanilla	100	2.5	19
Sugar Free: Chocolate	70	3	14
Caramel; Vanilla	60	3	10
Juicy Gels: Lemon Lime, 5.5 oz	150	0	38
Strawberry, 5.5 oz	170	0	41
Sugar Free, Cherry, 3.25 oz	10	0	2
Naturals: Chocolate, 3.8 oz	130	2.5	24
Vanilla, 3.8 oz	130	3.5	22
Jell-O *(Kraft):*			
Gelatin, av. all flavors, 3.4 oz	70	0	17
Puddings: *4 Packs*			
Chocolate Vanilla Swirls, 3.5 oz	110	1.5	24
Strawberry Cheesecake, 3.5 oz	130	2	24
Fat Free, Chocolate, 3.5 oz	100	0	21
Sugar Free Puddings: *4 Packs*			
Chocolate, 3.6 oz	60	1.5	9
Rice Pudding, 3.6 oz	70	1.5	12
Temptations, Lem. Meringue Pie, 3.4 oz	80	1.5	18
Kozy Shack:			
Flan, Creme Caramel, 1 cup, 4 oz	160	4	28
Gluten Free Puddings:			
Chocolate, 4.6 oz	140	2.5	27
Cinn. Raisin Rice, 4.6 oz	140	2.5	26
French Vanilla Rice, 4.6 oz	140	2.5	24
Original Rice, 4.6 oz	130	2.5	24
Tapioca, 4.6 oz	130	2	25
Simply Well Puddings:			
Chocolate, 4 oz	90	2.5	13
Rice; Tapioca, 4 oz	90	1.5	14
Kroger: *Per Container*			
Puddings: *Per 3.5 oz*			
Butterscotch	110	2	22
Chocolate	110	2.5	21
Swiss Miss:			
Puddings: *Per 4 oz Cup*			
Classic Butterscotch	130	3.5	22
Creamy : Milk Choc.	150	3.5	27
Vanilla	140	3.5	24
Old Fashioned Tapioca	140	3.5	24
Triple Chocolate Dream	160	4	27

Homemade Puddings

	C	F	Cb
Apple Tapioca, $^1/_2$ cup	150	0	32
Bread Pudding, $^1/_2$ cup	250	8	40
Blancmange, $^1/_2$ cup	140	5	19
Chocolate, $^1/_2$ cup	190	6	30
Crème Brulée, $^1/_2$ cup	400	35	16
Plum Pudding, 2 oz	170	3	32
Rice, with Raisins, $^1/_2$ cup	200	4	38
Sponge Pudding, 3.5 oz	340	16	45
Tapioca Cream, $^1/_2$ cup	110	4	15
Trifle, $^1/_2$ cup	180	7	26

Custards

	C	F	Cb
Custard Mix *(Jello/Royal Flan)*, average:			
Dry, $^1/_4$ of 2.9 oz package, 0.7 oz	80	0	19
Prepared: whole milk, $^1/_2$ cup	155	4	25
2% milk, $^1/_2$ cup	140	2.5	25
Non-Fat milk, $^1/_2$ cup	125	0	25
Home Made Egg Custard:			
With Whole Milk, $^1/_2$ cup	170	8	18
With 2% Milk, $^1/_2$ cup	155	6.5	18

Gelatin • Parfait • Jell-O

	C	F	Cb
Jell-O:			
Gelatin Dessert Mix: *Dry Mix Only*			
All flavors, 0.8 oz	80	0	19
Sugar free, all flavors, 0.3 oz	10	0	0
Instant Pudding & Pie Filling: *Dry Mix Only*			
Chocolate/Fudge, 1 oz	100	0	25
Devil's Food, 1 oz	140	0	25
Oreo,			
Cookies 'N Cream, 1 oz	120	1	28
White Chocolate, 0.8 oz	90	0	23
Sugar free, Fat-Free:			
Chocolate var., 0.3 oz	35	0	8
Other flavors, 0.3 oz	25	0	6
No Bake Dessert Mix: *Dry Mix Only*			
Cheesecake: Real, 2 oz	290	15	39
Cherry, 2.2 oz	210	3.5	42
Strawberry, 2.4 oz	200	3.5	42
Oreo, 2 oz	280	8	48
Peanut Butter Cup, 2 oz	290	15	39
Pumpkin Style Pie, 1.2 oz	130	1.5	29
Ida Mae, Strawberry Parfait	90	2	18
Reser's, Parfaits, av. all flavors, 3.9 oz	105	2	19

Meringues

	C	F	Cb
Meringue Swirl, $^1/_2$ oz	50	0	8
Meringue Shell, 1 oz	100	0	16

Chicken Eggs

	C	F	Cb
Fresh Eggs:			
Raw:			
Small	55	4	0
Medium	65	4	0
Large	70	5	0
Extra Large	80	5.5	0
Jumbo	90	6	0
Egg Yolk, 1 extra large	55	4.5	0
Egg White, 1 extra large	17	0	0
Dried Egg Powder:			
Whole Egg: $^1/_4$ cup, 1 oz	170	12	0
1 Tbsp	30	2	0
Egg White, $^1/_4$ cup, 1 oz	105	0	0
Egg Yolk, $^1/_4$ cup, 1 oz	195	18	0

Egg Substitutes

$^1/_4$ Cup (Equivalent to 1 Egg) ~ Zero Cholesterol

	C	F	Cb
All Whites (Crystal Farms), 1.6 oz	25	0	0
Better 'n Eggs (Crystal Farms):			
Regular, $^1/_4$ cup, 2 oz	30	0	1
Egg Beaters (ConAgra):			
100% Egg White 3 Tbsp	25	0	0
Original, 3 Tbsp, 1.6 oz	25	0	0.5
Southwestern Style, 3 Tbsp, 1.6 oz	20	0	0.5
Egg Replacer (Ener-g), 1.5 tsp	15	0	4
Egg Substitute (Albertson's), $^1/_4$ cup	30	0	1
Naturegg (Burnbrae Farms),			
Simply Egg White, $^1/_4$ cup, 2 oz	30	0	0
Vegan Egg Substitute:			
Aquafaba, $^1/_4$ cup, 2 oz	10	0	2

Liquid from cooked/canned beans or chickpeas. Replaces eggs and egg whites in recipes.
Extra Info: www.aquafaba.com

Other Eggs

	C	F	Cb
Duck, 1 large, 2.5 oz	130	9.5	0
Goose, 1 large, 5 oz	280	19	0
Quail, 3 eggs, 1 oz	42	3	0
Turkey, 1 large, 3 oz	135	9.5	0
Turtle, 1 egg, 1.75 oz	75	5	0

Omega-3 Fat Enriched

	C	F	Cb
Egg·Land's Best, 1 large	60	4	0
Horizon Organic, 1 large	70	4.5	1

Note: Cholesterol content is the same as regular eggs.

Cooked Eggs

	C	F	Cb
Boiled Egg: *Same as Raw Egg*			
Hard-Cooked, Small, peeled	65	4	0
Fried Egg:			
With fat: 1 large egg	105	9	0.5
2 small eggs	175	13	1
No fat/nonstick pan, 1 large	75	5	0.5
Deviled Egg, 2 halves	145	13	0.5
Eggs Benedict, (2),			
on Toast or English Muffin	860	56	25
Eggs Florentine, (2),			
on Toast or English Muffin	890	59	25
Pickled Egg, 1 large	80	5.5	0
Poached Egg, 1 large	65	4	0
Quiche (Homemade):			
Egg & Bacon, 1 slice, 5.3 oz	580	43	27
Ham & Cheese, 1 slice, 5.3 oz	475	33	29
Scotch Egg, 1 egg	300	21	16
Scrambled Eggs:			
1 large egg:			
With 1 Tbsp milk + 1 tsp fat	120	9	1
With 1 Tbsp skim milk/no fat	85	5.5	1
2 large eggs:			
With 2 Tbsp milk + 2 tsp fat	260	20	2
With 2 Tbsp skim milk, w/o fat	180	11	2

Omelets

	C	F	Cb
1 Egg:			
Plain (with 1 tsp fat)	125	10	0.5
With: ½ oz cheese	175	15	0.5
$^1/_2$ oz cheese + $^1/_2$ oz ham	200	16	0.5
2 Eggs:			
Plain (with 2 tsp fat)	250	20	1
With: 1 oz cheese	360	29	2
1 oz cheese +1 oz ham	410	32	2
3 Eggs:			
Plain (with 1 Tbsp fat)	360	29	1.5
With: 2 oz cheese	580	47	2.5
2 oz cheese+2 oz ham	680	53	2.5
Extras, Tomato/Onion/Veggies, 2 oz	20	0	4.5
Egg Substitute (EggBeaters):			
2 eggs ($^1/_2$ cup) + 1 tsp fat	100	4	2
3 eggs ($^3/_4$ cup) + 2 tsp fat	160	8	3
Extras: 1 oz Cheese	110	9	1
1 oz Ham	50	3	1

Egg Nog

	C	F	Cb
Average all Brands,			
$^1/_2$ cup, 4 oz	170	9.5	17
Borden, Regular, 4 fl.oz	160	8	18
Hood, Golden, $^1/_2$ cup, 4 fl.oz	180	9	22
Horizon, Light/Low-Fat,	130	3	23

Breakfast Sides

	C	F	Cb
Toast:			
Plain, 1 thick slice	85	1	13
With: 2 tsp butter/marg.	155	9	13
3 tsp/1 Tbsp fat	190	13	13
English Muffin:			
Plain, 2 oz	130	1	26
With 3 tsp fat	230	12	26
Bacon, 2 strips	70	5	0
Ham, lean, 2 oz	100	3	0
Hash Brown:			
1/2 cup, 3 oz	125	6.5	14
1 cup serving, 6 oz	250	13	28
Sausages, 2 oz link	180	16	1.5

Frozen Egg Breakfasts

Jimmy Dean:

	C	F	Cb
Breakfast Sandwich: *Per Sandwich*			
Biscuit, Sausage, Egg & Cheese	410	29	26
Croissant, Egg, Red Peppers, Onions			
& Jack Cheese	290	16	27
Muffin, Meat Lovers	480	34	26
Omelets: *Per Omelet*			
Three Cheese	290	23	4
Ham & Cheese	250	19	4

MorningStar Farms,

	C	F	Cb
Breakfast Muffin Sandwich,			
Veggie Sausage, Egg & Chse	210	8	20

Pillsbury:

	C	F	Cb
Toaster Scrambles:			
Bacon	190	10	18
Bacon & Sausage	190	11	18
Ham	180	10	17

Red Baron:

	C	F	Cb
Biscuit Scrambles:			
Bacon (1), 5.85 oz	440	21	47
Sausage (1), 5.85 oz	430	20	47

Frozen Pancake/Waffles ~ *See Page 132*

Toaster Pastries ~ *See Page 64*

Frozen Egg Rolls

Kahiki: *Each, without sauce*

	C	F	Cb
Chicken; Vegetable, av., 2.3 oz	150	3.5	26
Pork, 2.8 oz	190	5	31

Lotus Restaurant:

	C	F	Cb
Imperial, Chicken/Pork (1)	160	6.5	24
Vegetarian, (1)	120	5	20

Pagoda Express: *Each, with Sauce*

	C	F	Cb
Chicken	160	4	24
Pork	180	7	23
Pork & Shrimp	180	7	23
Vegetable	140	4	24

Fast-Foods/Restaurants

	C	F	Cb
Arby's,			
Bacon, Egg & Cheese Croissant	440	27	29
Au Bon Pain, 2 Egg on Plain Bagel	390	11	51
Bob Evans:			
Omelets, Low Calorie:			
Border Scramble	840	53	55
Western	740	43	52
Bojangles: Cheddar 'Bo'	510	31	42
Bacon, Egg & Cheese Biscuit	480	28	42
Bruegger's:			
Bagel: Egg & Cheese, 6.8 oz	450	14	62
Western, 9.2 oz	560	25	64
Burger King:			
Burrito, Egg-Normous	910	55	73
Croissan'wich:			
Bacon, Egg & Cheese	340	18	30
Ham, Egg & Cheese	330	16	31
King, with Double Sausage	700	51	31
Carl's Jr:			
Burrito: Bacon & Egg	570	35	32
Big Country	740	45	55
Loaded Breakfast	760	48	46
Steak & Egg	630	36	37
Chick-fil-A, Chicken, Egg & Cheese,			
on Sunflower Multigrain Bagel	480	18	51
Del Taco, Bacon Breakfast Burrito	640	36	38
Denny's: *With Hashbrowns, Without Bread*			
Omelette:			
Loaded Veggie	600	43	25
Ultimate	820	66	25
Dunkin Donuts:			
Bagel, Bacon, Egg & Cheese	520	18	67
Croissant, Saus., Egg & Cheese	700	50	41
Eat 'N Park:			
Omelette:			
Ham & Cheese	535	35	5
Meat Lovers	725	55	3
Hardee's:			
Biscuit: Loaded Omelet	490	28	40
Sausage & Egg	560	39	39
IHOP: 2 Eggs, Scrambled	220	17	2
Omelette, Spinach & Mushroom	890	70	20
Jack in the Box:			
Biscuit: Bacon, Egg & Cheese	410	25	26
Saus., Egg & Cheese	535	38	27
McDonald's:			
Biscuit, Bacon, Egg & Cheese, reg.	450	24	40
McMuffin, Egg	300	12	30
Whataburger, Breakfast Platter,			
with Bacon	740	52	36

Quick Guide   C   F   Cb

Butter
Average All Brands

	C	F	Cb
Regular: 1 tsp, 0.2 oz	35	4	0
1 Tbsp, 0.5 oz	100	11	0
2 Tbsp, 1 oz	205	23	0
1 Stick, ½ cup, 4 oz	810	92	0
1 Pound, 2 cups, 16 oz	3255	368	0
Light: Regular, 40% Fat			
1 tsp, 0.2 oz	30	3	0
1 Tbsp, 0.5 oz	70	7.5	0
2 Tbsp, 1 oz	140	15	0
Whipped Butter: Regular			
1 tsp, 0.1 oz	20	2.5	0
1 Tbsp, 0.3 oz	65	7.5	0
1 Stick, 2.7 oz	545	62	0
Whipped Light Butter (Land O Lakes):			
1 tsp, 0.15 oz	15	1.5	0
1 Tbsp, 0.4 oz	45	5	0
2 Tbsp, 0.8 oz	90	10	0

Unsalted ~ *Same as Salted*

Flavored Butter/Spreads
Average All Brands

	C	F	Cb
Honey Butter, (60% Fat):			
1 Tbsp, 0.5 oz	90	8	4
Downey's, 2% Fat,			
1 Tbsp, 0.5 oz	60	1	11
Garlic Butter, (80% Fat):			
1 Tbsp, 0.5 oz	100	11	0
Sweet Cream Butter:			
Land O Lakes: Regual, 1 Tbsp	100	11	0
Honey Butter Spread, 1 Tbsp	70	6	4

Butter & Butter Blends
Per 1 Tablespoon

	C	F	Cb
Challenge: Stick, 0.5 oz	100	11	0
Tub, Whipped, 0.3 oz	70	7	0
Brummel & Brown,			
Spread Made with Yogurt, 0.5oz	45	5	0
Land O'Lakes:			
Sticks, Original, 0.5oz	100	11	0
Tubs, Butter With Olive Oil, 0.5 oz	90	10	0

Ghee (Clarified Butter)   C   F   Cb
(Example ~ *Purity Farms*)
Note: Ghee is 100% fat compared to regular butter (80% fat + 20% water)

	C	F	Cb
1 tsp, 0.2 oz	45	5	0
1 Tbsp, 0.5 oz	120	14	0

Light & Reduced Fat Spreads
Per Tablespoon

	C	F	Cb
bestlife,			
Buttery Spread, 0.5 oz	60	6	0
Benecol: Regular, 0.5 oz	70	8	0
Light, 0.5 oz	50	5	0
Blue Bonnet:			
Stick, Light Spread, 0.5 oz	50	5	0.5
Tub, Orig. Soft Spread, 0.5 oz	60	6	0.5
Country Crock (Shedd's): Stick, 0.5 oz	80	8	0
Tubs: Original Spread, 0.5 oz	50	6	0
Light Spread, 0.5 oz	35	4	0
Churn Style, 0.5 oz	50	6	0
Fleischmann's:			
Orig., Soft Spread, 0.4 oz	60	7	0
Olive Oil Spread, 0.4 oz	60	7	1
Unsalted Spread, 0.4 oz	60	7	0
I Can't Believe It's Not Butter!:			
Tubs: Original Spread, 0.5 oz	60	6	0
Light, 0.5 oz	40	4	0
Olive Oil Spread, 1 Tbsp	60	6	0
Parkay:			
Original Spread, 0.4 oz	70	7	0.5
Spray, 5 sprays	0	0	0
Squeeze Bottle, 0.5 oz	70	8	0
Promise: Activ, Spread, 0.5 oz	45	5	0
Buttery Spread, 0.5 oz	80	8	0
Light Spread, 0.5 oz	45	5	0
Smart Balance:			
Tubs, Buttery Spread:			
Original, 0.4 oz	80	9	0
EVOO, 0.4 oz	60	7	0
Light EVOO, 0.4 oz	50	5	0
Light with Flaxseed Oil. 0.5 oz	50	5	0
Omega 3: Reg., 0.5 oz	80	9	0
Light, 0.5 oz	50	5	0

Butter Substitutes

	C	F	Cb
Butter Buds:			
Butter Flavored: Mix, 1 tsp	5	0	2
Sprinkles, 1 tsp	10	0	2
Earth Balance,			
Original, 1 Tbsp	100	11	0
Molly McButter, 1 tsp	5	0	1
Sunsweet, (Butter/Oil Replacement),			
Lighter Bake, 1 Tbsp, 0.7 oz	35	0	9

F Fats ~ Spreads & Oils ◊ Mayo

Animal Fats/Lards C F Cb

Average All Types
Beef Tallow/Drippings, Lard (Pork),
Chicken, Duck, Goose, Turkey:

		C	F	Cb
1 Tbsp, 0.5 oz		115	13	0
2¼ Tbsp, 1 oz		255	28	0
1 cup, 7.3 oz		1850	205	0
½ pound, 8 oz		2040	227	0

Ghee/Butter/ Oil ~ *See Page 93*

Vegetable Shortening

Average All Types

		C	F	Cb
1 Tbsp, 0.5 oz		115	13	0
2¼ Tbsp, 1 oz		250	28	0
1 cup, 7.3 oz		1810	205	0

Vegetable Oils

Includes almond, avocado, canola, corn, coconut, flaxseed, grapeseed, linseed, mustard, olive, palm, peanut, rice bran, safflower, sesame, sunflower, soybean, wheat germ. Note: Oil is 100% fat.

		C	F	Cb
1 tsp, 0.2 oz		45	5	0
1 Tbsp, 0.5 oz		120	14	0
2 Tbsp, 1 oz		240	28	0
1 cup, 7.3 oz		1930	205	0

Fish Oils

Average All Types
(Includes Cod Liver, Herring, Salmon, Sardines): 1 Tbsp, 0.5 oz **125** **14** **0**

Cooking Sprays/Squeezes

Cooking Sprays: (PAM, Mazola, I Can't Believe It's Not Butter, Weight Watchers, Wesson):

	C	F	Cb
Pam: ¼ second spray	2	0	0
1-3 second spray	6	1	0
I Can't Believe It's Not Butter,			
Original Spray	0	0	0
Parkay, Buttery Spray	0	0	0

Olestra (Olean) C F Cb

Olestra *(Olean)* **0 0 0**
Note: Olean is Proctor & Gamble's brand name for Olestra – a no-calorie cooking oil that gives snacks (like potato chips, tortilla chips and crackers) taste and texture without adding fat or calories.
Examples:
• *Frito-Lay,* Light Products
  (Lays, Ruffles, Tostitos, Doritos)
• *Pringles,* Fat-Free Potato Crisps

Quick Guide C F Cb

Mayonnaise:
Regular: *Per 1 Tbsp, 0.5 oz Unless Indicated*

	C	F	Cb
Average All Brands	90	10	0
Best Foods; Hellman's; Kraft:			
Original/Real	90	10	0
½ cup, 4 oz	720	80	0
Hain, Safflower Mayonnaise	100	11	0
Spectrum, Canola Mayo	100	11	0
Light/Reduced Fat: *Per 1 Tbsp, 0.5 oz*			
Best Foods/Hellman's	35	3.5	1
Kraft, Light/Olive Oil	35	3	1
Smart Balance, Omega	50	5	0
Spectrum, Light Canola Mayo,			
Eggless	35	3.5	0.5
Fat Free:			
Kraft: Original, 1 Tbsp	10	0	2
½ cup, 4 oz	80	0	16
Sugar Free:			
Dukes Mayo, 1 Tbsp	100	12	0

Mayonnaise Style Dressing:
Per 1 Tbsp, 0.5 oz

	C	F	Cb
Best Foods, Sandwich Spread	60	5	2
Kraft:			
Miracle Whip Dressing:			
Original	40	3.5	1
Light	20	1.5	1
Fat Free	15	0	3
Mayo:			
Chipotle	35	3	1
Horseradish-Dijon	35	3	1
Sandwich Shop, Hot & Spicy	100	11	0
Nasoya, Egg & Dairy Free:			
Nayonaise: Regular/Whipped	40	3.5	1
Light	20	1.5	1
Sir Kensington's, Egg/Dairy Free			
Fabanaise (Vegan Mayo)	90	10	0

Quick Guide   C F Cb

Fresh Fish

Low Oil: *Less than 2.5% fat)*
White/Lightly-colored flesh. Examples:
Cod, Flounder, Haddock, Halibut, Mahi Mahi, Perch, Pike, Pollock, Snapper, Sole, Whiting.

	C	F	Cb
Raw, without bones, 4 oz	100	1	0
Steamed, broiled, baked, 4 oz	140	1.5	0
Fried: Lightly floured, 4 oz	210	8	3.5
Breaded, 4 oz	260	12	8
In Batter, 4 oz	320	16	27

Medium Oil: *2.5-5% fat*
Lightly-colored flesh. Examples:
Bluefin Tuna, Catfish, Kingfish, Orange Roughy, Salmon (Pink), Swordfish, Rainbow Trout, Yellowtail.

	C	F	Cb
Raw, without bones, 4 oz	145	7	0
Baked/Broiled, 4 oz	195	8	0
Fried, 4 oz	230	11	8

High Oil: *Over 5% fat*
Darker-colored flesh. Examples:
Albacore Tuna, Mackerel, Salmon (Atlantic/Chinook/Sockeye), Sardines, Trout.

	C	F	Cb
Raw, without bones, 4 oz	220	14	0
Baked/Broiled, 4 oz	275	17	0
Fried, 4 oz	340	23	12

Cooking Yields (Fin Fish):
4 oz Raw wt. = 3.5 oz Cooked weight
4 oz Cooked wt. = 5 oz Raw weight

Calorie & Fat Variations:
The amount of fat/oil in fish varies with the species, season and locality. Within the same fish, fat/oil content is generally higher towards the head.

Fish & Shellfish

Edible Weights: (no bones/shell)

	C	F	Cb
Abalone: Raw, 3 oz	90	0.5	5
Fried, 3 oz	160	6	10
Ahi Tuna, grilled, 6 oz fillet (w/o fat)	235	2	0
Anchovy: Paste, 1 Tbsp, 0.5 oz	45	3	0
Canned in oil, drained, (5), 0.7 oz	40	2	0
Barracuda (Pacific), raw, 4 oz	130	3	0
Basa/Swai, raw, 4 oz fillet	70	2	0
Bass:			
Sea: Raw, 4.6 oz fillet	125	2.5	0
Baked, 3 oz	105	2	0
Striped: Raw, 1 fillet, 5.5 oz	150	3.5	0
Baked, 3 oz	105	3	0
Freshwater: Raw, 3 oz	95	3	0
Baked, 3 oz	125	4	0

Fish & Shellfish (Cont)   C F Cb

Edible Weights: (no bones/shell)

	C	F	Cb
Calamari/Squid:			
Raw, 4 oz	100	1.5	3.5
Baked, 1 cup	190	6.5	5.5
Fried, 3 oz	150	6	7
Catfish:			
Farmed: Raw, 1 fillet 5.6 oz	190	9.5	0
Baked, 1 fillet 5 oz	205	10	0
Wild: Raw, 1 fillet, 5.6 oz	150	4.5	0
Baked, 1 fillet, 5 oz	150	4	0
Breaded, fried, 1 fillet, 3 oz	200	12	7
Caviar, black/red, 1 Tbsp, 16g	40	3	0.5
Clams: Raw (4 large/9 small), 3 oz	70	1	3
Breaded, fried (20 small), 6.6 oz	380	21	20
Canned, drained, $1/2$ cup, 2.8 oz	115	1	0
Steamed (10 small), 3.3 oz	140	2	5
Cod:			
Atlantic: Raw, 4 oz	95	1	0
Baked, 3 oz	90	1	0
Canned, solids & liquid	90	0.5	0
Pacific: Raw, 4 oz	80	0.5	0
Baked, 3 oz	70	0.5	0
Crab:			
Alaska King,			
1 leg, cooked, 4.7 oz	130	2	0
Blue: Raw, 1 crab, 6 oz	150	1	0
Steamed, 3 oz	70	0.5	0
Canned, drained, 6.5 oz can	105	0.5	0
Dungeness: Raw, 1 crab, 5.8 oz	140	1.5	0
Steamed, 4.45 oz	140	1.5	0
Crab Cakes *(Capt. D's)*, (1), 2.8 oz	250	16	16
Crayfish:			
Farmed: Raw, 3 oz	60	1	0
Steamed, 3 oz	75	1	0
Wild: Raw 3 oz	65	1	0
Steamed, 3 oz	70	1	0
Cuttlefish, raw, 3 oz	70	1	1
Dolphinfish ~ *See Mahi-Mahi*			
Eel: Raw, 3 oz	155	10	0
Baked, 3 oz	200	13	0
Fish & Chips *(Red Lobster)*, battered, without condiments	700	33	61
Fish Sandwich *(Burger King)*, without Tartar Sauce	340	9	49
Fish Oil, 1 Tbsp, 0.5 oz	125	14	0
Flounder/Sole:			
Raw, 4 oz	80	2	0
Baked, 3 oz	75	2	0
Frozen Fish ~ *See Pages 114-122*			

Fish & Shellfish (Cont) — C F Cb

Edible Weights: Without Bones or Shell

Item	C	F	Cb
Haddock: Raw, 4 oz	85	0.5	0
Baked, 3 oz	75	0.5	0
Smoked, 3 oz	100	1	0
Halibut:			
Atlantic: Raw, 4 oz	105	1.5	0
Baked, 1/2 fillet, 5.6 oz	175	2.5	0
Herring:			
Atlantic, raw, 4 oz	180	10	0
Canned: Plain, drained, 3 oz	130	8	0
In Tomato Sauce, 3.5 oz	140	8	2
Pickled, 2 pieces, 1 oz	75	5	3
Smoked, kippered, 4 oz	245	14	0
Jellyfish: Raw, 4 oz	30	0	0
Dried, Salted, 1 cup, 2 oz	20	1	0
Ling, raw, 4 oz	100	0.5	0
Lobster, Northern:			
1.5 lb Whole Lobster, edible portion:			
Raw, 6.3 oz	140	1.5	0
Boiled, 5 oz	140	1	0
Lobster Salads, average, 1/2 cup	220	13	5
Lobster Newberg, average, 3/4 cup	360	20	9
Lobster Thermidor, av., 1 serving	370	22	15
Lobster Tail (Rock)			
Red Lobster, grilled/roasted	230	6	2
Lox, Regular/Nova, 2 oz	65	2.5	0
Mackerel, Atlantic: Raw, 4 oz	230	16	0
Baked, 3 oz fillet	225	15	0
Pacific/Jack: Raw, 4 oz	180	9	0
Baked, 3 oz	170	9	0
Spanish: Raw, 4 oz	160	7	0
Baked, 3 oz	135	5.5	0
Mahi-Mahi/Dolphinfish:			
Raw, 4 oz	95	1	0
Baked, 4 oz	125	1	0
Monkfish: Raw, 4 oz	85	1.5	0
Baked, 3 oz	80	2	0
Mullet, Striped: Raw, 4 oz	135	4.5	0
Baked, 3 oz	130	4	0
Mussels:			
Raw: 4 oz (edible wt)	100	2.5	4
1 cup, 5.3 oz (edible weight)	130	3.5	5
Cooked, moist heat, 3 oz	150	4	6
Ocean Perch:			
Atlantic: Raw, 4 oz	90	2	0
Baked, 3 oz	80	1.5	0
Octopus:			
Common: Raw, 4 oz	95	1	3
Boiled, 3 oz	140	2	4
Orange Roughy:			
Raw, 4 oz	85	1	0
Baked, 3 oz	90	1	0

Fish & Shellfish (Cont) — C F Cb

Edible Weights: Without Bones or Shell

Item	C	F	Cb
Oysters, Common, Raw, 3 oz	70	2	4
Eastern:			
Farmed: Raw, 6 medium, 3 oz	50	1.5	5
Cooked, dry heat, 6 med., 2 oz	45	1.5	5
Wild: Raw, 6 medium, 3 oz	45	1.5	3
Cooked, dry heat, 6 med., 2 oz	45	1.5	3
Breaded & Fried, 6 med., 3 oz	175	11	10
Pacific: Raw, 1 medium, 1.8 oz	40	1	3
Steamed, 1 medium, 0.8 oz	40	1	3
Perch ~ *See Ocean Perch*			
Pike: Northern: Raw, 4 oz	100	1	0
Baked, 3 oz	95	1	0
Walleye: Raw, 4 oz	105	1.5	0
Baked, 3 oz	100	1.5	0
Pollock, Atlantic: Raw, 4 oz	105	1	0
Baked, 3 oz	100	1	0
Pompano, Florida, raw, 4 oz	185	11	0
Red Snapper ~ *See Snapper*			
Roe, raw, 2 Tbsp, 1 oz	40	2	0.5
Sablefish: Raw, 4 oz	220	17	0
Smoked, 3 oz	220	17	0
Salmon:			
Atlantic, Farmed: Raw, 4 oz	235	15	0
Baked, 3 oz	175	10	0
Steaks: Raw, 7 oz	410	27	0
Baked, 6 oz	365	22	0
Atlantic, Wild: Raw, 4 oz	160	7	0
Baked, 3 oz	155	7	0
Steaks: Raw, 7 oz	280	13	0
Baked, 6 oz	310	14	0
Chinook: Raw, 4 oz	205	12	0
Baked, 3 oz	195	11	0
Smoked, 3 oz	100	3.5	0
King: Raw, 3.5 oz	185	12	0
Kippered, 3.5 oz piece	265	16	0
Smoked & canned, 3.5 oz	150	6	0
Coho:			
Farmed: Raw, 4 oz	180	8.5	0
Baked, 3 oz	150	7	0
Wild: Raw, 4 oz	165	6.5	0
Steamed, 3 oz	155	6.5	0
Pink/Chum: Raw, 4 oz	145	5	0
Baked, 3.5 oz	155	5.5	0
Canned: Drained solids, 11 oz	435	16	0
Without skin & bones, 8.5 oz	330	10	0
Sockeye: Raw, 4 oz	160	6.5	0
Baked, 3 oz	145	5.5	0
Canned, Drained solids, 3 oz	140	6.5	0
Smoked, 3.5 oz	205	7.5	0
Salmon Cake (1), 3 oz	240	15	6

Fish & Shellfish (Cont) — C, F, Cb

	C	F	Cb
Sardines: Canned, Average all Brands			
Drained of Oil:			
1/4 cup drained, 2.2 oz	130	9	0
3.75 oz can, drained, 3.3 oz	190	11	0
1 large/2 medium, 3/5", 0.8 oz	50	3	0
in Tomato Sauce, 3.8 oz	150	8	3
Sashimi ~ See Japanese Foods, Page 171			
Scallops: Raw, 6 lge/15 small, 3 oz	65	0.5	3
Breaded, Fried (6), 5 oz	385	20	39
Steamed, 3 oz	95	0.5	0
Sea Bass ~ See Bass			
Seafood Salad, Deli Style,			
1/2 cup, 3.5 oz	250	21	11
Shark: Raw, 4 oz	145	5	0
Baked, 4 oz	185	7	0
Batter-dipped, fried, 4 oz	260	16	7
Shrimp:			
Raw: Small/Medium (4), 0.8 oz	15	0	0
Large (4), 1 oz	20	0	0
Breaded & Fried, 4.8 oz	395	24	27
Steamed, in shell, 3 oz	100	1.5	0
Canned, 1 can, 4.5 oz	130	2	0
Snapper: Raw, 4 oz	115	1.5	0
Baked: 3 oz	110	1.5	0
6 oz fillet	220	3	0
Sole: Raw, 4 oz	80	2	0
Baked, 3 oz	75	2	0
Squid ~ see Calamari			
Surimi, (Imitation Crab), 4 oz	110	0.5	17
Swai/Basa, raw, 4 oz	70	2	0
Swordfish: Raw, 4 oz	165	7.5	0
Medium Steak, 6 oz	250	11	0
Baked: Small Steak, 4 oz	205	7	0
Medium Steak, 6 oz	290	13	0
Tilapia: Raw, 4 oz	110	2	0
Baked: 3 oz	110	2.5	0
Trout, Rainbow:			
Farmed: Raw, 4 oz	160	7	0
Baked, 3 oz	145	6.5	0
Wild: Raw, 4 oz	135	4	0
Baked, 3 oz	130	5	0
Tuna:			
Raw: Bluefin, 4 oz	165	5.5	0
Skipjack, Yellowfin, av., 4 oz	120	1	0
Baked: Bluefin, 3 oz	155	5.5	0
Skipjack, Yellowfin, av., 3 oz	110	1	0
Canned: in Water, drained			
Chunk Light: 2 oz	50	1	0
3 oz can	75	1.5	1
5 oz can	125	2.5	1.5

Tuna (Cont): in Water, drained (Cont)	C	F	Cb
Solid White: 2 oz	60	0.5	0
5 oz can	150	1.5	0
7 oz can	210	2	0
in Oil, drained:			
Chunk Light: 2 oz can	80	4	0
5 oz can	200	10	0
Solid White: 2 oz can	90	4	0
6 oz can	270	12	0
Whitefish: Raw, 4 oz	150	6.5	0
Baked, 3 oz	145	6.5	1
Smoked, 3 oz	90	1	0
Whiting: Raw, 4 oz	100	1.5	0
Baked, 3 oz	100	1.5	0
Yellowtail: Raw, 4 oz	165	6	0
Grilled, 3 oz	160	6	0

Other Canned/Packaged Fish

	C	F	Cb
Bumble Bee: Skinless, Boneless			
Mackerel, in oil, drained, 1.9 oz	160	15	0
Pink Salmon, in oil, drained, 2 oz	60	1.5	0
Red Salmon, in oil, drained, 2.2 oz	100	5	0
Sardines, in oil, drained, 3 oz	210	15	0
Tuna Ready-To-Eat Kits: with Crackers:			
Sensations, Tuna Medley:			
Tom. & Basil, 3 oz can & 3oz Crackers	150	2.5	16
Thai Chili, 3 oz can & 3oz Crackers	180	2.5	23
Tuna, Snack on the Run!: with Crackers Kit			
Tuna Salad, 2.9 oz can, w/- Crackers	300	23	18
Tuna, Fat Free w/ Wheat Crackers,			
2.9 oz can	130	2.5	20
Tuna, White Albacore:			
Pouch, in water, 2 oz	70	1.5	0
Solid, in oil, drained, 2 oz	80	2.5	0
Chicken of the Sea:			
Pink Salmon: Skinless/boneless: 3 oz	80	2	0
Traditional, 14.75 oz can, 2.1 oz serve	90	5	0
Sardines, in oil, smoked, 3.75 oz can	150	10	0
Tuna: Lunch Solutions,			
Tuna Salad Cup & Crackers, 3.4 oz	80	0.5	7
To-Go-Cups, Tuna Salad, 2.8 oz	80	0.5	7
Starkist:			
Pouch: Per 2.6 oz Pouch			
Albacore White Tuna in water	80	1.5	0
Chunk, Light, Tuna in water	70	0.5	0
Lunch-To-Go Kit, Chunk Light Tuna			
with Light Mayo & Crackers, 4 oz	230	9	20
Tuna Creations: Per 2.6 oz			
Bold Hot Buffalo Style	70	1	0
Bold Thai Chili Style	90	1	7

Flours & Grains	C	F	Cb
Amaranth Flour, $^1/_2$ cup, 3.5 oz	365	6.5	65
Arrowroot Flour, $^1/_2$ cup, 2.3 oz	230	0	56
Barley: Grain, regular, $^1/_2$ cup, 2.6 oz	255	1	55
Pearled, raw, 3.5 oz	350	1	78
Buckwheat: Grain, $^1/_2$ cup, 3 oz	290	3	61
Flour, whole-groat, $^1/_2$ cup, 2 oz	200	2	42
Groats: Roasted, dry, $^1/_2$ cup, 3 oz	285	2	62
Roasted, cooked, 3.5 oz	80	0.5	17
Bulgur: Dry, $^1/_2$ cup, 2.5 oz	240	1	53
Cooked, $^1/_2$ cup, 3.2 oz	75	0.5	17
Carob Flour, $^1/_2$ cup, 1.8 oz	115	0.5	46
Corn Kernels, cooked, av., $^1/_2$ cup	80	0.5	18
Corn Bran, $^1/_2$ cup, 1.3 oz	85	0.5	33
Corn Flour/Masa, $^1/_2$ cup, 2 oz	215	2.5	43
Corn Grits:			
Dry, $^1/_2$ cup, 2.8oz	290	1	62
Cooked, $^1/_2$ cup, 4.3 oz	70	0.5	15
Corn Germ, toasted, $^1/_2$ cup, 4 oz	100	1.5	22
Cornmeal, average all varieties:			
3 Tbsp, 1 oz	105	0.5	22
$^1/_2$ cup, 2.5 oz	255	1	54
Mixes, same as above	230	1	48
Cornstarch: 1 Tbsp, 0.3 oz	30	0	8
$^1/_2$ cup, 2.3oz	245	0	58
Couscous: Dry, 1 oz	110	0	22
Cooked, 1 cup, 5.5 oz	175	0.5	37
Farina: Dry, $^1/_2$ cup, 3 oz	325	0.5	69
Cooked, $^1/_2$ cup, 4 oz	55	0	12
Flaxseed: Whole, 1 T., 0.3 oz	45	3.5	2
Ground, 2 Tbsp, 0.3 oz	60	4.5	4
Garbanzo, (Chick Pea), $^1/_2$ cup, 1.6 oz	180	3	27
Gluten Free Flour, 3 Tbsp	100	0	24
Matzo Meal, $^1/_2$ cup, 2.2 oz	230	0.5	48
Millet: Raw, $^1/_2$ cup, 3.5 oz	380	4	73
Cooked, $^1/_2$ cup, 3 oz	105	1	21
Oat Bran: Raw, $^1/_3$ cup, 1 oz	75	2	21
Cooked, $^1/_2$ cup, 3.8 oz	45	1	13
Oats, Rolled/Oatmeal:			
Dry/Groats, $^1/_2$ cup, 1.5 oz	160	3	28
Cooked, $^1/_2$ cup, 4.2 oz	75	1	13
Polenta ~ See Cornmeal			
Potato Flour, $^1/_2$ cup, 2.8 oz	285	0.5	66
Psyllium Husks, 1 Tbsp, 0.2 oz	10	0	4
Quinoa: Dry $^1/_2$ cup, 3 oz	320	5	59
Cooked, $^1/_2$ cup, 3.8 oz	130	2	24
Rice Bran, $^1/_2$ cup, 2 oz	180	12	28
Rice Flour, $^1/_2$ cup, 2.8 oz	290	1	63

Flours & Grains (Cont)	C	F	Cb
Rice Polish, $^1/_2$ cup, 3.5 oz	360	0.5	80
Rye Flour:			
Dark, $^1/_2$ cup, 2.3 oz	210	2	44
Light, $^1/_2$ cup, 1.8 oz	190	1	41
Medium, $^1/_2$ cup, 1.8 oz	180	1	40
Rye Grain: $^1/_2$ cup, 3 oz	280	2	59
Flakes, $^1/_4$ cup, 1 oz	100	0.5	21
Semolina Flour, $^1/_2$ cup, 3 oz	300	1	61
Sorghum, $^1/_2$ cup, 3.4 oz	325	3	72
Soy Flour:			
Defatted, 1 cup, 3.5 oz	330	1	38
Low-Fat, 1 cup, 3 oz	325	6	33
Full-Fat, 1 cup, 3 oz	365	17	29
Soy Meal, defatted, 1 cup, 4.3 oz	415	3	49
Spelt Flour, $^1/_2$ cup, 2 oz	190	1	41
Tapioca Pearl:			
Dry, $^1/_2$ cup, 2.7 oz	270	0	67
3 Tbsp, 1 oz	100	0	25
Teff Seed Flour, 2 oz	215	2	42
Tortilla Flour Mix,			
$^1/_2$ cup, 2 oz	220	6	37
Triticale:			
$^1/_2$ cup, 3.4 oz	325	2	70
Flour, wholegrain, $^1/_2$ cup, 2.3 oz	220	1	48
Wheat Bran, unprocessed, $^1/_2$ cup, 1 oz	65	1	19
Wheat Flakes, $^1/_2$ cup, 1.5 oz	160	1	35
Wheat Germ:			
Raw, $^1/_4$ cup, 1 oz	105	3	15
Toasted, $^1/_4$ cup, 1 oz	110	3	14
Wheat Flour:			
White, All Purpose/Self-Rising:			
1 level Tbsp, 0.3 oz	30	0	6
$^1/_2$ cup, 2.2 oz	230	0.5	48
1 cup, 4.4 oz	455	1.5	95
Whole Wheat, 1 cup, 4.2 oz	405	2	87

FRUIT
TIME

Fruit ~ Fresh

Weights As Purchased

	C	F	Cb
Apples, all varieties, average:			
Whole, with skin:			
1 small, 4 oz	55	0	14
1 medium, 5.5 oz	75	0	19
1 large, 8 oz	110	0	28
1 extra large, 11 oz	145	0	36
Flesh only, no skin or core: 1 oz	15	0	3.5
Slices, 1 cup, 4 oz	55	0	14
Candy/Caramel Apple, 1 med., 6.5 oz	245	4	54
Chiquita, Apple Bites, 14 slices, 5 oz	80	0	20
Apricots: 1 small, 1.5oz	20	0	4
1 medium, 2 oz	25	0	6
1 large, 3 oz	40	0	10
1 extra large, 4 oz	50	0	12
Asian Pear, (Nashi Fruit), 1 med., 7 oz	85	0	21
Avocado:			
Fuerte (Florida) variety:			
1/4 medium, 2.7 oz pulp	90	7.5	6
1/2 medium, 5.4 oz pulp	180	15	12
Mashed, 2 Tbsp, 1 oz	35	3	2
Hass variety (Californian/Mexican):			
Cubes, 1/2 cup, 2.5 oz	120	11	6
Mashed: 2 Tbsp, 1 oz	50	4	2
1/4 cup, 2 oz	95	8	5
Pulp: 1/4 medium, 1.5 oz	70	6.5	3
1/2 medium, 3 oz	140	13	7
1 medium (8.5 oz whole), 6 oz	280	26	14
Salad slices (3), 1 oz	50	4	2

Note: The fat of avocados is heart-healthy. Avocados are very low in carbs ~ most is fiber. This benefits blood sugar and cholesterol levels. Use in place of butter and other high-fat spreads.

	C	F	Cb
Banana:			
Weight with skin:			
1 baby, 3 oz	50	0	12
1 small (5"), 4 oz	65	0	16
1 medium (7"), 5 oz	80	0	20
1 large (8"), 8 oz	120	0	30
1 extra large (9"), 9 oz	135	0	34
Flesh only, weight without skin:			
Mashed, 1/2 cup, 4 oz	100	0	25
Slices, 1/2 cup, 2.5 oz	65	0	16
Green Bananas, weight with skin:			
1 medium (7"), 5 oz	75	0	18
1 large (8"), 7 oz	110	0	27
Blackberries, 1 cup, 5 oz	60	0.5	14
Blueberries: 1/4 cup, 1 oz	15	0	4
1 cup or 1/2 pint container, 5 oz	80	0	20
1 pint container, 10 oz	160	0	40

	C	F	Cb
Boysenberries, 1 cup, 4.5 oz	60	4.5	14
Breadfruit, 1/2 cup, 4 oz	115	0	30
Cactus Fruit:			
1 small, 2 oz	15	0	4
1 medium, 5 oz	40	0	9
1 large, 7 oz	55	0	13
Pulp, no skin, 1 cup, 5.3 oz	60	0	14
Cantaloupe: Flesh, without skin, 1 oz	10	0	2
Pieces/Balls, 1 cup, 5.5 oz	55	0	13
Slices, 1/2 circle, without rind:			
1 thin (buffet), 1/8", 0.5 oz	5	0	1
1 medium (1/4"), 1 oz	10	0	2
1 thick (1/2"), 2 oz	20	0	5
Wedges, length cut, without skin:			
1 thin, 1/16 medium, 2 oz	20	0	5
1 thick, 1/8 medium, 4 oz	40	0	9
Whole, weight with seeds and skin:			
1/2 small, 20 oz	195	1	46
1/2 medium, 28 oz	270	1.5	65
1/2 large, 2.5 lb	370	2	90
Cape Gooseberries, 1 cup, 5 oz	70	1	15
Cherimoya: Pulp, 1/2 cup, 3 oz	60	0	14
1 Fruit (11 oz), 8 oz edible	170	1	40
Cherries, (Red/White), sweet, raw:			
6 medium or 4 large, 2 oz	30	0	7
1 cup, 4.5 oz	75	0	18
1/2 lb quantity	130	0	32
Sour, red, raw, 1 cup, 4 oz	50	0	12
Clementine, 1 medium, 2.6 oz	35	0	9
Coconut, raw:			
Young, sweet,			
Pieces: 1 piece (2" x 2"), 1.5 oz	35	2	4
1/2 cup, 3.5 oz	80	5	9
Mature, hard, 1 piece (2"x 2"), 1.5 oz	160	15	6
Crabapples, slices, 1/2 cup, 2 oz	40	0	11
Cranberries, fresh, 1/4 cup, 1 oz	25	0	6.5
Custard Apple ~ *See Cherimoya*			
Dates: Medium (1), 0.3 oz	20	0	5
Large Medjool (1), 0.5 oz	40	0	10
Extra Large Medjool (1), 0.9 oz	65	0	16
Chopped, 1/2 cup, 3 oz	240	0	58
Dragon Fruit, (Pitahaya):			
1 medium, 4"long, 12 oz	60	0	12
1 large, 5"long, 16 oz	80	0	18
Durian, pulp, 4 oz	165	6	31
Elderberries, 1/2 cup, 2.5 oz	55	0.5	13

Weights As Purchased	C	F	Cb
Feijoa, (Pineapple Guava), 1 medium, 2 oz	30	0.5	5.5
Figs, green/black:			
1 medium, 2 oz	40	0	10
1 large, 3 oz	60	0	15
Gooseberries, raw, 1 cup, 5 oz	65	1	15
Grapefruit, all varieties, average:			
1/2 fruit, 10 oz (6 oz flesh)	55	0	13
1 cup sections w/ juice, 8 oz	75	0	18
Grapes: Average, 1 cup, 5.5 oz	105	0	28
1 small bunch, 4 oz	80	0	20
1 medium bunch, 7 oz	140	0	36
1 large bunch, 16 oz	315	0	82
Granadilla, pulp, 1/2 cup, 4 oz	110	0	27
Guanabana, pulp, 1/2 cup, 4 oz	75	0	19
Guava, 1 medium, 4 oz	80	1	16
Honeydew:			
1 slice, 3/4" thick, 3 oz	30	0	7
1 wedge (1/8 of 7" diameter), 12 oz (with rind)	80	0	20
Cubes/Balls, 1 cup, 6 oz	60	0	14
1/2 small (41/2 lb whole)	180	0.5	42
1/2 medium (6lb whole)	230	1	56
Honey Murcots, 1 only, 5 oz	45	0	11
Jaboticaba, 1 cup, 5.5 oz	55	0	14
Jackfruit, flesh, 1/8, 4 oz	105	0	27
Kiwano, 1/2 medium, 5 oz	35	0	8
Kiwifruit:			
1 Medium, 2.7 oz	45	0	11
1 Large, 3.2 oz	55	0	13
Langsat, Duku, 1 medium, 2 oz	25	0	5
Lemons: 1 medium, 5oz	20	0	4
1 wedge, 1 oz	5	0	1
Limes, 1 medium, 2.4 oz	20	0	7
Loganberries, frozen, 1/2 cup, 2.5 oz	40	0	9
Longans, 5 fruit, 0.5oz	10	0	2.5
Loquats, 4 fruit, 2.3 oz	30	0	8
Lychees, 4 fruit, 2.3 oz	30	0	7
Mamey Apple, cubes, 1 cup, 6 oz	85	1	20
Mandarin Orange:			
1 small, 3 oz	35	0	9
1 medium, 4 oz	45	0	11
1 large, 6 oz	50	0	13
Mango:			
Slices, 1/2 cup, 3 oz	55	0	14
1 small mango, 7 oz	90	0.5	24
1 medium: 10 oz	130	0.5	34
Side cheek, 4 oz	60	0	14
1 large, 17 oz	220	1	58
1 extra large, 24 oz	310	1.5	82
Marionberries, 1 cup, 5 oz	75	1	15

Weights As Purchased	C	F	Cb
Melons, all varieties, average, cubes/balls, 1 cup, 6 oz	60	0	14
Mulberries, 20 fruit, 1 oz	15	0	3
Nashi Fruit/Asian Pear, 1 med. 7 oz	85	0	21
Nectarines: 1 medium, 5oz	60	0	14
1 large, 7 oz	80	0	18
Oheloberries, 1/2 cup, 2.5 oz	20	0	5
Olives, Pickled: Green, 10 lge, 1.5 oz	60	6.5	1.5
Ripe, Greek Style, 10 medium, 1 oz	70	6	4
Ripe (Black) Californian:			
1 small/medium	5	0	0.2
1 large/extra large	6	0.5	0.5
1 jumbo	7	0.5	0.5
1 colossal	11	1	0.5
Oranges, all varieties, average, weights with skin:			
1 small, (2.5" diam.), 5 oz	45	0	11
1 medium (3") 7 oz	75	0	18
1 large, (3.5") 10 oz	105	0	25
1 extra large, (4"), 14 oz	130	0	30
Flesh/Pulp only, 1 cup, 6 oz	85	0	21
Peel, 1 Tbsp	0	0	0
California Navel (3"), 7 oz	70	0	17
California Valencia, 1 medium (23/4" diam.) 6 oz	60	0	14
Florida Orange, 1 med., 7 oz	70	0	17
Sunkist Navel, large, 14 oz	130	0	30
Papaya:			
1" pieces, 1 cup, 5 oz	60	0	15
1 medium, 16 oz	120	0	30
Green (unripe), 1/2 cup, 3.5 oz	20	0	5
Passionfruit:			
1 small, 1.5 oz	15	0	3
1 large, 2.7 oz	30	0	6
Pulp, 1/2 cup, 4 oz	110	0	27
Peaches: 1 baby/donut, 3 oz	30	0	7
1 small, 5 oz	50	0	12
1 medium, 6 oz	60	0	14
1 large, 7 oz	70	0	16
1 extra large, 9 oz	90	0	21
Pears, all varieties, average:			
1 mini, 2.5 oz	35	0	8
1 small, 5 oz	75	0	18
1 medium, 7 oz	100	0	25
1 large, 9 oz	130	0	33
1 extra large, 12 oz	170	0	42
Pepino, 1/2 medium, 4 oz	20	0	4
Persimmons: Native, 1 oz	35	0	9
Japanese (21/2"d. x 21/2"h), 7 oz	120	0	30
Maui, seedless, 1 medium, 5 oz	100	0	25

Weights As Purchased	C	F	Cb
Pineapple, average all varieties:			
Weights without skin:			
1 thin slice ($^1/_2$"), 2 oz	30	0	7
1 thick slice ($^3/_4$"), 3 oz	40	0	10
1 cup, chunks, 6 oz	80	0	20
Whole fruit, wt with skin:			
Baby/Mini, 16 oz	150	0	39
Medium size, 3 lbs	450	1	118
Canned ~ *See Page 102*			
Pitanga, (Surinam-Cherry) (5), 1.2 oz	10	0	2
Plaintain:			
Fresh/Raw, weight with skin:			
1 medium, 10 oz	220	0	55
Slices, 1 cup, 5 oz	180	0	44
Cooked:			
Mashed, $^1/_2$ cup, 3.5 oz	115	0	30
Slices, 1 cup, 5.5 oz	180	0	47
Fried in oil: 10 slices ($^1/_4$"), 2 oz	160	6	26
1 cup, 4.2 oz	360	14	58
Plums, all varieties, average:			
1 mini/Damson, (1" diam), 0.5 oz	10	0	1.5
1 small (2"), 2.3oz	30	0	7
1 medium ($2^1/_2$"), 3.5 oz	45	0	10
1 large (3"), 5 oz	60	0	14
Plumcot, 1 medium, 6 oz	75	0	18
Pomegranate:			
1 small (3"), 5.5 oz	70	1	15
1 medium ($3^1/_2$"), 10 oz	125	2	27
1 large (4"), 16 oz	230	3	50
Seeds/Arils, $^1/_4$ cup, 2 oz	40	1	10
Pomelo, flesh, $^1/_2$ cup, 3.5 oz	35	0	9
Prickly Pear ~ *See Cactus Fruit*			
Quince, 1 medium, 3.5 oz	55	0	14
Rambutan/Rambotang,			
Red/Yellow, 1 medium, 2 oz	15	0	4
Raspberries: $^1/_2$ cup, 2 oz	30	0	7
10 raspberries, 0.8 oz	10	0	2
1 cup, 4.3 oz	65	1	15
1 pint, 11 oz	160	2	37
Sapodilla: 1 medium, 6 oz	140	2	34
Pulp, 1 cup, 8.5 oz	200	2.5	45
Sapote:			
Black: 1 medium, 4.5 oz	60	0	14
Pulp only, $^1/_2$ cup, 4 oz	100	1	22
Mamey, piece, 1 cup, 6 oz	220	1	50
Satsuma Tangerine, 1 medium, 3 oz	45	0	11
Soursop, pulp, 1 cup, 8 oz	150	0.5	38
Starfruit, (Carambola):			
1 medium, ($3^1/_2$" long), 3 oz	30	0	6
1 large ($4^1/_2$"), 4.5 oz	40	0	8
Strawberries: 1 cup, 5.5 oz	50	0.5	12
6 medium/3 large, 2 oz	20	0	4
1 pint container, heaping, 16 oz	130	0	32
Chocolate dipped, 1 large	45	2.5	6

Weights As Purchased	C	F	Cb
Sugar-Apple (Sweetsop),			
pulp, $^1/_2$ cup, 4 oz	120	0	28
Sugar Cane:			
Unpeeled, 1 baton (7" long), 4 oz	30	0	7
Peeled, 1 small stick (3"), 2 oz	35	0	8
Tamarillo, 1 medium, 3 oz	20	0	3
Tamarind: 1 fruit (3"x1")	5	0	1.5
Pulp, $^1/_2$ cup, 2 oz	140	0.5	37
Tangelo: 1 small, 4 oz	55	0	13
1 medium, 5 oz	70	0	17
1 large, 7 oz	95	0	23
Tangerine, 1 med., ($2^1/_2$" diam.), 4 oz	50	0	13
Tangor, 1 medium, 4 oz	35	0	7
Tomatillos:			
3 medium, 3.5 oz	35	0.5	6
1lb (16 oz) quantity	160	2	27
Tomatoes:			
1 small ($2^1/_4$" diameter), 3 oz	15	0	3
1 medium ($2^3/_4$"), 5 oz	25	0	5
Sliced: 2 thin slices, 1 oz	5	0	1
2 thick ($^3/_8$"), 2 oz	10	0	2
Wedge, $^1/_4$, 1.3 oz	6	0	1
1 large ($3^1/_2$"), 8 oz	40	0.5	9
1 extra large (4"), 12 oz	60	0.5	14
Cherry: 4 medium, 2 oz	10	0	2
1 cup, 5 oz	25	0	6
Grape, 5 medium, 2 oz	10	0	2
Yellow Tear Drop, 3 medium, 1 oz	5	0	2
Canned Tomatoes/Products ~ *See Page 144*			
Tree Tomato/Tamarillo, 3 oz	20	0	5
Ugli Fruit, Tangelo type, 5 oz	40	0	8
Watermelon:			
Flesh only, weights without skin:			
1 thin slice ($^1/_2$"), $^1/_4$ circle, 3 oz	25	0	6
1 thick slice (1"): $^1/_4$ circle, 6 oz	50	0	12
$^1/_2$ circle, 12 oz	100	1	24
Buffet Slice, small, thin, 1 oz	8	0	2
Cubes or Balls, 1 cup, 5.5 oz	45	0	11
Round Seedless Melon, weight with skin:			
Medium size, 13 lb, (8" diam.):			
whole melon, 13 lb	1160	5	280
wedge, $^1/_8$ whole, 26 oz	145	1	35
Mini size, 6 lb, (6.5" diam.):			
whole melon, 6 lb	480	2.5	110
wedge, $^1/_8$ whole, 12 oz	60	0	14

Dried Fruit

	C	F	Cb
Apples, 5 rings, 1 oz	80	0	19
Apricots, 8 halves, 1 oz	65	0	16
Banana Chips, 1/3 cup, 1 oz	180	9	16
Banana Flakes, 4 Tbsp, 1 oz	80	0	20
Cranberries (Craisins):			
Original, 1/4 cup	130	0	33
Reduced Sugar, 1/4 cup	100	0	31
Chocolate Covered, 1/4 cup, 2 oz	180	8	28
Dates ~ See Dates in Fresh Fruit			
Figs, 3 medium figs, 1 oz	90	0	23
Goji Berries, 3 Tbsp, 1 oz	100	0	21
Mango Slices, 5 pieces, 1.4 oz	25	0	6
Papaya Spears, 2 pieces, 1.4 oz	120	0	30
Peaches, 2 halves, 1 oz	60	0	15
Pears, 3 halves, 2 oz	140	0.5	34
Plums (Sunsweet), (5), 1.4 oz	100	0	24
Prunes/Dried Plums:			
with pits, 3 medium, 1 oz	70	0	17
without pits, 4 medium, 1 oz	70	0	17
Cooked: with sugar, 1/2 cup, 5 oz	155	0	38
without sugar, 1/2 cup, 4.5 oz	135	0	33
Raisins: 2 Tbsp, 1 oz pack	85	0	20
1/2 cup, 2.8 oz	220	0.5	56
White Mulberries, 1 oz	90	0.5	22

Candied/Glazed Fruit

	C	F	Cb
Apricot, 1 medium, 1 oz	70	0	17
Cherry, Maraschino (1)	8	0	2
Citron/Fruit Peel, 1 oz	85	0	20
Ginger, 1 oz	90	0	21
Pineapple, 1 slice, 1.3 oz	120	0	29
Tamarind, dried, sweetened, 1 oz	70	0	17

Fruit Leather Rolls

	C	F	Cb
Betty Crocker: Fruit By The Foot,			
1 roll, 0.8 oz	80	0	17
Fruit Gushers, 1 oz	90	1	20
Fruit Roll-Ups, 1 roll	50	1	12
Stretch Island, Leathers, 1 pouch, 0.5 oz	45	0	12

Canned/Bottled Fruit

Solids & Liquids:
Per 1/2 Cup, 4 1/2 oz Unless indicated

	C	F	Cb
Apricots/Peaches/Pears:			
in juice, light	60	0	15
in heavy syrup	105	0	28
in water/diet	35	0	8
Black/Blueberries:			
in heavy syrup	120	0	30
in light syrup	110	0	26

Canned/Bottled Fruit (Cont)

	C	F	Cb
Cherries, pitted:			
in heavy syrup	105	0	27
in light syrup	85	0	22
in water	55	0	15
Maraschino, 1 oz	50	0	12
Fruit Cocktail/Salad:			
in heavy syrup	95	0	25
in juice, light	60	0	16
in water/diet	35	0	10
Gooseberries, light syrup	90	0	24
Grapefruit, in light syrup	75	0	20
Lychees, 1/2 cup, 4.5 oz	105	0	26
Mixed Fruit: in fruit juices/light syrup	70	0	18
in heavy syrup	90	0	24
in water/diet	40	0	10
Pineapple, all varieties:			
in heavy syrup, 4.3 oz	110	0	26
in own juice, 4 oz	60	0	15
Prunes: with syrup, 3 oz	90	0	23
Stewed in water, 1/2 cup	135	0	35

Fruit Snack Cups

	C	F	Cb
Deli/Take-Out: Small, 6 oz	70	0	16
Large, 12 oz	140	0	32
Yogurt and Fruit Cup, 15 oz	380	4.5	75
Del Monte:			
Fruit & Veggie Fusions, all flav., 4 oz	70	0	17
Fruit Refreshers, average, 7 oz	95	0	24
Fruit Snack Cups in Gel, av., 4.5 oz	80	0	20
Light Fruit Cups, in Gel, av.,4.5 oz	50	0	12
Dole:			
Fruit Bowls In 100% Juice: *Per 4 oz Container*			
Diced Pears	90	0	22
Mixed Fruit	80	0	19
Fruit in Gel: *Per 4.3 oz Container*			
Mixed Fruit, in Black Cherry Gel	90	0	24
Average other fruits, in various Gels	95	0	24

Apple & Fruit Sauces

	C	F	Cb
Apple Sauce:			
Regular/sweetened, 2 Tbsp, 1 oz	20	0	6
4 oz package	90	0	22
Cranberry, Jellied, 1/4 cup	110	0	25
Fruit Sauces & Purees:			
All fruit types, average: 2 Tbsp, 1 oz	25	0	6
1/2 cup, 4 oz	100	0	24
Mott's:			
Apple Sauce: Orig., sweeetened, 4 oz	90	0	24
Other Fruit Flavors, sweetened, 4 oz	90	0	23
Unsweetened Apple, 3.9 oz	50	0	13
Ocean Spray,			
Jellied Cranberry Sce, 3.5 oz	160	0	40

Quick Guide

Ice Cream
Average all Flavors:

Regular (10% fat):
Examples: Dreyer's Grand, Hood, Friendly's

	C	F	Cb
½ cup, 4 fl.oz	140	7	16
1 cup, 8 fl.oz	280	14	32
1 pint, 16 fl.oz	560	28	64

Rich/Premium (16-17% fat):
Examples: Baskin Robbins, Ben & Jerry's, Haagen-Dazs

½ cup, 4 fl.oz	250	16	24
1 cup, 8 fl.oz	500	32	48
1 pint, 16 fl.oz	1000	64	96

Reduced-Fat/Light (5% fat):
Examples: Breyers ½ The Fat, Friendly's Light, Hood Light

½ cup, 4 fl.oz	140	5	21
1 cup, 8 fl.oz	280	10	42
1 pint, 16 fl.oz	560	20	84

Fat-Free:
Example: Breyers

½ cup, 4 fl.oz	90	0	21
1 cup, 8 fl.oz	180	0	42
1 pint, 16 fl.oz	360	0	84

Scoop Shops:
Average all Brands
Add extra for cone (see next column)

Kids, 3 fl.oz	125	8	12
Regular, 6 fl.oz	250	16	24
Large, 9 fl.oz	375	24	36

Soft Serve:
Average all Brands

Regular: ½ cup, 4 fl.oz	255	15	25
1 cup, 8 fl.oz	510	30	50
Light: ½ cup, 4 fl.oz	145	3	25
1 cup, 8 fl.oz	290	6	50

Quick Guide

Frozen Yogurt
Average all Brands

	C	F	Cb
Hard: Low-Fat, ½ cup	110	3	19
Non-Fat, ½ cup	110	0	24
Soft: Low-Fat, ½ cup	120	4	17
Non-Fat, ½ cup	100	0	30

Brands ~ *See Ice Cream & Novelties Section*

Quick Guide

Gelato/Ices/Frozen Custard
Gelato: *Per ½ Cup*

	C	F	Cb
Milk base: Vanilla	160	6	25
Chocolate Hazelnut	230	15	21
Water base, ½ cup	100	0	26

Frozen Custard, Choc./Vanilla, av:

½ cup	210	11	23
Single Scoop, 5 oz wt	300	15	38
Double Scoop, 10 oz wt	600	30	76

Ice (Milk base): *Average all flavors*

Hard (4% fat), ½ cup	100	3	15
Soft Serve (3% fat), ½ cup	110	2	19
Shaved Ice, average, 12 fl.oz	160	0	40
Sherbet, average, ½ cup	110	1.5	22
Sorbet, Fruit, fat free, ½ cup	70	0	19
Fruit Ice Pops	80	0	20

Sundaes

Baskin Robbins:

Classic: Banana Royale	680	33	90
Brownie	810	42	100
Classic Banana	970	39	146
Denny's,			
Banana Split, 15 oz	760	30	116

Toppings ~ *See Page 195*
McDonald's:
Sundaes:

Hot Caramel, 6.4 oz	380	11	51
Hot Fudge, 6.3 oz	380	14	43
Toppings, Peanuts, 0.3 oz	50	4	2

Ice Cream Cones & Cups

Average all Brands

Wafer Cone/Cup, average	20	0	4
Sugar Cone, average	50	0	14
Waffle Cone:			
Small	50	1	10
Large	90	0.5	19
Brands:			
Comet, Sugar Cone	50	0	11
Keebler, Sugar Cone	50	0	10
Oreo, Chocolate Cone	50	1	10

Ice Cream ~ Brands ⓒ ⓕ ⓒᵇ

Amy's:

Non Dairy Frozen Dessert: *Per ½ Cup*

	C	F	Cb
Chocolate; Vanilla, average, 3.3 oz	175	12	15
Mint /Mocha Choc. Chip, av., 3.5 oz	230	16	20

Baskin-Robbins ~ *See Fast-Foods Section*

Ben & Jerry's:

Scoop Shop Ice Cream: *Hand Scooped, 3 oz Serving*

	C	F	Cb
Americone Dream	240	13	26
Bourbon Brown Butter	240	13	27
Butter Pecan	250	19	17
Choc. Chip Cookie Dough	230	13	26
Chocolate Fudge Brownie	220	11	26
Chunky Monkey	240	15	24
Coconut Seven Layer Bar	250	16	24
Coffee, Coffee, BuzzBuzzBuzz	260	17	23
Mint Chocolate Chunk	220	14	22
Strawberry Cheesecake	200	12	22
Sweet Cream & Cookies	210	12	23
Vanilla Toffee Bar Crunch	260	17	22

Ice Cream, 1 Pint Tubs: *Per ½ Cup*

	C	F	Cb
Banana Split	250	14	28
Cherry Garcia	260	15	27
Chubby Hubby	340	21	33
Everything But The; PB FudgeCore, av.	305	19	29
Milk & Cookies	280	17	28
Peanut Butter Cup	370	26	29
Salted Caramel Core	270	14	31
Red Velvet Cake	260	14	29
S'mores	310	16	36
Strawbery Cheesecake	260	15	28
Triple Caramel Chunk	270	15	32
Vanilla Caramel Fudge	290	16	33

Non Dairy: Chunky Monkey

	C	F	Cb
Chunky Monkey	260	14	31
Chocolate Fudge Brownie	200	11	23
Coffee Caramel Fudge	240	12	31
PB & Cookies	290	17	31

Fro Yo Frozen Yogurt: *Per ½ Cup*

	C	F	Cb
Cherry Garcia	170	3	32
Chocolate Fudge Brownie	180	2.5	35
Half Baked	180	3	35
Pfish Food, 3.6 oz	250	7	42
Greek: Peach Melba	130	4	22
Raspberry	140	5	21
Sorbet, all flavors	80	0	20

Blue Bunny: ⓒ ⓕ ⓒᵇ

Premium Ice Cream: *Pint Container*

	C	F	Cb
Banana Split, 2.65 oz	160	7	23
Bunny Tracks, 2.6 oz	190	11	22
Chocolate, 2.3 oz	130	7	17
Cocoa Bunny, 2.6 oz	170	8	22
Cookies 'n Cream, 2.3 oz	150	7	20

Sweet Freedom: *Per ½ cup*

	C	F	Cb
Bunny Tracks, 2.5 oz	140	7	23
Butter Pecan, 2.53 oz	110	4.5	19
Double Strawberry, 2.53 oz	90	2.5	20

Note: Carbohydrate figures include 4-6 g sugar alcohols

Frozen Yogurt: *Per ½ cup*

	C	F	Cb
Caramel Praline Crunch	130	4	21
Strawberry Banana	100	2	20
Vanilla Bean, 2.32 oz	100	2.5	18

Bars/Pops ~ *See Page 108*

Breyers:

Original Ice Cream: *Per ½ cup*

	C	F	Cb
Butter Pecan, 2.2 oz	140	6	18
Cherry Van.; Cookies & Crm, av., 2.3 oz	130	4	22
Chocolate Truffle, 2.36 oz	170	9	21
Mint Chocolate Chip, 2.4 oz	150	8	17
Nat. Strawberry, 2.3 oz	110	5	14
Salted Caramel, 2.2 oz	130	3.5	23
Vanilla, Chocolate, 2.2 oz	130	7	16
Fat Free, av. all flavors	90	0	21

Half The Fat: *Per ½ Cup*

	C	F	Cb
Cookies & Cream, 2.1 oz	120	4	20
Creamy Vanilla, 2 oz	100	3	17

No Added Sugar Dairy Dessert: *Per ½ cup*

	C	F	Cb
Butter Pecan, 2 oz	100	5	13
Salted Caramel Swirl, 2 oz	90	4	16
Vanilla Chocolate Strawberry, 2 oz	85	3.5	14

Note: Carbohydrate figures include 1-6g sugar alcohol and 0-2g fiber

Blasts!: *Per ½ Cup*

	C	F	Cb
Girl Scout Cookies, Thin Mint, 2.2 oz	140	4.5	23
Mrs Field's, 2.1 oz	140	5	23
Oreo, Cookies & Cream Mint, 2.1 oz	130	4.5	22
Waffle Cone, w/ Choc. Chips, 2.2oz	140	5	23
CarbSmart, average all flav., ½ cup	115	6	14

Note: Carbohydrate figures include 5g sugar alcohol and 4g fiber

Bruster's:

	C	F	Cb
Ice Cream, Banana; Black Raspb., av., 5 oz	285	14	37

Fat Free, No Added Sugar:

	C	F	Cb
Coffee; Sea Salt Caramel, av., 5 oz	175	0	36
Fudge Ripple,; Mint with Fudge, 5 oz	200	0	43
Vanilla, Caramel Swirl, 5 oz	170	0	36

Frozen Yogurt: Chocolate, 5 oz

	C	F	Cb
Mint Chip; Peanut Butter, 5 oz	175	7	24

Ice Cream ~ Brands (Cont)   C   F   Cb

Carvel Ice Cream ~ *See Fast-Foods Section*
Coldstone Creamery ~ *See Fast-Foods Section*
Dairy Queen/Brazier ~ *See Fast-Foods Section*
Dannon:

	C	F	Cb
Oikos Greek Frozen Yogurt: *Four Pack*			
Key Lime, 5.3 oz	150	4.5	16
Lemon Meringue, 5.3 oz	150	4.5	15
Average other flavors	150	5	15
YoCream Frozen Yogurt(Yogurt Shops): *Small 3 oz Cup*			
Premium, Peanut Butter	120	4	19
Custard, Vanilla	170	9	18
Low Fat: Chocolate Caramel Turtle	120	1.5	25
Dulce De Leche; Dutch Choc., av.	110	1.5	22
French Vanilla; Sweet Coconut, av.	110	1.5	21
Fudge Brownie Batter	110	0.5	24
No Sugar Added Nonfat:			
Cheesecake	80	0	18
Praline	90	0	18
Raspberry	80	0	17
Strawberry Banana	80	0	18

Note: Carbohydrate figure includes 0-5g sugar alcohol

Dippin' Dots:

	C	F	Cb
Original Dots: *Per ½ Cup*			
Banana Split	160	8	20
Caramel Brownie Sundae	190	9	23
Cookies 'n Cream	200	11	22
Cotton Candy	160	8	18
Mint Chocolate	170	8	21
Strawberry	160	8	18
Vanilla	160	8	18

Dove:

	C	F	Cb
Ice Cream: *Per ½ Cup*			
Mint/Vanilla Choc. Chunk	180	11	17
Unconditional Chocolate	200	12	23

Dreyer's/Edy's:

	C	F	Cb
Classic Ice Cream: *Per ½ Cup*			
Chocolate; Vanilla, av.	140	7	16
Kit Kat	170	9	20
Mint Chocolate Chip	160	8	19
Mocha Almond Fudge	160	8	19
Rocky Road	160	8	20
Slow Churned, ½ The Fat: *Per ½ Cup*			
Butter Pecan	130	5	17
Chocolate	100	3.5	15
Coffee; Neapolitan	100	3	15
Neapolitan	120	4.5	17
Strawberry	100	3	16

Friendly's: C   F   Cb

	C	F	Cb
Pure & Simple: *Per ½ Cup*			
Chocolate	160	10	15
Chocolate Fudge	160	9	18
Chocolate Peanut Butter	200	13	16
Rich & Creamy Ice Cream: *Per ½ Cup*			
Butter Crunch; Classic Chocolate, av.	150	7	18
Chocolate Almond Chip	160	9	17
Coffee	130	7	15
Strawberry; Vanilla, av.	140	7	16
Vienna Mocha Chunk	170	9	19
Light: *Per ½ Cup*			
Pistachio Almond	120	4.5	17
Vanilla	110	3.5	17
SundaeXtreme: *Per ½ Cup*			
Chocolate Fudge Brownie	150	5	25
Choc. Chip Cookie Dough	170	6	26
Chocolate P'nut Butter	190	9	22
Sherbet, Rasp Orange Lemon, ½ cup	130	1.5	28
Yogurt Frozen,			
Regular, average, ½ cup	140	4.5	23

Gelati-da:

	C	F	Cb
Gelato: *Per ½ Cup*			
Amaretto Chocolate	150	4.5	23
Choc Mint Milano	120	2.5	22
Coffee Fudge Latte	130	2	22
Limoncello; Vanilla Marsala, average	120	3	21
Red Raspberry	130	1.5	25

Great Value *(Walmart):*

	C	F	Cb
Ice Cream: *Per ½ cup*			
Chocolate Chip Cookie Dough	150	8	19
Coffee	130	7	15
Decadent Fudge Tracks	180	10	20
Homestyle Vanilla	140	7	17
Peanut Butter Cup	160	9	17
Sherbet, average all flavs	110	0	26

Haagen-Dazs:

	C	F	Cb
Tubs, Regular: *Per ½ Cup*			
Butter Pecan	300	22	20
Chocolate Peanut Butter	330	22	25
Dulce de Leche	270	16	28
White Chocolate Raspberry Truffle	280	16	31
Sorbet: *Per ½ Cup*			
Mango	150	0	38
Orchard Peach	140	0	34

Healthy Choice,

	C	F	Cb
Greek Frozen Yogurt,			
average all varieties,	105	2	19

Bars ~*See Page 109*

Ice Cream ~ Brands (Cont)

Hood:

	C	F	Cb
Classic: *Per ¹/₂ Cup*			
Chocolate	140	6	18
Classic Trio	140	7	17
Cookie Dough	170	8	21
Cookies 'N Cream	150	8	19
Creamy Coffee	140	7	16
Fudge Twister	140	6	20
Golden/Natural Vanilla; Patchwork	140	7	17
Maple Walnut	150	9	17
Churned, Light: *Per ¹/₂ Cup*			
Chocolate Chip	120	4.5	18
Coffee	100	3	16
Moosehead Lake Fudge	160	7	21
Under The Stars	160	8	18
Vanilla	110	3	16
Frozen Fat-Free Yogurt: *Per ¹/₂ Cup*			
Chocolate; Strawberry, av.	85	0	19
Mocha Fudge	100	0	22
Strawberry	80	0	19

New England Creamery ~ www.CalorieKing.com

Jerseymaid *(Vons): Per ¹/₂ Cup*

Ice Cream:

	C	F	Cb
Cookies & Cream	160	8	18
Choc Chip; Mint Choc Chip	150	9	16
Heavenly Hash	165	9	19
Mocha Almond Fudge; Chocolate	150	9	16
Neapolitan; Real Vanilla	140	8	15
Strawberry	130	6	17

Oberweis:

Super Premium Ice Cream: *Per ¹/₂ Cup*

	C	F	Cb
Chocolate, 2.85 oz	480	31	43
Choc. Peanut Butter, 3 oz	280	19	21
Cookie Dough, 2.8	220	13	22
Espresso Caramel Chip, 3 oz	230	14	27
Mango Pomegranate, 2.9 oz	210	12	24
Vanilla, 2.75	210	14	18

Oikos ~ *see Dannon*

Pinkberry:

Frozen Yogurt: *without Toppings*

	C	F	Cb
Original: Mini, 3.2 oz wt	90	0	19
Small, 4.9 oz wt	140	0	29
Medium, 8 oz wt	230	0	48
Large, 13 oz wt	370	0	78
Chocolate Hazelnut, 13 oz	560	15	96
Cookies & Cream, 13 oz	520	7.5	96
Mango, 13 oz	405	0	89

Red Mango:

	C	F	Cb
Frozen Yogurt: *No Toppings included*			
Original: 3.3 oz wt	80	0	19
Small, 4.7 oz wt	120	0	27
Regular, 7.5 oz wt	190	0	43
Large, 11.4 oz wt	290	0	65
Blueberry: 3.3 oz wt	100	0	23
Small, 4.7 oz wt	150	0	33
Regular, 7.5 oz wt	230	0	53
Large, 11.4 oz wt	350	0	81
Dulce de Leche: 3.3 oz wt	80	0	18
Small, 4.7 oz wt	120	0	27
Regular, 7.5 oz wt	190	0	43
Large, 11.4 oz wt	290	0	65
Pomegranate: 3.3 oz wt	90	0	21
Small, 4.6 oz wt	130	0	30
Regular, 7.5 oz wt	210	0	48
Large, 11.4 oz wt	320	0	73

Rice Dream:

Frozen Dessert: *Per ¹/₂ Cup*

	C	F	Cb
Cocoa Marble Fudge	170	6	31
Mint Carob Chip	180	7	28
Strawberry	170	6	30
Vanilla	160	6	26

Bars ~ *See Page 110*

Skinny Cow:

Bars/Sandwiches/Cones ~ *See Page 110*

So Delicious: *Per ¹/₂ Cup*

	C	F	Cb
Almond Milk: Choc.; Mint Chip, av.	135	8	16
Mocha Almond Fudge	150	8	17
Vanilla	120	7	14
Cashew Milk: Cappuccino	150	7	21
Dark Choc. Truffle; Snickerdoodle, av.	185	9	24
Coconut Milk: Choc.; Coconut, av.	140	8	21
Choc. P'Nut Butter Swirl	200	14	22
Mocha Almond Fudge	160	8	23
No Sugar Added: Mint Chip	120	11	18
Vanilla Bean	100	8	18
Note: Carbohydrate Figure Includes 3g Sugar Alcohol			
Soy Milk: Chocolate Velvet	130	3.5	23
Cookie Dough	170	7	29
Creamy Van.; Neapolitan	120	3	24
Peanut Butter Zig Zag	210	11	28

Ice Cream ~ Brands (Cont)

	C	F	Cb
Soy Dream:			
Frozen Dessert: *Per 1/2 Cup*			
Butter Pecan	190	11	23
French Vanilla	170	9	21
Vanilla Fudge Swil	170	9	23
Stonyfield Farm:			
Frozen Yogurt: *Per 1/2 Cup*			
After Dark Chocolate	100	0	21
Creme Caramel	130	1.5	26
Gotta Have Vanilla	100	0	20
Stop & Shop:			
Ice Cream: *Per 1/2 Cup*			
Chocolate	150	8	18
Neapolitan; Vanilla, average	140	7.5	17
Vanilla Fudge Swirl	140	7	18
Light: Moose Tracks	130	5	18
Vanilla	100	3	17
Premium:			
Cookies & Cream	170	9	21
Mint Chocolate Chip	160	9	18
Simply Enjoy:			
Chocolate	210	12	22
Strawberry; Vanilla, average	225	13	25
Tasti D-Lite:			
Soft Serve: *Per 3 oz Wt*			
Banana	70	1	14
Blueberry Cheesecake	90	1.5	17
Brownie Batter Chocolate	90	2	16
Buttercrunch Mania	110	4	16
Coffee 'n Cream	80	1.5	16
Marshmallow Vanilla	90	1.5	17
Peanut Butter Fudge	90	3	15
Tofutti:			
Premium Pints: *Per 1/2 Cup*			
Better Pecan	250	15	27
Chocolate	210	13	20
Vanilla	210	13	21
Vanilla Almond Bark	240	15	24
Van. Fudge; Wild Berry Supreme, av.	190	9	25
TCBY ~ *See Page 250*			
Turkey Hill: *Per 1/2 Cup*			
All Natural:			
Chocolate/Mint Chip	175	10	18
Salted Caramel	160	8	20

	C	F	Cb
Turkey Hill (Cont): *Per 1/2 Cup*			
Light: Extreme Cookies 'n Cream			
Moose Tracks	140	6	20
Vanilla Bean	100	2	17
No Sugar Added:			
Dutch Chocolate; Vanilla Bean, av.	70	0	20
Premium Ice Cream:			
Black Cherry	130	6	18
Butter Pecan; Choco Mint Chip, av.	160	10	16
Chocolate Peanut Butter Cup	180	11	18
Cookies 'n Cream; Tin Roof Sundae	150	8	19
Rocky Road	170	8	23
Vanilla Bean	130	7	16
Stuff'd, average all flavors	145	6	22
Frozen Yogurt: *Per 1/2 Cup*			
Mint Cookies 'n Cream	110	1.5	22
Fat-Free: Chocolate Marshmallow	110	0	24
Other flavors	90	0	19
Sherbet, Fruit Rainbow	120	1	26
Wawa:			
Premium Ice Cream: *Per 1/2 Cup*			
Butter Pecan; Mint Choc. Chip, av.	180	10	20
Chocolate; Vanilla Bean, average	160	8	20
Cookies & Cream	180	9	21
Strawberry Shortcake	160	7	22
Wegmans: *Per 1/2 Cup*			
Regular: Chocolate	130	7	15
French Van./ Vanilla, average	145	7	19
Light Extra Churned: Cookie Dough	130	3	23
French Vanilla	120	3.5	19
Yoplait:			
Go-Gurt!, average all flavors, 2.3 oz	60	0.5	12
Frozen Yogurt: *Per 1/2 Cup*			
Original Fruit flavors, average	115	2	21
Vanilla	110	2.5	19
Greek:			
Fruit Flavors, average	130	2	21
Honey Caramel	140	2.5	22
Vanilla	100	2	18

Ice Cream Bars & Pops ~ Brands

Per Bar/Serving Unless indicated   **C**   **F**   **Cb**

	C	F	Cb
Ben & Jerry's:			
Slices:			
Am. Dream; Choc Chip Cookie Dough, av.	285	18	30
Chocolate Fudge Brownie	250	16	27
Vanilla Peanut Butter Cup	300	22	24
Big Bear ~ *See Klondike*			
Blue Bunny:			
Single Bars: Big Alaska Bar, 3.3 oz	250	15	27
Chocolate Eclair, 2.8 oz	210	9	29
Cookies 'n Cream, 3 oz	240	11	33
Heath Bar, 3 oz	290	20	26
Hot Fudge Bar, 3.6 oz	360	24	33
Strawberry Shortcake, 2.8 oz	200	10	27
Turtle Bar, 3.5 oz	350	23	33
Tweety Bar, 2.8 oz	90	0	22
Snacks, Choc. Chip Cookie, 1.7 oz	150	8	19
Cones, 6 Pack:			
Caramel Lovers, 3.4 oz	310	16	38
Chocolate Lovers, 3.2 oz	270	12	36
Cookies 'n Cream, 3.2 oz	270	13	37
Big Dipper:			
Cookies 'n Cream, 3 oz	260	12	35
Chocolate Lovers, 3 oz	260	12	36
Big Swirls, Choc., Van., 3 oz	250	12	32
Ice Cream Sandwiches:			
Singles: Chips Galore, 3.4 oz	310	14	43
Cookies 'N Cream, 3 oz	240	10	37
8 Pack, Birthday Party, 2.6 oz	170	5	30
Big: Bopper, 5 oz	450	20	63
Double Strawberry, 3.9 oz	250	7	42
Mississippi Mud, 4 oz	280	8	47
Breyers:			
Carb Smart, 6 Pack:			
Fudge Bar, 1.7 oz	70	3	11
Vanilla Ice Cream Bar, 2 oz	150	11	13
Vanilla & Almond Ice Cream Bar, 2 oz	160	12	13
Note: Carbohydrate figure includes 4-5g sugar alcohol			
Butterfinger *(Nestle)*,			
Loaded Ice Cream Bar	280	18	27

Per Bar/Serving Unless indicated   **C**   **F**   **Cb**

	C	F	Cb
Cool Classics:			
Arctic Blasters:			
Crispy Bar	160	11	15
Fudge Bar	100	1	21
Ice Cream Bar	150	10	13
Orange Cream	100	2.5	18
Strawberry Shortcake	150	8	20
Toffee Bar	160	11	14
Icepix: Grape; Cherry; Orange	35	0	8
Honeydew; Watermelon; Cantelope	35	0	9
Swirl Pops, Mango-Cherry	80	0	20
Creamsicles: *Per Bar*			
Box of 12, 100 Cal. Orange Crm Pops	100	1.5	19
Box of 18, Sugar-Free Cream Pops	30	0	6
Note: Sugar-Free carbohydrate figures include 5g Sucralose sweetener			
Diana's Bananas:			
Banana Babies:			
Milk/Dark Chocolate (1)	130	6	18
Milk Choc. & Peanuts (1)	215	13	21
Banana Bites, (5), 2 oz	130	8	16
Dove:			
Single Bars: *Per 2.6 oz Bar*			
Milk Chocolate Vanilla	250	16	24
And Almonds	250	17	21
Caramel Swirl & Cashews	250	16	23
Dark Chocolate Vanilla	250	17	24
Miniatures, Variety Pack,			
w/ Milk/Dark Choc., 5 pieces, av.	330	21	32
Sorbet Bars: Dark Chocolate Raspb.	150	8	19
Milk Chocolate Strawberry	150	7	20
Drumstick *(Nestlé)*:			
Classic Cones: Vanilla	290	15	34
Vanilla Caramel	300	15	38
Super Nugget: Van. Fudge	320	17	37
Strawberry	310	17	34
S'mores, Toasted Marshmallow	270	12	39
Strawberry, with Fudge	300	15	37
King Size: Triple Chocolate	350	14	51
Vanilla with Chocolate Layers	360	16	49
Lil' Drums: Choc. w/ Choc Swirls	130	6	16
Average other varieties	110	6	18
Simply Dipped: Mint	260	12	37
Vanilla	260	12	37

Ice Cream Bars & Pops

Ice Cream Bars/Pops ~ Brands (Cont)

Per Bar/Serving

	C	F	Cb
Edy's ~ See Dreyer's			
Eskimo Pie (Nestle):			
Milk Chocolate, Vanilla	150	10	14
Dark Chocolate, No Sugar Added	150	10	13
Fat Boy:			
Sundae On A Stick:			
Nut Sundae	270	20	23
Toffee Crunch	280	20	26
Vanilla Dipped	260	19	22
Sandwiches: Chocolate, 3 oz	210	9	31
Cookies 'n Cream, 3 oz	220	8	34
Mint Chocolate Chip, 3 oz	220	9	33
Prem. Van.; Key Lime, 3 oz	210	8	31
Raspberry Cheesecake, 3 oz	210	7	35
Strawberry, 3 oz	210	7	35
Fresh & Easy, Vanilla Sundae Cone	260	15	29
Fudge Bar (Nestle), Regular, 2.8 oz	110	2	21
Fudgesicle:			
100 Calorie: Fudge Bar	100	2	17
Low Fat Fudge Bar	60	1.5	12
No Sugar Added	80	1.5	19
Good Humor:			
Dessert Bars, Singles:			
Original Vanilla, 2.8 oz	240	14	27
Birthday Cake, 2.6 oz	200	10	25
Chocolate Eclair, 2.6 oz	190	9	27
Oreo 2.6 oz	210	11	26
Toasted Almond, 2.6 oz	200	11	24
Cones:			
Singles: Giant King Cone,			
Vanilla Chocolate, 5 oz	390	22	44
King Cone, Vanilla, 2.7 oz	230	14	25
4-Packs:			
Dessert Oreo Cone, 2.65 oz	200	9	29
King Cones, Vanilla, 3 oz	240	12	31
Sandwiches:			
Single, Giant, Neapolitan; Van., av.	220	5	40
4-Pack, Choc. Chip Cookie, 2.7 oz	250	10	40
Stickless: *4 or 6-Pack*			
Reese's PB Dessert Cup Bar: 2.4 oz	260	17	25
2.7 oz	280	19	22
Haagen-Dazs:			
Dark Chocolate Bar, Chocolate	280	20	22
Milk Chocolate Bars:			
Coffee & Almond Crunch	290	21	22
Vanilla & Almonds	290	21	21
Vanilla	270	19	22
Snack Size:			
Coffee & Almond Crunch	190	14	15
Vanilla & Almonds	195	15	13
Gelato, Vanilla Caramel Pizzelle	290	19	25

Per Bar/Serving

	C	F	Cb
Healthy Choice: Fudge Bar	80	0.5	15
Smoothie Bars:			
Mango Peach	70	0.5	14
Raspberry	80	0.5	15
Strawberry	70	0.5	13
Hershey's:			
Bars, Gluten Free: Banjo	170	11	17
Fudjo	120	0	24
Orange Blossom	80	2.5	13
Cones: Incredible	290	14	38
Moose Tracks	480	28	52
P-Nutty	260	15	30
Low fat, Cookies & Cream; Crazy, av.	120	1.5	25
Pops, all flavors	35	0	10
Sandwiches:			
99 Cent Vanilla Ice Cream	210	9	30
Giant:			
Andes Creme de Menthe	350	16	48
Neopolitan	320	14	43
Vanilla, 6 oz	300	12	43
Signature Bars: Chocolate Eclair	220	10	30
Cotton Candy	280	15	32
Strawb. Shortcake	240	11	32
Hood:			
Bars: Ice Cream Bar	130	7	14
Orange Cream	90	1.5	18
Hoodsie:			
Cups, Chocolate; Vanilla, 3 oz	100	5	12
Sundae Cups, 3 oz	120	5	19
Sandwich, av. 2.2 oz	175	6	29
Klondike:			
Bars:			
Single, Orig. Vanilla, 5.5 oz	300	17	34
4-Pack: Krunch, 3 oz	250	14	29
Mint Choc. Chip, 2.8 oz	230	14	26
Oreo Cookies & Cream, 2.6 oz	250	15	27
8-Count Snack Size: Orig., 1.4 oz	120	7	13
English Toffee, 1.3 oz	115	7	12
Choco Taco, Original, 4 oz	250	12	34
Kandy: Caramel & Peanuts, 3.5 oz	250	14	28
6 Pack: Cookies & Cream, 2.15 oz	200	10	24
Mint Fudge, 2.15 oz	190	11	23
Triple Chocolate, 2 oz	180	10	22
Sandwiches:			
Single: Mrs Fields, 3.9 oz	340	2	55
Oreo, 4.5 oz	220	7	37
4-Pack: Mrs Fields, 2.3 oz	210	8	34
Oreo, 2.4 oz	210	7	35
6-Pack, Vanilla, 2.7 oz	180	5	31

Updated Nutrition Data ~ www.CalorieKing.com
Persons with Diabetes ~ See Disclaimer (Page 22)

Ice Cream Bars & Pops

Ice Cream Bars/Pops ~ Brands (Cont)

Per Bar/Serving	C	F	Cb
Luigi's:			
Real Italian Ice: Cherry; Mango	100	0	26
Chocolate Fudge	150	0	36
Watermelon; Blue Raspberry	160	0	39
M&M's:			
Cone, Single, 2.6 oz	240	11	32
Cookie Ice Cream Sandwich, 2.9 oz	250	13	34
Magnum:			
Singles: Almond	270	18	25
Double Caramel	270	17	29
Minis, Classic	150	10	14
Multipacks: Dark Chocolate	240	16	23
Infinity Chocolate	270	18	25
White	240	15	24
Double: Choc. Hazelnut	280	19	26
Double Raspberry	260	16	28
Minute Maid, Juice Bars, 2.25 fl.oz	40	0	10
Nestlé:			
Bars: Crunch Bar	180	11	19
Orange & Cream	90	1.5	18
Strawberry Shortcake	210	9	31
Cones, Magical Minis	110	3.5	19
Dibs, Crunch, 4 oz container	340	24	30
Drumsticks ~ See Page 109			
Ice Pop, Wildberry & Zesty Lemon	90	0	22
Outshine Fruit Bars:			
Creamy Coconut	120	3	20
Peach	90	0	23
Other Fruit Flavors, av.	70	0	16
Sandwich, Vanilla	160	3.5	29
Toll House,			
Choc. Chip Cookie Sandwich	380	15	57
Popsicle:			
Firecracker, all flavors (1)	35	0	9
Hello Kitty; Scribbles (2)	60	0	14
Marvel Avengers Assemble (1)	40	0	10
SpongeBob Pop-Ups (1)	80	1	11
Slow Melts, Mighty Minis, 5 pieces	60	0	11
Reese's *(Good Humor),*			
P'nut Butter Ice Cream Cup, 2.4 oz	260	17	25
Skinny Cow: *Per Item*			
Bars: Fudge	110	1	22
Chocolate Truffle	100	2.5	19
Vanilla Almond Crunch	190	11	19
Candy Bars, av. all flavors	155	9	17
Cones, average all flavors	155	3	28
Sandwiches, all flavors	180	9	22
Snickers:			
Bars: Regular, 1.8 oz	180	11	18
Mini Bar, 1 piece, 0.9 oz	90	6	9
Cone, 2.9 oz	250	13	29
Ice Cream Brownie, 3.3 oz	300	13	41

Per Bar/Serving	C	F	Cb
Snow Cone *(Wonder)*, av. all, 7 fl.oz	60	0	15
So Delicious *(Turtle Mountain):*			
Almond Based Minis:			
Bars, Mocha ALm. Fudge (1), 1.8 oz	150	10	14
Sandwich, Vanilla, 1.3 oz	90	3.5	13
Coconut Based Minis:			
Bars: Almond, 1.8 oz	180	13	17
Simply Strawberry, 2 oz	80	3.5	14
Soy Based Minis:			
Sandwiches, av. all varieties, 1.4 oz	90	2	18
Soy Dream: Almond Bar (1), 3 oz	140	16	24
Bites, Choc/Vanilla/Coconut, 15 pcs	140	16	22
Lil' Dreamers, Vanilla	100	4	15
Tampico, Freezer Pops, all var., 1.4 oz	30	0	7
Tofutti: *Per Item*			
Bars:			
Chocolate Fudge/Coffee Break Treats	30	0	6
Hooray Hooray Bar	120	8	8
Marry Me Bar	170	8	22
Totally Fudge Pops	95	1.5	19
Note: Carb figures include 0-7g sugar alcohols			
Cones, all flavors	220	13	24
Cuties, average all flavors	130	6	18
Turkey Hill:			
Bar, Vanilla Ice Cream, 3.3 oz	320	23	26
Sandwiches: Double Decker, 2.5 oz	190	7	30
Vanilla Bean, 2.5 oz	190	7	29
Sundae Cone, Van. Fudge	320	18	33
Twix, Ice Cream Bar, 3.3 oz	350	20	38
Wegmans:			
Bars: Fudge, low fat	100	1	20
Peanut Butter Sundae Crunch	200	11	22
Vanilla, Choc Coated, 2 oz	160	11	14
Sandwiches: Vanilla	160	5	26
Light Vanilla	150	3	29
Weight Watchers: *Per Item*			
Bars:			
Dulce de Leche, 1.83 oz	120	4.5	19
English Toffee Crunch (2), 2.4 oz	200	6	13
Giant, Chocolate Fudge Bar, 2.6 oz	90	1	21
Cones, Double Caramel Swirl, 1.45 oz	90	2	17
Sandwiches: Cherry Chseecake, snack	90	1	19
Round: Giant Vanilla	140	2	31
Mint	140	1.5	31
Yoplait ~ *See Frozen Yogurt*			
Yosicle, Swirlz, average all flavors, (1)	45	1	7

Canned & Packaged Meals ~ Brands

Amy's: Per Serve **C** **F** **Cb**
Frozen:
Asian Meals:

	C	F	Cb
Stir-Fry Asian Noodle,10 oz	300	7	50
Sweet & Sour Asian Noodle, 8 oz	250	3	46
Bowls: Baked Ziti, 9.5 oz	390	12	62
Broccoli & Cheddar Bake, 9.5 oz	420	20	44
Pesto Tortellini, 9.5 oz	450	20	50
Burritos: Bean & Cheese, 5.5 oz	280	5	49
Bean & Rice, 5.5 oz	240	6	38
Breakfast Burrito, 6 oz	270	8	38
Entrees: Cheese Enchilada, 4.5 oz	240	14	18
Cheese Lasagna, 10.3 oz	410	16	46
Macaroni & Cheese, 8 oz	290	5	43
Roasted Vegetable Tamale, 10.3 oz	280	7	44

Light & Lean: Per 8 oz Serve

	C	F	Cb
Black Bean & Cheese Enchilada	250	5	44
Mattar Paner	260	6	42
Soft Taco Fiesta	230	4.5	40

Pot Pies:

	C	F	Cb
Broccoli, 7.5 oz	460	24	50
Vegetable, 7.5 oz	430	20	54
Snacks: Cheese Pizza, 5-6 pieces	210	9	25
Nacho, Cheese & Bean, 5-6 pcs	220	9	25
Swirls: Artichoke & Parmesan (2)	200	11	20
Cheddar Jalepeno (2)	210	9	25
Mushroom & Cheese; Pesto (2)	190	9	20

Veggie Burger Patties:

	C	F	Cb
All American	140	3.5	14
Black Bean	140	4.5	19
California	110	4	16

Wraps:

	C	F	Cb
Indian Samosa, 5 oz	250	9	35
Teriyaki, gluten free, 5.5 oz	250	6	38
Tofu Scramble B'fast, gluten free, 5.5 oz	300	13	35

Atkins: Per 9 oz Tray/Bowl
Frozen:

	C	F	Cb
Beef Merlot	310	21	9
Chicken & Broccoli Alfredo	330	21	10
Chili Con Carne	320	21	8
Crustless Chicken Pot Pie	320	22	8
Italian Style Pasta Bake	320	15	17
Meatloaf w/ Portobello Mshrm Gravy	340	22	12

Bagel Bites:
Frozen:

	C	F	Cb
Cheese, Sausage & Pepperoni, 4 pcs	200	6	28
Supreme; Three Cheese, av., 4 pcs, 3 oz	195	5	31

B&M: **C** **F** **Cb**

Baked Beans: Per 16 oz Can, ¹/₂ cup, 4.6 oz

	C	F	Cb
Original	170	2	31
Boston's Best	170	1.5	32
Maple Flavor	150	1	28
Vegetarian	160	1	25
Brown Bread, Raisin, ¹/₂ slice, 2 oz	130	0.5	29

Banquet:

Homestyle Bakes: 1 Cup, Prepared

	C	F	Cb
Cheeseburger Mac Bake	240	6	36
Chicken Taco Bake	280	7	41
Creamy Turkey & Stuffing	240	10	29
Pizza Pasta Bake	280	6	46

Frozen:

	C	F	Cb
Meals: Boneless Pork Rib, 10.5 oz	370	14	45
Cheesy & Macaroni & Beef, 7 oz	230	9	27
Chicken: Fingers, 6.5 oz	310	12	33
Fettuccine Chicken Alfredo, 8 oz	300	12	36
Fried Chicken, 10 oz	330	14	40
Parmesan, 8.5 oz	320	11	41
Strip Meal, 8.9 oz	440	19	45
Fish Sticks, w/ Mac & Cheese,7.5 oz	330	11	46
Homestyle Patty, 10 oz	340	17	32
Lasagna, with Meat Sauce	250	9	31
Meatloaf, 9.5 oz	330	11	43
Pepper Steak, 10 oz	320	13	39
Rigatoni & Italian Sausage, 8 oz	300	12	35
Salisbury Steak w/ Mshd Pot., 9.5 oz	350	14	44
Spaghetti & Meatballs, 10 oz	320	14	34
Spaghetti & Chicken Nuggets, 7 oz	230	7	32
Sweet & Sour Chicken, 8 oz	420	10	70
Turkey, 10 oz	280	11	29

Family:

	C	F	Cb
BBQ Seasoned Chicken Patty & Sce	140	4	16
Chicken Alfredo, with Broccoli & Noodles, 8 oz	210	6	29
Salisbury Steak & Gravy, 4.5 oz	180	12	11

Pies: Per 7 oz
Breakfast Deep Dish:

	C	F	Cb
Cheesy Ham & Potato	440	25	46
Sausage & Gravy	450	33	44
Pot Pie: Chicken; Turkey, average	335	19	32
Chicken & Broccoli	330	18	31

Barilla:	C	F	Cb
Microwaveables: *Per 9 oz Container*			
Ital. Ssg; Meat Sauce Gemelli, av	350	7	60
Marinara/Tomato & Basil Penne, av.	310	4	60
Betty Crocker:			
Bowl Appetit:			
Herb Chkn Flav. Veggie Rice	250	3	51
Pasta Alfredo	350	9	55
Three-Cheese Rotini	340	7	59
Hamburger Helper: *Per 1 Cup, Prep'd*			
Bacon Cheeseburger Macaroni	320	14	27
Beef Pasta	280	12	24
Four Cheese Lasagna	300	12	24
Potato Stroganoff	290	12	27
Salisbury	280	11	27
Strogaoff	310	12	30
Three Cheese	320	13	30
Tomato Basil Penne	300	11	32
Potatoes: *Per Serving, Prepared*			
Casserole: Au Gratin, 1/2 cup	150	6	24
Cheddar & Bacon, 1/2 c.	150	6	24
Roasted Garlic, 1/2 cup	130	4	21
Scalloped, 2/3 cup	130	3	24
Sour Cream and Chives, 2/3 cup	130	3	24
Mashed Potatoes:			
Hearty Four Cheese, 2/3 cup	150	6.5	17
Homestyle Butter & Herb, 2/3 cup	150	7	17
Savory Roasted Garlic, 2/3 cup	150	6.5	18
Sweet Potato, 1/2 cup	200	8.5	27
Tuna Helper: *Per 1 Cup, Prepared*			
Creamy Pasta	250	10	27
Average other varieties	265	10	30
Ultimate Helper: *1 Cup Prepared*			
Cheddar Broccoli	310	10	27
Creamy Parmesan Alfedo	340	10	30
Three Cheese Marinara	360	14	36
Biggest Loser:			
Refrigerated:			
Simply Sensible: *Per 1/2 Package*			
Beef Pot Roast & Gravy	220	5	16
Beef Tips & Gravy	200	3.5	21
Lasagna	200	5	28
Mediterranean-Style Chicken	250	6	36
Zing Chicken	230	1.5	38

Birds Eye:	C	F	Cb
Frozen:			
Voila!: *Per 1 Cup Prepared Unless Indicated*			
Alfredo Chicken, 1 1/2 cups	280	12	37
Beef & Broccoli Stir Fry	160	6	13
Chicken Florentine	230	6	27
Chicken Parmesan	360	11	50
Garlic Shrimp	230	9	30
Shrimp Scampi	190	2.5	31
Sweet & Sour Chicken	200	1	38
Boca:			
Frozen:			
Burger:			
All American Flame Grilled, 2.5 oz	120	5	6
Cheeseburger, 2.5 oz	100	4.5	6
Grilled Vegetables, 2.5 oz	80	1	7
Original Vegan, 2.5 oz	70	0.5	6
Chik'n: Orig. Nuggets, 3 oz	180	7	17
Patties (1), 2.5 oz	160	6	15
Spicy Patties (1), 2.5 oz	160	6	15
Boston Market:			
Frozen:			
Dinners: Beef Steak & Pasta, 14 oz	470	14	52
Chicken Parmesan, 13 oz	500	13	70
Oven Roasted Chicken, 13 oz	280	7	32
Salisbury Steak, 14.5 oz	530	32	38
Swedish M'balls, 13 oz	570	26	55
Buitoni:			
Refrigerated:			
Ravioli: Four Cheese, 3.7 oz	330	12	42
Spinach & Artichoke, 3.8 oz	310	11	42
Tortellini: Mixed Cheese, 3.7 oz	320	8	47
Tortelloni, Chkn & Proscuitto, 3.8 oz	330	9	46
Other Pasta Dishes ~ *See Page 133*			
Bush's Best: *Per 1/2 Cup, 4.6 oz*			
Baked Beans: Original	140	1	29
Vegetarian	130	0	29
Average other varieties	150	1	32
Black Beans	100	0	18
Black Eyed Peas	80	0	15
Chili Beans, Pinto, medium	110	1	20
Dark Red Kidney Beans	120	0	22
Garbanzo Beans	120	2	20
Grillin' Beans:			
Bourbon & Brown Sugar	170	0.5	35
Smokehouse Tradition	160	1	33
Southern Pit	170	0.5	35
Steakhouse	180	0.5	39
Refried Beans: Cocina Latina, Trad.	150	3	23
Cocina Latina, Fat Free	130	0	24

Campbell's:	C	F	Cb
Pork & Beans, 11 oz can,			
4.6 oz serving	130	1	25
Chunky Microwaveable Bowls:			
Firehouse; Roadhouse,			
Chunky Beef & Beans Chili, 1 cup	240	7	30
Spaghetti O's: *Per 1 Cup*			
Original, 8.9 oz	170	1	35
With Meatballs, 8.9 oz	230	7	31
With Sliced Franks, 8.9 oz	210	6	29
Chef Boyardee:			
Canned: *Per Cup*			
Beefaroni, 8.8 oz	240	10	30
Lasagna, 8.8 oz	230	8	31
Ravioli in Tomato & Meat Sauce : *Per 1 Cup*			
Beef: Regular, 15 oz	370	11	53
Overstuffed, 9.2 oz	230	5	37
Cheese, 9 oz	210	2	40
Ital. Sausage, overstuffed, 9.2 oz	240	6	38
Spaghetti & M'balls, 9 oz	260	11	31
Microwaveable: *Per 7.5 oz Cup*			
Beefaroni	220	8	28
Beef Ravioli	200	7	28
Cheese Ravioli	190	5	28
Mini Micro Beef Ravioli	160	4	25
With Meatballs	250	10	32
Boxed Pizza Maker Kits: *Single Kits*			
Cheese, ¼ package, 4 oz	260	4.5	47
Pepperoni, ¼ package, 4 oz	280	8	42
Pizza Sauce, w/ Chse, ¼ c., 2 oz	35	1.5	4
Dennison's Chili: *Per Cup*			
Chili Con Carne:			
Original: w/ Beans, 9 oz	330	13	33
without Beans, 8.8 oz	310	16	20
Chunky, w/ Beans, 8.8 oz	300	10	32
Hot, with Beans, 9 oz	350	14	36
Vegetarian, 99% fat free, 9 oz	190	1.5	34
Devour ~ *See Heinz Page 114*			
Dinty Moore *(Hormel):*			
Big Bowl (Microwave): *Approx. ½ of 15 oz Bowl*			
Beef Stew, 8.3 oz	200	10	17
Chicken & Dumplings, 8.5 oz	220	7	29
Scalloped Potatoes & Ham, 8.7 oz	290	17	23

Dr. McDougall's: *Per 2 oz Package*	C	F	Cb
Asian Noodle Entree Cups,			
average all varieties	200	1.5	41
Quinoa Cups: Black Bean	320	4	57
Curry Almond and Br. Rice	260	3	51
Sweet Potato Kale	260	3.5	48
Eden Organics: *Per ½ Cup*			
Baked Beans, w/ Sorghum, 4.6 oz	150	0	27
Chili Black Beans & Quinoa, 4.4 oz	100	1	18
Lentils, w/ Onions & Bay Leaf, 4.6 oz	90	0	13
Refried Beans:			
Black Beans, 4.6 oz	110	1.5	18
Pinto; Kidney, av., 4.6 oz	85	1	17
Farmhouse:			
Rice: *Per 1 Cup, Prepared*			
Long Grain & Wild Herbs & Butter	250	7	44
Mexican	230	5	42
Roasted Chicken Flavor	230	5	44
French's:			
French Crispy Fried Onions:			
Original; White Cheddar:			
2 Tbsp, 0.3 oz	45	3.5	3
¼ cup, 0.5 oz	90	7	6
1 cup, 2 oz	360	28	24
GardenBurger:			
Veggie Burger: *Per Burger*			
Original	110	3	16
Black Bean Chipotle	90	3	16
Portabella	100	2.5	16
Garden Lites:			
Entrees: *Per 7 oz Serving*			
Cheddar Broccoli	210	6	29
Kale & Quinoa Souffle	200	6	23
Mac & Cheese	240	10	26
Roasted Vegetable Souffle	170	3	28
Veggie Bites:			
Broccoli & Brown Rice (4)	130	5	16
Cornbread (4)	170	2.5	31
Italian (4)	130	5	16
Kale & Brown Rice (4)	130	5	17
Gorton's:			
Battered Pollock Fillets,			
Crispy (2), 3.8 oz	230	13	24
Breaded Pollock Fillets:			
Crunchy/Lemon Herb (2), av., 3.8 oz	225	9	26
Gourmet,			
Signature Seasoned Salmon, 3.5 oz	90	2	2
Grilled Fillets: *Per Fillet*			
Garlic/Lemon Butter Pollock, 3.5 oz	85	3	0
Signature Tilapia, 3.2 oz	80	2	2

Gorton's (Cont):	C	F	Cb
Shrimp:			
Crispy Beer Batter Shrimp (5), 3.5 oz	250	14	23
Crunchy Butterfly Shrimp (5), 3.5 oz	250	12	25
Garl. Butter Shrimp Scampi (6), 4 oz	120	5	9
Simply Bake: Salmon, 4.4 oz	140	2.5	8
Hadddock Garlic Herb Butter, 4.9 oz	130	2.5	7
Tilapia, Signature Seasoning, 5.2 oz	130	3	6
Skillet Crisp, Lightly Battered,			
Tilapia, Garlic Herb, .3.35 oz	180	8	15
Smart & Crunchy,			
Pollock Fish Sticks (5), 3 oz	170	4.5	24
Great Value *(Walmart):*			
Breakfast Bowls:			
Bacon, 7 oz	430	27	19
Sausage, 7 oz	390	25	22
Sausage & Gravy, 7 oz	360	24	21
Frozen Meals: *Per 10 oz Pkg*			
Chicken Parmesan & Penne	400	16	45
Meatloaf & Mashed Potatoes	370	21	29
Rstd Turkey Breast w/ Mshd Potatoes	260	11	23
Salisbury Steak with Potatoes	340	19	26
Skillet Meal, Parmig. & Penne, 12 oz	495	24	52
Health Valley:			
Vegetarian Chili: *Per 8.7 oz Cup*			
3 Bean Chipotle; Spicy Tomato, av.	195	3	37
Tame Tomato, no salt added	210	2.5	41
Healthy Choice:			
Cafe Steamers (Frozen):			
Beef Teriyaki, 9.5 oz	280	5	42
Chicken & Noodles, 10 oz	260	7	31
Crustless Chicken Pot Pie, 9.6 oz	300	6	40
Four Chse Ravioli & Chkn Marinara, 10 oz	270	6	34
General Tso's Spicy Chicken, 10.3 oz	290	3.5	47
Spaghetti & Meatballs, 9.5 oz	280	7	35
Sweet & Sour Chicken, 10 oz	390	8	65
Sweet Sesame Chicken, 9.7 oz	300	6	43
Classics: Chicken Parmig., 11.6 oz	360	12	47
Lemon Pepper Fish, 10.7 oz	290	4	50
Simply Steamers:			
Beef & Broccoli, 10 oz	280	7	32
Chicken & Vegetable Stir Fry, 9.2 oz	190	4	15
Gr. Chicken & Broccoli Alfredo, 9.1 oz	190	5	8
Gr. Chicken Pesto & Veggies, 9.1 oz	200	5	11
Honey Balsamic Chicken, 9.87 oz	210	2.5	28
Meatball Marinara, 10 oz	280	6	36

Extra Product Listings ~ *www·CalorieKing·com*

Heinz:	C	F	Cb
Beans, Vegetarian, ½ cup, 4 oz	140	0.5	27
Devour Frozen Meals: *Per Package*			
Angus Beef with Cornbread	750	34	83
Buffalo Chicken Mac & Cheese	460	30	24
Cheese Ravioli w/sundried Tom. Sce	490	19	59
Chicken & Waffles	620	21	83
Chicken Enchiladas Suiza	460	18	55
Deep Dish Honey BBQ Chkn Pizza	600	26	69
Deep Dish Three Meat Pizza	660	35	63
Italian Sausage Lasagna	470	23	41
Lasagna Alfredo w/Bacon & Ssg	570	37	33
Pesto Ravioli w/Spicy Italian Ssg	670	37	55
Pulled Chicken Burrito Bowl	450	15	46
White Chedd. Mac & Cheese w/Bacon	710	41	54
Hormel:			
Chili w/ Beans:			
Regular; Hot; Chunky, av. 8.7 oz	260	7	32
Turkey, 98% Fat-Free,8.7 oz	220	3	29
Vegetarian, 99% Fat Free, 8.7 oz	200	1.5	35
Chili w/out Beans:			
Regular, 8.3 oz	250	12	19
Hot; Chunky, average, 8.3 oz	255	13	19
Turkey, 98% Fat-Free, 8.3 oz	190	3	16
Compleats, Comfort Classics: *Per 7.5 oz*			
Beefy Mac & Cheese	220	4	35
Chicken & Noodles	180	6	20
Dumplings & CHicken	170	4	25
Noodles & Beef	150	2	26
Spaghetti & Meat Sauce	230	7	32
Compleats, Homesyle:			
Beef Pot Roast, 9 oz	230	6	22
Chicken Alfredo, 10 oz	340	18	28
Chkn Breast & Msh'd Pot., 10 oz	210	4.5	26
Meatloaf & Mashed Pot., 9 oz	280	12	27
Salisbury Steak, 9 oz	300	17	23
Swedish Mtballs, 9 oz	270	12	27
Refrigerated Meals: *Per Package*			
H'style Meat Loaf & Tom. Sce, 5 oz	220	9	14
Sliced Rst Turkey Brst & Gravy, 5 oz	110	2	3
Slow Simm. Beef Tips w/ Gravy, 4.3 oz	170	10	4
Side Dishes:			
Garlic Mashed Potatoes, 5 oz	140	7	17
HomeStyle Mashed Potatoes, 5 oz	160	9	18
Loaded Mashed Potatoes, 5 oz	190	11	18
Mashed Sweet Potatoes, 5 oz	170	6	27

Horizon Organic:	C	F	Cb
Mac & Cheese: *Per 1 Cup Prepared*			
Cheesy Mac:			
Macaroni & Mild Cheddar	350	11	53
Pasta Shells & White Cheddar	350	11	52
Organic Mac:			
Macaroni & Mild Cheddar	350	12	50
Pasta Shells & White Cheddar	360	12	50
Protein Mac, Mild Chedd. Cheese	355	12	47
Hot Pockets:			
Sandwiches: *Per Sandwich*			
Crispy Buttery Crust: BBQ Rcpe Beef	320	13	44
Cheddar Cheeseburger	290	11	39
Hickory Ham & Cheese	280	11	38
Crispy Crust:			
Five Cheese Pizza	350	18	37
Pepperoni Pizza	340	19	35
Croissant Crust:			
Hickory Ham & Cheddar	310	15	35
Philly Steak	320	16	35
Sausage, Egg & Cheese	320	17	35
Flaky Crust, Chicken Pot Pie	240	10	30
Garlic Buttery Seasoned Crust			
Four Cheese Pizza	320	13	39
Four Meat & Four Chse	310	14	37
Meatballs & Mozzarella	310	13	38
Pepperoni & Sausage Pizza	310	14	38
Pretzel Bread,			
Appwd Bacon Chedd. Chse Melt	310	13	36
Seasoned Crust,			
Philly Steak & Cheese	300	12	38
Hungry Jack:			
Casserole Potatoes:			
Cheddar & Bacon, prepared	160	7	20
CreamyScalloped, prepared	170	7	24
Hashbrowns:			
Original, 1/3 cup prepared	100	4.5	14
Cheesy, 1/2 cup prepared	140	7	17
Mashed Potatoes, average,			
Dry Mix only, 1/3 cup unprepared	80	0	19
Hungry Man:			
Dinners:			
Beer Battered Chicken	770	38	73
Boneless Fried Chicken	800	39	81
Boneless Pork Rib Shaped Patties	780	35	94
Country Fried Chicken	530	27	54
Grilled Beef Patty	450	22	39
Home-Style Meatloaf	650	32	64
Mexican Style Fiesta	570	18	90
Roasted Carved White Meat Turkey	420	11	60
Salisbury Steak	580	32	51

Hungry Man (Cont):	C	F	Cb
Selects: *Per Package*			
Classic Fried Chicken	940	56	58
Steak Strips	420	12	55
XXL Sandwiches: *Per Package*			
Angus Beef Charbroil	740	47	52
BBQ Pork Ribs	690	39	62
Chicken Parmesan	610	29	63
Crispy Fried Chicken	670	32	64
José Olé:			
Breakfast Burritos:			
Egg & Bacon, 4 oz	260	10	30
Egg & Sausage, 4 oz	240	10	28
Premium Burritos:			
Chicken Monterey (1)	270	7	39
Steak & Cheese (1)	310	11	40
Premium Chimichangas:			
Chicken & Cheese (1), 5 oz	330	13	42
Steak & Cheese (1), 5 oz	350	15	39
Snacks:			
Mini: Chimichangas,			
Steak & Cheddar (3)	370	20	36
Quesadillas,			
Chicken & Cheese (3)	210	8	25
Tacos, Beef & Cheese (4)	220	11	23
Taquitos: Chicken, Corn Tortillas, (3)	200	8	26
Beef & Cheese, Flour Tortillas, (2)	260	14	26
Kashi:			
Entrees: *Per 10 oz Package*			
Amaranth Polenta Plantain	340	9	59
Black Bean Mango	330	9	56
Chimichurri Quinoa	240	7	41
Sweet Potato Quinoa	270	6	48
Kid Cuisine: *Per Meal*			
All Star Chicken Breast Nuggets	440	1	55
Beef Patty with Cheese & Bun	350	10	53
Cheese Pizza	450	16	61
Fish Sticks	340	11	46
Fun Shaped Chicken Brast Nuggets	430	19	51
Mac. & Cheese	410	11	59
Mini Corn Dogs	490	15	75
Pepperoni Pizza, Reduced Fat	370	10	57
Popcorn Chicken	420	13	62
Spaghetti w/ Mini Meatballs	330	7	51

Knorr: *Sides, Dry Mix Only*

	C	F	Cb
Cajun: Dirty Rice, 2.3 oz	230	2	48
Red Beans & Rice, 2.3 oz	230	2	47
Fiesta: Mexican Rice, 2.3 oz	230	1	48
Taco Rice, 2.2 oz	220	1	46
Italian, Creamy Pesto Pasta, 2.2 oz	220	2	44
Pasta:			
Alfredo; Parmesan, av.	245	4	42
Alfredo Broccoli, 2.2 oz	240	3.5	43
Butter & Herb, 2.2 oz	230	1.5	46
Cheesy Bacon Macaroni, 2 oz	220	1.5	43
Chicken Flavor, 2.2 oz	230	2	44
Rice: Beef Rice, 2.3 oz	230	1	49
Chedd. Brocc./Chkn Rice, av., 2.3 oz	240	2	49
Creamy Chkn Rice, 2.3 oz	240	1.5	49
Garlic Parm. Rice, 2.4 oz	250	2	50
Herb & Butter Rice, 2.3 oz	230	1	49
Mushroom Rice; Rice Pilaf, 2.3 oz	230	1	47

Kraft:

Mac & Cheese Dry Mix: *Per 2.5 oz*

	C	F	Cb
Original; Chedd. Explosion, av.	260	3.5	48
Alfredo	250	2.5	48
Three Cheese; Thick 'N Creamy	250	2	48

Liquid: *Just Add Water*

	C	F	Cb
Deluxe Mac & Cheese:			
Orig. Chedd.; Four Chse, av., 3.5 oz	315	10	45
White Chedd. & Garlic Herb, 3 oz	280	9	45
Easy Mac Microcups,			
Extreme Cheese; Wh. Grain, 2 oz	210	3.5	39
Easy Mac Single Cup, Orig., 3.5 oz	440	8	81
Homestyle, all flavors, 3 oz	270	8	42

Velveeta: *Per Container*

	C	F	Cb
Cheesy Bowls: Chicken Afredo	330	12	36
Chicken Chili Cheese Mac	310	10	33
Lasagna, with Meat Sauce	350	17	36
Ultimate Cheeseburger Mac	380	17	39
Cheesy Potatoes:			
Au Gratin, 2 oz dry	180	7	24
Bacon Scalloped, 2.1 oz dry	190	7	24
Southwest Diced, 1.9 oz dry	170	7	24
Shells & Cheese Microcups:			
Original; Queso Blanco, 2.4 oz dry	220	8	30
2% Milk, 2.4 oz dry	180	3	30

Kroger:

Kitchen Creation Skillet Dinners: *Per Cup, Prepared*

	C	F	Cb
Creamy Broccoli; Creamy Pasta	300	12	33
Double Cheeseburger	320	13	30
Lasagna	280	12	26

Frozen:

Healthy Meals Made Simple: *Refrigerated, Per Cup*

	C	F	Cb
Braised Beef Pot Roast & Gravy	220	5	15
Lean Beef Tips & Gravy	210	4	20
Lem. Herb Chkn w/ Rice	170	1.5	23
Sweet & Spicy Chicken	270	1.5	48

Meals Made Simple:

	C	F	Cb
Beef Stir Fry, 1¾ cups	180	4	26
Chicken Florentine, 2¼ cups, 6.9 oz	320	18	22
Chicken Stir Fry, 1½ cups	180	2	25
Shrimp Fried Rice, 1¼ cups, 8 oz	240	0	44

Oven Ready:

	C	F	Cb
Breaded Calamari Rings (10), 3 oz	200	10	21
Coconut Shrimp (5), with 1 oz sweet Chili Sauce	350	20	34

La Choy:

Family Meals, Canned: *Per 1 Cup*

	C	F	Cb
Beef Pepper Oriental, 8.9 oz	80	1	11
Beef Chow Mein, 8.7 oz	80	1	11
Chicken Chow Mein, 8.8 oz	100	3	10
Sweet & Sour Chicken, 8.9 oz	120	1	22

Lean Cuisine:

Comfort: *Per Complete Meal*

	C	F	Cb
Baked Chicken	250	6	34
Cheddar Bacon Chicken	200	7	12
Chkn in Sweet BBQ Sce	280	8	33
Chicken Parmesan	310	9	39
Glazed Chicken	240	3	34
Glazed Turkey Tenderloins	270	5	41
Herb Roasted Chicken	170	4	17
Meatloaf w/ Mashed Potoes	230	6	24
Roasted Turkey Breast	260	3	45
Salisbury Steak with Mac & Cheese	270	9	25
Shrimp Alfredo	200	3	30
Steak Portabella	160	3	16

Craveables: *Per Package*

	C	F	Cb
Flatbread Melt, Chkn Ranch Club	370	9	52
Paninis: Chicken Club	350	9	45
Chicken, Spinach & Mushroom	350	9	45
Philly-Style Steak & Cheese	330	9	44
Spring Rolls: Garlic Chicken (3)	210	7	25
Thai- Style Chicken (3)	190	7	22

Lean Cuisine (Cont): C F Cb

Market Place:

	C	F	Cb
Butternut Squash Ravioli	260	4	46
Chicken Cashew Stir Fry	270	2	48
Chicken with Peanut Sauce	290	7	35
Creamy Basil Chicken w/ Tortellini	240	6	28
Fiesta Grilled Chicken	250	5	33
Garlic Sesame Noodles w/ Beef	300	6	46
Pomegranate Chicken	180	3	20
Ricotta Cheese & Spinach Ravioli	310	7	51
Spicy Beef & Bean Enchilada	310	6	50
Spicy Penne Arrabbiata	240	5	40
Spinach Artichoke Ravioli	280	7	41
Sweet & Spicy Korean-Style Beef	320	7	50
Sweet Sriracha Braised Beef	180	5	18

Pizzas ~ *See Page 136*

Extra Product Listings ~ *www.CalorieKing.com*

Lean Pockets:

Sandwiches: *Per Single Pocket*

Pretzel Bread:

	C	F	Cb
Chicken Japalpeno Cheddar	260	7	36
Roasted Turkey, Bacon & Cheese	260	8	36

Seasoned Crust,

	C	F	Cb
Four Cheee Pizza	260	6	42

Whole Grain Crust:

	C	F	Cb
Bacon, Egg & Cheese	260	8	35
Chicken, Broccoli & Cheddar	240	5	39
Garlic Chicken White Pizza	260	6	41
Hickory Ham, Egg & Cheese	250	8	35

Lightlife (Meatless):

	C	F	Cb
Bowls: Chickpea Curry, 8 oz	310	7	50
Southwestern Quinoa & Black Bean	270	5	47
Gimme Lean Beef, 2 oz	60	0	7
Pasta: Veggie Sausage Ravioli, 8 oz	540	16	77
Wild Mushroom Ravioli, 8 oz	390	2	77
Smart Dogs: Veggie Hot Dog (1)	50	2	2
Jumbo Dog (1)	100	3.5	4
Smart Grounds, Crumbles, 2 oz	65	0	6
Smart Menue, Veggie Meatballs (3)	100	1.5	9
Smart Patties: Black Bean Burger	100	2.5	11
Garden Veggie Tempeh Burger (1)	100	3	10
Smart Sausages: Chorizo	150	9	4
Harvest Apple	170	9	13
Italian	140	7	7

Lunchables: C F Cb

Convenience Meals: *Single Serve Package*

	C	F	Cb
Ham & American	340	16	37
Pepperoni & Mozzarella	250	14	20
Uploaded: 6-Piece Chicken Dunks	410	18	49
6" Ham & American Sandwich	510	19	68
Nachos Grande	380	15	55
Ultimate Deep Dish Pepp. Pizza	430	18	53

Lunchmakers (Armour): *Per Package*

	C	F	Cb
Bologna Cracker Crunchers	250	14	21
Cheese Pizza	210	9	25
Nachos	210	9	30
Pepperoni Pizza	220	10	25
Turkey Cracker Crunchers	210	10	22

Marie Callender's:

Beef: *Per Container*

	C	F	Cb
Beef & Broccoli	370	9	50
Meat Loaf & Gravy	500	26	45
Spaghetti w/ Meat Sce	540	18	75
Steak & Roasted Potatoes	330	10	41
Three Meat Four Cheese Lasagna	240	8	30

Chicken: *Per Container*

	C	F	Cb
Chicken Parmigiana	440	16	51
Cntry Fried Chkn & Gravy	560	27	61
Herb Roasted Chicken	450	20	35
Sweet & Sour Chicken	510	13	81

Fish, Golden Battered Fish Filet | 430 | 12 | 60

Pasta: *Per Container*

	C	F	Cb
Fettuccini Alfredo & Garlic Bread	610	31	59
Grilled Chicken Alfredo Bake	460	19	45

Pot Pies: *Per 1 Cup, 7 oz*

	C	F	Cb
Beef	400	21	40
Cheesy Chicken & Bacon	510	32	41
Chicken	430	25	39
Chicken Corn Chowder	460	28	38

Creamy:

	C	F	Cb
Mushroom Chicken	430	25	39
Parmesan Chicken	430	26	36
Turkey	480	28	46

Family size: *Per 1 Cup*

	C	F	Cb
Cheesy Chicken Lasagna, 8 oz	320	14	33
Vermont White Cheddar, Mac & Cheese, 6.3 oz	350	20	31

Maruchan:	C	F	Cb
Bowls, all var., 3.3 oz	380	16	50
Ramen, Noodle Soup, average all, 3 oz pkg	380	16	52
Instant Lunch, average, 1 package	290	11	39
Yakisoba: *Per 4 oz Pkg*			
Chicken/Teriyaki Beef Flavor, av.	520	21	72
Sweet & Sour Chicken	560	22	78
Michael Angelo's:			
Organic: Chicken Parmesan, 10 oz	360	6	47
Eggplant Parmesan, 10 oz	260	11	23
Four Cheese Lasagna, 10 oz	360	12	39
Lasagna with Meat Sauce, 10 oz	390	16	38
Signature: Chicken Alfredo, 11 oz	320	8	43
Four Cheese Lasagna, 11 oz	420	15	50
Shrimp Scampi, 10 oz	550	29	47
Minute Rice:			
Ready To Serve: *Per 4.4 oz Container, Prepared*			
Brown/Chicken Rice Mix, average	230	4	44
Fried/Yellow Rice Mix, average	220	2.5	44
Morningstar Farms (Meatless):			
Bowls: Ital. Sausage Bake Veggie	240	11	33
Tuscan Greens & Beans	270	15	28
Breakfast, Patties, all flavors (1)	70	3	3
Burgers:			
Grillers Original (1)	130	6	5
Medit. Chickpea (1)	200	9	22
Spicy Black Bean (1)	110	4	13
Chik'n:			
Buffalo Wings (5)	200	9	19
Nuggets (4)	180	8	18
Pot Pie, Veggie Bowl	330	15	37
Chik Patties,			
Original (1)	160	6	19
Progressive Options:			
Garden Veggie Nuggets (5)	160	10	14
White Bean Chili Burger (1)	150	9	14
Newman's Own:			
Complete Skillet Meal: *Per ½ of 22-24 oz Package*			
Beef & Broccoli	250	10	22
Chicken: Fajita	310	6	46
Fettuccini Alfredo	410	12	49
Florentine & Farfalle	370	10	42
Italian Ssg. & Rigatoni	510	28	48
Orange Chicken	420	16	52
Nissin:			
Chow Mein: *Per 4 oz Package*			
Chicken Flavor	520	20	72
Spicy Chicken Flavor	560	28	66
Teriyaki Beef	480	20	66
With Shrimp	540	24	68
Parmigiana & Penne	490	25	47

Nissin (Cont):	C	F	Cb
Cup Noodles, all flavors, 1 cup	290	11	42
Very Veggie: Per ½ Pkg			
Spicy Chicken, 2.75 oz	340	11	53
Other var., 2.75 oz pkg	330	11	49
Raoh, ½ container, 1.9 oz	180	2	37
Souper Meals,			
av. all flavors, ½ pkg, 2.15 oz	280	13	38
Top Ramen, all flavors, 3 oz pkg	380	14	52
Old El Paso:			
Dinner Kits: *Prepared with Chicken*			
Chicken Soft Taco	330	15	29
Enchilada	390	16	27
Fajita	340	13	33
Pasta Roni: *Per Cup, Prepared*			
Angel Hair Pasta, with Herbs	310	12	42
Butter & Herb Italiano	300	12	42
Chicken & Broccoli	360	15	47
Chicken Flavor	300	12	39
Fettuccine Alfredo	440	24	48
Tomato Parmesan	270	9	39
White Cheddar & Broccoli	310	13	39
P.F. Chang's: *Per ½ Package, 11 oz*			
Meals: Beef with Broccoli	350	17	27
General Chang's Chicken	380	13	47
Kung Pao Chicken	350	15	34
Mongolian Style Beef	340	11	42
Orange Chicken	420	15	54
Sesame Chicken	380	20	32
Shrimp Lo Mein	410	13	56
Sweet & Sour Chicken	350	11	48
Prego:			
Ready Meals: *Per Pouch*			
Creamy Three Cheese Alfedo Rotini	370	19	37
Creamy Tomato Penne	390	12	61
Marinara & Italian Sausage Rotini	350	9	55
Roasted Tomato &Vegetables Penne	320	4	60

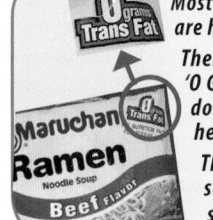

Most packaged noodle soups are high in calories and fat.

Their promotion of '0 Grams Trans Fat' does not make them heart-healthy.

They are still high in saturated fat as well as salt/sodium.

Rice-A-Roni:	C	F	Cb
Classic Favorites: *Per Cup, Prepared*			
Beef; Herb & Butter; Rice Pilaf, av.	310	9	52
Cheddar Broccoli	350	16	47
Chicken & Garlic	250	8	41
Spanish Rice	260	7	45
Microwave Cups:			
Cheddar Broccoli	230	4.5	41
Chicken Flavor	190	1	41
Four Cheese	240	6	43
Rosarita:			
Black Beans, 4.5 oz	110	0.5	19
Pinto Beans, 4.5 oz	120	0	22
Refried Beans:			
Traditional, 4.5 oz	120	2.5	18
No Fat, 4.5 oz	100	0	18
Safeway Select: *Per Tray*			
Frozen:			
Beef Salisbury Steak	400	25	23
Black Pepper Chicken	210	3.5	31
Chicken Cacciatore	290	10	34
Chicken Tikka Masala	260	5	36
Fettuccini Alfredo	480	15	75
H'style Baked Chicken	220	6	26
Lime Chili Chicken	260	3.5	43
Orange Chicken, Party Size, 6 oz	240	6	37
Penne Pasta, w/ Basil Cream Sauce	300	11	42
Pot Roast, w/ith Vegetables	200	6	22
S & W: *Per ½ Cup*			
Black Beans, 4.6 oz	120	0	22
Chili Beans,			
in Zesty Tom. Sauce, 4.6 oz	130	1.5	23
Kidney Beans, 4.6 oz	110	0	21
White Beans, 4.6 oz	100	0	19
Seapak ~ *See www.calorieking.com*			
Simply Asia:			
Noodle Bowls: *Per 8.5oz Bowl*			
Roasted Peanut	460	12	75
Sesame Teriyaki	390	3	82
Soy Ginger	420	6	84
Spicy Mongolian	430	6	86
Noodles & Sauce: *Per ⅓ Pkg*			
Sesame Teriyaki	300	3	60
Soy Ginger	320	4.5	60
Spicy Kung Pao	350	7	63
Quick Noodles: *Per 8.8 oz Tray*			
Honey Teriyaki	430	3.5	85
Pad Thai	460	3	93
Szechwan Garl. Chow Mein	460	7	83

Smart Ones *(Weight Watchers):*	C	F	Cb
Classic Favorites: *Per Meal*			
Angel Hair Marinara	180	2	34
Cheese Ravioli,			
in Mushroom Cream Sauce	230	5	35
Chicken Enchiladas Suiza	290	6	46
Lasagna Bake with Meat Sauce	250	5	39
Lasagna Florentine	310	9	45
Lemon Herb Chkn Piccata	210	2.5	32
Macaroni & Cheese	260	2	51
Pasta Primavera	200	2.5	35
Pasta w/ Ricotta & Spinach	290	5	44
Ravioli Florentine	210	3.5	37
Spagh. w/ Meat Sauce	280	3.5	50
Three Cheese Macaroni	300	6	48
Traditional Lasagna w/ Meat Sce	310	8	45
Tuna Noodle Casserole	250	3	44
Smart Anytime: *Per Meal*			
Brick Overn-Style Pepperoni Pizza	430	13	57
Chicken Quesadilla	170	6	17
Chicken Ranchero Mini Wrap	220	6	30
Chicken Slider	210	9	21
Spicy Chicken Slider	190	8	21
Smart Beginnings: *Per Meal*			
Breakfast Quesadilla	230	7	29
English Muffin S'wich,			
Egg White & Cheese	210	5	28
Three Cheese Omelet	200	7	20
Smart Creations: *Per Meal*			
Asian Style Beef & Broccili	160	4.5	16
Chicken Fettucini	300	4	45
Chicken Mesquite	250	3.5	33
Chicken Parmesan	280	5	37
Homestyle Turkey Breast,			
with Stuffing	280	6	36
Meatloaf	270	9	25
Teriyaki Chkn & Veggies	250	2.5	41
Stagg:			
Chili with Beans, 15 oz Can: *Per Cup*			
Classic,8.7 oz	330	17	28
Dynamite Hot, 8.7 oz	275	13	26
Turkey Ranchero,8.7 oz	340	17	30

Stouffers:

Classics: *Per Package*

	C	F	Cb
Baked Chicken Breast	240	8	17
Chicken a la King	360	12	44
Chicken Fett. Alfredo	570	27	55
Chicken Parmesan	410	14	47
Fettuccini Alfredo	630	35	63
Fish Filet with Mac & Cheese	400	19	35
Five Cheese Lasagna	330	14	33
Green Pepper Steak	240	4	32
Lasagna Bake with Meat Sauce	350	10	49
Macaroni & Beef	410	16	45
Macaroni & Cheese, w/ Broccoli	480	20	52
Meat Lovers Lasagna	420	19	41
Roast Turkey	270	9	30
Smoked Turkey Club Panini	380	15	37
Spagh. w/ Meatballs	360	12	45
Stuffed Pepper	210	9	23
Tuna Noodle Casserole	450	20	45
getable Lasagna	400	19	43
White Meat Chicken Pot Pie	670	38	64

Fit Kitchen: *Per Package*

	C	F	Cb
Bourbon Steak	410	13	48
Monterey Chicken	400	12	46
Rstd Red Pepper Chicken	370	10	42
Rotisserie Seasoned Turkey	330	10	37
Teriyaki Chicken	480	7	75

Satisfying Servings: *Per Package*

	C	F	Cb
Baked Ziti	520	18	68
Chicken Fettuccini Alfredo	840	38	94
Five Cheese Lasagna	660	28	66
Lasagna Italiano	580	24	60
Lasagna, w/ Meat Sce	260	9	28
Meatloaf	530	26	40
Meat Lovers Lasagna	620	28	32
Roast Turkey	440	16	47
Salisbury Steak	630	34	41

Simple Side Dishes: *Per Package*

	C	F	Cb
Cheddar Potato Bake	540	34	42
Creamed Spinach	400	32	16
Garlic Parmesan Mac & Cheese	680	30	72
Harvest Apple	380	6	80
Spinach Souffle	450	30	27
Welsh Rarebit	560	40	24
White Cheddar Mac & Cheese	640	32	62

Swanson:

Dinners: *Per Package*

	C	F	Cb
Chicken Nuggets	590	25	71
Rib Style Bnless Pork	540	23	71
Salisbury Steak	450	22	44

Skillets: *For Two*

	C	F	Cb
Alfredo Chicken	370	12	42
Beef Lo Mein	360	6	55
Chicken Parmesan	430	14	60
Garlic Chicken	420	15	51
Teriyaki Chicken	290	2.5	51

Tasty Bite:

Spice & Simmer: *Per ⅓ Pkg, 3.2 oz*

	C	F	Cb
Kashmir Curry	110	7	10
Korma	90	7	5
Tikka Masala	90	4	12

Thai Entrees: *Per ½ Pkg, 5 oz*

	C	F	Cb
Bangkok Vegetables	130	7	11
Cashew Curry	140	9	12
Penang Ginger Curry	100	6	10

Vegetarian Entrees: *Per ½ Pkg, 5 oz*

	C	F	Cb
Bengal Lentils	160	6	20
Bombay Potatoes	120	2	22
Jaipur Vegetables	180	11	12
Jodhpur Lentils	110	2.5	16
Madras Lentils	150	6	18
Punjab Eggplant	150	9	13

TGI Friday's:

	C	F	Cb
Cheese & Bacon Loaded Fries, 3 oz	200	11	20
Chicken Parmesan Sliders, 3 oz	260	13	27
Chkn Wings, Buffalo Style Sce, 4.2 oz	220	16	10
Cream Cheese Stuffed Jalap., 2.7 oz	220	11	20
Crispy Green Bean Fries & Sce, 3 oz	190	9	26
Dill Pickle Chips, w/ Horseradish Sce	200	11	22
Mozzarella Sticks (1), w/ Marinara Sauce	100	5	10
Potato Skins, Bacon Ranch(3)	140	8	15

Thai Kitchen:

Take-Out Meals: *Per ½ Package*

	C	F	Cb
Original Pad Thai	250	2	54
Thai Basil & Chili	250	3	50
Thai Peanut	270	5	51

Noodle Carts: *Per 9 oz Tray*

	C	F	Cb
Pad Thai	460	2	104
Thai Peanut	510	9	96

Rice Noodle Soup Bowls,

	C	F	Cb
average all varieties, 2.5 oz	240	2	50

Stir-Fry Rice Noodles: *Per ½ Package*

	C	F	Cb
Original Pad Thai	390	3.5	84
Thai Peanut	390	2	87

Tofurky: *Per Item*	C	F	Cb
Chick'n:			
Barbeque, 3.2 oz	200	5	14
Sesame Garlic, 3.2 oz	210	9	10
Tandoori, 3.2 oz	180	6	9
Pocket: Ham & Cheeses Style	230	7	40
Pepperoni Pizza Style	230	5	43
Turk'y Broccoli & Cheddar Style	220	5	41
Trader Joe's:			
Baked Beans, Organic, av., ¹/₂ cup	140	0	29
Black Beans:			
Regular, ¹/₂ cup	110	0	19
Cuban Style, ¹/₂ cup	100	0.5	19
Chicken Chili with Beans, 1 cup	290	9	32
Pasta, Shells & White Cheddar, 1 cup	280	6	47
Potatoes: Garlic Mashed, ¹/₂ cup	150	7	19
Cheddar Cheese Au Gratin, ¹/₂ cup	140	5	21
Turkey Chili w/ Beans, 1 cup	240	4.5	30
Frozen:			
Butter Chicken w/ Basmati Rice, 1 cup	270	8	33
Chicken Chow Mein, ¹/₃ pkg, 6.7 oz	210	2	35
Chicken Quesadilla (1), 6 oz	320	16	26
Citrus Glazed Chicken with Rice, 8 oz	270	5	40
Mac & Cheese: Regular, 1 cup, 7 oz	360	15	42
Reduced Guilt, 7 oz	270	6	40
Pies: Chicken Pot Pie, ¹/₂ pie, 8 oz	360	22	28
Shepherd's Pie, 1 cup, 8 oz	170	3	22
Shrimp Stir Fry, 6.4 oz	70	0.5	6
Spaghetti & Beef Meatballs, 1 cup, 9 oz	380	13	48
Spicy Beef & Broccoli, 1³/₄ cups	430	13	64
Thai Vegetable Kao Soi, 12.6 oz	430	20	55
Vegetable Pad Thai, 10.5 oz tray	520	21	74
Tyson:			
Any'tizers Snacks:			
Chicken Wings:			
Buffalo Style Hot Wings, bone-in, 3 oz	190	13	3
Honey BBQ, 3 oz	190	12	8
Hot & Spicy, 3 oz	190	13	1
Chicken Wyngz, Boneless:			
Buffalo Style, 3 pcs	150	7	8
Honey BBQ, 3 oz	200	8	20

Tyson (Cont):	C	F	Cb
Beef: Country Fried Steak, (1)	300	21	15
Steak Fingers (2)	250	18	14
Buffalo Style Chicken Strips, 3 oz	190	9	17
Chicken Patties, (1)	200	13	10
Crispy Chicken Strips, 3 oz	190	9	12
Fun Chiccken Nuggets, (4)	180	11	10
Grilled & Ready Chicken Breasts:			
Fajita Strips, 3 oz	110	4	1
Fillets (1)	110	2	2
Oven Roasted, Diced, 3 oz	100	2.5	1
Pulled, 2 oz	80	2.5	2
Southwestern, 3 oz	120	3	5
Sweet Teriyaki Fillets, 3 oz	140	6	4
Honey Batt. Chkn Brst Tenders, 3 oz	220	13	13
Honey BBQ Chicken Strips, 3 oz	200	8	20
Naturals, Chicken Breasts:			
Grilled Nuggets, 3 oz	110	3	2
Ital. Style Lightly Breaded Strips, 3 oz	150	7	7
Lightly Breaded Strips, 3 oz	150	7	7
Wh. Grain Breaded Chunks, 3 oz	210	10	12
Premium Selects, 3 oz	170	9	7
Southern Style Tenderloins, 3 oz	180	9	12
Spicy Chicken Breast Patties, (1)	200	13	10
Uncle Ben's:			
Country Inn: *Per Cup, Prepared with Water Only*			
Broccoli Rice Au Gratin	210	2.5	41
Chicken & Vegetable Rice	200	1.5	43
Chicken Flavored Rice	200	1.5	42
Rice Pilaf	200	1	43
Flavored Grains: *Dry Mix Only, as Directed*			
5 Grain Medley Quinoa Pilaf	200	1.5	41
Basmati Medley Savory Herb	200	0.5	43
Brown Rice Medley, Roasted Garlic & Herbs, 2 oz	200	2	40
Flav. Infusions, dry mix, av., 1.7 oz	155	0.5	34
Ready Rice: *Per Package, Heat & Serve*			
Butter & Garlic Flavored	220	4	41
Garden Vegetable	210	2.5	42
Roasted Chicken Flavored	210	3	42
Teriyaki Style	220	3	42
Van Camp's:			
Baked Beans: Orig., ¹/₂ cup, 4.8 oz	150	0.5	30
Bacon Flavored, ¹/₂ cup, 4.8 oz	170	1	32
Beanee Weenee, Original, 7.75 oz	260	8	33

Van De Kamp's:

	C	F	Cb
Appetizers:			
Crab Cakes, 3 oz	120	2	11
Crunchy Popcorn Fish, 4 oz	270	3	25
Fillets:			
Beer Battered/Crispy, 3.8 oz	210	10	21
Crunchy, 1.8 oz	90	4	13
Fish Sticks,			
Crunchy, 3.6 oz	220	10	20
Fish For Tacos & Sandwiches:			
Fish Tenders, 3.6 oz	230	11	21
Sandwich: Original Recipe, 3 oz	190	10	18
Spicy Recipe, 3 oz	170	9	19
Flavor Crusted Fillets:			
Black Pepper & Salt Salmon, 4.5 oz	230	8	20
Garlic Herb Cod, 5 oz	260	10	26
Lemon Pepper Cod, 5 oz	280	10	26
Mediterranean Tilapia,, 5 oz	270	10	26
Parmesan & Rstd Garlic Tilapia, 5 oz	280	1	26

Whole Foods (365):

	C	F	Cb
Chickenless Nuggets, breaded (4), 2.8 oz	180	7	16
Meatless Meatballs (4), 2 oz	110	4	9
Meatless Burgers (1), 2.5 oz	120	4.5	7
Pasta Rings in Tomato Sauce, 1 cup	150	1	31
Vegetarian Chili, 1 cup	130	2	25

Worthington/Loma Linda:

	C	F	Cb
Big Franks: 1 link, 1.8 oz	110	6	3
Low-fat, 1 link, 1.1 oz	45	1.5	3
Chili, 1 cup, 8.10 oz	280	10	25
Choplets, Low Fat, 2 slices, 3.2 oz	90	1	4
Diced Chik, Low Fat, 2 oz	50	0	2
Fishless Tuna, 1.5 oz drained	60	1	5
FriChik, 2 pieces, 3.2 oz	140	8	3
Linketts (1), 1.3 oz	70	4	1
Little Links (2), 1.6 oz	90	5	3
Redi-Burger, Low Fat, 3 oz	120	2.5	7
Saucettes (1), 1.35 oz	90	6	1
Super Links (1), 1.1 oz	45	1.5	3
Tender Rounds w/ Gravy (6), 2.8 oz	120	4.5	6
Vegetarian Burger, 1/4 cup, 1.9 oz	70	1.5	3
Veja-Links (1), 1.1 oz	45	1.5	3

Yves Veggie Cuisine *(Meatless):*

	C	F	Cb
Balls, Falafel (3)	150	7	17
Bites, Kale & Quinoa (4)	90	2.5	13
Breakfast, Veggie Patties (2)	80	2	5
Burgers: Gluten Free Veggie (1)	110	6	5
Kale & Root Vegetables (1)	110	6	5
The Good Veggie (1)	110	3.5	7
Deli Slices:	80	2.5	2
Bologna, 3 slices	60	1	2
Ham, 5 slices	80	1	5
Pepperoni, 10 slices	45	1	3
Salami, 5 slices	80	1	5
Turkey, 5 slices	80	1	4
Dogs: Good Dog (1)	45	1	2
Veggie (1)	50	0.5	3
Jumbo (1), 2.7 oz	110	2	4
Veggie Tofu (1)	50	1	2
Ground Rounds:			
Original, 1.9 oz	60	0.5	5
Garden Veggie Crumble, 1.95 oz	80	1.5	9
Taco Stuffers, 1.95 oz	80	3	6
Hot Dog:			
Good Dog (1), 2 oz	70	3.5	1
Hot Dog (1), 1.5 oz	50	0.5	2
Jumbo Hot Dog (1), 2.8 oz	110	3	5
Tofu Dog (1), 1.5 oz	45	1	2

Zatarain's:

New Orleans Style: *Per Dry Mix Only*

	C	F	Cb
Black Beans & Rice, Original, 2.3 oz	230	1	47
Caribbean Rice Mix, 2.5 oz	250	2	52
Chicken Flavor Rice, 2 oz	210	0.5	45
Creamy Parmesan Rice Mix, 2.3 oz	240	4	45
Garlic & Herb & Rice Mix, 1.5 oz	130	0.5	29
Rice Pilaf, 2 oz	210	0.5	45
Smothered Chicken Rice Mix, 1.6 oz	160	0.5	34
Yellow Rice, 2 oz	200	0.5	43

Frozen Meals: *Per Meal*

	C	F	Cb
Blackened Chicken Alfredo, 10.5 oz	500	21	56
Dirty Rice with Beef & Pork, 10 oz	430	13	64
Jambalaya Flavored w/ Ssg, 12 oz	490	10	86
Red Beans & Rice w/ Sausage, 12 oz	540	17	79
Shrimp Scampi with Pasta, 10.5 oz	350	10	49

Note: Cooking reduces weight of meat by 20-45% due to water and fat losses. Average weight loss is 30%. Actual loss depends on cooking method and cooking time.

Examples:

4 oz raw weight = approx. 3 oz cooked weight

4 oz cooked weight = approx. $5^1/_2$ oz raw weight

What 3 oz Cooked Meat Looks Like:

• Rectangular piece (4" x $2^1/_2$ " x $^1/_2$" thick)

• Deck of cards ($3^1/_2$" x $2^1/_2$" x $^5/_8$ " thick)

Quick Guide C F Cb

Sirloin (Choice Grade):
External fat trimmed to $^1/_2$"
Broiled, Edible Portion (no bone)

Small/Regular Serving, 3 oz, cooked weight:
(from 4-$4^1/_2$ oz raw)

Lean + external fat ($^1/_8$"), 3 oz	220	13	0
Lean + marbling, 3 oz	185	9	0
Lean only, 3 oz	160	6	0

(No external fat or marbling)

Medium Serving, 5 oz, cooked weight:
(from approximately 7 oz raw)

Lean + external fat ($^1/_8$"), 5 oz	365	22	0
Lean + marbling, 5 oz	310	15	0
Lean only, 5 oz	265	10	0

Large Serving, 8 oz, cooked weight:
(from approximately 11-12 oz raw)

Lean + external fat ($^1/_2$"), 8 oz	585	36	0
Lean + marbling, 8 oz	500	24	0
Lean only, 8 oz	425	15	0

Extra Large Serving, 12 oz, cooked weight:
(from approximately 16-17 oz raw)

Lean + external fat ($^1/_8$"), 12 oz	875	54	0
Lean + marbling, 12 oz	745	36	0
Lean only, 12 oz	640	22	0

Pan Fried:
Sirloin (Choice), medium serving,

Lean + external fat ($^1/_8$"), 5 oz	445	30	0

Other Steaks C F Cb

Filet Mignon (Tenderloin):
1 Medium steak, 6 oz raw weight:
Broiled, with $^1/_4$" fat trim:

Lean + fat ($^1/_4$"), 4 oz	360	27	0
Lean only, 3.5 oz	230	12	0

New York/Club Steak:
Top Loin/Short Loin:
1 steak, regular (9.25 oz raw, $^1/_4$" fat):
Broiled: Lean + fat ($^1/_4$"), 6.3 oz

Broiled: Lean + fat ($^1/_4$"), 6.3 oz	580	43	0
Lean + marbling, 5.5 oz	400	25	0
Lean only, 5.25 oz	360	20	0

Porterhouse Steak:
1 Medium, 6 oz raw weight, w/out bone, broiled:

Lean + fat ($^1/_4$"), 4.3 oz	410	33	0
Lean only, 3.5 oz	210	11	0

1 Large , 12 oz raw weight, without bone, broiled:

Lean + fat ($^1/_4$"), 8.5 oz cooked	820	66	0
Lean only, 7 oz cooked	420	22	0

T-Bone Steak: *Broiled or Grilled*
Medium Size: *8 oz raw weight, without bone*
Approximately 6 oz cooked:

Lean + Fat ($^1/_4$"), 5 oz	400	28	0
Lean only, 4 oz	265	12	0

Large Size: *12 oz raw weight*
Approximately 9 oz cooked:

Lean + fat ($^1/_4$"), 7 oz, without bone	560	39	0
Lean only, 6 oz, without bone	400	18	0

Extra Large Size: *20 oz raw weight*
Approximately 16 oz cooked:

Lean + Fat ($^1/_4$"), 12 oz, without bone	960	66	0
Lean Only, 10 oz, without bone	660	30	0

Also See Fast-Foods & Restaurants Section ~
Lone Star Steakhouse; Outback Steakhouse

M Meat & Beef

Beef – Individual Cuts   C F Cb

Average All Grades
Edible Weight, Without Bone

	C	F	Cb
Brisket, whole, braised:			
Lean + fat ($^1/_4$" trim), 3 oz	330	27	0
Lean + marbling, 3 oz	250	17	0
Lean only, 3 oz	185	9	0
Chuck Blade, braised:			
Lean + fat ($^1/_4$"), 3 oz	310	24	0
Lean + marbling, 3 oz	295	22	0
Lean only, 3 oz	245	13	0
Flank: Raw, 4 oz	175	8	0
Braised, 3 oz	225	14	0
Broiled, 3 oz	155	6	0
Round, bottom, braised:			
Lean + marbling, 3 oz	190	7.5	0
Lean only, 3 oz	185	6.5	0
Round, eye/tip, rstd:			
Lean + fat ($^1/_4$"), 3 oz	205	11	0
Lean, w/ marbling, 3 oz	150	5	0
Round, top: *Per 3 oz, Cooked Weight*			
Braised, Lean + fat	210	10	0
Lean only	170	4	0
Broiled, Lean + fat	180	8	0
Lean only	160	5	0
Pan-fried, Lean + fat	235	13	0
Lean only	195	7	0

Beef Ribs

Back Ribs: *7" long, visible fat trimmed to $^1/_4$"*
10.3 oz raw w/ bone or 3.5 oz cooked, braised, w/o bone

	C	F	Cb
1 average rib	410	34	0
3 ribs	1230	102	0

Short Ribs: *2$^1/_2$" long, visible fat trimmed to $^1/_4$"*
6 oz raw with bone or 2.52 oz cooked, braised, w/o bone

	C	F	Cb
1 average rib	320	28	0
3 ribs	960	85	0

Ground Beef

	C	F	Cb
Ground Beef, Raw: *Per 4 oz*			
70% lean (30% fat)	380	34	0
75% lean (25% fat)	335	29	0
80% lean (20% fat)	290	23	0
85% lean (15% fat)	245	17	0
90% lean (10% fat)	200	12	0
95% lean (5% fat)	155	6	0
Baked/Broiled: Regular (70%), 3 oz	230	16	0
Lean (80%), 3 oz	215	14	0
Extra lean (90%), 3 oz	185	10	0
Pan-Broiled:			
Regular (70%), 3 oz	230	15	0
Lean (80%), 3 oz	210	14	0
Extra lean (90%), 3 oz	195	10	0
Ground Beef Patties: *Average, 23% Fat*			
Raw, 4 oz	330	25	0
Broiled, 3 oz (from 4 oz raw)	250	19	0

Quick Guide   C F Cb

Roast Beef
Round (Eye/Tip, average): *Average All Cuts*
Small/Regular Serving: *3 oz*
(2 thin slices/1 thick slice)

	C	F	Cb
Lean + fat ($^1/_8$" fat trim)	180	9	0
Lean only	145	4	0
Medium Serving: *5 oz*			
(3-4 thin slices)			
Lean + fat ($^1/_8$" fat trim)	300	15	0
Lean only	245	6.5	0
Large Serving, 8 oz: *3 thick slices*			
Lean + fat ($^1/_8$" fat trim)	480	24	0
Lean only	385	11	0

Roast Dinner Extras

	C	F	Cb
Gravy: Thin, 2 Tbsp	20	0.5	3.5
Thick, 2 Tbsp	50	2	0.5
1 Ladle/4 Tbsp	100	4	1
Veggies: Beans, green, $^1/_2$ cup	20	0	5
Cauliflower with cheese sauce, 4 oz	135	9	15
Corn, kernels, $^1/_4$ cup	35	0	9
Carrots, $^1/_4$ cup	20	0	3
Peas, $^1/_4$ cup	35	0	6
Potato:			
Baked in jacket: Plain, 1 large	280	0	63
With sour cream, 2 Tbsp	270	5	64
With whipped butter, 1 Tbsp	350	8	63
Roasted with fat, 1 small	155	8	30
Sweet Potato/Yam, 1 medium	105	1	24
Yorkshire Pudding, 1 oz	90	3.5	11

	C	F	Cb
Beef Kebab: *Cooked*			
Beef & Veggies, 2 oz	160	10	4
If very lean meat	100	4	4

"347 ~ 348 ~ 349..."

124

Lamb

	C	F	Cb

Choice Grade:

Leg (Whole), roasted:
	C	F	Cb
Lean + fat, 3 oz	220	14	0
Lean only, 3 oz	160	7	0

Leg (Sirloin Half), roasted:
Lean + fat, 3 oz	250	18	0
Lean only, 3 oz	175	8	0

Leg (Shank Half), roasted:
Lean + fat, 3 oz	190	11	0
Lean only, 3 oz	155	6	0

Loin Chop, broiled:
1 chop (raw weight, 4.25 oz):
Lean + fat (2.25 oz edible)	180	12	0
Lean only (1.6 oz edible)	85	3.5	0

Rib Chop, broiled:
1 chop (raw wt., 3.5 oz):
Lean + fat (2.5 oz edible)	255	21	0
Lean only (1.75 oz edible)	105	6	0

Shoulder (Arm/Blade):
Braised: Lean + fat, 3 oz	295	21	0
Lean only, 3 oz	240	12	0
Broiled: Lean + fat, 3 oz	240	17	0
Lean only, 3 oz	170	8	0
Roasted: Similar to Broiled			

Cubed Lamb (Leg/Shoulder):
For stew or kebab:
Braised, lean only, 3 oz	190	8	0
Broiled, lean only, 3 oz	160	6	0

Veal

Edible Weights:
Leg (Top Round):
	C	F	Cb
Braised: Lean + fat, 3 oz	180	6	0
Lean only, 3 oz	175	5	0
Pan-fried, breaded:			
Lean + fat, 3 oz	195	8	9
Lean only, 3 oz	185	6	9
Pan-fried, not breaded:			
Lean + fat, 3 oz	180	7	0
Lean only, 3 oz	155	4	0
Roasted: Lean + fat, 3 oz	135	4	0
Lean only, 3 oz	130	3	0

Veal (Cont)

	C	F	Cb

Loin Chop: 1 chop, 7 oz raw weight
Braised: Lean + fat, 3 oz	240	15	0
Lean only, 3 oz	190	8	0
Roasted: Lean + fat, 3 oz	185	11	0
Lean only, 3 oz	150	6	0

Rib, roasted: Lean + fat, 3 oz
	195	12	0
Lean only, 3 oz	150	7	0

Shoulder, Arm/Blade, roasted:
Lean + fat, 3 oz	155	7	0
Lean only, 3 oz	140	5	0

Sirloin, roasted:
Lean + fat, 3 oz	170	9	0
Lean only, 3 oz	145	6	0

Cubed for Stew, braised:
Leg/Shoulder, lean only, 3 oz	160	4	0
(1 lb raw yields approximately 9.25 oz cooked)			

Pork

Fresh Pork: Cooked Weight, without bone):
4 oz raw weight = approx. 3 oz cooked weight

BBQ, Pulled:
	C	F	Cb
2 oz	90	2.5	10
4 oz	180	5	20
8oz	360	10	40

Blade Steak, broiled:
Lean + fat, 3 oz	220	15	0
Lean only, 3 oz	190	11	0

Country Style Ribs, broiled/roasted:
Lean + fat, 3 oz	280	22	0
Lean only, 3 oz	210	13	0

Spareribs, braised: Lean & fat, 6 oz
(from 1 lb raw weight)	675	52	0

Leg (Ham), whole, roasted:
Lean + fat, 3 oz	230	15	0
Lean only, 3 oz	180	8	0

Loin Chops, broiled: Average
(From 1 chop: 5 oz raw weight with bone or 4 oz raw weight, without bone)
Lean + fat, 3 oz	200	11	0
Lean only, 3 oz	165	7	0

Loin Roast, roasted:
Lean + fat, 3 oz	210	13	0
Lean only, 3 oz	180	8	0

Rib Chops, (Boneless), broiled:
Lean + fat, 3 oz	220	14	0
Lean only, 3 oz	185	9	0

Rib Roast:
Lean + fat, 3 oz	215	13	0
Lean only, 3 oz	180	9	0

Pork (Cont) | C | F | Cb

	C	F	Cb
Sirloin Chop, broiled:			
Lean + fat, 3 oz	180	8	0
Lean only, 3 oz	165	6	0
Sirloin Roast, roasted:			
Lean + fat, 3 oz	175	8	0
Lean only, 3 oz	170	7	0
Tenderloin (Boneless), roasted:			
Lean + fat, 3 oz	125	4	0
Lean only, 3 oz	120	3	0
Ground Pork:			
Raw, average, $1/4$ lb, 4 oz	300	24	0
Broiled, 3 oz	250	18	0
Pan-fried, drained, 3 oz	260	19	0

Bacon

	C	F	Cb
Raw: 1 med. slice, 0.75 oz	95	9	0
1 thick slice, 1.3 oz	175	17	0
(1 lb raw yields approximately 5 oz cooked)			
Broiled/Pan-Fried:			
1 medium slice, 0.3 oz	40	3	0
3 medium slices, 0.8	125	10	0
2 thin slices, 0.5 oz	75	6	0
1 thick slice, 0.9 oz	65	5	0
Canadian Bacon:			
Cooked: 1 slice, 1 oz	45	2	0.5
2 slices, 2 oz	90	4	1
Bacon Bits, 1 Tbsp, 0.3 oz	35	2	0
Breakfast Strips, Broiled, 1 sl., 0.4 oz	50	4	0

Ham

	C	F	Cb
Boneless Ham, cooked:			
Regular, (approximately 13% fat):			
Roasted, 3 oz	150	8	0
Extra Lean (5% fat),			
Roasted, 3 oz	125	5	0
Whole Ham, cooked:			
Lean + fat (as purchased)			
Roasted, 3 oz	210	15	0
Lean only, Roasted, 3 oz	135	5	0
Canned Ham: Similar to boneless ham			
Chopped, canned, 3 oz	200	16	0
Ham Patties, cooked, (1), 2.3 oz	220	20	1
Ham Steak, extra lean, 2 oz	70	2.5	0
Lunch Slices ~ See Deli Meats, Page 128			

Game & Other Meats | C | F | Cb

	C	F	Cb
Bison Steak,			
lean, 6 oz (raw)	205	4	0
Boar (wild), roasted, 3 oz	140	4	0
Buffalo Steak,			
New West Foods, 4 oz	70	3	0
Caribou, roasted, 3 oz	140	4	0
Deer/Venison, roasted 3 oz	135	3	0
Goat (Capretto):			
Raw, 3 oz	95	2	0
Roasted, 3 oz	120	2.5	0
Ostrich:			
Blackwing Ostrich Meats:			
Sausage Patties (2) 2 oz	60	0.5	0
Sport Jerky, 0.5 oz piece	25	0	0
New West Foods:			
Ground Ostrich, 4 oz	165	7	0
Ostrich Steak, 4 oz steak	130	2.5	0
Rabbit: Roasted, 3 oz	165	7	0
Stewed, 1 cup, diced, 5 oz	290	12	0

Variety & Organ Meats

	C	F	Cb
Brain (Lamb): Braised, 3 oz	125	9	0
Pan-fried, 3 oz	230	19	0
Chitterlings, pork, simmered, 3 oz	260	25	0
Ears, pork, simmered, 1 ear, 4 oz	185	12	0
Feet, Pork: Simmered, 3 oz	200	14	0
Cured, pickled, 3 oz	170	14	0
Hormel, 2 oz	80	6	0
Head Cheese (Pork Snouts/Ears/Vinegar/Spices),			
1 oz slice	50	4	0
Heart, Beef, braised, 3 oz	140	4	0
Jowl, pork, raw, 4 oz	750	80	0
Kidneys, braised, 3 oz	140	5	0
Liver (beef): Raw, 4 oz	150	4	4
Braised, 3 oz	140	4	3
Pan-fried, 3 oz	185	7	7
Pancreas, pork, braised, 3 oz	185	8	0
Pork Cracklins, 0.5 oz	80	6	0
Pork Hocks, 1 piece, 6 oz	340	23	0
Scrapple, pork, 2 oz	120	8	8
Spleen, pork, braised, 3 oz	130	3	0
Stomach, pork, raw, 4 oz	185	12	0
Sweetbreads:			
Beef,/Lamb, cooked, 3 oz	125	9	0
Tail, pork, simmered, 3 oz	340	31	0
Tongue: Raised Veal, 3 oz	170	9	0
Beef/Lamb/Pork, av., 3 oz	235	17	0
Tripe, beef, raw, 3 oz	85	3.5	0

Quick Guide   Ⓒ Ⓕ Ⓒ♭

Franks & Weiners
Average All Brands
Regular (Pork Mix): *Per Frank*

	C	F	Cb
Regular, 1.5 oz	140	13	1
Bun Length/Jumbo, 2 oz	185	17	2
Extra Long, 2.75 oz	255	24	2
Small/Cocktail, each	30	3	0.5

Beef Franks: *Per Frank*

Regular, 1.5 oz	140	13	2
Bun Length/Jumbo, 2 oz	175	17	2.5
1/4 lb Dog, 4 oz	375	33	5

Franks & Weiners

Ball Park: *Per 2 oz Frank Unless Indicated*
Angus Beef:

	C	F	Cb
Original; Bun Size, 2 oz	170	15	3
Lean, 1.8 oz	70	5	2
Beef: Original, Bun Size, 2 oz	190	16	4
Deli Style, Regular, 1.8 oz	150	12	2
Grillmaster, Hearty, 3 oz	250	21	3
Lean, 1.76 oz	80	5	2
Park's Finest, 2 oz	170	15	2
Foster Farms, Chicken; Turkey, 2 oz	140	12	1

Hebrew National: *Per Frank*
Beef: Regular, 1.7 oz

Regular, 1.7 oz	150	13	2
1/4 Pounder, 4 oz	350	31	4
Jumbo, 3 oz	260	23	3
97% Fat-Free, 1.6 oz	45	1	2
Bun Length Beef Frank, 2 oz	170	15	2

Jennie-O: *Per Frank*
Turkey Franks:

1.2 oz	70	6	1
Jumbo, 2 oz	120	10	1
Turkey Bratwurst, 3.8 oz	170	10	2

Oscar Mayer: *Per Frank*
Angus Beef:

Classic, 1.5 oz	130	12	1
Bun Length, 1.76 oz	170	15	2
Turkey, Classic, 1.6 oz	100	7	2

Shelton's: *Per Frank*

Chicken, uncured, 1.2 oz	80	7	0
Turkey, Regular, 1.2 oz	60	4.5	1
Zacky Farms, Chkn; Turkey, av, 2 oz	115	10	4

Quick Guide   Ⓒ Ⓕ Ⓒ♭

Fresh Sausages
Pork/Beef: *Average All Types*

	C	F	Cb
Small: Raw, 4" link, 1 oz	85	7.5	0
Broiled/Pan-fried	80	7	0
Medium: Raw, 2 oz	170	15	0
Broiled/Pan-fried	165	14	0
Large: Raw, 3 oz	255	22	0
Broiled/Pan-fried	245	21	0
Italian: Raw, 3.2 oz	315	28	1
Cooked, 2.4 oz	230	18	3
Chorizo: Beef Chorizo, 2.5 oz piece	250	23	5
Pork Chorizo, 2 oz piece	250	23	5

Note: Fat is lost in broiling/pan frying.
Cooked weight = approx. 60-70% raw weight

Smoked Sausages

Per Link:

	C	F	Cb
Butterball, Turkey, 2 oz	100	6	4
Eckrich:			
Original (1)	230	18	6
Cheddar (1), 2.36 oz	210	18	3
Hillshire Farm:			
Cheddarwurst, 2 oz	180	16	2
Chicken Hardwood, 2 oz	100	7	3
Polska Kielbasa, 2 oz	180	16	0

Johnsonville ~ *See CalorieKing.Com*

Breakfast Sausages/Patties

Butterball: *Fully Cooked*

Turkey: B'fast Sausage Links (3), 2 oz	90	5	0
Patties (2), 2 oz	90	5.5	0

Jimmy Dean: *Fully Cooked*
Heat 'N Serve Sausage Links:

Pork, Regular (3), 1.9 oz	210	19	2
Turkey (3), 2 oz	130	8	2

Heat 'N Serve Sausage Patties:

Pork, Original (2), 1.8 oz	200	17	2
Turkey (2), 1.8 oz	120	8	1
Maple Pork Sausages,(3), 2.4 oz	260	22	3
Pork Patties, (2), 2.3 oz	270	24	2

Breakfast Sandwiches ~ *See Page 92*
Jones Dairy Farm:
Golden Brown Sausages: *Fully Cooked*

Mild Pork Sausages (3), 2 oz	250	24	1
Maple Pork Sausages (3), 2 oz	240	22	2

Vegetarian Patties:
Boca ~ *See Page 117*
GardenBurer ~ *See Page 114*

Bagel, Corn & Hot Dogs   C   F   Cb

Hot Dogs, Ready-To-Go:
Includes Ketchup/Relish

	C	F	Cb
Regular, 1.5 oz frank, 1.5 oz bun	260	15	22
Bun Length, 2 oz frank, 1.5 oz bun	290	18	21
Jumbo Dog, 2 oz frank, 2 oz bun	360	20	36
¼ lb Beef Dog, 2 oz bun	480	15	36
Mile Long Dog, 2.6 oz dog, 1.5 oz bun	360	24	23

Corn Dogs:
Beef/Pork Frank, average, 2.6 oz	170	10	16
Foster Farms:			
Corn Dogs:			
Chili Cheese (1), 2.7 oz	190	9	21
Honey Crunchy:			
Regular (1), 2.7 oz	190	9	18
Jumbo (1), 4 oz	280	14	27
Mini (4), 2.7 oz	220	13	19
State Fair: *Per Dog*			
Beef Corn Dog, 2.7 oz	230	11	26
Classic Corn Dog, Reg., 4 oz	330	11	34
Mini Classic (5), 3.3 oz	270	14	29

Bagel Dogs:
Hebrew National:			
Beef Bagel Dogs, 4 pieces, 2.75 oz	240	13	22
Schwanns, Bagel Dogs,			
with Cheese, 1 piece, 4.5 oz	370	16	40
Vienna Beef:			
Bagel Dog: 5.5 oz	410	19	44
6.5 oz	490	19	58
Mini (5), 4.6 oz	310	18	31

Hot Dog Toppings/Extras:
American Cheese, 1 slice, 1 oz	110	9	1
Chili Con Carne, ¼ cup	50	2	5.5
Ketchup, 1 Tbsp	15	0	4
Mustard, 1 Tbsp	20	0	1
Onions, chopped, 1 Tbsp	5	0	1
Pickle Relish, 1 Tbsp	20	0	5
Sauerkraut, ½ cup	20	0	5

Deli/Lunch Meats & Sausage

	C	F	Cb
Beef Jerky/Meat Snacks,			
Berliner (pork/beef), 1 oz	65	5	1
Beerwurst (Beef):			
Small (2¾"diam), 1/16" slice	20	2	0
Large (4" diam), 1/8" slice	75	7	0.5
Beerwurst (Pork):			
Small (2.75"diameter), 1/16" slice	15	1	0
Large (4"diameter), 1/8" Slice	55	4	0.5
Blood Sausage, 1 oz	100	9	0.5

Deli/Lunch Meats & Sausages (Cont)

Bologna: C   F   Cb

	C	F	Cb
Beef Bologna: 1 slice, 1 oz	90	8	0
Light, 1 slice, 1 oz	60	4	2
Oscar Mayer: Regular, 1 oz	90	8	1
98% Fat Free, 1 oz	40	1.5	1
Light, 1 slice, 1 oz	60	4	1
Boar's Head, Ring, 2 oz	150	13	1
Pork Bologna: 1 Slice, 1 oz	65	6	1
Fat-Free, 1 slice, 1 oz	20	0	2
Turkey Bologna, average, 1 oz	60	5	0.5
Bratwurst: Average, 1 oz	80	7	1
Bob Evan's, Beer B'wurst, 2.2 oz link	170	14	0
Braunschweiger, (Pork/Liver/Sausage),			
Oscar Mayer, 2 oz slice	190	17	0
Chicken, average:			
1 thick or 2 thin slices, 1 oz	30	1	1
2 oz slice	60	2	2
Hillshire Farm,			
Rotiss. Seas'nd Chicken Breast, 2 oz	50	0.5	2
Corned Beef, average, full fat, 1 oz	60	5	0.5
Ham, Sliced:			
Baked/Broiled, 1 oz slice	35	1	1
Oscar Mayer, Baked, Lean,			
3 slices, 2.3 oz	80	2.5	1
Honey/Brown Sugar, av., 1 oz	35	1	1
Prosciutto, average, 1 oz	70	5	0
Ham & Cheese Loaf, average, 1 oz	70	5	1
Italian Sausage, 2.6 oz	250	20	3
Kielbasa: Polish Sausage, 2 oz	65	5	1
Beef, 2 oz link	190	17	1
Knockwurst, av., 1 oz	90	8	0.5
Linguica *(Gaspar's),* 2 oz	130	9	1
Liverwurst, 1 oz	65	5	2
Liver Pate, fresh, average, 1 oz	90	8	1
Mortadella, 1 oz	105	9	0
Olive Loaf: Average, 1 oz	70	5	3
Oscar Mayer, 1 oz	80	6	1
Pancetta, *Boars Head,* 1 slice	50	4.5	0

Deli/Lunch Meats & Sausages (Cont)

	C	F	Cb
Pastrami (Beef):			
Boar's Head:			
1st cut Brisket, 2 oz	90	4	2
Cap-Off Top Round, 2 oz	80	3	1
Hillshire, Deli Select,			
Ultra Thin. 2 oz	60	1.5	0.5
Peppered Beef, 1 oz slice	40	2	1
Pepperoni, 5 slices, 1 oz	140	13	0
Pickle Loaf, average, 1 oz	70	5	5
Pickle & Pepper Loaf,			
Boars Head, 2 oz	150	13	2
Proscuitto/Proscuitti, av., 1 oz	70	5	1
Roast Beef, Lean, 1 oz	40	2	0
Salami: Beef, av., 1 oz	80	7	1
Oscar Mayer, Hard, 1 slice, 1.8 oz	100	8	0.5
Beer Salami, average, 1 oz	50	4	0.5
Oscar Mayer: Cotto, 1 slice, 1 oz	70	6	0.5
Beef Cotto, 1 slice, 1 oz	60	5	0.5
Dry, Hard, average, 4 slices, 1 oz	100	8	1
Genoa: Average, 1 oz	100	8	1
Stick, 1.8 oz	175	14	2
Bridgford, Italian, 1 oz	120	11	0
SPAM (Hormel): *Per 2 oz*			
Classic: 2 oz serving	180	16	1
7 oz can	630	56	3.5
12 oz can	1080	96	6
Spam Lite: 2 oz	110	8	1
12 oz can	660	48	6
Other Spam Products: *Per 2 oz*			
Hickory Smoked	180	16	1
Hot & Spicy	160	16	2
Oven Roasted Turkey	80	4.5	1
Spam Spresd	140	12	1
Spam with Bacon	180	16	1
Spam with Cheese	170	15	1
25% Less Sodium	180	16	1
Spam Singles: *Per 3 oz*			
Classic, 2.5 oz package	210	18	2
Lite, 2.5 oz package	130	9	2

Deli/Lunch Meats & Sausages (Cont)

	C	F	Cb
Summer Sausage:			
Armour, Beef, 2 oz	190	17	2
Hillshire Farm, 2 oz	190	16	1
Treet *(Armour),* Luncheon Loaf,			
Original, 2 oz	140	11	4
Turkey, average: 1 oz slice	30	1	0.5
0.8 oz slice	22	0.5	0.5
Turkey Breast:			
Butterball, Oven Roasted:			
1 slice 1 oz	30	0.5	1
Deli Inspirations,			
Extra Thin Slices, 4 slices, 2 oz	50	1	3
Hillshire, Deli Select,			
Oven Roasted, 6 slices, 2 oz	50	0.5	2
Turkey Ham, 1 slice, 1 oz	35	1.5	0.5
Turkey Loaf, 1 oz	30	1	0.5
Turkey Pastrami, 1 oz	35	1.5	1
Turkey Roll, 1 oz	40	2	0.5
Vegetarian Deli ~ *See Page 118*			

Meat Spreads

	C	F	Cb
Average All Brands:			
Chicken, white meat, 2.1 oz	140	11	2
Corned Beef, 2.1 oz	140	11	1
Ham, Deviled, 2.1 oz	180	15	1
Liverwurst	160	13	4
Roast Beef	130	10	2
Turkey	110	7	2
Underwood: *Per 2 oz*			
Chicken, White Meat	140	11	2
Deviled Ham	180	15	1
Liverwurst	160	13	4
Roast Beef	130	10	2

Paté

	C	F	Cb
Les Trois Petit Cochons: *Per 2 oz*			
Pate: de Campagne 2 oz	240	22	2
de Canard a l'Orange; Forestier, 2 oz	210	18	3
Paysan, 2 oz	150	12	2
Rustique, 2 oz	240	22	2
Venison, 2 oz	200	16	2
Wild Boar, 2 oz	180	15	4
Old Wisconsin Pate,			
Braunschweiger, 2 oz	210	18	3

Nuts	**C**	**F**	**Cb**

Per 1 oz Unless Indicated

	C	**F**	**Cb**
Acorns, raw 1 oz	110	7	12
Almonds: Dried/Dry Roasted:			
Whole: 12 medium size, 0.5 oz	85	7.5	3
23-25 medium size, 1 oz	170	15	6
$^1/_2$ cup, 2.5 oz	420	37	13
Ground, 1 cup, 3.4 oz	545	47	20
Sliced, $^1/_2$ cup, 1.6 oz	260	22	10
Slivered, $^1/_2$ cup, 2 oz	310	27	12
Chocolate Coated (5-6), 1 oz	150	10	15
Honey Roasted, 1 oz	170	14	8
Oil Roasted (*Blue Diamond*), 1 oz	170	16	5
Brazil Nuts, 8 medium, 1 oz	185	19	3.5
Cashews, dry or oil roasted:			
14 large/18 med./26 small: 1 oz	165	14	9
$^1/_2$ cup, 2.4 oz	375	31	20
Honey Roasted, 1 oz	165	13	10
Chestnuts:			
Average, dried, 1 oz	105	1	22
Raw/Fresh, 5-6 nuts, 1 oz	60	0	13
Canned, water chestnuts,			
sliced/whole/drained, 1 oz	30	0	7
Coconut, Fresh:			
1 piece, 2″x2″x $^1/_2$″, 1 oz	185	18	7
Shredded, fresh, $^1/_2$ cup, 1.4 oz	140	13	6
Dried (Desiccated):			
Sweetened: Shredded, 1 oz	145	10	14
Grated, $^1/_2$ cup, 1.3 oz	185	13	18
Unsweetened, 1 oz	185	18	7
Cream (canned), $^1/_2$ cup, 5.2 oz	285	26	12
Milk (canned), unsweetened,			
$^1/_4$ cup, 2 fl.oz	100	10	3
Water (center liquid), $^1/_2$ cup, 4.3 oz	25	0	4.5
Filberts or Hazelnuts:			
Shelled, 18-20 nuts	180	17	4.5
Chopped, $^1/_4$ cup, 1 oz	180	18	5
Ground, $^1/_4$ cup, 0.6 oz	120	12	3
Ginkgo Nuts, canned, 14 med., 1 oz	32	0.5	6.5
Hickory,			
30 small nuts, 1 oz	200	18	5
Macadamia Nuts, Shelled:			
Raw or Dry Roasted, avg:			
12 small or 8 med., 1 oz	200	21	4
6-7 large, 1 oz	200	21	4
$^1/_2$ cup, 2.3 oz	480	51	10
Mixed Nuts: Raw, 18-22 nuts, 1 oz	170	15	7
Oil Roasted, all types	170	16	6
Sweet Roasts, 26 pieces, 1 oz	160	12	10
Planters, Dry Roasted/Honey	160	12	9
Nut Toppings, chopped, 1 Tbsp, 0.3 oz	40	4	1.5

Per 1 oz Unless Indicated

	C	**F**	**Cb**
Peanuts:			
Dry or oil roasted, average:			
Small handful, 0.5 oz	85	7	3
$^1/_5$ cup, 1 oz	165	14	6
$^1/_2$ cup, 2.5 oz	415	35	15
3 oz bag	500	42	18
7 oz bag	1160	98	42
Raw: Shelled, 1 oz	160	14	4.5
In shell, 1 oz	115	110	3
Planters:			
Cocktail, all varieties	170	14	5
Honey Roasted	160	13	7
Spanish Redskins	170	15	4
Sweet N' Crunchy	140	8	15
Japanese Style Peanuts,			
Coated in Crunchy Shell	150	8	13
Pecans, roasted:			
10 halves, 0.5 oz	95	10	2
20 Halves, 1 oz	195	20	4
1 cup, halves, 3.5 oz	680	71	14
Pilinuts, dried, 1 oz	215	24	1
Pine Nuts,			
dried, 1 Tbsp, 0.3 oz	70	7	1.5
Pistachios, raw:			
Shelled, 45 nuts, 1 oz	160	13	8
Unshelled, 2 oz	165	14	7
Lance, Roasted, 1.5 oz	120	9	6
Sesame Nut Mix, 1 oz	160	13	9
Soy Nuts: Dry Roasted	130	6	9
$^1/_2$ cup, 3 oz	390	18	28
Dr Soy, Chocolate coated, 1 oz pkg	140	7	13
Trail Mix *(Planters):*			
Daybreak, Berry Almond, 1.5 oz	180	7	27
Energy Mix, 1.5 oz	250	20	14
Fruit & Nut	140	9	14
Nut & Chocolate, 1.3oz	150	9	14
Nuts, Seeds & Raisins, 1 oz	160	11	11
Spicy Nuts & Cajun Sticks	150	11	10
Sweet & Nutty, 1 oz	150	9	13
Walnuts, average all types:			
7-10 halves, 0.5 oz	90	9	2
15-20 halves, 1 oz	175	17	3
Chopped, $^1/_2$ cup, 2.2 oz	380	36	6
Ground, $^1/_4$ cup, 0.7 oz	130	13	3

Quick Guide   C F Cb

Peanut Butter: *Average All Brands*

	C	F	Cb
1 level tsp, 0.2 oz	35	3	1
1 level Tbsp, 0.6 oz	100	8.5	3.5
1 oz Quantity	165	14	6
$^1/_2$ cup, 5 oz	835	72	29

Peanut Butter ~ Brands

	C	F	Cb
Jif: Regular, all varieties, 2 Tbsp	190	16	8
Natural, average all varieties, 2 Tbsp	185	15	10
Reduced Fat, all varieties, 2 Tbsp	190	12	15
To Go: Crmy/Crunch, av.,1.5 oz cup	250	21	11
Chocolate Silk, 1.5 oz cup	250	18	18
Whipped: Creamy, 2 Tbsp	140	12	6
Chocolate flavored, 2 Tbsp	150	11	11
Laura Scudder's, Natural, Smooth; Nutty, average, 2 Tbsp	190	16	5
Peter Pan:			
Natural, Creamy/Crunchy, av., 2 T.	205	17	6
Creamy/Crunchy, Red.-Fat, 2 Tbsp	200	13	14
Plus Creamy, 2 Tbsp	210	17	7
Planters, Creamy/Crunchy, 2 Tbsp	180	15	8
Smucker's, Goober, Grape/Srawberry, 3 Tbsp. 2 oz	240	13	24
Skippy: Natural, Creamy/Chunky, 2 T.	190	16	6
Reduced Fat, all varieties, 2 Tbsp	180	12	15
PB Bites, average all, 15 pcs, 1 oz	160	10	14

Peanut Butter & Jelly Sandwich

1 sandwich: *With 2 oz Bread*

	C	F	Cb
Thin Spread, 1 Tbsp Peanut Butter + 1 Tbsp Jelly	310	10	48
Thick Spread, 2 Tbsp Peanut Butter + 2 Tbsp Jelly	480	19	67

Nut & Chocolate Spread

Nutella:	C	F	Cb
1 Tbsp, 0.7 oz	110	6	11
2 Tbsp, 1.3 oz	200	11	22

Note: Nutella contains approx. 50% sugar & 13% hazelnuts

Other Nut & Seed Butters

Per 1 Tbsp, 0.5 oz

	C	F	Cb
Almond Butter	100	10	3.5
Cashew Butter	95	8	4.5
Hazelnut Butter; Pecan Butter	110	10	2
Pistachio Butter	90	6.5	4.5
Sesame Butter (Tahini)	90	8	3
Soy Nut Butter	75	5	4

Seeds   C F Cb

	C	F	Cb
Alfalfa Seeds, sprouted, $^1/_2$ cup, 0.5 oz	5	0	1
Caraway/Fennel, 1 tsp	7	0.5	1
Chia Seeds: 1 Tbsp, 0.4 oz	45	3	4
3 Tbsp, 1 oz	140	8.5	12
Cottonseed Kernels, roasted, 1 Tbsp	50	3.5	2
Flax Seeds, 3 Tbsp, 1 oz	140	9	9
Lotus Seeds, dried, $^1/_2$ cup, 0.5 oz	55	0.5	10
Poppy Seeds, 1 tsp	15	1	1
Pumpkin/Pepita Seeds, whole:			
Roasted/Tamari: 1 oz	150	12	4
$^1/_2$ cup, 4 oz	590	48	15
Dried (hulled), $^1/_4$ cup, 1 oz	155	13	5
Safflower Kernels, dried, 1 oz	150	11	10
Sesame Seeds:			
Dried, 1 Tbsp, 0.3 oz	50	4.5	2
Roasted/Toasted, 1 oz	160	14	7.5
Sunflower Kernels/Seeds:			
Dried, $^1/_4$ cup w/out hulls, 0.3 oz	200	18	7
Dry Roasted: 1 Tbsp, 0.3 oz	45	4	2
$^1/_4$ cup, 1 oz	165	14	7
Oil Roasted, $^1/_5$ cup, 1 oz	170	14	6.5
Watermelon Seeds, dried, $^1/_4$ cup, 1 oz	150	13	4

*N*ut eaters are healthier and live longer, say scientists.

Nuts are a nutritious source of protein, vitamins, minerals, fiber, healthy fats, and antioxidants.

The fat and fiber of nuts can help reduce blood cholesterol. Their protein and fiber also promotes meal satiety (fullness) and reduces hunger levels – of benefit in weight control.

Eat nuts instead of high-sugar snacks, candy and soft drinks. Add chopped nuts to breakfast cereals.

Quick Guide

	C	F	Cb
Pancakes:			
Plain: *Average All Types*			
Small (3" diameter), 0.8 oz	50	2	6
Medium (4" diameter), 1.3 oz	85	3.5	11
Large (6" diameter), 2.5 oz	175	7.5	22
Add Extra for Syrups/Butter			
Pancake Syrup: Regular, 1 Tbsp	50	0	12
$^1/_4$ cup, 4 Tbsp	185	0	49
Lite, 1 Tbsp	25	0	6.5
$^1/_4$ cup, 4 Tbsp	100	0	27
Butter/Margarine:			
Regular, 1 Tbsp	100	11	0
Whipped, 1 Tbsp	65	7.5	0
Waffles:			
Homemade, 7" waffle, 2.5 oz	220	11	25
Frozen + Toasted, (4" diam.), 1 oz	105	3	16

Pancake Brands

Prepared as Directed

	C	F	Cb
Aunt Jemima: *Prepared*			
Mixes: *Makes 4" Pancakes*			
Original (4)	250	8	36
Original Complete (2)	160	1.5	32
Buttermilk (4)	160	3	27
Whole Wheat Blend (3)	200	6.5	30
Bisquick: *Prepared with Water*			
Pancake/Waffle Mix: *Makes 3 Pancake*			
Complete, Buttermilk, 2 oz	200	3	40
Shake 'n Pour, Buttermilk, 2.2 oz	230	3.5	45
Hungry Jack:			
Pancake & Waffle Mixes: *Makes 4" Pancake*			
Complete Mixes: Just Add Water			
Chocolate Chip (3)	190	2.5	39
Extra Light & Fluffy (3)	180	1	38
Wheat Blends (3)	180	1.5	39
Easy Packs: *Dry Mix Only*			
Buttermilk, 1.9 oz	190	1	39
Chocolate Chip, 1.9 oz	190	2.5	39
Traditional: *Dry Mix Only*			
Original, 1.7 oz	160	1	34
Buttermilk, 1.7 oz	160	1	34
Extra Light & Fluffy, 1.6 oz	150	1	32
Northern Pines,			
Premium Mix (3), 4", 3.5 oz, prep'd	200	3.5	38

Frozen Breakfasts

	C	F	Cb
Aunt Jemima:			
French Toast: Cinnamon, 2 slices	210	4	35
Homestyle, 2 slices	210	4	34
Sticks, Cinnamon (4)	260	10	39
Pancakes: Blueberry (3)	260	6	45
Buttermilk (3)	260	7	44
Homestyle (3)	240	6	41
Mini Pancakes (10)	280	8	45
Low-Fat (3)	200	3	39
Eggo *(Kellogg's):*			
French Toaster Sticks: Original (2)	220	6	35
Cinnamon (2)	220	6	38
Pancakes: Blueberry (3)	260	8	42
Choc. Chip (3)	270	9	42
Waffles: Buttermilk (2)	190	8	27
Strawberry (2)	180	6	29
Krusteaz:			
French Toast, Cinnamon Swirl,			
Regular Cut, 3 slices	320	7	53
Pancakes:			
Blueberry (3)	290	4	55
Buttermilk (3)	290	3.5	57
Pillsbury:			
Pancakes,			
Buttermilk; Homestlye, (3)	230	4	45

Frozen Waffles

	C	F	Cb
Aunt Jemima: Buttermilk (2)	190	5	29
Homestyle (2)	180	5	30
Eggo *(Kellogg's):*			
Blueberry (2)	180	6	29
Chocolatey Chip (2)	200	7	31
Strawberry (2)	180	6	29
Nutri-Grain:			
Blueberry (2)	180	6	30
Whole Wheat (2)	170	6	27
Kashi, all varieties (2)	150	5	26
Nature's Path:			
Ancient Grains (2)	180	6	30
Buckwheat Wildberry (2)	190	7	33
Chia Plus; Homestyle; Maple Syrup, (2)	210	7	34
Dark Chocolate Chip (2)	220	7	34
Flax Plus (2)	190	8	27
Van's: 8 Wh. Grains, Multigrain, 2.7 oz	150	5	25
Belgian, Homestyle (2)	250	10	37
Gluten Free,			
Apple Cinnamon (2)	200	6	35
Mini, Chocolate Chip (8), 2 oz	160	5	29

Spaghetti/Pasta   Ⓒ Ⓕ Ⓒb

- Pasta includes all shapes and sizes; (e.g. spaghetti, fettuccini, elbows, shells, twists, sheets, cannelloni, linguini, tubes, ziti).
- All regular pasta products have the same cals/fat/carbs on a weight basis.
- 1 oz Dry = approximately 2.5 -3 oz cooked.

Dry Spaghetti/Pasta

	C	F	Cb
1 oz quantity	105	0.5	21
1lb box/pkg, 16 oz	1685	7	339
Elbows, 1 cup, 4 oz	380	2	80
Shells, small, 1 cup, 3.3 oz	330	1.5	69
Spirals, 1 cup, 3 oz	305	1.5	64

Cooked Spaghetti/Pasta

	C	F	Cb
Plain, All Types (no added fat):			
Firm/Al Dente (8-10 minutes), 1 oz	42	0.5	8.5
Medium (11-13 minutes), 1 oz	37	0.5	7.5
Tender (14-20 minutes), 1 oz	32	0.5	7
Longer cooking increases water absorbed			
Spaghetti: ¹/₂ cup, 2.5 oz	90	0.5	18
Medium serving, 1 cup, 5 oz	225	1.5	44
Large serving, 2 cups, 10 oz	450	3	88
Extra large, 3 cups, 15 oz	675	5	132
Elbows/Spirals, 1 cup, 5 oz	220	1.5	43
Small Shells, 1 cup, 4 oz	180	1	36
Protein-fortified: Dry, 1 c., 3.4 oz	350	2	63
Cooked, 1 cup, 5 oz	230	0.5	45
Spinach/Vegetable: Dry, 1 cup, 3 oz	310	1	61
Cooked, 1 cup, 5 oz	180	0.5	38
Whole-wheat: Dry, 1 cup, 3.8 oz	365	1.5	79
Cooked, 1 cup, 5 oz	175	1	37

Fresh Pasta (Refrigerated)

	C	F	Cb
Average All Brands:			
Plain/Spinach/Tomato:			
As purchased, 4.5 oz	370	3	70
Cooked, 1 cup, 5 oz	185	1.5	35
Home-made, w/o egg, cooked, 1 c. 5 oz	175	1	35
Buitoni:			
Cut Pasta:			
Angel Hair, 3 oz	230	2	43
Fettuccine/Linguine, 3 oz	240	2	45
House Foods:			
Tofu Shirataki Noodles:			
Angel Hair/Fettuccini,			
Macaroni/Spaghetti, 4 oz	20	0.5	3
Nasoya,			
Shirataki Spaghetti,			
Pasta Zero, ²/₃ cup, 4 oz	15	0	4

Buitoni: *Per 1 Cup Unless Indicated* Ⓒ Ⓕ Ⓒb

	C	F	Cb
Agnolotti, Mushroom, 3.8 oz	280	10	34
Ravioli, Four Cheese3.7 oz	330	12	42
Tortellini: Mixed Cheese, 3.7 oz	320	8	47
Spinach Cheese, 3.7 oz	320	7	49
Tortelloni: Swt Italian Sausage, 4 oz	350	10	51
Cheese & Roasted Garlic, 3.7 oz	280	8	39
Other Varieties ~ *See Page 112*			
Pasta Sauces ~ *See Page 144*			

Macaroni & Cheese

	C	F	Cb
Packaged (Kraft) ~ *See Page 116*			
Restaurant: *Average*			
Side Serve, 6 oz	265	13	26
Medium serve, 1 cup, 9 oz	350	17	34
Large serve, 2 cups, 18 oz	700	34	68

Noodles

	C	F	Cb
Plain/Egg: Dry, 1 oz	110	1.5	20
1 cup, 1.4 oz	145	1.5	27
Cooked: 1 oz	40	0.5	7
¹/₂ cup, 2.8 oz	110	1.5	20
1 cup, 5.5 oz	220	3.5	40
Stir-Fried: 1 cup, 5.5 oz	270	9	40
2 cup serving, 11 oz	540	18	80
Low Carb Noodles,			
Quest Pasta, 4 oz	10	0	3
Note: Carbs are from glucomannan fiber			
Yolk Free (Cooked):			
Manischewitz, Yolk Free, 2 oz	200	1	41
Chinese: Cellophane/Rice, dry, 1 oz	100	0	25
Chow Mein/hard, dry, 1 oz	150	9	16
Japanese: Soba: Dry, 1 oz	95	0.5	21
Cooked, 1 cup, 4 oz	115	0.5	24
Somen: Dry, 1 oz	100	0.5	21
Cooked, 1 cup, 6 oz	230	0.5	49
Japanese Style Pan Fried,			
Yaki-Soba (*Maruchan's*), av., 5.6 oz	260	3	50
Ramen Noodles ~ *See Page 118*			
Rice Noodles: Dry, 3.5 oz	365	0.5	83
Cooked, 1 cup, 6.2 oz	190	0.5	44
Yakisoba, Stir Fry, 3.5 oz	430	6	52
House Foods, Tofu Shirataki, 4 oz	20	0.5	3
Chikara, Udon, average, 7.5 oz pkt	250	1	52
Simply Asia/Thai Kitchen ~ *See Pages 119 & 121*			

Egg Roll/Won Ton Wrappers

	C	F	Cb
Egg/Spring Roll (1), 0.8 oz	65	0	15
Won Ton Wrapper (1), 0.3 oz	20	0	4

Quick Guide	**C**	**F**	**Cb**
Fruit Pies: *Average All Brands, 9" Pie*			
Apple; Blueberry; Cherry:			
Small Serving,			
$^1/_8$ pie, 4.8 oz	350	16	49
Medium Serving,			
$^1/_6$ pie, 6.5 oz	465	22	65
Large Serving			
$^1/_4$ pie, 9.5 oz	700	33	98
Whole Pie (9"), 38 oz	2800	131	392
Other Pies: *Per Serving, $^1/_6$ of 9" Pie*			
Chocolate Cream Pie	345	22	38
Custard: Egg Pie	220	12	22
Coconut Pie	330	18	35
Lemon Meringue Pie	305	10	53
Peach Pie	260	12	39
Pecan Pie	440	23	57
Pumpkin Pie	315	14	41
Shoo-Fly Pie	400	13	70

Dessert/Fruit Pies ~ Brands			
Hostess:			
Cherry Pie, 4.5 oz	480	20	69
Lemon Pie, 4.5 oz	510	25	65
Marie Callender's:			
Banana Cream, 4.2 oz slice	310	18	35
Peach Cobbler, 4 oz slice	350	19	43
Pumpkin, 4.5 oz	340	14	49
Turtle, 4.7 oz	560	36	55
Mrs Smith's:			
Original Flaky Crust: *Per $^1/_8$ Pie*			
Apple, 4.6 oz	340	17	45
Cherry, 4.4 oz	350	17	47
Peach, 4.6	340	19	41
Pumpkin, 4.6 oz	300	13	42
Very Berry, 4.4 oz	340	17	44
Sara Lee:			
Creme Pies:			
Chocolate, $^1/_5$ pie, 3.9 oz	450	27	50
Coconut, $^1/_6$ pie, 4.5 oz	370	20	44
Key Lime, $^1/_5$ pie	410	17	60
Oven Fresh Pies: *$^1/_8$ pie, 4.27 oz Unless Indicated*			
Apple	320	16	41
Cherry	330	16	43
Dutch Apple	320	14	46
Pumpkin Pie, 4.4 oz	250	10	37
Southern Sweet Potato	270	9	43
Tastykake: Apple (1), 4 oz	270	11	40
Tasty-Klair (1), 4 oz	308	21	48

Croissants	**C**	**F**	**Cb**
Average all Brands			
Plain/Butter/Cheese: Mini, 1 oz	115	6	13
Small, 1.5 oz	170	9	19
Medium, 2 oz	230	12	26
Large, 2.5 oz	290	15	32
Sweet Croissants:			
Almond Filled, 3 oz	330	18	39
Chocolate Filled, 3 oz	360	19	43
Dunkin' Donuts, Plain Croissant	340	18	37
Sara Lee:			
French Style: Original, 1.8 oz	185	9	21
Mini, 1 oz	230	11	26
Croissant Sandwiches ~ *See Page 165*			

Pastry & Pie Crust	**C**	**F**	**Cb**
Pie Crust, Baked, 9" diameter shell:			
1 Pie Shell, 6.5 oz	970	64	87
2-crust Pie, 9", 11.3 oz	1660	109	150
Filo Pastry: 4 sheets, 2.5 oz	210	2.5	40
Athens, Filo Dough, 5 sheets, 2 oz	170	1	36
Puff:			
Pepperidge Farm: $^1/_2$ sheet	480	30	48
Bake & Fill Shell (1)	180	11	18
Arrowhead Mills,			
Graham Cracker Pie Crust, $^1/_8$ of 9"	110	5	14
Keebler:			
Ready Crust: *Per $^1/_8$ of 9" Crust*			
Chocolate	100	4.5	14
Graham: Regular	100	5	14
Reduced Fat	100	3.5	15
Shortbread Crust	100	5	14
Marie Callenders,			
Pie Crust, $^1/_8$ pie, 1 oz	130	9	12
Mrs Smith's,			
Deep Dish, $^1/_8$ pie, 1 oz	130	7	14
Nabisco:			
Honey Maid,			
Graham Cracker, $^1/_6$ pie, 1 oz	150	5	14
Nilla, Pie Crust,			
$^1/_6$ of Pie, Crust, 1 oz	140	6	13
Pillsbury,			
Rolled, $^1/_8$, 0.9 oz	100	6	12
Trader Joe's, Pie Crust, $^1/_8$ pie, 1.2 oz	190	13	17

Pie Fillings ~ Canned	**C**	**F**	**Cb**
Apple/Blueb./Cherry/Strawb., average:			
Sweetened: $^1/_3$ cup, 3.2oz	90	0	22
1 cup, 9.5 oz	270	0	66
1 can, 21 oz	600	0	150
Light/Lite, $^1/_3$ cup, 3.2 oz	60	0	15
Unsweetened, $^1/_3$ cup, 3.2 oz	35	0	8
Lemon Crm/Creme, $^1/_3$ cup, 3.2 oz	130	1.5	28

Pizzas ~ Ready to Eat

Figures Based On Pizza Hut Unless Indicated

Cheese

Medium Size (12"):
Hand Tossed Crust:

	C	F	Cb
$1/8$ Pizza (1 slice)	210	8	26
$1/2$ Pizza (4 slices)	840	32	104
Whole Pizza (8 slices)	1680	64	208
Original Pan: $1/8$ Pizza (1 slice)	240	10	28
$1/2$ Pizza (4 slices)	960	40	112
Whole Pizza (8 slices)	1920	80	224
Thin 'N Crispy Crust:			
$1/8$ Pizza (1 slice)	180	7	22
$1/2$ Pizza (4 slices)	720	28	88
Whole Pizza (8 slices)	1440	56	176

Ham & Pineapple

Figures Based On Domino's
Medium Size (12"):
Hand Tossed Crust:

	C	F	Cb
$1/8$ Pizza (1 slice)	210	6	28
$1/2$ Pizza (4 slices)	840	24	112
Whole Pizza (8 slices)	1680	48	224
Handmade Pan: $1/8$ Pizza (1 slice)	290	13	31
$1/2$ Pizza (4 slices)	1160	52	124
Whole Pizza (8 slices)	2320	104	248
Thin Crust:			
$1/8$ Pizza (1 slice)	145	6.5	15
$1/2$ Pizza (4 slices)	580	26	60
Whole Pizza (8 slices)	1160	52	120

MeatZZA

Medium Size (12"):
Hand Tossed Crust:

	C	F	Cb
$1/8$ Pizza (1 slice)	270	12	27
$1/2$ Pizza (4 slices)	1080	48	108
Whole Pizza (8 slices)	2160	96	216
Handmade Pan: $1/8$ Pizza (1 slice)	350	19	30
$1/2$ Pizza (4 slices)	1400	76	120
Whole Pizza (8 slices)	2800	152	240
Thin Crust: $1/8$ Pizza (1 slice)	215	13	15
$1/2$ Pizza (4 slices)	860	52	60
Whole Pizza (8 slices)	1720	104	120

Pepperoni

Medium Size (12"):
Hand Tossed Crust:

	C	F	Cb
$1/8$ Pizza (1 slice)	220	9	26
$1/2$ Pizza (4 slices)	880	36	104
Whole Pizza (8 slices)	1760	72	208
Handmade Pan: $1/8$ Pizza (1 slice)	300	15	29
$1/2$ Pizza (4 slices)	1200	60	116
Whole Pizza (8 slices)	2400	120	232
Thin Crust: $1/8$ Pizza (1 slice)	160	9	14
$1/2$ Pizza (4 slices)	640	36	56
Whole Pizza (8 slices)	1280	72	112

Large Pizzas

Large (14")
Hand Tossed Crust:

	C	F	Cb
Cheese: $1/8$ Pizza (1 slice)	290	10	36
$1/2$ Pizza (4 slices)	1160	40	144
MeatZZA: $1/8$ Pizza (1 slice)	370	17	37
$1/2$ Pizza (4 slices)	1480	68	148
Pepperoni: $1/8$ Pizza (1 slice)	300	12	35
$1/2$ Pizza (4 slices)	1200	48	140

Extra Large, Single Slice

Figures Based On Sbarro

	C	F	Cb
Cheese	430	15	51
Ham & Pineapple	490	16	60
Sausage	520	24	50
X-Treme Pepperoni	620	32	53

Individual Personal Pizzas

Pan (6"): Figures Based On Pizza Hut

	C	F	Cb
Buffalo Chicken	640	24	72
Cheese	600	24	68
Pepperoni	640	28	68
Supreme	720	36	68
Veggie Lovers	560	20	72

Chicago-Style Deep Dish: Individual
Figures Based On Uno Pizzeria

	C	F	Cb
Cheese & Tomato, 18.8 oz	1700	115	110
Chicago Classic, 25.8 oz	2220	157	112
Prima Pepperoni, 18.5 oz	1720	118	110
Sausage& Spinach Alfredo, 22.7 oz	1900	143	79

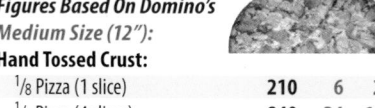

Frozen Pizzas

	C	F	Cb
Amy's: *Per 1/3 Pizza*			
Cheese Pizza	290	12	33
Margherita	280	12	32
Mushroom & Olive	260	10	33
Pesto	310	12	39
Roasted Vegetable	280	9	42
California Pizza Kitchen:			
Crispy Flatbreads: *Per Piece*			
BBQ Recipe Chicken, 3.3 oz	200	6	24
Margherita, 3 oz	190	8	20
Sicilean Recipe, 4.3 oz	210	9	22
Crispy Thin Crust: *Per 1/3 Pizza*			
Margherita	320	16	31
Sicilian Recipe	360	18	30
Signature Pepperoni	350	19	29
White	320	17	30
Gluten-Free:			
BBQ Recipe Chicken, 1/2 pizza	330	11	43
Margherita, 1/3 pizza	220	9	27
Organic: Five Cheese & Tomato	270	10	33
Mushroom & Green Onion	240	8	33
Celeste: *Per Pizza*			
Pizza For One: Original	320	14	42
Deluxe	340	15	42
Four Cheese	330	15	38
Pepperoni	340	13	43
Sausage & Pepperoni	380	19	41
Zesty Four Cheese	350	16	43
Daiya *(Vegan):*			
Cheese Lovers, 1/3 pizza	390	17	54
Mushroom & Garlic, 1/3 pizza	390	14	58
Pepperoni Style, 1/3 pizza	470	21	64
Supreme, 1/4 pizza	340	14	45
DiGiorno: *Per Slice, Unless Indicated*			
Cheese Stuffed Crust:			
Bacon Cheeseburger, 1/6 pizza, 4.5 oz	300	11	33
Five Cheese, 1/5 Pizza, 5.3 oz	370	15	41
Pepperoni, 1/5 pizza, 5.3 oz	380	16	41
Three Meat, 1/6 pizza 4.8 oz	300	12	31
Supreme, 1/6 pizza, 5 oz	350	16	35
Classic Thin Crust, Supreme, 1/5 pizza, 5 oz	320	15	32

DiGiorno (Cont):	C	F	Cb
Garlic Bread: *Per 1/6 Pizza*			
Pepperoni, 5 oz	360	14	41
Supreme, 4.3 oz	280	12	32
Original Rising Crust: *Per 1/6 Pizza*			
Four Cheese, 4.7 oz	290	10	36
Italian Sausage, 5 oz	330	14	37
Spicy Chicken Supreme, 5.3 oz	290	8	37
Small Pizzas: *Per 1/2 Pizza*			
Cheese Stuffed Crust:			
Four Cheese, 4.2 oz	330	15	33
Pepperoni, 4.2 oz	330	16	33
Three Meat, 4.6 oz	360	18	34
Traditional Crust:			
Pepperoni, 4.6 oz	360	17	41
Three Meat, 4.7 oz	370	17	43
Freschetta:			
Brick Oven: *Per 1/5 Pizza Unless Indicated*			
5 Italian Cheese, 1/4 Pizza, 5.2 oz	380	18	40
Chicken Club, 1/4 Pizza, 5.5 oz	360	15	41
Pepp. & Italian Style Cheese, 4.6 oz	340	17	33
Roasted M'shrms & Spinach, 4.6 oz	270	10	34
Three Meat Medley, 4.6 oz	350	18	33
Zesty Italian Supreme, 4.6 oz	310	14	34
Naturally Rising: *Per 1/6 Pizza Unless Indicated*			
4 Cheese Medley, 1/5 Pizza, 5 oz	380	14	47
Canada Style Bacon P'apple, 4.5 oz	290	9	40
Classic Supreme, 5 oz	350	15	41
Old Fashioned Sausage, 4.7 oz	340	13	40
Signature Pepperoni, 4.5 oz	330	13	40
Jeno's: *Per Pizza*			
Crispy 'N Tasty:			
Cheese, 5 oz	310	14	38
Pepperoni, 5 oz	340	17	37
Kroger:			
3 Minute Microwave: *Per 8 oz Pizza*			
3-Meat	500	17	64
Cheese	490	16	66
Combination	520	20	64
Pepperoni	530	20	65
Supreme	490	18	63
French Bread, Pepperoni, 5 oz	380	17	42

Frozen Pizzas (Cont) | C | F | Cb

Lean Cuisine:

	C	F	Cb
Craveables: Four Cheese, 6 oz	380	7	60
Pepperoni, 6 oz	410	9	61
Supreme, 6 oz	330	7	49
Deep Dish:			
Three Meat, 6 oz	420	9	62
Spinach & Mushroom, 6 oz	350	7	54
Thin Crust: BBQ Chicken, 6 oz	390	9	55
Margherita, 6 oz	320	4	55

Red Baron:

Brick Oven: *Per ¼ Pizza*

	C	F	Cb
Cheese Trio, 4.4 oz	320	14	36
Meat Trio, Pepperoni,4.6 oz	340	16	36
Sausage Supreme, 4.7 oz	320	14	37

Classic Crust: *Per ¼ Pizza*

	C	F	Cb
4 Cheese, 5.2 oz	390	17	42
Sausage & Pepp., 5.3 oz	400	19	42
Supreme, 4.7 oz	320	15	34

Deep Dish Minis:

	C	F	Cb
Cheese, 4 pieces, 5.4 oz	390	14	50
Pepperoni, 4 pieces, 5.6 oz	430	20	50

Deep Dish Singles: *Per Pizza*

	C	F	Cb
Hawaiian Style, 5.3 oz	350	13	48
Meat-Trio, 5.6 oz	400	17	48
Sausage, 5.8 oz	420	19	48
Scrambles: Bacon, 5.85 oz	440	21	47
Sausage, 5.85 oz	430	20	47

Thin & Crispy Crust: *Per ⅓ Pizza*

	C	F	Cb
5 Cheese, 5 oz	360	16	40
Pepperoni, 5.3 oz	390	19	41
Supreme, 4.4 oz	300	15	31

Safeway Select:

Pizzeria Crust:

	C	F	Cb
Cheese Trio, ¼ pizza	340	15	34
Fajita Chkn Ole, ⅕ pizza	250	10	29
Pepperoni & Sausage, ⅕ pizza	320	17	30

Self Rising: *Per ⅙ Pizza*

	C	F	Cb
Four Cheese	300	9	41
Pepperoni	350	14	41
Sausage & Pepperoni	340	13	41

Smart Ones *(Weight Watchers):*

	C	F	Cb
Classic Favorites, Thin Crust,			
Cheese Pizza, 6 oz	290	6	42
Smart Anytime, Brick Oven Style,			
Pepperoni Pizza, 6 oz	430	13	57

Stouffer's: | C | F | Cb

French Bread Pizzas:

Two Per Box:

	C	F	Cb
Deluxe (1)	430	21	44
Grilled Vegetable (1)	340	12	44
Sausage & Pepperoni (1)	460	24	43
Three Meat (1)	470	25	43

Nine Per Box:

	C	F	Cb
Cheese (1)	380	16	43
Pepperoni (1)	430	21	44

Tombstone:

Original: *Per ¼ Pizza*

	C	F	Cb
Canadian Style Bacon	310	11	35
Five Cheese	350	16	34
Pepperoni	360	18	35
Pepperoni & Sausage	350	16	35

Brick Oven Thin Crust:

	C	F	Cb
Cheese, ⅓ Pizza	330	14	36
Pepperoni; Supreme, av.,¼ pizza	310	16	27

Garlic Bread Crust:

	C	F	Cb
Pepperoni, ⅙ pizza	340	15	39
Supreme, ⅙ pizza	330	13	40

Roadhouse:

	C	F	Cb
Bring on The Meat, ⅕ pizza	330	21	20
Double Down Deluxe, ⅕ pizza	310	18	21
Piled High Pepperoni, ⅕ pizza	330	21	20

Tony's:

Pizzeria Style Crust: *Per ¼ Pizza*

	C	F	Cb
Bacon Cheeseburger, 4.8 oz	360	16	39
Cheese, 4.8 oz	330	13	41
Meat Trio, 5 oz	360	16	41
Pepperoni, 4.7 oz	330	14	40
Sausage & Pepperoni, 4.87 oz	350	15	41
Supreme, 5.3 oz	350	15	42

Totino's:

Crisp Crust Party Pizza: *Per ½ Pizza*

	C	F	Cb
Canadian Bacon	320	14	37
Cheese	310	14	37
Combination	350	17	37
Hamburger	340	16	37
Pepperoni	350	18	37
Pepperoni Trio	350	18	37
Sausage	350	17	37
Triple Meat	340	16	37

Pizza Rolls:

	C	F	Cb
Pepperoni (6), 3 oz	220	9	29
Pepperoni Trio (6), 3 oz	230	10	29
Other var., (6), 3 oz	210	8	29

Trader Joe's:

	C	F	Cb
3 Cheese, ⅓ pizza	310	9	42
Parlanno, ¼ pizza	340	16	34
Pizza 4 Formaggi, ⅓ pizza	310	9	42
Spinach, ⅓ pizza	300	12	38

Quick Guide

C F Cb

Chicken
From 3lb ready-to-cook chicken
Breast/Wing Quarter:

	C	F	Cb
Roasted: with skin	300	15	0
without skin	185	5	0
Fried, batter dipped	530	30	17

Leg Quarter:
Thigh & Drumstick:

	C	F	Cb
Roasted: with skin	270	16	0
without skin	185	8	0
Fried, batter dipped	435	25	15

KFC ~ See Fast-Foods Section

Per 4 oz Edible Portion

Average of Light Meat: *Per 4 oz without Bone*

	C	F	Cb
Roasted: with skin	250	12	0
without skin	175	4.5	0
Stewed: with skin	230	12	0
without skin	180	4.5	0
Fried: Batter-dipped, with skin, 4 oz	315	17	11
Flour-coated, with skin, 4 oz	280	14	2

Average of Dark Meat: *Per 4 oz without Bone*

	C	F	Cb
Roasted: with skin	290	18	0
without skin	235	11	0
Stewed: with skin	265	17	0
without skin	220	10	0
Fried: Batter-dipped, with skin, 4 oz	340	21	11
Flour-coated, with skin, 4 oz	325	19	5

Chicken Parts

Broilers or Fryers: *Edible Weights (no bone)*
Breast: *Per ½ Breast*

	C	F	Cb
Raw: with skin, 5 oz	250	14	0
without skin, 4.25 oz	140	3	0
Roasted: with skin, 3.5 oz	195	8	0
without skin, 3 oz	140	3	0
Stewed: with skin, 4 oz	200	8	0
without skin, 3.3 oz	145	3	0
Fried: Batter-dipped, w/ skin, 5 oz	365	19	13
Flour-coated, with skin, 3.5 oz	220	9	2

Drumstick: *Per Drumstick*

	C	F	Cb
Roasted: with skin, 2 oz	115	6	0
without skin, 1.5 oz	75	2.5	0
Stewed: with skin, 2 oz	115	6	0
without skin, 1.5 oz	80	3	0
Fried: Batter-dipped, w/ skin, 2.5 oz	195	11	6
Flour-coated, with skin, 1.8 oz	120	7	1

Chicken Parts (Cont)

C F Cb

Broilers or Fryers (Cont): *Edible Weights (no bone)*
Thigh Portion:

	C	F	Cb
Raw: with skin, 3.3 oz			
(4¼ oz with bone)	200	14	0
without skin, 2.4 oz	80	3	0
Roasted: with skin, 2.3 oz	155	10	0
without skin, 2 oz	110	6	0
Stewed: with skin, 2.5 oz	160	10	0
without skin, 2 oz	105	5	0
Fried: Batter-dipped, with skin 3 oz	240	14	8
Flour-coated, with skin, 2.3 oz	165	9	2

Wing: *Per Wing, Bone In*
Raw Weight, 3.2 oz

	C	F	Cb
Raw: with skin	110	8	0
without skin	35	1	0
Roasted: with skin	100	7	0
without skin	45	2	0
Fried: Batter-dipped, with skin	160	11	5
Flour-coated, with skin	105	7	1
Stewed, with skin, 4 oz	100	7	0

Buffalo Wings ~ See Fast-Foods Section

	C	F	Cb
Neck: Simmered, with skin	95	7	0
without skin	30	2	0

Skin Only: *Skin from ½ Chicken*

	C	F	Cb
Raw skin, 3 oz	275	26	0
Roasted skin, 2 oz	255	23	0
Stewed skin, 2.5 oz	260	24	0
Fried, flour-coated, 2 oz	280	24	5
Fried, batter-dipped, 6.8 oz	750	55	44

Roasters: *Average of Light & Dark Meat*

	C	F	Cb
Roasted: with skin, 4 oz	250	15	0
without skin, 4 oz	190	8	0
Dark Meat, without skin	200	10	0
Light Meat, without skin	175	5	0

Stewing Chicken: *Per 4 oz, average of Light & Dark Meat*

	C	F	Cb
Stewed: with skin	325	22	0
without skin	270	14	0
Dark Meat, without skin	290	17	0
Light Meat, without skin	240	9	0

Capon Chicken:

	C	F	Cb
Roasted: with skin, 4 oz	260	13	0
½ Chicken, with skin, 22.5 oz	1460	74	0

Chicken Offal & Stuffing:

	C	F	Cb
Giblets: Simmered, 1 cup	230	7	0.5
Fried, flour-coated, 1 cup	400	20	6
Gizzard, simmered, 1 cup	210	4	0
Heart, simmered, 1 cup	270	12	0.2
Liver: Raw, 4 oz	130	5.5	4
Simmered, 1 cup	215	8.5	1
Liver Pate, fresh, 1 Tbsp, 0.5 oz	30	2	1
Stuffing, average, ½ cup	180	9	22

Chicken Products | C | F | Cb

Bumble Bee:
Chicken In Water: *Per 2 oz Drained*

	C	F	Cb
Premium White	70	1.5	0
Premium Breast	70	1	1

Foster Farms:

	C	F	Cb
Chicken Breast Strips, grilled, 3 oz	100	2	1
Wings: Chipotle, 3 wings, 3 oz	190	13	4
Honey BBQ Glazed, 3 wings, 3 oz	190	11	7
Hot 'n' Spicy, 3 wings, 3 oz	190	14	1

Tyson:
Anytizers, Frozen:
Wings:

	C	F	Cb
Hot Wings, Buffalo Style (3)	190	13	1
Honey BBQ Seasoned (3)	190	12	8

Wyngz, Boneless:

	C	F	Cb
Buffalo Style, 3 pieces, 3 oz	150	7	8
Sweet Garlic Glazed, 3 pcs, 2.8 oz	130	5	10

Duck, Goose, Quail

Duck, Roasted:

	C	F	Cb
with skin, 3 oz	290	24	0
without skin, 3 oz	170	10	0
½ duck, with skin, 13.5 oz	1290	108	0
Goose: Roasted with skin, 3 oz	260	19	0
without skin, 3 oz	200	11	0
Pheasant, cooked, 3 oz	210	10	0
Quail, cooked, 1 whole, 6 oz	385	24	0

Turkey

Fryer-Roasters: *Per 3 oz Serving*
Roasted:

	C	F	Cb
Light Meat: with skin	140	4	0
without skin	120	1	0
Dark Meat: with skin	155	6	0
without skin	140	4	0

½ of Whole Turkey: (Approx. 3.3 lbs raw weight without neck and giblets; 1.8 lbs cooked weight)

	C	F	Cb
Roasted: with skin	1650	74	0
without skin	1125	31	0

Ground Turkey, raw: (4 oz raw wt. = 3 oz ckd wt.)

	C	F	Cb
85% lean, regular, 4 oz	170	10	0
93% lean: Average, 4 oz	160	8	0
Jennie-O, 4 oz	170	8	0
Trader Joe's, 4 oz	150	8	0
94% lean,			
Foster Farms, 4 oz	150	7	0
Breast, no skin, 4 oz	115	1	0
Patties: Small, 3 oz	130	7	0
Medium, 4 oz	170	10	0

Turkey Parts | C | F | Cb

Roasted, Edible Weights, without bone:
Breast, (½), (from 17.3 oz raw weight with bone):

	C	F	Cb
with skin, 12 oz (no bone)	525	11	0
without skin, 10.8 oz	415	2	0
Back (½): with skin, 4.5 oz	265	13	0
without skin, 3.5 oz	165	6	0

Leg (Thigh & Drumstick):
(from 1 lb raw weight with bone)

	C	F	Cb
with skin, 8.5 oz (without bone)	410	13	0
without skin, 7.8 oz (w/out bone)	355	8.5	0

Wing: (From 7.3 oz raw weight)

	C	F	Cb
with skin, 3 oz (without bone)	185	9	0
without skin, 2 oz (w/out bone)	100	2	0
Neck: Simmered, 1 neck, 9 oz (with bone)	275	11	0
Giblets, simmered, 1 cup, 5 oz	240	7	3

Young Hens (Roasted)

Light Meat:

	C	F	Cb
with skin, 3 oz	175	8	0
without skin, 3 oz	135	3	0
Dark Meat: with skin, 3 oz	200	11	0
without skin, 3 oz	165	7	0

Young Toms ~ *Similar to Young Hens*

Turkey Products

	C	F	Cb
Foster Farms, Meatballs, cooked, Homestyle (3)	160	9	3
Hormel, Canned Turkey Breast, in water, 2 oz	50	1	0
Jennie-O:			
Bacon, 1 slice, 0.5 oz	30	2.5	0
Bratwurst, lean, raw, 1 link, 3.85 oz	170	10	2
Burgers, raw, All Natural, White Meat, 5.3 oz	200	10	0
Meatballs, Fully Cooked: Italian, 3 oz	180	13	2
Home Style, 3 oz	180	13	3
Spam, Oven Roasted Turkey, 2 oz	80	4.5	1
Trader Joe's,			
Italian Turkey Meatloaf, 3 oz	140	8	5
Valley Fresh, 100% Natural, Canned White Turkey Breast, in water, 2 oz	50	1	0

White Rice — **C** **F** **Cb**

	C	F	Cb
Raw:			
Glutinous, 1 cup, 6.5 oz	685	1	151
Long Grain, 1 cup, 6.5 oz	675	1	148
Short Grain, 1 cup, 7 oz	715	1	158
Wild Rice, 1 cup, 5.5 oz	570	2	120
Cooked Rice: *Boiled/Steamed*			
Short/Medium Grain:			
½ cup, 3.3 oz	140	0	30
1 cup (½ Pint), 7.2 oz	265	0.5	59
2 cups (1 Pint), 13 oz	480	1	106
Long Grain: ½ cup, 2.8 oz	100	0	22
1 cup, 5.5 oz	205	0.5	44
Glutinous/Sticky, 1 cup, 6 oz	170	0.5	37
Parboiled, ½ cup, 3 oz	105	0.5	22
Precooked/Instant:			
Dry, ½ cup, 3.5 oz	380	1	82
Cooked, ½ cup, 3 oz	95	0.5	21
Wild Rice,			
Cooked, 1 cup, 5.8 oz	165	0.5	35

Brown Rice

Average of Short or Long Grain

	C	F	Cb
Raw/Dry: ½ cup, 3.3 oz	340	2.5	71
1 cup, 6.5 oz	685	5.5	143
Cooked: ½ cup, 3.5 oz	110	1	22
1 cup, 7 oz	220	2	46

Rice Dishes — **C** **F** **Cb**

	C	F	Cb
Chinese Fried Rice:			
½ cup, 2.5 oz	140	4.5	21
1 cup, (½ Pint), 5 oz	280	9	42
2 cups, (1 Pint), 10 oz	565	18	84
Mexican Style Rice:			
Taco Time, Seasoned, 4.6 oz	200	3	40
Rice-A-Roni ~ *See Page 119*			
Rice with Raisins/Pinenuts, 1 cup	400	11	60
Rice Pilaf: Restaurant, 1 cup	275	7.5	46
O'Charley's, side dish, 1 portion	160	4	27
Rice Pudding,			
Kozy Shack, Original, 1 pudding cup	130	2.5	24
Risotto, 1 cup	420	12	70
Saffron Rice, 4 oz	175	7	25
Spanish Rice: 1 cup, 5 oz	390	9	72
El Pollo Loco, Small, 4.5 oz	170	2.5	33
Sticky Rice, 1 cup, 5 oz	155	0.5	34
Sushi Rice: 1 Tbsp	25	0	5
1 cup, 5.2 oz	390	0	77
Other Packaged Rice Products:			
Uncle Ben's / Zatarain's ~ *See Page 121*			

CalorieKing.com Recipes

See the CalorieKing website for a salubrious selection of healthy recipes – all analyzed for calories, fat, protein, carbohydrate, fiber and sodium.

Choose from:
- **Starters/Appetizers**
- **Salads**
- **Entrees: Meat, Fish and Chicken**
- **Vegetarian**
- **Desserts**
- **Cakes, Cookies**
- **Drinks**

www.CalorieKing.com/recipes

HEALTHY RECIPE TIPS

- **Use non-fat milk** in place of whole or 2% milk
- **Use low-fat yogurt** in place of sour cream
- **Skim fat** from surface of soups and casseroles after cooling
- **Add extra vegetables** to soups and hot entreés
- **Cakes/cookies/muffins:** Replace most or all the fat/oil with applesauce and/or prune puree (Example, *Sunsweet Lighter Bake*)
- **Drinks:** Replace sugar with no-calorie sweeteners such as *Equal, Stevia, Splenda and Sweet 'N Low*

Deli Salads

Average All Outlets	C	F	Cb
Antipasto Salad, 1/2 cup	135	8	13
3-Bean Salad, 1/2 cup	90	4.5	12
Bulgur Salad, 1/2 cup	70	2	12
Caesar Salad, Classic, 1 cup	200	14	15
Side Salad, without Dressing	25	0	6
Carrot Raisin: with Dressing, 1/2 cup	135	12	6
without Dressing, 1/2 cup	20	0	5
Chef's Salad: Regular, w/o Dressing	620	37	8
with 2 oz Thousand Island Drssng	860	61	8
Chicken Salad, 1/2 cup/scoop, 4 oz	280	21	2
Coleslaw: Traditional, 1/2 cup	150	8	18
w/ Low Cal Dressing, 1/2 c.	50	2	8
Corn, Mexican, 1/2 cup	240	12	33
Cucumber: Non-Oil Dressing, 1/2 cup	60	0	14
with Oil Dressing, 1/2 cup	140	12	8
Eggplant Salad, 1/2 cup	75	5	7
Fettucini, with veges, 1/2 cup	135	6	16
Garden Salad, without Dressing, 1 cup	10	0	2
Greek Salad, 1 cup	105	8	7
Greek Vegetables, 1 cup	110	8	6
Lobster Salad, 1/2 cup, 4 oz	250	21	11
Macaroni Salad, 1/2 cup, 5 oz	360	26	26
Nicoise, 1 cup	450	32	18
Pasta Salad, 1/2 cup	200	11	19
Potato Salad: Dijon, 3 oz	120	7	13
with Mayonnaise, 1/2 cup, 4 oz	215	15	17
Lowfat, 1/2 cup	110	1.5	21
Rice Salad, 1/2 cup	150	10	13
Saffron Rice, 4 oz	175	7	25
Spinach Salad, 1 cup	180	13	13
Tabouli, 1/2 cup	125	7	13
Three Bean Salad, 1/2 cup	90	4.5	12
Tomato & Mozzarella, 1/2 cup	180	14	10
Tortellini, with Basil Pesto, 1/2 cup	150	9	15
Waldorf, with Mayo, 1/2 cup	110	7	12

Signature Salads: Per 6 oz Serving
(Supplied to Deli's and Institutions)

	C	F	Cb
Antipasto Salad	510	50	4
Artichoke Salad, marinated	400	41	8
California Medley	120	7	15
Cheese Agnolotti	250	8	23
Chicken Salad	420	33	11
Crabmeat Flavored	450	38	20
Egg Salad	300	23	14
Fresh Button Mushroom	190	16	6

Signature Salads (Cont): Per 6 oz	C	F	Cb
Fresh Button Mushroom	190	16	6
Ham Salad	400	32	14
Prima Pasta Salad	360	30	18
Seafood Pasta Del Mar	170	10	21
Seafood, Crab & Shrimp	420	34	20
Shrimp Salad	360	32	8
Tuna Salad	450	36	14

~ Also See Fast-Foods & Restaurants Section

Fresh Salad Packs

Pre-Packaged (Supermarkets):
Dole:

Kits: Per 3.5 oz, with Dressing	C	F	Cb
Caesar: Original	150	12	8
Kale	210	15	11
Chopped:			
Chipotle & Cheddar	120	9	10
Sesame Asian	160	16	13
Southwest	120	9	9
Salad Blends: Without Dressing			
American; Mediterranean, 3 oz	15	0	3
Arugula; Baby Spinach, 3 oz	20	0	3

Fresh Express:

Complete Salad Kits: Per 3 1/2 oz, Prepared	C	F	Cb
Asian	120	5	17
Caesar: Classic	150	12	7
Lite	90	6	7
Supreme	160	14	6
Pear Gorgonzola	130	6	17
Gourmet Cafe: Per Package			
Chopped Santa Fe	290	19	18
Tuscan	330	28	9

Ready Pac:

Bistro Bowls: Per Container, with Dressing	C	F	Cb
Apple Bleu Pecan, 4.5 oz	230	14	23
Caprese, 5 oz	210	17	12
Cranb. Walnut, 4.5 oz	210	9	26
Kale, Apple Veggie, 5.5 oz	240	13	31
Spinach Dijon, 4.76 oz	280	19	20
Turkey & Bacon Cobb, 7.3 oz	290	22	6

Salad Toppings

	C	F	Cb
Bac'n Pieces,			
McCormick, 1Tbsp, 0.3 oz	30	1	2
Bacon Bits (Hormel), 1Tbsp	25	1.5	0
Bac-Os, Bits (Betty Crocker), 1 Tbsp	30	1	2
Chow Mein Noodles,			
dry, 1/2 cup	120	7	13
Croutons, 2 Tbsp, 0.3 oz	40	1	7
Salad Toppins,			
McCormick, 4 tsp	35	1.5	3
Sunflower Seeds, 1 Tbsp, 0.3 oz	45	4	1.5
Toasted Sliced Almonds, 2 T., 0.5 oz	85	7	3

Quick Guide   C   F   Cb

Salad Dressings
Average All Brands: Per 2 Tbsp, Approx 1 fl.oz

	C	F	Cb
Balsamic Vinaigrette:			
Regular	90	9	3
Light, 2 Tbsp	45	4	2
Fat Free, 2 Tbsp	25	0	6
Blue Cheese: Regular, 2 Tbsp	145	15	1.5
Regular, ¼ cup, 2 oz	280	30	3
Light, 2 Tbsp	30	1	4
Caesar: Regular, 2 Tbsp	165	17	1
Regular, ¼ cup, 2 oz	310	34	2
Light, 2 Tbsp	35	1.5	5.5
Coleslaw: Regular, 2 Tbsp	125	11	8
Regular, ¼ cup, 2 oz	245	21	15
Light, 2 Tbsp	110	7	14
French: Regular	145	14	5
Regular, ¼ cup, 2 oz	260	25	9
Light, 2 Tbsp	65	4	9
Fat/Oil-Free, 2 Tbsp	40	0	10
Italian: Regular, 2 Tbsp	85	8.5	3
Regular, ¼ cup, 2 oz	165	16	6
Light, 2 Tbsp	55	5.5	2
Fat/Oil-Free, 2 Tbas	15	0	2.5
Ranch: Regular, 2 Tbsp	145	16	2
Regular, ¼ cup, 2 oz	290	30	4
Light, 2 Tbsp	60	4	6.5
Fat-Free, 2 Tbsp	35	0.5	8
Thousand Island: Reg., 2 T.	115	11	4.5
Regular, ¼ cup, 2 oz	210	20	9
Light, 2 Tbsp	60	3.5	7
Fat-Free, 2 Tbsp	40	0.5	10

Enjoy a healthy salad but don't drown it in high-fat salad dressings.

Use 'light' dressings to halve the fat and calories.

Brands ~ Salad Dressings

	C	F	Cb
Annie's Naturals: *Per 2 Tbsp*			
Organic: Goddess Dressing	120	12	2
Green Garlic	80	8	2
Papaya Poppy Seed	90	8	5
Thousand Island	90	8	5
Vinaigrettes:			
Red Wine & Olive Oil	140	15	0
Sesame Ginger	90	8	4
Shitake & Sesame	120	13	1
Bernstein's: *Per 2 Tbsp*			
Creamy Caesar	120	13	1
Herb Garden French	130	12	6
Italian	110	12	1
Restaurant Recipe Italian	120	12	1
Fat-Free, Cheese & Garlic Italian	10	0	2
Light Fantastic: Cheese Fantastico	25	1.5	3
Roasted Garlic Balsamic	45	3.5	3
Best Foods: *Per 1 Tbsp Unless Indicated*			
Dijonnaise, 1 tsp	5	0	0
Mayonnaise: Real	100	11	0
Light	35	3.5	1
Low-Fat	15	1	2
Canola	40	4	0.5
with Olive Oil	60	6	0.5
Mayonesa, Lemom-Lime	100	10	0
Cardini's: *Per 2 Tbsp*			
Aged Parmesan Ranch	150	16	1
Caesar: Original	160	17	1
Fat-Free Caesar	40	0	9
Garlic Lemon	90	9	2
Light Caesar	80	7	5
Honey Mustard	120	11	6
Roasted Asian Sesame	120	10	6
Vinaigrette, Balsamic:			
Regular	100	8	5
Lite	50	3	5
Great Value *(Walmart): Per 2 Tbsp*			
Caesar	120	12	2
Ranch: Bacon	140	14	1
Buttermilk	110	11	2
Chipotle	120	13	2
Classic	130	14	1
Zesty Italian	60	6	3
Hampton Creek *(Vegan): Per 1 Tbsp*			
Just Mayo:			
Original	90	10	0
Chipotle; Sriracha	90	10	1
Garlic	100	10	0

Brands ~ Salad Dressings (Cont)

Hidden Valley:	C	F	Cb
Greek: Creamy Caesar; Cucumber Dill	60	5	3
Lemon Garlic	60	5	4
Ranch	60	5	3
Ranch: Bacon	140	14	1
Buffalo	110	1	2
Fiesta Salsa, Light	60	5	3
Ranch	60	5	3
Southwest Chipotle	100	10	2

Kraft: *Per 2 Tbsp*

Regular Dressings:			
Asian Toasted Sesame	80	6	6
Blue Cheese	120	12	3
Buttermilk Ranch	120	12	3
Catalina Classic	90	6	9
Classic Caesar	110	11	3
Creamy Balsamic	90	8	3
Creamy Italian	80	7	3
Cucumber Ranch	110	11	3
Honey Mustard	90	6	9
Zesty Catalina	90	6	9
Zesty Italian	60	4.5	3
Fat Free: Classic Caesar	50	0	11
French Style	45	0	11
Italian	15	0	3
Thousand Island	45	0	10
Lite: Asian Toasted Sesame	45	1.5	6
Creamy French	70	4.5	9
Creamy Caesar	40	2	3
Zesty Italian	25	1.5	3

Seven Seas:			
Green Goddess	100	8	6
Viva Italian Anything	50	4.5	3

Marie's: *Per 2 Tbsp*

Caesar	170	19	1

Classics:			
Chunky Blue Cheese	160	17	1
Coleslaw	140	13	7
Creamy Italian Garlic	180	19	1
Creamy Ranch	180	19	1
Thousand Island	150	15	3
Premier Super, Blue Cheese	160	17	1
Ranch: Buttermilk	150	16	1
Parmesan	170	19	1
Specialty: Honey Mustard	140	13	6
Poppy Seed	150	13	8

Marzetti's:	C	F	Cb
Organic: Blue Cheese	130	14	1
Caesar	140	15	1
Parmesan Ranch	130	14	2
Chunky Blue Cheese	150	15	1
Classic Ranch	160	17	1
Honey Dijon	130	12	6

Newman's Own: *Per 2 Tbsp*

Regular: Balsamic Vinaigrette	90	9	3
Creamy Caesar	170	18	1
Family Recipe Italian	130	13	1
Olive Oil & Vinegar	150	16	1
Parmesan & Rstd Garlic	110	11	2
Ranch	150	16	2
Raspberry & Walnut Vinaig.	70	5	7
Light: Balsamic Vinaigrette	45	4	2
Italian	60	6	1

Wish-Bone: *Per 2 Tbsp*

Creamy: Chunky Blue Cheese	150	14	1
Caesar	180	18	1
Deluxe French	120	11	5
Italian	110	10	4
Ranch	130	13	2
Russian	110	6	14
Sweet 'n Spicy French	140	12	7
Thousand Island	130	12	5
Light: Blue Cheese	70	6	2
Creamy Caesar	70	6	2
Honey Dijon	70	5	6
Italian	35	2.5	3
Parmesan Peppercorn Ranch	60	5	2
Ranch	70	5	4
Thousand Island	60	5	4
Light Vinaigrette: Balsamic & Basil	50	4	3
Asian with Sesame & Ginger	70	5	5
Raspberry Walnut	70	4	7
Fat-Free:			
Chunky Blue Cheese	30	0	7
Ranch	30	0	6
Oil & Vinegar:			
Balsamic Vinaigrette	60	5	3
House Italian	110	10	3
Red Wine Vinaigrette	70	5	6
Robusto Italian	80	7	4

Gravy

	C	F	Cb
Homemade Gravy, average:			
Thin, little fat,			
2 Tbsp, 1 oz	20	1	3
Thick: 2 Tbsp, 1.3 oz	50	2	9
¼ cup, 2.5 oz	100	4	18
McCormick:			
Brown, 1 Tbsp	25	0.5	3
Turkey, 1 Tbsp	20	0.5	4

Gravy-In-Jars

	C	F	Cb
Boston Market,			
Classic Beef, ¼ cup, 2 oz	30	1	4
Campbell's,			
Beef/Chicken/Turkey, ¼ cup, 2 oz	25	1	3
Heinz: *Per ¼ Cup, 2 oz*			
Homestyle: Bistro Au Jus	20	0.5	2
Classic Chicken	30	2	3
Pork; Rich Mushroom	20	0.5	3
Roasted Turkey	25	1	3
Savory Beef	30	1	4
Safeway, all varieties, ¼ cup, 2 oz	20	0.5	4

Tomato Products

	C	F	Cb
Whole/Chopped/Crushed/Diced:			
Regular: 1 cup, 8.5 oz	50	0	10
In Aspic, ½ cup	50	0	12
with Green Chili, 1 c., 8.5 oz	60	0	16
Stewed, ½ cup, 1.7 oz	40	1.5	7
Wedges in Tomato Juice, 1 cup	70	0.5	18
Salsa, average, 2 Tbsp, 1 oz	25	0	6
Tomato Ketchup:			
Regular: 1 Tbsp, 0.5 oz	15	0	4
Single Serve, 1 packet	10	0	3
Heinz, Simply Heinz			
1 Tbsp, 0.5 oz	15	0	4
Tomato Paste:			
Regular: 2 Tbsp, 1 oz	25	0	6
¾ cup, 6 oz	140	1	32
Tomato Puree, ½ cup, 4.5 oz	50	0	10
Tomato Sauce:			
Regular, ½ cup, 4.4 oz	50	0	11
Spanish Style, ½ cup, 4.3 oz	40	0	9
with Mushr., ½ cup, 4.3 oz	45	0	10
with Onions, ½ cup, 4.3 oz	50	0	12
Tomato Seasoning, 3 tsp	20	0	4
Sundried Tomatoes:			
Natural, 5-6 pieces, 0.4 oz	20	0	5
In Oil, drained, 6 pieces, 0.5 oz	40	2.5	4

Sauces ~ Brands

	C	F	Cb
A-1:			
Marinades: *Per Tbsp, ½ oz*			
Chicago Steakhouse	20	1	3
Classic	15	0	4
New Orleans Cajun	25	0	6
New York Steakhouse	20	0	5
Steak Sauce: Original	15	0	3
Bold & Spicy	20	0	4
Cracked Peppercorn	15	0	3
Thick & Hearty	25	0	6
Barilla:			
Pasta Sauces:			
Chunky Traditional, 4.8 oz	60	1	13
Creamy Alfredo, 2.15 oz	70	6	4
Garlic Alfredo, 2.15 oz	60	5	4
Marinara, 4.8 oz	70	1	14
Meat Sauce;Mushroom, 4.8 oz	60	1	13
Sun-Dried Tomato Pesto, 2.1 oz	200	18	7
Traditional Basil Pesto, 2.1 oz	200	19	5
Bertolli:			
Alfredo Sauces: *Per ¼ Cup*			
Creamy Basil	100	10	2
Garlic Romano w/ Parmesan	100	10	2
Mushroom	80	7	2
Traditional: *Per ½ Cup*			
Arrabbiata Pasta Sauce	60	1.5	11
Five Cheese	90	3.5	14
Italian Vodka	150	9	11
Vidalia Onion	80	2.5	14
Vineyard, Marinara; Portobello Mshrm	80	2.5	13
Best Foods/Hellmann's:			
Relish Sandwich Spread, 1 T.	60	6	2
Tartar Sauce, 2 Tbsp	70	6	4
Buitoni:			
Pasta Sauces:			
Alfredo: Regular, ¼ cup	140	12	4
Light, ¼ cup	90	6	4
Marinara: Regular ½ cup	70	3	10
with Roasted Garlic, ½ cup	60	1	10
Pesto: with Basil, ¼ cup	270	26	4
Reduced Fat, ¼ cup	230	17	8
Bull's-Eye: *Per 2 Tbsp*			
BBQ Sauce: Original	50	0	12
Hickory Smoke	60	0	15
Regional, average all varieties	50	0	11
Catelli: *Per ½ Cup*			
Pasta, Garden Select Six Vegetable:			
Country Mushroom	70	1.5	11
Diced Tomato & Basil	70	1	12
Meat Sauce	80	2.5	11
Pizza Sauce, all varieties	60	1.5	11

Sauces ~ Brands (Cont)

	C	F	Cb
Cento:			
Arrabbiata Sauce, 4.4 oz	50	3	6
Red Clam Sauce, 4.3 oz	60	2	6
Italiano Sauce, 2.2 oz	25	0	6
Marinara Sauce, 4.37 oz	60	3	6
Porcini Mushroom Sauce, 4.37 oz	60	4	6
Rustica Passata, 4.2 oz	20	1	9
Vodka Pasta Sauce, 4.4 oz	120	9	5
Classico:			
Alfredo: Per 1/4 Cup			
Creamy	60	4.5	3
Roasted Red Pepper	60	4	4
Family Favorites:			
Pesto: Per 1/4 Cup			
Basil Pesto	240	24	5
Sun-Dried Tomato Pesto	100	6	9
Red Sauces: Per 1/2 Cup			
Family Favorites: Meat	60	1	10
Parmesan & Romano	70	2	10
Traditional	80	2.5	13
Riserva: Arrabbiata, 4.4 oz	60	1	11
Eggplant & Artichoke, 4.4 oz	60	1.5	10
Tomato Cream Collection:			
Creamy Tomato & Roasted Garlic	35	1.5	5
Four Cheese Tomato	40	2	5
Spicy Tomato & Parmesan	40	2	5
Colgin, Liquid Smoke, 1 tsp	0	0	0
Contadina:			
Pizza Sauce: Per 2.2 oz			
Flavored with Pepperoni	35	1	6
Original; Four Cheese	30	0.5	6
Tomato Sauce, average	20	0.5	4
Crosse & Blackwell:			
Meat: Ham Glaze, 1 Tbsp	25	0	7
Mint Meat Sauce, 1 tsp	5	0	2
Seafood:			
Cocktail, 1/4 cup, 2.5 oz	90	0	21
Shrimp Sauce, 1/4 cup, 2.5 oz	90	0	21
Dave's Gourmet: Per 1/2 Cup			
Pasta Sauce:			
Butternut Squash, 4.23 oz	100	4	17
Organic: Red Heirloom, 4.4 oz	45	1.5	7
Rstd Garlic & Sweet Basil, 4.23 oz	70	4.5	8
Del Monte:			
Pasta Sauces: Per 1/2 Cup			
Four Cheese; Traditional, av.	60	1	12
Mushroom	60	1	11
Average other varieties	60	1	13
Sloppy Joe Sauce, Orig., 1/4 cup	60	0	13

	C	F	Cb
Emeril's:			
Alfredo, Four Cheese Sauce, 1/4 cup	60	5	4
Pasta Sauces: Per 1/2 Cup			
Homestyle Marinara	90	3	14
Kicked Up Tomato	80	3.5	11
Roasted Gaaahlic	80	3.5	12
Roasted Red Pepper	70	3.5	9
Vodka Sauce	110	7	12
Francesco Rinaldi:			
Alfredo, all flavors, 2.1 oz	90	8	2
Cheese,			
Three Cheese, 4.37 oz	70	1	15
Garden, all var., 4.37 oz	60	1	12
Meat: Meat Flavored, 4.37 oz	90	3.5	14
Sicilian Family, Sausage, 4.37 oz	70	2.5	11
Pizza, 2.15 oz	20	0	4
Tomato, Marinara, 4.37 oz	60	1	12
French's,			
Worcestershire Sce, 1 Tbsp	5	0	1
Heinz: Per 1 Tbsp			
57/Steak Sauce	20	0	4
Chili Sauce	20	0	5
Cocktail Sauce, Original,			
1/4 cup, 2.2 oz	70	0	18
Horseradish Sauce	75	6	3
Tomato Ketchup: Regular	20	0	5
Reduced Sugar	5	0	1
Worcestershire Sauce	5	0	1
House of Tsang:			
Bangkok Peanut Sce, 1.16 oz	40	2	4
Classic Sauce, 0.6 oz	25	0.5	5
Ginger Sriracha Sauce, 1.23 oz	15	0	4
General Tsao, 0.67 oz	45	0.5	10
Green Thai Curry Sauce, 1.1 oz	60	4	6
Korean Teriyaki Sauce, 0.67 oz	35	1	6
Oyster Flavored Sauce, 0.63 oz	30	0	7
Saigon Sizzle Sauce 0.63 oz	45	1	8
Sweet & Sour Sauce, 0.63 oz	35	0	8
Hunt's:			
BBQ Sauce, Original, 2 Tbsp	60	0	15
Hickory & Brown Sugar BBQ Sce, 2 Tbsp	70	0	18
Manwich, Sloppy Joe Sauce,			
Original, 1/4 cup, 2.3 oz	35	0	8
Pasta Sauce: Per 1/2 Cup			
Four Cheese	60	1	10
Garlic & Herb	40	1	8
Meat Flavor	60	1	10
Mushroom	50	0.5	10
Traditional	60	1	11

Brands (Cont)

	C	F	Cb
Kikkoman: *Per Tablespoon*			
Marinade: Honey & Mustard	30	0	6
Teriyaki Marinade & Sauce	15	0	2
Toasted Sesame	40	0.5	8
Sauce: Black Bean & Garlic	25	0	4
Ponzu Lime	10	0	2
Soy/Low Sodium	10	0	1
Steak; Sweet & Sour, average	20	0	5
Tamari	15	0	1
Knorr:			
Classic Sauce: *Per Whole Package*			
Bernaise, dry mix only	100	0	20
Hollandaise, dry mix only	100	0	20
Kraft:			
Barbecue Sauces, av., 2 Tbsp	50	0	12
Specialty Sauce: Cocktail, 2 Tbsp	60	0.5	11
Coleslaw Dressing, 1.2 oz	110	8	9
Horseradish, 1 oz	100	9	4
Sandwich Spread, 1 Tbsp	35	2.5	3
Tartar, Original, 1 Tbsp	60	5	4
Las Palmas:			
Green Enchilada Sauce, all varieties, 2 oz	25	1.5	3
Red Enchilada Sauce, 2 oz	15	0.5	3
La Victoria,			
Red/Green Enchilada Sauce, av., 2 oz	15	0.5	3
Lawry's:			
30 Minute Marinade: *Per Tbsp*			
Caribbean Jerk	30	0	7
Herb & Garlic; Lemon Pepper	10	0	2
Mesquite, w/ Lime Juice	10	0	2
Sesame Ginger, w/ Mandarin	30	0	7
Steak & Chop, w/ Garl. Pepp.	5	0	0.5
Packet Seasonings: *Dry*			
Fajitas; Taco, average, 2 tsp	15	0	3
Other varieties, average, 2 tsp	20	0	4
Lea & Perrins:			
Marinade for Chicken, 1 Tbsp	15	0	1
Steak Sauce, Bold, 1 Tbsp	20	0	5
Worcestershire Sauce, Original			
1 tsp, 5 ml	5	0	1
McCormicks:			
Seafood Sauces: *Per 2 Tbsp*			
Asian	50	1.5	7
Cajun Style	15	0	3
Lemon Butter Dill	100	9	4
Lemon Herb	140	15	0.5
Mediterranean; Santa Fe Style	20	0	4
Scampi	160	17	2

	C	F	Cb
Mrs. Dash:			
Marinades: *Per 1 Tbsp*			
Garlic Herb	15	0	3
Lemon Pepper	10	0	2
Lime Garlic	15	0	3
Sweet Teriyaki	35	0	9
Newman's Own: *Per 1/2 Cup*			
Pasta Sauce: Five Cheese	80	2	11
Fra Diavolo	80	3	10
Marinara; Sockarooni	70	1	12
Roasted Garlic & Peppers	70	1.5	11
Tomato & Basil Bombolina	80	2	13
Vodka	120	5	13
0 Organics *(Von's): Per 1/2 Cup*			
Marinara; Roasted Garlic, av.	60	1.5	9
Mushroom; Tomato Basil	50	1.5	8
Old El Paso:			
Enchilada Sauce:			
Green, 1/4 cup, 2.15 oz	25	1.5	4
Red, 1/4 cup, 2.1 oz	20	0	4
Taco Sauce, all varieties, 1 Tbsp	5	0	1
Pace: *Per 2 Tbsp*			
Picante Sauce	10	0	3
Salsa: Thick & Chunky, av.	10	0	2
Fire, Chipotle & Jalapeno	10	0	2
Restaurant Style, Peach Mango	15	0	4
Prego: *Per 1/2 Cup*			
Alfredo, average all varieties	150	14	6
Classic Italian:			
Fresh Mushroom; Traditional	70	1.5	13
Marinara	80	3	10
Tomato, Basil Garlic	80	2.5	12
Farmers Market: Classic Marinara	90	4.5	10
Four Cheese; Roasted Garlic, av.	80	3.5	11
Garden Vegetable	60	2	9
Mushroom; Trad. Basil, average	75	3	11
Pizza Sauce, Pizzeria Style	70	2	12
Pemium Pasta: Creamy Vodka	140	7	15
Flav. with Bacon & Provolone	100	3	15
Pesto Marinara	90	3.5	12
Spicy Sausage	110	4	15
Premier Japan,			
Hoisin; Teriyaki, 1 Tbsp	15	0	3

Brands (Cont)   C   F   Cb

Ragu:

Cheesy: *Per ¼ Cup*

	C	F	Cb
Classic Alfredo	90	8	2
Creamy Mozzarella	80	7	2
Creamy Tomato	90	8	4
Double Cheddar	100	9	2
Four Cheese	80	8	2
Light Parmesan Alfredo	60	4	2
Roasted Garlic Parmesan	100	9	3
Six Cheese	90	2.5	14

Chunky: *Per ½ Cup*

	C	F	Cb
Roasted Garlic	90	2.5	14
Average other varieties	90	2.5	14

Old World Style: *Per ½ Cup*

	C	F	Cb
Flavored with Meat	80	2.5	10
Marinara	80	2.5	11
Traditional	80	2	13

Pizza: Homemade Style, ¼ cup — 30 / 1 / 5
Quick Sauce, Traditional, ¼ cup — 45 / 1.5 / 6

Safeway Select:
Salsa, all varieties, average, 2 Tbsp — 15 / 0 / 3

Select Sauces: *Per ½ Cup*

	C	F	Cb
Arrabbiata	110	8	10
Artichoke Pesto	60	2	9
Four Cheese	80	3.5	11
Marinara	60	2	10
Spicy Red Bell Pepper	50	1	9
Sundried Tomato & Olive	60	1.5	11
Tomato Alfredo; Vodka	130	10	9

Taco Bell, Creamy Jalapeno Sauce,
1 Tablespoon, 0.5 oz — 70 / 7 / 1

Tony Roma's:
Bold & Spicy BBQ Sauce, 2 Tbsp — 50 / 0 / 12
Carolina Honeys BBQ Sauce,
2 Tablespoons — 70 / 0 / 18

Trader Joe's:
BBQ Sauce,
Kansas City Style, 2 Tbsp — 60 / 0 / 15
Tomato Basil Marinara, ½ cup — 80 / 4.5 / 10

Walnut Acres,
Organic Pasta Sauces,
average all var., ½ cup, 4.5 oz — 50 / 1 / 9

Seasonings & Flavorings   C F Cb

	C	F	Cb
Auromatic Bitters *(Angostua)*, 1 tsp	15	0	4
Bacon Bits, average, 1 Tbsp	35	2	2
Bacon Chips *(Durkee)*, 1 Tbsp	30	1	2
Bac-Os *(Betty Crocker)*, 1Tbsp	30	1.5	2
Blends *(Mrs Dash)*, 1 tsp	0	0	0
Butter Buds, 1 tsp	5	0	2
Flavor Enhancer *(Accent)*, 1 tsp	0	0	0
Flavor Sprinkles *(Molly McButter)*, Natural/Cheese, 1 tsp	5	0	1
Garlic Bread Sprinkle, 1 tsp	8	0.5	1
Garlic Salt, 1 tsp	2	0	0
Italian Seasoning, 1 tsp	4	0	1
Lemon Pepper Seasoning, 1 tsp	7	0	1
Meat Tenderizer, av., 1 tsp	7	0	1
Salad Crunchies *(McCormick)*, 1 tsp	10	0.5	2
Salt, Reg., Sea Salt, Lite Salt	0	0	0
Seasoning *(Old Bay)*, ¼ tsp	0	0	0
Seasoning Mix *(Vegit)*, ¼ tsp	0	0	0
Seasoning Mixes, av., ¼ pkg	70	1	9
Taco Seasoning, av., ¼ pkg	30	0.5	4
Bragg's, Liquid Aminos	0	0	0
Old El Paso: Chili Season. Mix, 1 Tbsp	8	0.5	1.5
Cheesy Taco Seasoning Mix, 1 Tbsp	10	0.5	2
Taco/Burrito Seasoning Mix, 2 tsp	15	0	4
Fajita Seasoning Mix, 1 tsp	5	0	1.5

Spices & Herbs

	C	F	Cb
Average all types, 1 tsp	5	0	1
All Purpose, 1 tsp	0	0	0
Allspice, ground	5	0	1
Chili Powder	8	0	1
Cinnamon, ground	6	0	2
Curry Powder	6	0	1
Garlic Powder	9	0	2
Nutmeg, ground	12	0	1
Onion Powder	7	0	2
Parsley, dried	4	0	1
Pepper, average	6	0	1
Saffron	2	0	0
Salt-Free Blends, 1 tsp	0	0	0
Tumeric, ground	8	0	1
Seeds: Fenugreek	12	1	2
Mustard, Poppyseed	15	1	1
Other varieties, average	7	0	1

Home-Popped Popcorn

	C	F	Cb
Popping Corn Kernels,			
2 Tbsp, 1 oz	110	1	26
(makes approximately 5 cups)			
Air-popped, without oil: Plain, 1 oz	110	1	22
1 cup, 0.2 oz	20	0	5
Oil-popped: Plain, 1 oz	145	8	16
1 cup, 0.4 oz	55	3	6
Popcorn Oil, 1 Tbsp	120	14	0

Microwave Popcorn

	C	F	Cb
Average all Brands: *Per 1 Cup Popped, Unless Indicated*			
Butter: Regular, 1 cup	35	2	4
Light, 1 cup	25	1	4
Act II Popcorn:			
Butter: 1 cup	25	1	4
4¹/₂ cups, 1 oz	130	6	19
94% Fat-Free Butter:			
1 cup	20	0.5	4
6¹/₂ cups, 1 oz	130	2	27
Butter Lovers: 1 cup	25	1	4
4¹/₂ cups, 1 oz	140	7	19
Xreme Butter: 1 cup	25	1	4
4¹/₂ cups	160	9	19
BodyKey *(Amway)*, Slim Popcorn,			
Sea Salt, 1 bag	110	7	10
Jolly Time:			
Blast O Butter, 1 cup	45	3	4
Crispy & Light Butter, 1 cup	25	1	4
Xtra Butter: 1 cup	40	2.5	4
4 cups	160	10	16
Newman's Own:			
Butter Flavor, Microwave:			
Regular, 3¹/₂ cups	130	5	18
Light, 3¹/₂ cups	120	4	19
Butter Boom, 3¹/₂ cups	130	5	18
Orville Redenbacher's: *Popped*			
Butter: 4 cups	170	12	17
Light, 6 cups	160	6	26
Movie Theater Butter, 5 cups	160	10	18
Ultimate Butter, 4¹/₂ cups	160	9	19
Naturals, Lime & Salt, 5 cups	220	15	21
Sweet & Savory: Caramel, 3 cups	170	8	26
Cheddar Cheese, 4¹/₂ cups	180	14	16
Pop Secret: *Per Cup*			
94% Fat-Free, Butter	20	0	3
Double Butter	40	2	3

Bagged Popcorn

	C	F	Cb
Average All Brands (Ready-to-Eat)			
Regular/Plain: ¹/₂ oz package	80	5	8
1 oz package	160	10	16
4 oz package	640	40	64
2 oz Box (store/airport)	320	16	32
3 oz Bag (9" high x 5" wide)	480	24	48
Caramel Popcorn,			
with nuts, 1 cup, 1.5 oz	230	12	39

Bagged Popcorn ~ Brands

	C	F	Cb
Boston's, Lite, 3¹/₂ cups, 1 oz	130	4.5	20
Cracker Jack: Original, 1 cup, 2 oz	240	4	46
Chocolate & Caramel, 1 cup, 2 oz	220	1	50
Crunch 'N Munch:			
Buttery Toffee: ²/₃ cup, 1.1 oz	150	5	24
1 cup, 1.65 oz	225	7.5	36
Caramel: ²/₃ cup, 1.1 oz	160	7	22
1 cup, 1.65 oz	240	10	33
12 oz box	1745	76	240
Fiddle Faddle:			
Average all varieties: 1 oz	120	2	24
1 cup, 2 oz	240	4	48
6 oz box	720	12	144
Popcorn Indiana:			
Kettlecorn,			
Original, 2 cups, 1 oz	130	5	21
Popcorn:			
Aged White Cheddar, 2.5 cups, 1 oz	150	9	14
Chicago Fair,			
Caramel & Cheese, 1 cup, 1 oz	140	6	20
Movie Theater, 2 cups, 1 oz	160	12	13
Seasalt, 3.5 cups, 1 oz	140	6	17
Poppycock:			
Bags: Cashew Lovers, ¹/₂ cup, 1 oz	150	6	20
Chocolate Lovers, ¹/₂ cup, 1.2 oz	160	7	22
Cannisters, Orig./Pecan Delight, av:			
¹/₂ cup, 1 oz	155	7	20
1 cup, 2 oz	310	14	40

Movie Theater Popcorn

	C	F	Cb
Small, (7 cups): Plain	385	21	44
with Butter (3 pumps, 0.8 oz)	570	42	44
Medium, (15 cups): Plain	825	45	94
with Butter (4 pumps, 1 oz)	1075	73	94
Large, (20 cups): Plain	1100	60	124
with Butter (6 pumps, 1.5 oz)	1485	102	124
Butter: 1 Pump, 0.3 oz	65	7	0
4 Pumps (2 Tbsp), 1 oz	250	28	0

Corn & Tortilla Chips Ⓒ Ⓕ Ⓒb

Average All Brands
Corn Chips:

	C	F	Cb
Average all types: 1 oz	150	8	18
8 oz bag	1200	64	144
Fritos, Original, 32 chips, 1 oz	160	10	15
Tortilla Chips: Average, 1 oz	140	7	18
(1 oz = approx. 12 chips or 13 strips)			
Doritos: Original, 1 oz	140	7	18
Nacho Chse; Salsa Verde, av., 1 oz	140	8	18
Popchips: Chili Limon, 1 oz	120	4	19
Nacho Cheese, 1 oz	130	5	18
Snyder's:			
El Restaurante, all flavors, 1 oz	150	8	17
Yellow Corn/White, av., 1 oz	135	5	21
Tostitos:			
Average all flav., 1 oz	145	7	19
Baked! Scoops, 1 oz	120	3	22
Utz: Multigrain, 1 oz	150	8	16
Baked, 1 oz	120	2	23
Other flavors, 1 oz	140	8	18

Potato Chips/Crisps

Average All Brands
Regular:

	C	F	Cb
Plain or flavored, (4 chips)	30	2	3
1 oz package (20 chips)	150	10	15
4 oz quantity	600	40	60
14 oz package	2100	140	210

Chips/Crisps ~ Brands

	C	F	Cb
Hippeas, Chick Pea Puffs,			
average all flavors, 0.78 oz	90	4	11
Lay's *(Fritolay):*			
Classics; Wavy Originals, 1 oz	160	10	15
Kettle Cooked, Original, 1 oz	150	9	17
Pringles:			
All Flavors: 1 oz	150	9	16
Large can, 6 oz	900	54	96
Stix, To Go Pak, Baked Cheese	80	3	10
Ruffles: Regular, av. all flavors, 1 oz	160	11	15
Reduced Fat, 1 oz	140	7	18
Simply7, Hummus/Lentil Chips,			
average all flavors, 1 oz	135	5	19
Sun Chips, Original, 16 crisps, 1 oz	140	6	18

Pretzels Ⓒ Ⓕ Ⓒb

Average All Brands
Hard-Baked Pretzels: *Each*

	C	F	Cb
1 oz quantity	110	1	23
Sticks, thin, 2¼" (9/oz)	12	0	3
Twists, thin, ¼" thick, (5/oz)	25	0	5
Dutch (2¾"x 2⅝"), 0.5 oz	55	1	11
Snyders, Sourdough, 0.8oz	100	0	22
Soft Pretzel Twists, average: *Each*			
Plain: Small, 2 oz	210	2	43
Medium, 4 oz	390	3.5	80
Large, 5 oz	485	4.5	100
Big Cheese, 1.8 oz	130	3	22
New York Street Vendors, 7 oz	660	6	135
Trader Joe's, Peanut Butter filled, 1 oz	140	8	14
Snyder's: Milk Chocolate Dips, 1 oz	140	6	19
White Creme Dips, 1 oz	130	6	19

Pretzels ~ Brands

	C	F	Cb
Flipz: Milk Choc, 8 pieces, 1 oz	130	5	20
White Fudge, 7 pcs, 1 oz	130	5	20
Rold Gold *(Frito-Lay):*			
Braided Twists,			
Honey Wheat (8), 1 oz	110	1	24
Pretzel, Sourdough (1)	90	1	19
Pretzel Thins (9), 1 oz	110	1	23
Rods (3), 1 oz	110	1	22
Tiny Twists (18), average, 1 oz	110	0	23
Sticks, 1 oz	100	0	23
Snyder's of Hanover:			
Butter Snaps (24), 1 oz	120	1	25
Choc Dipped Minis, av., 1 oz	135	6	20
Gluten Free Pretzel Sticks (30)	110	1.5	25
Pieces, average, 1 oz	140	8	16
Sticks (28), average, 1 oz	110	1	23
Thins (11), 1 oz	110	0	23
Twists (7), average,1 oz	120	2	24
Special K,			
Choc. Coated, av., all flavors, 1 oz	100	3.5	15
SuperPretzel:			
6 Count Soft, Original (1), 2.3 oz	160	1	34
Bites (5), 1.9 oz	140	0.5	32
Softstix, Cheese (2), 1.76 oz	130	3	22
Utz:			
Pretzels: Original; Extra Dark, 1 oz	110	1	21
Sourdough, Hard (1)	90	0	18

Snacks

Snacks	C	F	Cb

Note: Actual weight of packaged snacks is usually 5-10% more than label Net Wt. For accuracy, weigh snack and allow extra calories, fat and carbs for any extra weight.

	C	F	Cb
Apple Chips (Seneca), av., 1 oz	140	7	20
Bagel Crisps (N.Y. Style), 6 crisps, 1 oz	130	6	17
Baguette Chips (Pillsbury), av., (21)	130	5	19
Banana Chips (T.Joe's), 13 chips, 1 oz	160	11	13
Beef Jerky (Jack Link's), av., 1 oz	80	1	5
Beef Sticks: (Slim Jim), Giant, 1 oz	140	11	4
Jack Link's, Original, 1.5 oz	160	13	2
Beet Chips (Rhythm), Sea Salt, 1oz	130	4	20
Trader Joes, 1.3 oz	140	0.5	29
BodyKey (Amway):			
Mixed Nuts & Pumpkin Seeds, 1 bag	200	16	8
Whole Grain Tortilla Chips, 1 bag	210	11	24
Bugles, Original; Nacho Cheese, 1 oz	160	9	18
Cheese Balls (Utz), 1 oz serving	130	7	16
Cheese Bites (Tr. Joes), 1 oz	170	12	0.5
Cheese Nips, 1.3 oz package	170	7	22
Cheese Puffs, average, 1 oz	160	10	15
Cheetos:			
Crunchy: Av. all flavors, 1 oz	155	11	13
4 oz package	640	40	60
Baked!; Fantastix, av., 1 oz	130	5	19
Simply Puffs, Wh. Cheddar, 1 oz	150	9	16
Cheez-It (Sunshine):			
Snack Mix: Classic, 1/2 cup, 1 oz	140	4.5	20
Double Cheese, 3/4 cup, 1 oz	130	5	19
Sriracha, 1/2 cup, 0.9 oz	120	5	17
Sweet & Salty, 1/2 cup, 1oz	140	5	21
Chester's: Fries, Flamin' Hot, 1 oz	150	8	17
Puffcorn, Cheese, 1 oz	160	11	14
Chex Mix, (General Mills),			
Traditional, 1 oz	120	3.5	22
Chicharrones ~ See Pork Skins			
Crackers (Tr. Joes), Mini Edaname (28)	120	2	21
Churros (Rubio's), Cinnamon, 2 oz	240	13	30
Combo, Crackers, av., 1/3 cup, 1 oz	140	6	18
Cool Cuts, Carrot & Ranch, 2.3 oz	70	5	5
Corn Chips ~ See Page 149			
Corn Nuts: Av all flav., 1 oz	130	4.5	20
1.7 oz bag	210	8	34
Corn Puffs/Twists, (32), 1 oz	160	11	15
Dunkin Stix (Dolly Madison), (3)	490	25	63
Edamame,			
Seapointe, Dry Roasted, 1 oz	130	4	11
Fritos: Corn Chips, all varieties, av., 1oz	160	10	15
Flavor Twists, Honey BBQ, 1 oz	150	9	16

Snacks (Cont)	C	F	Cb
Fruit Snacks ~ See Page 102			
Funyuns, Onion Flavored, 1 oz	130	6	16
Goldfish, Crackers, av., 1 oz	140	5	20
Gold-n-Chees (Lance):			
Snack Mix, 1 oz	150	8	17
Tube, 1 oz	130	6	18
Gripz (Sunshine), Mighty Tiny (1)	120	6	15
Flamin Hot Peanuts (Munchies), 1 oz	180	14	6
Kale Chips (Rhythm),			
Roasted Garlic & Onion, 1 oz	160	11	14
Trader Joes, average, 1 oz	150	10	9
Lance, Sandwich Crackers (6), av.	200	9	25
Munchies (Frito-Lay),			
Snack Mix, all flavors, 1 oz	140	7	18
Munchos (Fritolay), all flavors, 1 oz	160	10	16
Newtons:			
Single Serve: 2 oz pkg	200	4	40
Fat-Free, 2 oz package	200	0	46
Nutella, w/ Breadsticks/Pretzels (1)	270	14	35
Nutter Butter, Sandwich Cookies:			
1.87 oz Package	250	10	37
Bites, Go-Pak, 3.5 oz	490	21	74
Onion Rings (T.G.I. Friday), 1 oz	140	7	16
Oreo Cookies, all Creme Fillings:			
Double Stuf (2), 1 oz	140	7	21
Mini Bite Size: 1 oz	130	6	21
Go-Pak, 3.5 oz	455	21	74
Oreo Cakesters, Golden, Soft, 0.9 oz	110	5	16
Oriental Mix Rice Snacks, 1 oz	125	3.5	21
Peanut Butter Nuggets, (10), 1 oz	140	6	15
Pepitas, dried or roasted,			
1/4 cup, 1 oz	155	14	3
Pirate's Booty:			
Aged White Cheddar, 4 oz	560	24	72
Veggie, 4 oz bag	560	28	72
Pita Chips (9), average, 1 oz	130	4	18
Plaintain Chips (Goya), 1 oz	150	8	19
PopCorners, Butter/Kettle, 1 oz	125	3.5	20
Popcorn ~ See Page 148			
Pork Cracklins, 1 oz	160	12	0
Pork Skins/Rinds: 1 oz	160	10	0
Baken-ets, Traditional, 0.5 oz	80	5	0
Mission, Chiccarones, 4 oz package	640	40	0
Potato Chips ~ See Page 149			
Potato Skins (TGI Friday),			
all flavors, 16 chips, 1 oz	140	8	15
Puffed Wheat,			
Sabritones, Chili & Lime, 1 oz	140	8	16
Pretzels ~ See Page 149			

Snacks (Cont)

	C	F	Cb
Rice Cakes:			
Lundberg, (1), average	80	0.5	17
Quaker: Plain, lightly salted (1)	35	0	7
Chocolate Crunch (1)	60	1	12
Rice Chips,			
Lundberg, average, 1 oz	140	7	18
Sandwich Crackers:			
Austin, Cheese Crackers:			
with Cheddar, 1.4 oz	190	10	23
with Peanut Butter, 1.3 oz	190	10	23
PB & J Flavored, 1.4 oz	190	8	26
Lance: Nip Chee, 6 pieces	190	9	24
Toasty, 6 pieces	180	9	21
Toast Chee, PB, 1.5 oz	220	1	25
Ritz Bits: Cheese (12), 1 oz Pkg	150	8	17
3 oz Pak	450	25	50
P'nut Butter: 1.5 oz pkg	210	11	24
Big Bag, 3 oz	420	22	48
Sesame Sticks, Salted,			
SunRidge Farm, 1 oz	170	12	14
Smart Puffs,			
Pirates Booty, 1 oz	140	7	16
Soybeans in Pods,			
AFC, ½ cup, 3.2 oz	90	5	3
Soy Crisps, average, 1 oz	120	3	17
Soy Nuts: Dry Roasted, ¼ cup, 1 oz	130	6	9
Choc-coated, 1 oz	140	7	13
Sun Chips,			
Fritolay, average, 1 oz	140	6	19
Takis: Crunchy Fajitas, 1 oz	140	8	16
4 oz package	560	32	64
Tings (Robert's), 2 oz bag	300	16	36
Toasted Chips (Ritz), av. all, 1 oz	130	5.5	20
Tortilla Chips,			
Garden of Eatin, Chili & Lime, 1 oz	140	7	18
Trail Mix (Nuts/Seeds/Dried Fruit):			
Regular, 3 Tbsp, 1 oz	140	9	13
Tropical, 3 Tbsp, 1 oz	130	7	16
Turkey Jerky: Teriyaki, 1 oz	80	1	8
Trader Joe's, Original, 1 oz	60	0.5	6
Veggie Crisps,			
Snyder's, 1 oz	140	6	18
Wheat Thins (Nabisco), av. all, 1 oz	135	5	21
Woats, Oatsnack, av., ¼ cup, 1 oz	120	5	17
Yogurt Pretzels, 1.5 oz	190	8	28
Yogurt Raisins, Vanilla,			
Sun-Maid, 1 oz	120	4.5	20

Fruit Snacks

	C	F	Cb
Betty Crocker: Fruit Gushers, 0.9 oz	90	1.5	21
Fruit by the Foot, 1 roll, 0.8 oz	80	1	17
Fruit Roll Ups, 1 roll, 0.5 oz	50	1	11
Fruit Flavored Shapes, all varieties, 0.9 oz	80	0	19
Sunkist:			
Fruit Lover's Trail Mix: B'fast Espresso, 1.5 oz	190	9	27
Other flavors, 1 oz	120	4	20
Fruit Snack Cups ~ See Page 102			

Vending Machines

	C	F	Cb
Bugles, Nacho Cheese, 1 oz	160	9	18
Cheese Balls (Utz), 1 oz	130	7	16
Cheetos, Crunchy, 1 oz	150	10	13
Cheeze-It, Snack Mix, 1.5 oz	195	6.5	30
Chester's, Flamin' Hot Fries, 1 oz	150	8	17
Choc Chip Cookies:			
Chips Ahoy, 1.2 oz	160	8	22
Famous Amos, (4), 1 oz	150	8	18
Grandma's, (1), 1.4 oz	200	10	25
Chocolate Bars:			
Hershey's, Milk Choc.,1.6 oz	220	13	22
Kit Kat, 1.5 oz	210	11	25
Snickers, 1.9 oz bar	250	12	33
Donut, plain cake, 1.4 oz	160	9	18
Doritos, av. all flavors, 1 oz	145	8	18
Fritos, Corn Chips, Orig., 1.8 oz	280	17	26
Fruit Pie,			
Hostess, Lemon, 4.5 oz	510	25	65
Granola/Cereal Bars, av., 1 oz	140	3	26
M & M's:			
Milk Chocolate, 1.7 oz	240	10	34
Peanuts, 1.8 oz	250	13	30
Oreo Cookies, 2 oz	270	11	41
Peanut Butter Cups,			
Reese's, 1.5 oz	210	12	24
Popcorn, plain, 1 oz	160	10	16
Pop Chips, 0.8 oz	100	3	16
Pork Skins, 1.5 oz	240	15	0
Potato Chips: 1 oz	150	10	15
Baked! (Ruffles), Orig.,1 oz	120	3	22
Potato Skins (TGI Friday's), all flavors, 1 oz	140	8	15
Pretzels (Snyder's), Olde Tyme, 1 oz	120	1	24
Raisins, 0.5 oz package	45	0	11
Rice Krispies Treat	90	2	17
Skittles, 2 oz	230	2.5	52
Starburst, Fruit Chews, Orig., 1.4 oz	130	0	31
Tortilla Chips, 1 oz	140	7	18

Homemade & Restaurant

Restaurant & Take-Out: *Average All Preparations: Per 8 fl.oz*	C	F	Cb
Bean Medley	200	3	34
Beef Consomme	30	0	2
Borscht, with Sour Cream	130	8	14
Bouillabaisse	400	15	10
Chicken & Corn	290	14	20
Chicken & Wild Rice	80	4	9
Chicken Consomme	50	0	2
Chicken Curry	180	8	18
Chicken Jambalaya	160	7	8
Chicken Noodle	80	2	12
With Chicken	160	4	12
Chicken Soup	80	2	6
Chili with Beans	250	12	25
Clam Chowder	240	15	17
Corn & Crab	120	3	18
Corn Chowder	150	8	16
Cream of Broccoli	200	12	20
Cream of Potato	150	6.5	17
Cream of Mushroom	200	13	15
Fish Chowder	220	15	6
French Onion	420	15	25
Gazpacho	50	0	5
Lentil Soup	250	9	28
Lobster Bisque	320	15	10
Matzo Ball, with 1 large ball	180	7	24
Minestrone	125	2.5	20
Mulligatawny	300	15	8
Pea & Ham	240	10	25
Potato & Bacon	170	7	19
Pumpkin, Creamy	210	10	26
Shark Fin Soup	100	4	8
Spicy Shrimp Soup, 1 bowl	160	7	10
Split Pea Soup	180	2.5	30
Vegetable (Fat Free)	75	0	18
Vegetable Beef	80	2	10
Vichyssoise	200	9	15
Watercress	90	4	13

Other Soups ~ *See International & Fast-Foods Sections (Arby's, Au Bon Pain, Boston Market, Dunkin' Donuts, Denny's, Schlotzsky's, Sizzler, Souplantation, Sweet Tomatoes, Zoup!)*

Homemade Soups: *Calculate calories, fat and carbohydrates from recipe ingredients.*

Bouillon Cubes & Powders

Bouillon Cubes: *Average all types*	C	F	Cb
Regular, 1 cube	5	0	1
Extra Large, 1 cube	20	1	1
Powders, average, 1 tsp	10	0	1
Herb-Ox:			
Instant Broth & Seasoning,			
Beef, 1 envelope, 0.14 oz	5	0	1
Chicken, 1 envelope, 0.14 oz	5	0	1

Soup ~ Brands

Amy's:

Heat & Serve (Organic): *Per 1 Cup, Unless Indicated*			
Alphabet	80	0	16
Chunky Vegetable	80	1.5	13
Cream of M'shrm, $^3/_4$ cup	150	9	13
Curried Lentil	230	9	30
Lentil	180	5	25
Lentil Vegetable	160	4	24
Rustic Italian Vegetable	140	6	18
Split Pea	110	1	19
Thai Coconut	140	10	9
Tuscan Bean & Rice	160	4.5	25

Andersen's: *Per 1 Cup*			
Split Pea	130	0	24
Split Pea flavored with Bacon	140	1	23

Bertoli: *Per ½ Carton, 12 oz*			
Meal Soups: Ricotta & Lobster Ravioli,			
in Seafood Bisque	380	16	41
Tomato Florentine			
& Tortellini with Chicken	410	19	36

Campbell's:

Chunky: *Per 8 fl.oz Cup*			
Baked Potato w/ Ched. & Bacon Bits	180	9	21
BBQ Seasoned Pork	160	1	28
Beef Burrito	170	6	19
Beer-n-Cheese, with Beef & Bacon	190	9	21
Chicken Corn Chowder	190	10	20
Classic Chicken Noodle	120	3	14
Healthy Request:			
Beef w/ Country Veggies	110	1.5	17
Chicken Corn Chowder	140	3	22
Chicken Noodle	110	3	14
New England Clam Chowder	130	3	20
Split Pea & Ham, Smoke Flavor	160	2.5	22
Mushroom Swiss Burger	160	7	16
Sausage & Pepper Rigatoni	200	8	23

Campbell's (Cont):

	C	F	Cb
Chunky (Cont): *Per 8 fl.oz Cup*			
Hearty: Beef Noodle	120	2.5	17
Cheeseburger Soup	200	13	14
Italian Style Wedding, with M'balls & Spinach	120	3	15
Condensed Soup: *Per ½ Cup, 4 fl.oz*			
Bean with Bacon	160	3	26
Beef with Veggies & Barley	80	1	15
Cheddar Cheese	100	5	14
Cream of Broccoli	90	5	9
Cream of Celery	100	7	8
Cream of Potato	90	2	16
Homestyle Chicken Noodle	70	2	10
Old Fashioned Tomato Rice	125	1.5	25
Split Pea w/ Ham & Bacon	180	2	29
Tomato	90	0	20
Go Soups: *Per 8 fl.oz Cup*			
Chicken & Quinoa with Chilies	140	1.5	22
Coconut Curry w/ Chicken & Shitaki Mushrooms	130	5	16
Creamy Red Pepper with Smoked Gouda	210	14	14
Golden Lentil w/ Madras Curry	140	6	18
Moroccan Style Chicken w/ Chickpeas	170	2	28
Spicy Chorizo, Chkn & Black Beans	200	6	25
Homestyle: *Per 8 fl.oz Cup*			
Butternut Squash Bisque	130	5	18
Chicken Noodle	90	2.5	10
Country Chicken Noodle	120	3	16
Creamy Chicken & Herb Dumplings	160	9	14
Creamy Gouda Bisque with Chicken	190	11	16
Harvest Tomato with Basil	110	1	23
Italian-Style Wedding	120	3.5	15
Maryland-Style Crab Soup	80	0.5	14
Mexican-Style Chkn Tortilla	130	2	20
Minestrone	100	1	18
Potato Broccoli Cheese	170	10	16
Southwest-Style White Chkn Chili	130	2.5	20
Vegetable Medley	90	0.5	18
Zesty Tomato Bisque	110	2	19
Light: Chicken Noodle	70	1	9
Baked Pot. w/ Bacon & Cheddar	100	3	15
Italian-Style Wedding	80	1.5	11
New England Clam Chowder	100	1.5	16
Southwestern-Style Vegetable	50	0	10

Campbell's (Cont):

	C	F	Cb
Slow Kettle Style: *Per 8 fl.oz*			
Braised Beef Stew	150	3	19
Portobello Mushroom & Madeira Bisque	240	18	16
Southwest Style Chicken Chili with Black Beans	190	2.5	28
Tomato & Sweet Basil Bisque	290	16	33
Tuscan Style Chicken & White Bean	140	2.5	17
Health Valley Organics: *Per 8 fl.oz Cup*			
40% Less Sodium:			
Chicken Noodle	80	2.5	11
Garden Vegetable	80	0	18
Broth, Chicken, no salt added	35	1.5	0
Creamed:			
Cream of Chicken	110	3	15
Cream of Celery	100	2	17
Cream of Mushroom	90	2	14
No Salt Added: Fagoili	130	3	21
Lentil	140	1.5	27
Minestroni	90	2	16
Potato Leek	100	2	20
Healthy Choice:			
Canned: *Per Cup*			
Bean & Ham, 8.8 oz	180	2.5	28
Chkn & Dumplings, 8.9 oz	150	3	22
Chicken Tortilla, 8.4 oz	140	1.5	23
Chicken with Rice, 8.4 oz	110	3	15
Country Vegetable, 8.7 oz	110	0.5	21
Split Pea & Ham, 8.4 oz	160	2.5	27
Vegetable Beef, 8.8 oz	130	1.5	20
Microwaveable Bowls: *Per Cup*			
Cheese Tortellini, 8.6 oz	110	1.5	17
Chicken Tortilla, 8.6 oz	150	2	23
Chicken with Rice, 8.5 oz	90	2.5	12
Country Vegetable, 8.6 oz	100	0.5	20
Hearty Vegetable Barley, 8.8 oz	140	1.5	28
Imagine:			
Broths, Organic: *Per Cup*			
Beef Flavor	20	1	2
Free Range Chicken	20	0.5	2
Vegetable	20	0	4
Vegetarian, No-Chicken	15	0	2
Chunky Style, Organic: *Per Cup*			
Chicken & Dumplings	120	4.5	16
Ginger Miso	70	1.5	11
Ital. Vegetables & Beans	130	1.5	25

Continued Nex Page...

Imagine (Cont):

	C	F	Cb
Creamy: *Per 8 fl.oz Cup*			
Butternut Squash	100	1.5	21
Cauliflower & Potato	70	1	14
Portobello Mushroom	80	2.5	12
Sweet Pea	80	1.5	14
Tomato Basil	80	1	15
Kettle Cuisine: *Per 8 oz*			
Angus Steak Chili with Beans	250	7	20
Beef, Barley & Vegetable	110	2.5	14
Broccoli Cheddar	320	24	15
Caribbean Jerk Chicken	220	5	31
Carrot Ginger	110	4.5	18
Chicken Tortilla	120	3	15
Chipotle Sweet Potato	140	7	20
Cream of Crab	290	22	15
Lobster Bisque	270	18	18
Manhattan Clam Chowder	120	3	16
North Atlantic Haddock Chowder	260	17	14
Knorr:			
Cubes: *Per ½ Cube, 1 Cup, Prepared*			
Beef; Chicken, average	15	1.5	1
Vegetable	20	1	1
Homestyle Stock: *Per 1 Tsp*			
Beef	10	0.5	1
Chicken	10	1	0.5
Lipton:			
Cup-a-Soup: *Per Envelope*			
Chkn Noodle, White Meat	50	1	8
Cream of Chicken	70	1.5	12
Recipe Secrets: *Per 1 Tbsp Dry Mix*			
Onion	20	0	4
Onion Mushroom	35	0	7
Savory Herb with Garlic	35	0	6
Manischewitz:			
Canned: *Per 1 cup*			
Broth, Chicken	15	0	2
Chicken Consomme, Clear	30	0	4
Chicken Noodle	180	2	20
Glass Jar: *Per 1 Cup*			
Matzo Ball	120	5	15
Reduced Sodium	130	6	17
Matzo Ball in Broth	180	8	23
Reduced Sodium	180	8	21
Maruchan:			
Instant Lunch,			
average all flavors, 1 pkg	290	12	38
Ramen, all flavors, 1 pkg, 3 oz	380	14	52

Nissin:

	C	F	Cb
Souper Meal: *Per ½ of 4.3 oz Ctn*			
Chicken Flavor, with Veggie Medley	280	13	37
Picante Shrimp Flavor, Hot & Spicy	290	13	37
Top Ramen, all flavors, 3 oz pkg	380	14	53
Pacific Foods:			
Condensed:			
Cream of Chicken, ½ cup	90	3.5	10
Cream of Mushroom, ½ cup	100	2.5	18
Hearty Organic: *Per 1 Cup*			
Butternut Squash Bisque	110	3.5	18
Cashew Carrot Ginger Bisque	130	5	20
Spicy Black Bean & Kale	120	0	24
Split Pea & Uncured Ham	160	2.5	26
Vegetable Quinoa	90	2	18
Progresso:			
Broths: Beef, 1 cup	20	0	3
Chicken, 1 cup	20	0	1
Hearty Classics: *Per Cup*			
Smokehouse Port & Beef Chili, with Beans	300	17	24
S'West Style White Chkn Chili, with Beans	180	3.5	22
Rich & Hearty: *Per 1 Cup*			
Chkn & Hm'style Noodles	100	2	14
Chicken Corn Chowder	190	8	23
New Engl. Clam Chowder	180	8	22
Savory Beef Barley Vegetables	100	2	16
Sirloin Steak & Vegetables	90	1.5	15
Traditional: *Per ½ Can, 1 Cup*			
Chickarina with Meatballs	110	4	12
Chicken & Sausage Gumbo	110	2.5	17
Potato Broccoli N Cheese Chowder	210	13	18
Vegetable Classic: *Per 1 Cup*			
French Onion	50	1	9
Garden Vegetable	90	0	20
Minestrone, 99% Fat Free	100	1	19
Tomato Basil	150	3	28
Light: *Per 1 cup*			
Beef Pot Roast	80	1.5	12
Chicken & Dumpling	70	1	10
New England Clam Chowder	100	2.5	15
Italian Style Vegetable	70	0	15

Safeway (Vons):	C	F	Cb
Signature Soups: *Per Cup*			
Broccoli & Cheesy Cheddar	250	18	12
Chunky Chicken Noodle	160	5	14
Fiesta Chicken Tortilla	110	2	15
Italian-Style Wedding	120	4	14
Pacific Coast Clam Chowder	320	20	27
Tuscan Tomato & Basil Bisque	290	22	20
Swanson:			
Broth: *Per 8 fl.oz Cup*			
Beef	15	0	1
Chicken	10	0.5	1
Organic Chicken	15	0.5	1
Vegetable	10	0	2
Infused: Beef	15	0.5	2
Thai Ginger	30	0.5	5
Tuscan Chicken	20	0.5	2
Tabatchnick:			
Frozen:			
Dairy: *Per 7.5 oz Pouch*			
Corn Chowder	130	4.5	21
Cream of Mushroom	100	5	11
New England Potato	130	14.5	20
Gluten Free: *Per 7.5 oz Pouch*			
Southwest Bean	220	5	36
Split Pea	140	0	34
Vegetarian Chili	200	3.5	32
Low Sodium: *Per 7.5oz Pouch*			
Barley & Mushroom	80	1	17
Split Pea	140	0	34
Vegetable	90	1.5	17
Meat: *Per 7.5 oz Pouch*			
Frenchman's Onion	60	1.5	11
Wilderness Wild Rice	90	0.5	19
Pareve: *Per 7.5 oz Pouch*			
Black Bean	220	2.5	39
Minestrone	110	1.5	20
Shelf Stable: *Per 2/3 Cup, 5.3 fl.oz*			
Broth: Classic Chicken	5	0	0
Other Chicken Flavors	10	0	1
Gourmet Beef	5	0	0
Soup, Creamy Tomato	70	2	14
Thai Kitchen:			
Rice Noodle Soup Bowls: *Per Bowl*			
Hot & Sour	250	4	51
Lemongrass & Chili	250	3.5	52
Roasted Garlic	250	3	52
Spring Onion	260	4.5	50
Thai Ginger	260	3	52

Trader Joe's:	C	F	Cb
28 fl.oz Cans: *Per Cup*			
Chunky, Low Fat:			
Lentil with Vegetables	140	3	21
Minestrone	110	2.5	19
14.5 oz Cans: *Per Cup*			
Organic: Black Bean	140	1.5	26
Lentil Vegetable	160	4	24
Split Pea	100	0	19
10.75 oz Can,			
Low Sodium, Minestrone	200	4	37
15 oz Can,			
Low Fat, Chicken Noodle, 1 cup	90	1	14
32 fl.oz. Cartons: *Per Cup*			
Butternut Squash	90	2	16
Carrot & Ginger	80	1	17
Creamy Corn & Rstd Pepper	110	2	23
Latin Style Black Bean	70	1	12
Sweet Potato Bisque	130	1	28
Organic: Butternut Squash	70	0	17
Tomato & Rstd Red Pepper	100	3.5	15
Low Sodium, Creamy Tomato	90	3.5	15
17.6 fl.oz Cartons: *Per Cup*			
Beef, Barley with Veggies	100	0.5	16
Chicken Noodle with Veggies	100	1	16
Whole Foods: *Per Cup*			
365 Organic:			
Chicken Noodle	100	1.5	12
Lentil	70	0	15
Minestrone	140	1.5	23
Southwestern Black Bean	120	1	23
Tomato Basil	90	2	16
Wolfgang Puck: *Per Cup*			
Organic:			
Butternut Squash	140	11	10
Chicken & Dumplings	140	7	14
Classic Minestrone	120	2.5	20
Corn Chowder	210	13	20
Free Range Chkn with Rice	110	4	15
New Engl. Clam Chowder	150	7	18
Signature Tortilla	140	3.5	21
Thick Hearty Lentil & Veggie	160	1	29
Thick Hearty Garden Vegetable	120	4	20
Tomato Basil Bisque	150	6	21

Soybean Products   C   F   Cb

	C	F	Cb
Cheeses (Soy) ~ *See Page 78*			
Miso Soy Bean Paste:			
Cold Mountain: Light Yellow, 1 tsp	10	0	1
Mellow Red, 1 tsp	15	0	3
Red, 1 tsp	10	0	1
Miso Soup (dry mix):			
1 Tbsp., dry mix	35	1	5
1 cup, prepared	35	1	5
Natto, ½ cup, 3 oz	160	7	14
Okara (Tofu fiber residue), ½ c., 2 oz	47	1	8
Tempeh: 1 piece, 3 oz	180	8	12
Fried, 3 oz	250	14	14
Seitan *(Westsoy)*, Strips, 3 oz	120	2	4
Soybean Protein *(TVP)*, 1 oz	95	0	8
Soy Bean Paste, 1 tsp	10	0	2
Soy Beans ~ *See Page 160*			
Soy Drinks ~ *See Page 49*			

Tofu ~ Brands

	C	F	Cb
Azumaya Tofu:			
Extra Firm; Firm, av., 3 oz	70	4	2
Soft (Silken), 3.2 oz	45	2	1
House Foods: *Per 3 oz*			
Premium Tofu: Extra Firm	80	4.5	2
Firm	70	4	2
Medium Firm	60	3.5	2
Soft (Silken)	60	3	2
Organic Tofu: Firm	70	4	2
Extra Firm	70	3.5	2
Ethnic: Tokusen Kinugoshi, Extra Soft	80	4	3
Sukui; Soon (Extra Soft)	45	2	2
Yaki Tofu (Broiled)	90	5	2
Mori-Nu Tofu:			
Morinaga Silken:			
Soft, 3 oz, 1" slice	45	2.5	1
Firm, 3 oz, 1" slice	50	2.5	2
Extra Firm, 3 oz, 1" slice	50	2	1
Organic Silken, Firm, 3 oz, 1" slice	50	2.5	1
Lite, Firm, 3 oz, 1" slice	30	1	1
Nasoya: Extra Firm, 3 oz	80	4	3
Firm, 3 oz	70	3.5	2
Silken, 3.2 oz	45	2	1
Soft, 2.8 oz	60	3	1
Tofuplus:			
Extra Firm, 3 oz	80	4	2
Firm, 3 oz	70	3	2
Sprouted, Super Firm, 3 oz	100	5	3

Supplements   C   F   Cb

	C	F	Cb
Aloe Vera Juice, undiluted, 2 fl.oz	5	0	1
: Tablets, 2 tabs	4	0	0.5
Flakes, 1 heaping Tbsp, 0.3 oz	30	0.5	4
Powder, 1 heaping Tbsp, 0.5 oz	50	0.5	6
Calcium Chews: CVS, 1 chew	20	0	3
Trader Joe's, Chocolate,1 chew	20	1	3
Cod Liver Oil, 1 Tbsp	125	13	0
Fiber Choice, 2 tabs	15	0	4
Fiber,			
Fibersure, 1 heaping tsp	25	0	6
Fish Oil Capsules, (1), av.	10	1	0
Flax Oil:			
Capsules (2)	10	1	0
Barlean's, softgels (3)	110	11	0
Garlic Tablets/Capsules, each	3	0	0
Glowelle:			
Beauty Drink, 8 fl.oz	100	0	24
Powder Stick (1)	50	0	12
Lecithin Granules, 1 Tbsp	55	4	0.5
Metamucil, Powder:			
Orange (Smooth Texture),			
1 rounded Tbsp	45	0	12
Sugar-Free, 1 rounded tsp	20	0	5
Pink Lemonade, Sugar-Free,			
1 rounded tsp	20	0	5
Capsules: Heart & Digestive (6)	10	0	3
Strong Bones (1)	10	0	3
Meta, Fiber Wafers (2)	100	4.5	16
Protein, Powders, av., 1 oz	100	0.5	0
Seaweed: Dried, 1 oz	85	0.5	22
Soaked, drained, 1 oz	15	0.5	3
Spirulina, 1 tablet	2	0	0.5
Vitamins/Minerals: Tabs/Caps (1)	2	0	0
Vitamin E Capsules, each	5	0.5	0
Viactiv Chews, Choc. (1)	20	0.5	4

Cough & Pharmaceutical

	C	F	Cb
Antacids: Av., 1 tablet	4	0	1
Liquid, 1 Tbsp	6	0	1
Antacid Sodium Counts ~ *See Page 280*			
Cough/Cold Syrups:			
Regular: With sugar, 1 Tbsp	35	0	9
With alcohol, 1 Tbsp	46	0	9
Diabetic Tussin, Sugar Free, 1 T.	0	0	0
Cough Drops/Lozenges ~ *See Page 75*			
Sudafed, Syrup 1 tsp	14	0	3
Tylenol, Liquid: Child, 1 tsp	17	0	4
Extra Strength, 1 tsp	11	0	3

Sugar

	C	F	Cb
White Sugar, granulated:			
1 level teaspoon, 4g	15	0	4
1 heaping teaspoon, 6g	25	0	6
1 Tablespoon, 12g	50	0	12
1 ounce, 1 oz	110	0	28
1 cup, 7 oz	775	0	200
1 lb (16 oz)	1760	0	454
Single Portion Packages:			
1 stick	15	0	4
1 packet	15	0	4
1 cube	10	0	2.5
Brown Sugar: 1 Tbsp	50	0	13
1 ounce, 1 oz	110	0	28
1 cup, not packed, 5 oz	550	0	140
1 cup, packed, 7.8 oz	835	0	216
Powdered Sugar:			
Sifted, 1 cup, 3.5 oz	390	0	100
Unsifted, 1 cup, 4¼ oz	470	0	120
Coconut Palm Sugar, 1 tsp, 4g	15	0	4
Dextrose, 1 tsp	12	0	3
Fructose, powder, 1 tsp	12	0	3
Glucose Powder, 1 oz	110	0	27
Glucose Tablets, (1)	20	0	5
Palm Sugar, 3 Tbsp	45	0	11
Piloncillo, (Brown Sugar), 3oz	325	0	81
Turbinado Sugar, 2 Tbsp, 1 oz	110	0	27

Sugar Substitutes

	C	F	Cb
Agave, 1 Tbsp, 0.7 oz	60	0	16
DiabetiSweet, 1 teaspoon	9	0	4.5
Note: Carb figure includes 4.5 g sugar alcohol			
Domino, Light, ½ tsp	5	0	2
Equal: Tablet (2)	0	0	0
Granular, 1 tsp	0	0	0
Packet (1)	0	0	0
Next, 1 packet	0	0	0
Nectresse, 1 packet	0	0	0
NutraSweet, 1 tsp	0	0	0
Splenda, Granulated No Calorie Sweetener:			
1 tsp	0	0	0
1 cup	95	0	24
Packets, all flavors	0	0	0
Sugar Blend,Orig/Brown, ½ cup	385	0	96
Stevia, single serving	0	0	0
Sugar Twin, 1 packet	0	0	0
Sweet 'N Low, 1 packet	0	0	0
Truvia, 1 packet	0	0	0
Walgreens, Wal-Sweet, 1 packet	0	0	0
Whey Low, 1 tsp	4	0	1

Syrups, Molasses, Agave

Syrups· Plain: *Average All Brands (Corn/Rice/Maple/Pancake/Sundae/Waffle) Includes Aunt Jemima, Cary's, Karo, Hershey's, Hungry Jack, IHOP, Log Cabin, Mrs Butterworth's*

	C	F	Cb
Regular/Dark/Light Color:			
1 Tbsp, 0.5 fl.oz	55	0	14
¼ cup (4 Tbsp)	220	0	55
Single Portion, 1.5 oz pkg	170	0	42
Lite, 1Tbsp, 1 oz	25	0	6
Sugar-Free: 2 Tbsp, 1 oz	18	0	5
Maple Grove, Cozy Cottage, 2 Tbsp	10	0	3
IHOP, 4 Tbsp, 2 oz	20	0	7
Fruit Syrups, (IHOP), ¼ cup, 2 oz	200	0	52
Honey Cream Syrup, ¼ cup, 2 oz	220	0	55
Molasses: Dark/Light: 1 T, 0.7 oz	60	0	15
1 cup, 12 oz	975	0.5	252
Blackstrap, 1 Tbsp, 0.8 oz	47	0	13
Agave Nectar, av. all flavors,			
1 Tablespoon, 0.8 oz	60	0	15

Flavored Syrups/Ice Cream Toppings

Hershey's: *Per 2 Tbsp*

	C	F	Cb
Double Chocolate,	105	0	26
Other Flavors, average	90	0	23
Lite	45	0	12
Smuckers: *Per 2 Tbsp*			
Magic Shell, average all flavors	220	17	16
Spoonables: Reg., average all flavors	115	1	28
Sugar Free: Caramel; Hot Fudge	90	0	24
Strawberry	30	0	9
Note: Carb figures include 8g-17g sugar alcohol			
Sundae Syrups: Regular, av. all flavors	105	0	25
Sugar Free, average all flavors	90	0	24
Note: Carb figures includes 15g sugar alcohol			

Honey, Jam, Preserves

Average all Brands

	C	F	Cb
Honey: 1 tsp, 0.23 oz	20	0	5.5
1 Tbsp, 0.7 oz	60	0	17
1 oz	85	0	24
½ cup, 6 oz	515	0	145
Single Portion, 0.5 oz package	45	0	12
Jams/Jellies/Marmalade/Preserves:			
Regular: 1 tsp, 0.3 oz	20	0	5
1 Tbsp, 0.8 oz	55	0	14
1 ounce, 1 oz	80	0	20
Single Portion, 0.5 oz pkg	40	0	11
Apple/Fruit Butters, 1 T., 0.6 oz	20	0	5
Fruit Spreads: Regular, 1 tsp	15	0	4
Low Sugar, 1 tsp	8	0	2
Jelly: Regular, average, 1 tsp	18	0	4.5
Imitation, Low Calorie, 1 tsp	4	0	1

Vegetables	C	F	Cb
Alfalfa Sprouts, ¹/₂ cup, 0.5 oz	5	0	0.5
Artichokes, Globe/French:			
1 medium, 4.5 oz	60	0	13
1 large, 5.7 oz	75	0	17
Artichoke Heart, plain, 2 pieces	15	0	3
Asparagus, raw/frozen:			
Cuts & Tips, ¹/₂ cup, 4.3 oz	20	0	3
Spears, 3 medium	10	0	2
Bamboo Shoots, cooked, ¹/₂ cup, 2 oz	7	0	1
Beans, Green/Snap/String:			
10 beans (4" long), 2 oz	20	0	4
Pieces, ¹/₂ cup, 3 oz	30	0	7
Dried Beans (Kidney, Brown, Lima, Navy, Pinto, White):			
Raw: 2 Tbsp, 1 oz	95	0.5	18
1 cup, 7 oz	665	3	126
Cooked: 1 oz	35	0	7
¹/₂ cup, 3 oz	105	0	21
Bean Sprouts, average, ¹/₂ cup, 2 oz	15	0	3.5
Beets (Beetroot):			
Raw, 1 beet (2" diam.), 4 oz	35	0	8
Cooked, 1 cup, slices, 3 oz	35	0	8
Canned ~ See Page 161			
Beet Greens, cooked, ¹/₂ cup, 2.5 oz	20	0	4
Bell Pepper ~ See Peppers			
Bitter Melon/Gourd, 1 cup, 1.5 oz	15	0	1.5
Blackeye Peas, cooked, ¹/₂ cup, 3 oz	100	0.5	18
Bok Choy (Chinese Chard),			
cooked, 3 oz	10	0	1.5
Breadfruit, ¹/₄ small fruit, 3 oz	100	0	26
Broadbeans (Fava Beans):			
Green, raw, (in pod): 4 pods			
(3.5 oz with shells, 1.2 oz beans)	30	0	6
1 cup beans, without shell, 4.5 oz	110	1	22
Mature Seeds: Raw, 1 cup, 5.3 oz	510	2.5	87
Cooked, ¹/₂ cup, 3 oz	95	0	17
Broccoflower, ¹/₅ head, 3.5 oz	35	0	7
Broccoli: Raw, chopped,1 cup, 3 oz	30	0	6
3 Florets, 2.5 oz	25	0	5
1 Spear (5" long), 1.oz	10	0	2
1 Whole: Medium, 14 oz	135	1.5	26
Large, 21 oz	205	2	40
1 Head (no stalk), 11 oz	105	1	21
1 Stalk, small (5" long), 5.3 oz	50	0.5	10
Brocco Sprouts, ¹/₂ cup, 1 oz	15	0	2
Brussels Sprouts:			
Cooked, ¹/₂ cup, 2.8 oz	30	0.5	6
2 Sprouts, 1.5 oz	15	0	3
Butterbeans, cooked, ¹/₂ cup, 3 oz	90	0	16
Cabbage, average other flavors:			
Raw: 1 leaf, large, 1 oz	5	0	2
Shredded, 1 cup, 2.5 oz	15	0	4
¹/₂ large head (7" diam), 22 oz	150	1	35
Cooked, shredded, ¹/₂ cup, 2.5 oz	15	0.5	3.5

Vegetables (Cont)	C	F	Cb
Cactus Leaf (Nopales):			
1 leaf, 4.5 oz	20	0	4
1 cup (slices), 3 oz	15	0	3
Carrots, regular thick variety:			
1 small, 4 oz	45	0	11
1 medium, 6 oz	70	0	16
1 large, 8 oz	95	0	22
Chopped, 1 cup, 4.5 oz	50	0	12
Grated, 1 cup, 4 oz	45	0	11
Slices, 1 cup, 4.5 oz	50	0	12
Sticks (4"), 4-5, 1.5 oz	20	0	4
Long thin variety, 1 medium, 2.2 oz	25	0	6
Baby: Snack size, 3 medium, 1 oz	10	0	2.5
Snack Pack, 3 oz	30	0	7
Cassava, raw, 1 cup, 2.5 oz	330	0.5	78
Cauliflower, raw:			
Pieces, 1 cup, 3.5 oz	25	0	5
¹/₂ medium head, 10 o_	70	0	15
Cooked, 3 florets, 2 oz	10	0	2
Celeriac, ¹/₂ cup, raw, 2.8 oz	35	0	7
Celery: 1 large stalk, 11", 2.2 oz	10	0	2
4 Strips, thin sticks, 0.5 oz	5	0	1
Chopped, 1 cup, 3.5 oz	15	0	3
Chard (Swiss), ¹/₂ cup, cooked, 3 oz	20	0	3.5
Chayote Squash:			
1 medium, 7 oz	40	0	9
Pieces, 1 cup, 4.5 oz	25	0	6
Chickpeas, (Garbanzo Beans):			
Dry, 1 cup, 7 oz	730	12	121
Cooked, 1 cup, 5.8 oz	270	4	45
Chicory Greens, 1 cup, 1 oz	7	0	1.5
Chili Peppers ~ See Peppers			
Chinese Long Bean, slices, 1 cup, 3.2 oz	45	0	8
Chives, chopped, 1 Tbsp	1	0	0
Choy Sum, 3 oz	15	0	3
Cilantro, (Coriander), 1 cup	5	0	0.5
Collards, cooked, ¹/₂ cup, 3 oz	25	0	5
Corn, Yellow/White:			
Raw: Kernels, ¹/₂ cup, 3 oz	80	0.5	19
Ear (5"x 1³/₄"), 5.5 oz	155	1	37
Cooked: Kernels, ¹/₂ cup, 3 oz	77	0.5	18
Cob, small, 2.3 oz	60	0.5	14
Ear, large, 5.5 oz	120	1	28
Cress, garden, raw, 1 cup, 1.8 oz	15	0	3
Cucumber, average other flavors:			
Slices, ¹/₂ cup, 2 oz	10	0	2
Green, 1 medium (9"), 11 oz	45	0	11
Persian, 1 medium (8"), 6 oz	25	0	5
Daikon Radish, ¹/₂ cup, slices, 2 oz	9	0	2
Dandelion Greens, raw, ¹/₂ cup, 1 oz	10	0	2.5
Edamame, (Immature green soybeans):			
Shelled, ¹/₂ cup, 2.6 oz	110	5	8
With shells, 10 pods, 1.3 oz	30	1	3

Vegetables (Cont)	C	F	Cb
Eggplant, raw: 4 oz	30	0	7
½ cup, 1" pieces, 1.5 oz	10	0	2
1 slice, fried, 1 oz	75	4	10
Endive, Belgian/French: Raw,			
1 medium head (6"), 2.5 oz	12	0	3
Fennel, 1 cup, sliced, 3 oz	25	0	7
Gai Choy Cabbage, cooked, 1 cup, 6 oz	20	0	3
Gai Lan, (Chinese Kale), cooked, 1 cup	35	0.5	7
Garbanzo Beans ~ See Chick Peas			
Garlic, 1 clove	4	0	1
Ginger: ¼ cup slices, 1 oz	20	0	5
Crystallized (sugared), 7 pieces, 1.5 oz	130	0	35
Horseradish, raw, 1 pod, 0.5 oz	5	0	1
Jerusalem Artichoke, raw, ½ cup	55	0	13
Jicama, raw, sliced, ½ cup, 2.3 oz	25	0	6
Kale, 1 cup, chopped, 2.5 oz	35	0.5	7
Kohlrabi, cooked, ½ cup, 1.8 oz	17	0	5
Leek, cooked, 1 whole, 4.5 oz	40	0	9
Lentils, green/brown: Dry, 1 oz	100	0.5	17
1 cup, 6.8 oz	675	3	115
Cooked, ½ cup, 3.5 oz	115	0.5	20
Lettuce, 1 cup, chopped/shredded, 2 oz	7	0	1
Butterhead, 2 leaves, 0.5 oz	2	0	0.5
Cos/Romaine, shredded, 1 cup	10	0	2
Iceberg: 1 outer leaf, 0.5 oz	2	0	0.5
1 medium head, 16 oz	75	1	16
Lima Beans, baby, cooked, ½ cup, 3 oz	105	0	20
Lotus Root, cooked, 10 slices, 3 oz	60	0	14
Mung Bean Sprouts, ½ cup, 2 oz	15	0	3
Mushrooms, average all varieties:			
Raw, diced/siced, 1 cup, 3 oz	20	0	3
Pieces, 1 cup, 1.3 oz	8	0	1
Fried/Sauteed, 6 oz	220	16	10
Grilled, pieces, ½ cup, 2.5 oz	20	0.5	4
Shitake, dried, 1 oz package	90	0	22
Mustard Greens, raw, ½ cup, 1 oz	7	0	2
Okra: Raw, 8 pods, 4 oz	30	0	7
Cooked, ½ cup, 2.8 oz	20	0	4
Onions, Raw: 1 small, 2.5 oz	30	0	7
1 medium, 4 oz	50	0	11
1 large, 5.5 oz	65	0	15
1 jumbo, 16 oz	190	0.5	46
Chopped, ½ cup, 3 oz	35	0	8
1 Tbsp, 0.4 oz	5	0	1
Slices: 1 cup, 4 oz	50	0	12
1 medium slice (⅛"), 0.5 oz	5	0	1
1 large slice (¼"), 1.3 oz	15	0	4
Flakes, dried ¼ cup, 0.5 oz	50	0	12
Rings, breaded & fried, 2 rings	80	5	9
Scallions, ½ cup, 2 oz	15	0	3
Spring, chopped, ½ cup, 2 oz	15	0	3

Vegetables (Cont)	C	F	Cb
Parsley, chopped, ½ cup, 1 oz	10	0	2
Parsnip: 1 medium, 4 oz	85	0	20
Cooked, slices, ½ cup, 2.8 oz	55	0	13
Peas: Green, raw, ¼ cup, 1.5 oz	30	0	5
With pods, 0.5 lb	70	0	13
Snow Peas, 10 pods, 1.2 oz	15	0	3
Split: Dry, hulled, 1 oz	100	0.5	17
Cooked, 1 cup, 7 oz	230	1	42
Peppers:			
Sweet, 1 medium, 4.2 oz	30	0	7
Bell: 1 medium, 4.2 oz	30	0	7
raw, chopped, ½ cup, 2.5 oz	20	0	5
2 rings (5" diam. x ¼" thick)	3	0	1
Chili: Green/Red, 1.5 oz	20	0	5
Habanero, 1 only, 0.3 oz	10	0	2
Pigeon Peas, cooked, ½ cup, 3 oz	95	1	17
Pimientos, 3 medium, 3.5 oz	25	0	5
Poi, ½ cup, 4.2 oz	135	0	33
Potatoes:			
Raw (with skin):			
1 baby, 2 oz	45	0	10
1 small, 6 oz	135	0	30
1 medium, 8 oz	180	0	40
1 large, 12 oz	270	0	60
1 extra large, 16 oz	360	0	80
Baked, (no added fat), large, 10 oz (raw wt):			
Plain: With skin, 7 oz (cooked wt)	185	0	42
W/o skin, 5.5 oz (cooked wt)	145	0	34
With Skin/Toppings:			
With 2 tsp fat	270	8	58
With Grated Cheese, 1 oz	370	9	58
With Plain Yogurt, 2 Tbsp	260	1	60
With Sour Crm & Chives, 2 Tbsp	320	6	60
Mashed:			
With milk plus fat, ½ cup, 4 oz	120	4.5	18
KFC Style without gravy, 4 oz	90	3	15
Loaded (fat/cream/cheese/bacon):			
Side serving, 6 oz	180	9	22
Large serving, 12 oz	360	18	44
Potato Skins, baked w/ cheese topping,			
½ whole, 4.3 oz	240	13	22
French Fries: Small serving, 2.6 oz	250	13	30
Medium serving, 4 oz	380	20	47
Frozen, uncooked, 18 fries, 4 oz	165	5.5	28
Oven-heated, 18 fries, 4 oz	165	5.5	28
Take-Out, 1 cup, 5 oz	440	25	60
Au Gratin, ½ cup, 4.3 oz	160	9	14
Pancakes, 2 small, 2 oz	120	6.5	12
Puffs, fried, 4 puffs, 1 oz	55	2.5	8
Scalloped, 8.5 oz	220	9	26

Vegetables (Cont)

	C	F	Cb
Pumpkin:			
Raw, 1" cubes, 1 cup, 4 oz	30	0	7
Cooked:			
Baked, without fat, 4 oz	90	7	9
Mashed: 1 scoop, 2 oz	10	0	2
¹/₂ cup, 4.3 oz	25	0	6
Pumpkin Flowers, 1 cup, 1.2 oz	5	0	1
Purslane: Cooked, ¹/₂ cup, 2 oz	10	0	2
Raw, 1" cubes, 1 cup, 1.5 oz	5	0	1.5
Radicchio: 2 leaves, 0.5 oz	5	0	1
Shredded, 1 cup, 1.5 oz	20	0	4
Radishes: 1 small	0	0	0
10 medium/5 large, 1.6 oz	5	0	1
Slices, ¹/₂ cup, 2 oz	10	0	2
Rhubarb, raw, ¹/₂ cup, 2 oz	15	0	3
Rutabaga, cubes, cooked, ¹/₂ cup, 3 oz	30	0	7
Salsify, cooked, slices, ¹/₂ cup, 2.5 oz	50	0	11
Sauerkraut, ¹/₂ cup, 2.5 oz	15	0	3
Seaweed: Dried, 1 oz	5	0	2
Soaked, drained, 1 oz	15	0	4
Nori/Laver, dried, 6 sheets, 0.5 oz	35	0	5
Shallots, chopped, 1 Tbsp, 0.5 oz	5	0	1
Sorrel, raw, ¹/₂ cup, 4 oz	20	0	4
Soybeans: Dry, ¹/₂ cup, 3.3 oz	390	18	28
Mature, dry, 1 oz	120	5.5	9
Cooked, ¹/₂ cup, 3 oz	150	7.5	8
Soy Products/Tofu/Tempeh ~ *See Page 156*			
Spinach: Cooked, ¹/₂ cup, 3 oz	20	0	4
Creamed, average, ¹/₂ cup, 4.5 oz	190	15	8
Raw: 3 leaves, 1 cup, 1 oz	7	0	1
1 Bunch, 12 oz	80	1.5	12
Squash:			
Summer: Raw, ¹/₂ cup, 2.5 oz	10	0	2
Cooked, slices, ¹/₂ cup, 3 oz	15	0	3
Winter, cooked:			
Acorn: Cubes, ¹/₂ cup, 3.5 oz	35	0	9
¹/₂ medium (10 oz raw weight)	115	0	30
Butternut: Cubes, ¹/₂ cup, 3.5 oz	40	0	10
¹/₄ medium (9 oz raw weight)	115	0	30
Spaghetti, ¹/₂ cup, 1.8 oz	15	0	3
Succotash, cooked, ¹/₂ cup, 3.3 oz	110	1	23
Sweetcorn ~ *See Corn*			
Sweet Potatoes:			
Cooked with skin (w/o fat),			
1 medium, 4 oz	105	0	24
Without skin, mashed, ¹/₂ cup, 5.5 oz	125	0	29
Fries (Alexia, Julienne syle),			
approximately 12 pieces, 3 oz	140	5	24

Vegetables (Cont)

	C	F	Cb
Swiss Chard, cooked, chopped, 1 c., 6 oz	35	0	7
Taro, cooked, ¹/₂ cup, 2.3 oz	95	0	23
Tomatoes: 1 small (2¹/₄" diam.), 3 oz	15	0	3
1 medium (2³/₄" diameter), 5 oz	25	0	5
1 large (3¹/₂" diameter), 8 oz	40	0.5	9
1 extra lge (4" diam.), 12 oz	60	0.5	14
Chopped, 1 cup, 6.5 oz	35	0.5	7
Tomatillo: 1 medium, 1.2 oz	10	0	2
1lb quantity for recipe	135	4.5	27
Turnip: Cooked, ¹/₂ cup, 2.8 oz	15	0	4
Greens, cooked, ¹/₂ cup, 2.5 oz	15	0	3
Water Chestnuts: 5-6 nuts, 1 oz	56	0.5	13
Raw, slices, ¹/₂ cup, 2.3 oz	60	0	15
Canned, 1 oz	15	0	3
Watercress, 10 sprigs, 1 oz	3	0	0.5
Yams: Cooked, steamed, ¹/₂ cup, 2.5 oz	80	0	19
Baked:			
1 medium (6") 8 oz	265	0.5	63
1 large (9") 12 oz	400	0.5	94
Yardlong Bean, 1 pod, 0.5 oz	5	0	1
Yucca Root, raw, ¹/₂ cup, 3.5 oz	165	0	39
Zucchini: Raw, 1 medium, 7 oz	30	0.5	7
1 large, 12 oz	60	1	12
Cooked, slices,			
¹/₂ cup, 3 oz	15	0	4

Frozen Vegetables

	C	F	Cb
Birds Eye:			
Mixtures & Blends:			
Broccoli, Cauliflower & Carrots, 3 oz	35	0	5.5
Stir-Fry: Broccoli, 3.4 oz	35	0	6
Crisp Green Bean, 5.5 oz	60	0	11
Sugar Snap, 3.4 oz	40	0	7.5
Pure & Simple:			
Baby: Broccoli Florets, 1 cup, 3 oz	35	0.5	4.5
Gold & White Corn, ²/₃ cup, 3.2 oz	105	1	22
Sweet Peas, ²/₃ cup, 3 oz	80	0	14
Recipe Ready:			
Chopped Green Peppers & Onions, 2.8 oz	25	0	5
Southwest Blend, 3.3 oz	80	0.5	15
Sauced & Seasoned: *Per 1 Cup*			
Green Beans & Spaetzle,			
in Bavarian Sauce	95	4.5	10
Pasta & Veggies in Creamy Cheese Sauce	125	3	20
Steamfresh:			
Pure & Simple Blends:			
Baby Broccoli Blend, 1 cup	65	1.5	8
Baby Potato Blend, ³/₄ cup	50	0	10
Brocc. & Cauliflower, 1 cup, 3.4 oz	30	0.5	4.5

Frozen Vegetables (Cont) — C F Cb

Green Giant:

	C	F	Cb
Mashed Cauliflowe: Original, 4.2 oz	80	5	7
Cheddar & Bacon, 4.2 oz	90	6	6
Riced Cauliflower/with Brocc., 3 oz	20	0	4
Roasted Veggies: Broccoli, 3 oz	30	0	6
Brussels Sprouts, 3 oz	30	0	6
Carrots, 3 oz	30	0.5	7
Cauliflower, 3 oz	20	0	3
Corn, 3 oz	120	1.5	25
Sautes:			
Fire Roasted, Prepared:			
Corn, Peppers & Onions, 1/2 cup	80	0.5	16
Root Veggies w/ Red Onions, 2/3 c.	60	0	14
Tri color Peppers, 1/3 cup	25	0	5
Zucchini, Carrots & Onions, 1/3 cup	20	0	4
Kits: Herb B'Nut Squash Medley, 4.3 oz	35	1	7
Chipotle Harvest, 1 cup prepared	280	3	25
Thai Coconut, 1 cup prepared	210	4	18
Steamers: Corn Niblets, 1/2 cup	90	1	19
Backyard Gr. Potatoes, 1/2 cup prep.	110	3	20
Creamed Spinach, 3.8 oz	70	2	9
Veggie Tots: Broccoli & Cheese, 3 oz	130	6	14
Brocolli; Cauliflower, 3 oz	110	4.5	15

Ore-Ida: *Per 3 oz Unless Indicated*

	C	F	Cb
Fries:			
Bold & Crispy: Chili Cheese Crinkle	160	7	22
Garlic Black Pepper Steakhouse	180	8	25
Zesties, Seasoned	180	7.5	26
Zesty, Seasoned Curly	185	9	24
Classic: Golden Crinkles	120	4.5	19
Golden	130	3.5	21
Steak	110	3	19
Extra Crispy Easy, Golden Crinkles	170	6	25
Extra Crispy:			
Fast Food Fries	150	6	24
Golden Crinkles	160	7	22
Seasoned Crinkles	150	6	22
Premium: Crispers	230	14	23
Country Style French	130	4.5	20
Golden Twirls	150	6	23
Texas Crispers	150	7	20
Hash Browns: Golden Patties (1)	140	8	15
Potatoes O'Brien	60	0	13
Shredded Hash Browns Pattie (1)	70	0	16
Mashed Potato Bites:			
Four Cheese, 2.5 oz	180	10	18
Loaded Baked, 2.5 oz	170	10	18
Onion: Chopped, 3 oz	20	0	5
Gourmet Rings, 2.7 oz	185	9	24
Onion Ringers, 3 oz	180	10	21
Steam n' Mash, Cut Russet, 3.5 oz	70	0	16
Tater Tots, Reg., Crispy Crowns,av.	165	9	20

Canned/Bottled — C F Cb

Solids & Liquid

	C	F	Cb
Artichoke Hearts:			
Fancifoods: Plain, 1 oz (1)	8	0	1
Marinated, 1/4 bottle, 1 oz	25	1.5	2
Asparagus: Drained, 3 spears	10	0	1.5
Pieces, 1/2 cup, 4.3 oz	25	0.5	3
Bamboo Shoots, 1 cup, 4.5 oz	25	0	4
Bean Salad, 1/2 cup, 4.4 oz	90	0	20
Beans: Baked, 1/2 cup, 4.5 oz	120	0.5	27
Butter, 1/2 cup, 4.5 oz	90	0	16
Green, 1/2 cup, 2.5 oz	15	0	3
Italian, 1/2 cup, 4.5 oz	30	0	6
Kidney, 1/2 cup 3.5 oz	105	0.5	19
Lima, 1/2 cup, 4.5 oz	80	0	15
Pinto, 1/2 cup, 4.5 oz	105	1	18
Beets: Sliced, 1/2 cup, 3 oz	25	0	6
Crinkle/Pickled, 1/2 cup	80	0	20
Carrots: Sliced, 1/2 cup, 2.5 oz	20	0	4
Del Monte, Honey Glazed, 1/2 cup	75	0	18
Corn: Kernels, 1/2 cup, 4.5 oz	80	0.5	18
Creamed style, 1/2 cup, 4.5 oz	90	0.5	23
Garbanzo/Chick Peas, 1/2 c, 4.2 oz	145	1.5	27
Hearts of Palm, (1), 1.2 oz	7	0	1
Mushrooms: 1/2 cup, 2.5 oz	20	0	4
In Butter Sauce, 2 oz	20	1	2
Onions: Cocktail (1)	0	0	0
Pickled, 1 medium, 0.5 oz	10	0	2
Peas, 1/2 cup, 3 oz	60	0.5	10
Peppers: Hot Chili, Jalapeno (1), 1 oz	5	0	1
Red/Green, 1 oz	5	0	1
Sweet, undrained, 2.5 oz	13	0	3
Jalapeno, with liquid,			
1/2 cup chopped	20	0.5	3
Fried, drained, 2 Tbsp, 1 oz	60	5	3
Salsa, average all varieties, 2 Tbsp	10	0	2
Sauerkraut, drained, 1 cup, 5 oz	25	0	6
Spinach, 1/2 cup, 3.5 oz	25	0.5	3.5
Succotash: Cream Style, 1/2 cup	100	0.5	23
w/ whole kernels, undrained, 1/2 cup	80	0.5	18
Sweetcorn ~ *See Corn*			
Sweet Potato, 1/2 cup, 3.5 oz	90	0	24
Tomatoes, Sundried: Nat., 5-6 pieces	20	0	5
In Oil, drained, 6 pieces, 0.5 oz	40	2.5	4
Tomato Products ~ *See Page 144*			
Vegetables, mixed, 1/2 cup, 4 oz	45	0	8
Yams: In Light Syrup, 1/2 cup, 4 oz	105	0	25
Candied, 1/2 cup, 5 oz	170	0	46
Zucchini, in Tomato Sauce, 1/2 cup, 4 oz	30	0	8

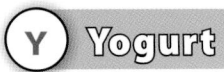

Quick Guide | C | F | Cb

Yogurt: *Average All Brands: Per 8 oz Container*

	C	F	Cb
Plain Yogurt: Whole	140	8	10
Low-Fat	145	3.5	16
Fat-Free	125	0.5	17
Fruit Flavored: Whole	225	8	32
Low-Fat	230	3	43
Fat-Free, regular	215	0.5	43
Fat-Free, no sugar added	80	0	15

Yogurt Parfait/Deli Cups:

With Fruit Pieces: ($2/3$ Yogurt + $1/3$ Fruit)

	C	F	Cb
Small, 8 oz cup	140	3	20
Large, 12 oz cup	210	4.5	30

With Fruit + Granola:

	C	F	Cb
Small, 8 oz cup (+ 0.75 oz Granola)	235	7	30
Large, 12 oz cup (+ 1.3 oz Granola)	400	13	58

Yogurt ~ Brands

Activia:

	C	F	Cb
4 oz Containers: Fiber with Fruit, av.	105	1.5	19
Fruit/Fusion, average all flavors	90	1.5	16
Lactose Free, average	95	2	16
Light, nonfat, all flavors	60	0	10
Greek, nonfat, 5.3 oz Ctn:			
Regular, average all flavors	125	0	20
Light, Strawberry; Blueberry	80	0	8

Almond Dream *(Non Dairy): Per 6 oz Ctn*

	C	F	Cb
Low-Fat: Plain	150	3	30
Mixed Berry; Strawberry; Vanilla	160	3	33

Alpina:

	C	F	Cb
Artisan Granolas: Plain, 6 oz	170	4.5	18
Blueberry, av., 6 oz	240	4	38
Strawberry; Vanilla, 6 oz	190	3.5	26
Greek, Non-Fat, av., 5.3 oz	125	0	19

Amande:

	C	F	Cb
Almond Milk Yogurt: Plain, 8 oz	170	9	19
Fruit Flavors, 6 oz	150	6	23
Vanilla, 8 oz	220	8	26
Coconut, Plain, 6 oz	170	8	23

Axelrod:

	C	F	Cb
32 oz Ctn: Regular Plain, 8 oz	160	8	15
Low Fat, Plain, 8 oz	140	2.5	18
Nonfat, Plain, 8 oz	140	0	21
6 oz Containers:			
Low Fat, Fruit flavors, average	180	1.5	36
NonFat, Fruit flavors, average	90	0	17

Brown Cow:

Cream Top, On The Bottom: *Per 5.3 oz Ctn*

	C	F	Cb
Whole Milk: Apricot Mango	150	5	22
Cherry Vanilla; Strawberry, av.	160	5	25
Chocolate	170	5	26

Brown Cow (Cont): | C | F | Cb

Cream Top: *Per 5.3 oz Ctn*

	C	F	Cb
Whole Milk: Plain	110	6	9
Cherry Vanilla	160	5	25
Coffee; Vanilla, av.	150	6	19

Specialties: *Per 5 oz Ctn*

	C	F	Cb
Cafe Mocha	140	5	20
Marbled Chocolate Raspberry	150	5	22
Vanilla Salted Caramel	150	5	2

Cabot: *Per 8 oz Serving*

	C	F	Cb
Greek Style, 32 oz Ctn: Plain	310	22	12
Lowfat (2%): Plain	180	5	10
Honey	230	4.5	29
Strawberry; Van. Bean	240	4	34

Chobani Greek Yogurt: *Per 5.3 oz Ctn*

	C	F	Cb
Blended: Coconut	140	4	15
Coffee	160	2.5	22
Fruit Flavors, average	135	2.5	15
Plain: Whole Milk	130	6	6
Non Fat	80	0	6
Flip: Almond Coco Loco	230	10	25
Coffee Brownie Bliss	180	4	24
Fruit On The Bottom:			
2% Fat, Fruit Flav., av.	140	3	18
Fat Free, Fruit Flav., av.	125	0	20
Kids: Fruit Flavors, average: 3.5 oz	90	2	11
2 oz	50	1	6
Smooth, Low-Fat:			
Fruit Flavors	120	1.5	16
Vanilla	120	2	15
Tots, Whole Milk, average	95	4.5	10

Coconut Dream *(Non Dairy): Per 6 oz Ctn*

	C	F	Cb
Plain	120	4	24
Berry varieties, aveage	135	3	28
Vanilla	120	3	28

Dannon:

Activia ~ *See Activia*

	C	F	Cb
All Natural, Plain: Lowfat, 8 oz	150	3.5	19
Nonfat, 8 oz	120	0	18
Whole Milk, 8 oz	175	8	18
Creamy, Strawberry, 4 oz	70	0	14
Fruit On The Bottom, av, 5.3 oz	130	1.5	26
Lowfat: Coffee; Vanilla, av., 5.3 oz	135	2	22
Vanilla, 6 oz	130	2	21
Whole Milk, all flav., 5.3 oz	140	4.5	20

Fage: *Per 5.3 oz Ctn*

Crossovers:

	C	F	Cb
Caramel, w/ Honey Rstd Almonds	220	8	23
Maple Syrup with Granola	190	5	21

Total Split Cups:

	C	F	Cb
Whole Milk: Fruit Flav., av.	150	6	13
Honey	210	6	29
2% Milk, Fruit Flav., av.	125	2.5	14
0% Fat, Fruit Flavors	105	0	14

Yogurt Brands (Cont) C F Cb

Fage (Cont):

	C	F	Cb
Total, Plain: Whole Milk, 7 oz	190	10	8
2%, Single Serve, 7 oz	150	4	8
0%, 6 oz	100	0	7

Great Value *(Walmart):*
Original Low Fat, 32 oz Containers:

	C	F	Cb
Fruit Flavors, average, 8 oz	200	2	38
Vanilla, 8 oz	190	2	38
Light, Vanilla, 8 oz	110	0	20

Greek:

	C	F	Cb
Fat-Free: 32 oz Ctn., Plain, 8 oz	120	0	9
Blended Strawberry, 5.3 oz	160	4.5	20
Lowfat, Key Lime Pie, 6 oz	150	1.5	29

Horizon Organic:
Whole Milk:

	C	F	Cb
32 oz Ctn: Plain, 8 oz	170	8	14
Vanilla, 8 oz	210	6	30
6 oz Ctn, average all flavors	170	5	25

Kemps,

	C	F	Cb
Light, 80 Calories, all flavors, 6 oz	80	0	15

La Yogurt: *Per 6 oz Container*

	C	F	Cb
Low Fat: Orig., Fruit Flavors, av.	155	1.5	30
Rich & Creamy, Fruit Flav., av.	180	1.5	35
Sabor Latino, Low Fat, Fruit	185	1.5	37

LALA:

	C	F	Cb
32 oz Tubs, Plain, 8 oz	130	2.5	17
Singles, Fruit Flav., av., 6 oz	150	1.5	30

Lucerne:

	C	F	Cb
Greek Nonfat, Plain, 8 oz	130	0	13
Low-Fat, av. all flavors, 6 oz	170	2	32
Light Nonfat, Vanilla, 6 oz	100	0	19
Non-Fat: Plain, 8 oz	120	0	21
Light, Vanilla, 8 oz	130	0	23

Mountain High: *Per 8 oz*
32 oz Containers:

	C	F	Cb
Whole Milk Original: Plain	170	7	15
Strawberry; Vanilla	200	7	28
Lowfat, Plain	150	3	16
Nonfat: Plain	120	0	17
Vanilla	160	0	30

Nancy's:

	C	F	Cb
Natural Whole Milk: Fruit flav., av	225	5	39
Honey, 8 oz	170	8	17

Organic Whole Milk: *Per 8 oz Container*

	C	F	Cb
Plain	180	8	16
with Fruit on Top, average	230	5	40
Organic Lowfat, Plain	140	3	16
Organic Nonfat: Plain	120	0	17
with Fruit On Top, average	155	0	28
Organic Soy: Plain, 6 oz	150	3	25
Plain, unsweetened, 6 oz	80	3.5	6

Oikos *(Dannon):*
Crunch:

	C	F	Cb
Vanilla Almond, 5 oz	180	7	18
Av. other flavors, 5 oz	170	3	25

Greek Whole Milk: *Per 5.3 oz Ctn*

	C	F	Cb
Coffee	160	4	20
Fruit flavors, average	155	4	18
Mayan Chocolate	150	4.5	15
Non Fat: Plain, 5.3 oz	80	0	6
Fruit flavors, 5.3 oz	110	0	15
Triple Zero Greek, all flavors, 5.3 oz	120	0	14
O Organics, Blended Low-Fat, av. 8 oz	160	2.5	26
Publix: Fat Free, Light, av., 6 oz	110	0	19
Premium Greek, av., 5.3 oz	130	0	18
Schnucks, Light/Nonfat, av., 6 oz	110	0	20

Siggi's:
Skyr: *Per 5.3 oz Unless Indicated*

	C	F	Cb
0%: Plain	90	0	6
Fruit Flavors, average	120	0	13
Vanilla	110	0	12
2%: Coconut	170	5	16
Fruit Flavors, average	140	2.5	12
4%: Fruit Flavors, 4.4 oz	140	4.5	12
Fruit, no added sugar, av., 4.4 oz	115	4	10

Silk: *Per 5.3 oz Containers*

	C	F	Cb
Almond Yogurt: Plain	180	13	10
Fruit flavors, average	180	11	18
Vanilla	200	11	21
Soy Yogurt: Fruit flavors, av	140	3.5	21
Vanilla	140	3.5	20

So Delicious:
Cultured Coconut Milk:

	C	F	Cb
Plain, 8 oz	170	7	25
Blueb./Strawb. 5.3 oz	140	4	24
Chocolate, 5.3 oz	150	5	27
Vanilla, 8 oz	190	6	33
Unsweetened: Plain, 8 oz	110	7	10
Vanilla, 8 oz	110	7	12

Stonyfield Organic:

	C	F	Cb
Double Cream, Vanilla on Bottom, Madagascar Vanilla, 5 oz	160	8	19

Fat Free Fruit On Bottom: *Per 5.3 oz*

	C	F	Cb
Blueberry	90	0	17
Chocolate Underground	110	0	22

Smooth & Creamy (32 oz Ctn):

	C	F	Cb
Fat Free: Plain, 8 oz	100	0	15
French Vanilla, 8 oz	140	0	27
Lowfat: Plain, 8 oz	110	2	14
French Vanilla, 8 oz	150	2	25
Whole Milk, French Vanilla, 8 oz	200	7	27

Yogurt Brands (Cont)

	C	F	Cb
Trader Joes:			
Organic: Banana; Vanilla, 4 oz	100	3	15
Cream Top, Whole Milk, Plain, 8 oz	160	9	9
Low Fat, Fruit Flavors, 6 oz	145	2.5	25
Nonfat: Plain + Vit D, 8 oz	100	0	16
Strawb. + Vit D, 4 oz	90	0	17
Vanilla, 5.3 oz cup	120	0	16
European: Lowfat, Choc./Mocha, 5.3 oz	135	3	21
Smth & Crmy: Whole Milk, Plain, 8 oz	170	7	14
Nonfat, Plain, 8 oz	120	0	17
French Village: Cream Line, Plain, 8 oz	180	10	13
Nonfat: Apricot Mango/Strawb., 6 oz	130	0	25
32 oz Ctn, Plain, 8 oz	120	0	17
Greek, 2% Low Fat, Plain, 8 oz	170	4.5	10
Whole Milk: Plain, 8 oz	280	22	12
Apricot Mango; Honey, av., 8 oz	300	18	27
0% Non Fat: Plain, 8 oz	120	0	7
Fruit Flavors; Honey, 5.3 oz	120	0	17
Vanilla Bean, 5.3 oz	130	0	20
Goats Milk, Plain ¾ cup, 6 oz	100	4.5	7
Voskos (Greek):			
Original: Plain, 8 oz	280	20	15
Fruit On The Bottom, av., 6 oz ctn	150	0	21
Honey, 8 oz	290	14	32
Nonfat: Plain, 8 oz	140	0	9
Fig, 5.3 oz ctn	160	0	28
Average other Fruit Flavors, 5.3 oz	120	0	18
Wallaby Organic, Blended,			
Low-Fat, Fruit Flavors, average, 6 oz	140	2.5	24
Wegmans:			
Fruit On The Bottom, Lowfat:			
Blueberry, 6 oz	160	2	29
Average other Fruit Flavors, 6 oz	165	2	31
Greek, Non-Fat: Plain, 5.3 oz	80	0	5
Fruit flavors, av., 5.3 oz	120	0	16
Vanilla Flavored, 5.3 oz	100	0	13
Whole Foods (365):			
32 oz Ctn, Plain: Whole Milk, 8oz	160	9	13
Low-Fat, 8 oz	120	2	15
Fat-Free, 8 oz	120	0	17
6 oz Ctn: Blueberry Lemon	160	1.5	31
Peach Melba	140	1	27
Greek, 0% Nonfat, Plain, 6 oz			
YoCrunch: *Per 6oz Container*			
Lowfat Vanilla Yogurt:			
with M&M's toppings	180	4	32
with Oreo Cookies toppings	170	3	31
with Snickers toppings	180	4	31
with Twix toppings	180	4	32

Yogurt Brands (Cont)

	C	F	Cb
Yoplait:			
Original, Fruit Flavors, av.	150	2	25
Custard, all flavors, 5.3 oz	170	5	24
Greek:			
100 Calories, average, 5.3 oz	100	0	11
Dippers, Rasp. Choc Chunk,			
w/ Choco-Drizzled Pretzels, 4.6 oz	240	5	38
Regular, fruit flavors, 5.3 oz	135	0	21
Whips: 2%, all flav., 4 oz	120	2	17
Fat Free, all flavors, 4 oz	100	0	15
Kids: Whole Milk, Strawb. Ban., 4 oz	110	3.5	14
Low Fat, average fruit flavors, 4 oz	100	0.5	20
Lactose Free, all flavors, 6 oz	150	2	25
Light: Fruit flavors, 6 oz	90	0	16
Thick & Creamy, 6 oz	100	0	19
Mix-Ins: Cherry Choc. Almond, 5.3 oz	200	8	26
Salted Caramel Pretzel, 5.3 oz	180	4.5	29
Very Berry Crisp, 5.3 oz	180	4	31
Thick & Creamy, all flavors, 6 oz	180	2.5	31
Trix, all flavors, av., 4 oz	100	0.5	20
Whips!: Chocolate, 4 oz	160	4	25
Fruit flavors, 4 oz	140	2.5	25

Yogurt Drinks & Probiotics

	C	F	Cb
Dannon:			
Activia, av. all flavors, 7 fl oz	165	3	27
DanActive, fruit flavors, 3.1 fl.oz	70	1	14
Danimals Smoothies,			
average all flavors, 3.1 fl.oz	60	0.5	10
Dan-o-nino, all flav., 3.1 fl.oz	70	0.5	15
Light & Fit, all flavors, 7 fl.oz	90	0	14
Glen Oaks, av. all flavors, 8 fl.oz	150	2.5	27
LaLa:			
5G Prot. Smoothies, average, 7 fl.oz	150	4	24
Greek Smoothies, all flav., 6.7 fl.oz	160	2.5	20
Lifeway Kefir:			
Whole Milk, Original, 8 fl.oz	150	8	12
Lowfat: Plain, 8 fl.oz	110	2	12
Chocolate Truffle, 8 fl.oz	140	2	20
Other flavors, 8 fl.oz	140	2	20
Bio, Nonfat, all flavors, 3.5 fl.oz	60	0	13
Perfect 12, all flavors, 8 fl.oz	110	2	12
Protein 40g, all flavors, 8 fl.oz	160	0	20
With Oats, all flavors, 8 fl.oz	160	2	24
Stonyfield Organic,			
Smoothies, av. all flav., 10 fl.oz	230	3	40
Yakult:			
Regular, 2.7 fl.oz bottle	50	0	12
Light, 2.7 fl.oz	30	0	6

Cafeteria-Style Foods   C   F   Cb

Average All Preparations:

	C	F	Cb
Beef Stroganoff, 5 oz	195	13	7
Beef Stroganoff, with 4 oz noodles	350	14	36
Chicken Lasagna, 1 piece	300	11	32
Chicken Chop Suey, with 4 oz rice	245	4	37
Deep Dish Burrito, 7 oz	265	13	20
Ground Beef Casserole, 2 scps, 6 oz	245	13	17
Italian Meat Sce, for Spaghetti, 5 oz	150	9	9
with 5 oz Spaghetti	350	10	49
Lasagna, 1 piece	275	11	25
Meatloaf, 3 oz	205	13	4
Ranch Beans, 2 scoops, 6 oz	350	11	45
Red Beans & Rice, 7 oz	280	9	37
Scalloped Potato/Ham, 2 scoops, 6 oz	160	6	20
Stuffed Shells in Sauce, (1)	105	3	17
Swedish Meatballs, (3)	205	12	9
Sweet & Sour Pork/Rice, 9 oz	240	3	40
Swiss Steak, w/ Mushroom Gravy, 6 oz	280	11	4
Tator Tot Casserole, 2 scoops, 6 oz	260	15	20
Tenderloin Tips/Mshrm Gravy: 5 oz	210	13	3
With 5 oz noodles	395	15	38
Tuna Noodle Casserole, 2 scoops, 6 oz	180	6	17
Turkey Tetrazzini, 2 scoops, 6 oz	195	7	17
Vegetable Lasagna, 1 piece	250	13	21

Croissants

	C	F	Cb
Unfilled, medium 1.5 oz	180	10	21
Filled: With Ham (2 oz), garnish	280	14	24
With Ham (2 oz), Cheese (2 oz)	470	30	20
With Chick (2 oz) Cheese (2 oz)	470	30	20
With Turkey/Ham/Cheese (2 oz ea.)	580	36	20
Au Bon Pain: Ham & Cheese	390	21	35
Spinach & Cheese	290	17	28

7-Eleven ~ *See Page 236*

Bagels

	C	F	Cb
Plain: Large, 4 oz (without filling)	320	2	65
With 2 oz Cream Cheese	500	27	54
With 2 oz Lox (Smoked Salmon)	400	4	65

Also see Bagels Section ~ *Page 54*
Fast-Foods Restaurants ~ *Page 175*
Au Bon Pain ~ *Page 179*
Bruegger's ~ *Page 185*
Einstein Bros Bagels ~ *Page 199*

Sandwiches   C   F   Cb

No Spreads Unless Indicated:
Includes 2 Slices Bread ~ 3 oz

	C	F	Cb
BLT, (5 strips Bacon, 2 Tbsp Mayo)	600	40	46
Breaded Chicken & Garnish	540	28	46
Chicken Salad, with Mayo., 5 oz	580	30	49
Chopped Liver, Egg Mayonnaise	630	25	44
Corned Beef with Mustard, 5 oz	560	28	44
Egg Salad, with Mayonnaise	570	29	49
Egg Salad Club, with Bacon & Mayo,	780	53	49
Grilled Cheese, (3 oz)	540	30	44
Ham, (4 oz), Cheese (4 oz), & Mayo.	910	56	44
Lobster Salad, (4 oz), w/ Mayo.	530	25	45
Overstuffed Tuna Salad, (7 oz)	870	39	75
Philly Cheese Steak Sandwich	550	23	42
Reuben, (6 oz Beef/Pastrami,			
2 oz Cheese, 2 Tbsp Dressing)	920	60	28
Roast Beef, (4 oz), with Mustard	460	12	45
Roast Pork, (4 oz), with Apple Sauce	500	16	55
Shrimp Salad Club, w/ Bacon & Mayo	800	57	48
Sloppy Joe with Sauce, (7 oz)	600	30	45
Steak Sandwich, (5 oz cooked)	680	32	41
Triple Cheese Melt, (4 oz)	720	45	46
Tuna Salad, (5 oz), with Mayonnaise	610	30	49
Turkey Breast, (5 oz), w/ Mayo.	460	18	44
Turkey Breast, (5 oz,) with Mustard	360	7	44
Turkey Club, with Bacon & Mayo.	830	38	31
Vegetarian, with Avocado & Cheese	820	49	72

7-Eleven ~ *Page 236*
Schlotzsky's ~ *Page 237*
Subway ~ *Page 245*

Wraps & Roll-Ups

Average All Types
Meat/Chicken/Fish/Veggie:

	C	F	Cb
Small, approximately 9 oz	500	25	48
Regular, approximately 15 oz	830	40	80
Large, approximately 22 oz	1400	70	134

Fast-Foods Restaurants ~ *Page 175*
Au Bon Pain ~ *Page 179*
Sonic Drive-In ~ *Page 241*
Subway ~ *Page 245*
WAWA ~ *Page 254*

Fair & Carnival Foods | C | L | CP

	C	L	CP
Barbeque Chicken/Meats:			
Chicken, 1/2 chicken, 15 oz	740	24	34
Grilled Chicken Pita, with dressing	680	19	82
Teriyaki Chicken, on stick, w/ dress.	250	6	4
Pork Ribs, 18 oz	1360	68	21
Turkey Leg: Regular, 19 oz	1135	54	0
Caveman (2lb Turkey Leg, with 1lb Bacon)	2360	177	3
Bacon: Fried, on-a-stick, with syrup	230	16	5
Choc-covered Bacon, 4.5 oz dish	640	43	30
Beef Stew over Rice, 2 cups	440	14	61
Butter Balls, deep fried, 4 Balls	460	38	24
Cheese Curds, Breaded & fried, Culver's, 6.7 oz	670	38	54
Corn Dogs: Regular, 4 oz	250	14	23
Jumbo, 6 oz	375	21	36
Pretzel-Wrapped Dog	300	16	30
Papa Pup, on-a-stick	400	24	32
Pronto Pup, on-a-stick	170	9	16
Corn On The Cob, 8" (1), 16 oz	200	1	42
Finger Foods:			
Artichoke, fried, 9 pieces	250	14	24
Chicken Nuggets, (6)	340	17	26
Chicken Strips, (4), 4.5 oz	445	21	33
Onion Rings, 3 rings	310	13	40
Onion Flower	1320	72	140
Shrimp, Fried, 10-12 pieces, 5 oz	555	30	36
Spam, deep-fried in batter, 2 pieces	330	24	18
Gator:			
Big Gator, Nuggets/Hushpuppies	550	31	54
Stick Gator, 1 sausage	250	20	4
Greek:			
Baklava, 2" square	245	13	32
Falafel, 11.6 oz	660	27	85
Greek Salad, 14 oz	520	48	17
Gyro, 7.5", 12 oz	680	40	55
Spanakopita, 8 oz	200	7.5	23
Hamburgers:			
1/3 Pound Burger, 7.5 oz	670	41	26
Cheeseburger, 6 oz	550	36	25
Hot Dogs: With Bun			
Regular: No extras	215	14	28
With Chili, 6 oz	450	32	32
With Chili & Cheese, 7.3 oz	500	36	31
1/3 Pound Hot Dog	550	41	31
Foot Long Hot Dog	470	26	41
Jumbo, Bratwurst/Kielbasa, average	800	60	28

Fair & Carnival Foods (Cont) | C | F | Cb

	C	F	Cb
Mexican:			
Burrito, with Bean/Beef, 17 oz	1100	41	104
Carne Asada, 14.5 oz	820	44	58
Cheese Quesadilla, 1.8 oz	480	27	40
Chicken Taco, 3.3 oz	210	12	16
Fish Taco, 5 oz	270	13	31
Jalapeno Pepper, choc-covered (3)	270	15	31
Nachos with Cheese, 9" plate	860	59	70
Tamale, 3.5 oz	180	8	21
Taquito, 5 oz	370	17	43
Pizza:			
Pizza Bread, Pepperoni, 1/2 loaf, 12 oz	1115	32	151
Pizza on-a-stick, 1 piece	535	28	55
Personal Pizza: Per 7"			
Cheese	670	24	80
Pepperoni	795	35	80
Ham & Pineapple	800	31	87
Potatoes & Fries:			
Australian Battered Potatoes	1290	66	155
Baked Potato, 14 oz	435	0.5	100
Fries: French, 7 oz	560	24	79
Cheese Fries, 10 oz	645	38	62
Chili Fries, 10 oz	700	36	83
Curly Fries, 7 oz	620	30	78
Jamaican Jerk Fries, 7 oz	640	34	77
Sweet Potato, baked, 14 oz	405	0.5	97
Tornado, on-a-stick	210	15	18
Salads/Sides:			
Chili, 1 cup	280	11	24
Cole Slaw, 5 oz	350	21	37
Pickle, whole (6")	30	0	8
Potato Salad, 5 oz	290	15	35
Sandwiches: 7 1/2" Roll			
Ham, 11 oz	645	39	47
Hot Pastrami, 9 oz	760	17	62
Roast Beef, 11 oz	620	36	46
Philadelphia Cheese Steak, 13 oz	680	36	49
Turkey, 11 oz	665	24	65
Drinks:			
Icee, 16 fl.oz	235	0	59
Shakes, average, 16 fl.oz	690	33	85
Slushies: Horchata, 16 fl.oz	280	8	50
Lemonade, 18 fl.oz	210	0	52
Orange Julius, 20 fl.oz	490	10	96
Strawberry Julius, 20 fl.oz	430	0	98
Soft Frozen Lemonade, 12 fl.oz	300	0	78
Smoothies, Berry Flavors, 16 fl.oz	350	1	80

Fair & Carnival Foods (Cont)

Cakes· Pastries:	C	F	Cb
Funnel Cake, Plain (1)	760	44	80
Toppings:			
Apple Cinnamon, 2 oz	85	3	16
Cinnamon & Sugar, 2 tsp	40	0	10
Strawberry & Cream, 2 oz	70	0	16
Cheesecake on-a-stick, 6 oz	655	47	56
Churro, (1), 9", 1.6 oz	170	8	22
Cream Puff, 4.3 oz	500	43	22
Fried Twinkie, (1)	420	34	45
Puff-on-a-Stick, (4), 8.6 oz	995	86	44
Strawberry Crepe, 4.3 oz	280	14	36
Twinkie Dog, (Sundae)	500	14	89
Candied Apple, 7 oz	330	0	80
Cookies:			
Sweet Martha, (1), 0.8 oz	90	4	14
Deep Fried: Oreos, tray (5)	890	48	108
Cookie Dough on stick, 3 pieces	670	32	89
Cotton Candy:			
Small, 1 oz	110	0	27
Large, 2.3 oz	250	0	62
Family Size, 5.5 oz	610	0	151
Dirt Dessert, 1 cup, 9.3 oz	405	12	69
Donuts, Jumbo Twist, (1), 7.5 oz	905	49	109
Fried Dough/FryBread:			
Plain: 7", 3.7 oz	390	19	47
9", 4³/₄ oz	510	25	61
Toppings: Cinnamon Sugar, 2 tsp	40	0	10
Butterscotch; Caramel, 2 Tbsp	115	0	29
Hot Fudge, average, 2 Tbsp	110	4	22
Cheese Powder, 2 tsp	70	3	2
Honey, 1 Tbsp, 0.8 oz	65	0	17
Fudge, 1.5 oz	200	11	25
Ice Cream & Frozen Treats:			
Deep-fried Klondike Bar, w/ syrup	430	16	18
Dippin' Dots Ice Cream, 6 oz cup	380	20	46
Frozen Banana, choc. coated, 5 oz	240	4	53
Frozen Yogurt, in sugar cone, 14 oz	475	2	94
Ice Cream: Small, sugar cone, 10 oz	775	42	83
Large, sugar cone, 14 oz	935	54	96
Sherbet, 8 oz	270	4	59
Snow Cone, with 3 oz syrup	270	0	68
Strawberry, Choc. Dipped, 1 piece	125	7	15
Popcorn:			
Plain: Small, 3 oz	450	24	48
Large, 6 oz	900	48	96
Kettle Corn: Small, 5 oz	600	15	110
Large, 10 oz	1200	30	220
Pretzels, Soft, 4.5 oz	340	2	70
S'more, on stick	275	16	27

Stadium Foods

	C	F	Cb
Burgers:			
Bacon Burger, 8.3 oz	470	25	34
Cheeseburger, 8.3 oz	450	23	33
Hamburger, 7.8 oz	400	19	33
French Fries, 6.4 oz	470	34	39
Fruit Cup, 6 oz	80	0	20
Hot Dogs:			
Chili Dog, 7.7 oz	520	29	45
Hot Dog, 6.4 oz	465	21	50
Jumbo Dog, 6 oz	440	25	38
Kraut Dog with Sauerkraut, 7.8 oz	490	27	41
Individual Pan Pizza (6"): *Per Pizza*			
BBQ Chicken	630	24	71
Cheese	630	27	71
Pepperoni	660	30	70
Nachos, 40 chips, with 4 oz cheese	1100	59	132
Sandwiches:			
Chicken: With Bacon, 8.3 oz	530	31	41
With Cheese, 8.3 oz	510	29	40
Without Cheese, 7.7 oz	460	25	40
Polish Sausage Sandwich, 7 oz	565	33	46
Snacks:			
Brownie, 2.5" x 4.5"	360	18	44
Cheese Sauce, 1.3 oz	100	8	4
Cheetos, 2.8 oz package	440	28	42
Chocolate Chip Cookie, 2.3 oz	280	12	40
Churro, (1), 10", 2 oz	210	10	26
Doritos, Nacho, 2.8 oz package	390	20	48
King Size Candy:			
Butterfinger, 3.8 oz	480	18	75
Nestle Crunch, 2.8 oz	390	21	85
Lay's, Chips, 2.8 oz package	440	28	42
Peanuts, in shell, 8 oz	930	80	24
Popcorn: Small (9 cup size)	575	35	56
Large (15 cup size)	950	58	93
Pretzel, Soft, Reg., 5.5 oz	490	3.5	101
Red Vines, 5 oz box	500	0	117
Snow Cone: With 3 oz syrup	270	0	68
With 6 oz syrup	540	0	136
Beverages:			
Orange Juice, 12 fl.oz	180	0	2
Beer:			
Heineken, 16 fl.oz	200	0	16
Miller: Draft, 16 fl.oz	195	0	17
Lite, 16 fl.oz	125	16	4
Jack Daniels, Punch, 12 fl.oz	235	0	34
Wine, White, 9 fl.oz	190	0	6
Soda, (with ¹/₂ ice), average:			
20 fl.oz	160	0	40
32 fl.oz	260	0	65
Starbuck's, Coffee, Frappuccino, 9.5 fl.oz	200	3	37

Asian & Chinese Dishes — C · F · Cb

Asian & Chinese Dishes	C	F	Cb
Appetizers:			
Crab Cake, 2.3 oz	125	10	1
Dumplings: *Per Dumpling*			
Pork: Steamed	80	4.5	5
Fried	90	6	5
Vegetable, steamed	35	1	5
Egg Rolls, Mini, 3 rolls	100	3	11
Spring Roll:			
Small, 1.5 oz	85	4	9
Medium, 3 oz	170	8	17
Large, 5 oz	290	15	29
Wonton, 1 only	75	4	5
Soup: Egg Flower, bowl 12 oz	90	2	16
Hot & Sour Soup, bowl 12 oz	110	3.5	14
Rice: Plain,1 cup, 6.5 oz	320	2	66
2 Cups, 13 oz	640	4	132
Fried: 1 cup, 5 oz	365	11	55
Large dish, 16 oz	950	28	67
Noodles, Chinese Egg, cooked, 1 cup	200	4	37
Entrees & Mains: *Per Serving*			
Almond Chicken, 6 oz	270	10	21
BBQ Pork, 5.5oz	440	23	15
Beef in Black Bean Sauce, 8.5 oz	390	17	17
Broccoli Beef, 6 oz	370	21	13
Chicken & Broccoli, 5.5 oz	160	8	10
Chicken Skewers, 3 oz	210	9	18
Chop Suey:			
Chicken, 5 oz	140	9	2
Pork, 5 oz	170	12	3
Chow Mein, Beef/Chicken, 8 oz	390	12	59
Crab Puff/Rangoon, 1 dumpling	190	11	13
Crispy Fried Chicken, 8 oz	485	33	12
Egg Drop Soup: With Noodles, 1 cup	110	3	16
Without Noodles, 1 cup	60	3	4
Egg Foo Yung with Sauce, 1 cup	270	15	16
Kung Pao Chicken, 5.5 oz	240	15	12
Lemon Chicken, 5 oz	525	21	57
Lo Mein, stir-fried, 8 oz	705	42	49
Omelet, Chicken/Shrimp, 16 oz	990	82	10
Orange Chicken, 5.5 oz	500	27	42
Steamed Whole Fish,			
½ Sockeye Salmon	646	36	23
Sweet & Sour:			
Fish, 20 oz	1160	58	106
Pork, 5.5 oz	400	23	35
Vegetable Combo, with oil, 6 oz	367	5	66
Vegetables, Steamed, without oil, 6 oz	135	1	29
Sauces: Mandarin Sauce 1.5 oz	70	0	17
Potsticker Sauce, 1.5 oz	35	0	8
Bubble Tea, average, 12 fl oz	280	0.5	68
Fortune Cookie, each	32	0.5	7

Cajun & Creole — C · F · Cb

Cajun & Creole	C	F	Cb
Alligator, cooked, 4 oz	160	2	0
Baked Herb Chicken, 1 serving	850	53	2
Bouillabaisse	400	15	10
Cajun Fried Turkey, 1 serving	630	25	0
Cocktail Sauce, 2 Tbsp	30	0	6
Couche-Couche, ½ cup	80	0	17
Crawfish Bisque, 1 serving	500	10	10
Crawfish, cooked, 2 oz	45	0.5	0
Creole Jambalaya, 1 serving	550	30	15
Frog Legs, steamed (2)	45	0	0
Guinea Fowl, flesh, 4 oz, cooked	160	4	0
Hogshead Cheese, ¼ cup	80	5.5	0
Jambalaya, Shrimp & Crabmeat	520	14	12
Red Beans & Rice, 1 serving	400	17	52
Roasted Quail, with Bacon, on Toast	550	25	15
Remoulade Sauce, 2 Tbsp, 1 oz	110	11	2
Shrimp Creole, 1 serving	450	20	10
Stuffed Smothered Steak, with 1 cup Rice	890	50	50
Turtle, cooked, 3 oz	120	3	0

Canadian Foods

Canadian Foods	C	F	Cb
Bagels, Montreal-Style:			
Plain, 100g/3.5 oz	300	2	60
Poppyseed, 100g/3.5 oz	310	4	58
Sesame, 100g/3.5 oz	320	6	56
Bannock: Plain 33g/1.2 oz	120	3	20
With currants/raisins, 85g/3 oz	215	9	32
Meals:			
Baked Beans in Maple Syrup, 1 cup, 250g/8.8 oz	320	1	62
Donnairs (*Pizza Delight*):			
Famous, regular, 250g/8.8 oz	510	21	60
Super, regular, 310g/11 oz	685	34	62
Poutine:			
A&W, 330g/12 oz	610	33	58
Boston Pizza, regular, 400g/14 oz	610	30	67
Burger King, Classic, 330g/11.6 oz	680	36	72
Harvey's, 240g/8.5 oz	730	41	63
McDonald's, 1 serving	510	29	44
Swiss Chalet, Chalet -Style, 340g/12 oz	150	12	195
Shish Taouk:			
Chicken: 1 skewer, 200g/7 oz	270	25	9
Wrap, 455g/16 oz	1150	12	195
Tassot:			
Beef, 283g/10 oz	430	28	12
Goat, 100g/3.5 oz	360	36	9
Toutiere, 170g/6oz	600	42	35

Canadian (Cont)

	C	F	Cb
Pastries:			
Beaver Tails:			
Cheese & Garlic, 80g/2.8 oz	390	30	28
Cinnamon & Sugar, 80g/2.8 oz	315	13	30
Butter Tart, mini, 1 tart	120	3	16
May West,			
Original, 54g/1.9 oz	240	11	34
Nanaimo Bar, 56g/2 oz	270	16	30
Snacks: Maple Syrup Taffy, 40g/1.4 oz	130	0	33
Potato Chips: Dill Pickle Flav., 40g	160	10	15
Ketchup Flavor, 50g/1.8 oz	260	16	26

French Foods

	C	F	Cb
Blanquette d'Agneau, (Lamb Stew)	800	30	17
Brioche, 1 cake	280	14	34
Bouillabaisse	400	15	10
Coq au Vin, leg/thigh	700	28	31
Coquilles St. Jacques	320	13	36
Crème Brulée, 1 serving	460	40	21
Baguette, 3 slices, 2.2 oz	150	1	35
Creme Caramel, (Caramel Custard)	260	10	38
Crepe Suzette, 1x6" crepe with sauce	220	10	13
Duck a l'Orange, ¼ duck, 22 oz	970	44	19
Escargot, (Snails), in garlic butter (6)	200	10	4
Frog Legs, fried, 4 medium pairs	400	20	10
Lamb Noisettes, fried, 2 chops	500	40	1
Potage Creme Crecy, (Carrot Soup)	360	18	14
Salade Nicoise, (Tuna/Olives/Vegs)	450	13	14
Veal Cordon Bleu, (Veal/Ham)	650	25	18
Vichyssoise, (Potato /Leek Soup), 1 c.	200	9	15
Baguette & French Stick ~ *Page 54*			

German Foods

	C	F	Cb
Beef: Goulash with Veggies	520	20	46
Weiner Schnitzel, 1 medium	750	35	38
Chicken: Fried, Viennese-style	530	20	28
Livers with Apple/Onion, 6 oz	460	28	10
Herring, pickled: Rollmops, 4 oz	260	16	3
With Sour Cream, 4 oz	310	20	3
Pork, Sauerbraten (Pot Roast)	650	35	15
Sausage: Bratwurst, grilled, 6 oz	450	37	2
Hot Sausage Curry	300	7	6
Cakes:			
Black Forest, 1 slice	380	16	30
Bavarian Bread Dumpling, 3 small	330	10	28
Kugelhupf Cake, 1 large slice, 4 oz	400	23	40
Torte: Linzer (Almond/Raspb. Jam)	430	18	58
Sacher (Chocolate/Apricot Jam)	260	12	23

Greek Foods

	C	F	Cb
Baklava Pastry: Small	240	13	32
Large, 3.8 oz	400	21	45
Calamari, deep fried, 1 cup	300	13	17
Chicken Kebob Plate	345	13	8
Dolmades, 2 rolls, 6 oz	200	5	13
Galactobureko, 1 only			
(Filo, Custard, Pastry in Syrup)	360	15	48
Greek Chicken Salad	400	18	9
Gyros: 6" Pita, 8 oz	475	32	35
7½" Pita, 12 oz	680	40	55
Hummus & Pita, 4 oz	260	12	30
Kataifi, (Filo, Nut, Pastry in Syrup)	350	11	56
Moussaka: Small serving, 8 oz	350	22	22
Large serving, 16 oz	700	44	44
Soup, Avgolemono (Egg & Lemon			
with Chicken & Rice), 1 cup	85	6	5
Souvlaki, (Lamb), each, 2 oz	120	6	1
Stuffed Tomatoes, (2)	250	12	17
Taramosalata, 1 T., 0.5 oz	40	3	2
Tyropita, (Filo/Egg/Cheese Pastry)	350	26	31

Hawaiian

	C	F	Cb
Ahi Tuna, grilled w/o fat, 6 oz fillet	220	2	0
Chicken Long Rice, 1 cup, 7 oz	240	14	12
Gyoza, 1 only	55	2	6
Haupia, (Coconut Pudd.), 1 pce, (4"x 2½")	120	6	17
Hawaiian Sweet Bread, ½" slice, 2 oz	180	4.5	29
Kalua: Chicken, 4 oz	280	16	0
Pork, 4 oz	350	24	0
Kim Chee, (pickled cabbage), ½ cup, 4 oz	20	0	5
Kulolo, (Taro Pudding), 1 slice	125	5	19
Lau Lau:			
Chicken (1), 7 oz	280	21	3
Pork (1), 7 oz	320	26	5
Loco Moco, (rice/burger/egg/gravy)	650	27	63
Lomi Salmon, ¼ cup, 4 oz	20	1	2
Malasadas, (Donut), 2 oz	240	13	26
Manapua, (Char Siu Pork Bun), 2.3 oz	180	8	25
Poi, (mashed cooked taro), 1 cup, 8.5 oz	270	0.5	65
Poke, average all types, 3 oz	90	1	0
Portuguese Sausage, 2 oz	180	15	2
Potato Salad, ½ cup, 5 oz	170	12	17
Shave Ice, (Matsumoto), all flavors:			
With Ice Cream, 1 large	300	4	64
With Beans, 1 large	290	0	72
Spam Musubi:			
With Regular Spam	265	11	34
(4 oz rice+1.3 oz Spam/7-Eleven Hawaii)			
Homemade, w/ Lite Spam (50% less fat)	220	5	34
Taro Pancake Mix, ⅓ cup (makes 2)	140	2	26

Hawaiian (Cont)   C F Cb

Plate Lunches:

	C	F	Cb
Chicken Katsu, (9 oz:) With Rice	1110	48	108
+ Macaroni Salad, ³/₄ cup	1360	68	123
or Tossed Salad + 2 T. French Dress.	1240	61	111
Hamburger, (5 oz): With Rice	710	24	81
Gravy + Macaroni Salad	1135	49	112
Mahi Mahi, (7 oz): With Rice	650	12	90
+ Macaroni Salad + Tartar Sce	1150	58	109
or Macaroni Salad, w/o Tartar ce	935	34	108
or Tossed Salad + 3 Tbsp Fr. Dress.	815	27	96
or Tossed Salad, without dressing	670	12	93
Teri Beef, (5 oz): With 2 scoops Rice	790	23	94
+ Macaroni Salad, ³/₄ cup	1095	47	113
or Tossed Salad, without dressing	800	23	95

Indian & Pakistani

Per Serving, Meat dishes allow 4 oz meat/serving

	C	F	Cb
Aloo Samosa, each	155	12	12
Alu Gosht Kari, (Meat/Potato Curry)	600	40	23
Chicken Korma	500	35	6
Chicken Pilaf	700	53	50
Chicken Tikka	260	16	2
Chicken Vindaloo	400	20	8
Chapati/Roti, 7" diameter, 1 piece	60	0.5	11
Dahl, (Lentil Puree):			
1 cup, without oil	230	1	37
1 Tbsp Tadka (oil topping)	120	13	0
Dhakla, (Lentil Dish), 1" square, 1 oz	105	5	13
Dhansak, ¹/₂ cup	105	3.5	11
Gosht Kari	460	25	17
Lamb Pilaf	520	35	40
Lassi, (Sweet or Mango), 1 cup, 8 oz	160	4	24
Masala Gosht, (Beef/Tomato/Gravy)	400	25	18
Mulligatawney Soup	300	15	8
Murgh Tikka, 1 cup	300	4	7
Naan Flatbread, 2 oz	160	3.5	29
Pappadum, 1 large/2 small	50	3	5
Pesrattu, (Lentil Crepe), 9", 2.6 oz	130	5	15
Pork Vindaloo Curry, without Rice	620	47	3
Rajmah, 1 cup	225	5	35
Rogan Josh,			
without Rice/Potatoes	500	30	3
Shahi Korma, (Braised Lamb)	430	28	3
Tandoori Chicken:			
Breast	260	13	5
Leg/Thigh portion	300	17	6

Italian Dishes   C F Cb

Entrees:

	C	F	Cb
Baked Ziti: Small	370	27	32
Regular	575	42	49
Breadstick, 2 oz piece	120	2.5	25
Broccoli Fettucine Alfredo, regular	815	23	125
Bruschetta, 2 slices	380	17	53
Calzones, av. all varieties	840	34	101
Cannelloni, 1 tube, 6 oz	280	15	18
Cheese Breadstick, 2.4 oz piece	180	8	20
Cheese Ravioli, with sauce	495	17	65
Chicken Alfredo	775	29	82
Chicken Parmigiana, 11 oz	520	22	16
Chicken Scallopine, dinner	1110	71	68
Eggplant Parmigiana	900	39	78
Fettucine Alfredo: Lunch, 9 oz	885	65	63
Dinner, 15 oz	1475	108	104
Linquine & Seafood, dinner	1130	71	79
Manicotti Formaggio	800	38	57
Meat Lasagne:			
Small, 10 oz	440	23	39
Large, 16 oz	700	36	60
Meat Ravioli	725	22	102
Minestrone Soup, 1 bowl	110	2	18
Penne Rustica: Lunch	1300	71	76
Dinner	1540	80	101
Ravioli, over-stuffed, average	990	67	57
Panini Sandwich:			
Chicken, 16 oz	900	38	81
Meats, average, 18 oz	940	39	81
Vegetarian, 15 oz	750	31	83
Pizza, Ready-To-Eat ~ *See Page 135*			
Spaghetti & Meatballs:			
With Tomato Sauce: Kids	500	20	58
Medium/Lunch	1080	63	89
Large/Dinner	1430	81	119
With Meat Sauce: Kids	550	25	56
Medium/Lunch	1300	79	84
Large/Dinner	1700	103	110
Veal Marsala, dinner	1320	66	132
Veal Parmigiana, dinner	1270	65	116
Vegetable Primavera	610	8	116
Salad,			
Caprese, 11 oz	445	34	10
Desserts:			
Gelato: Vanilla (Milk Base), ¹/₂ cup	200	15	18
Choc. Hazelnut (Milk), ¹/₂ cup	370	29	26
Water Base, ¹/₂ cup	100	0	25
Lemon Ice,	180	0	45
Tiramisu, 1 piece, 5 oz	400	29	30

Further listings ~ *See Fast-Foods Section*

Japanese

Item	C	F	Cb
Sashimi:(Sliced Raw Seafood/Beef)			
Ika (Squid), 4 oz	105	2	0
Hamachi (Yellowtail), 4 oz	165	6	0
Maguro (Yellowfin Tuna), 4 oz	120	1	0
Niku (Beef), 5 oz	200	10	0
Saba (Mackerel), 4 oz	160	7	0
Suzuki (Sea Bass), 4 oz	110	0.5	0
Tako (Octopus), 4 oz	95	1	0
Sushi Rice: Cooked, 1 Tbsp	25	0	5
1 cup, 5.3 oz	380	3	82
Sushi (Maki) Rolls: *Per Piece*			
Average all types (California Rolls; Cream Cheese with Crab; Eel; Salmon; Shrimp; Tuna; Yellowtail; Vegetable)			
Small (1.2″ diam. x 1.2″ high), 0.8 oz	25	0.5	3.5
Medium (1¾″ diam. x 1¾″ high), 1.6 oz	50	1	7
Large (2¼″ diam. x ⅞″ high), 2 oz	60	1.5	9
Sushi Packs: *Per Pack*			
Average all types: 6 large pieces	370	5	55
9 medium pieces	360	6	60
12 small pieces	265	3	45
Futomaki (thick roll), 6 pieces	380	5	72
Hand Roll (Cone), 4 oz	120	2	18
Inari (rice filled soybean pocket), 4 pces	420	9	73
Sushi-Nigiri, (fish on rice), average all varieties, 1 piece	70	0.5	12
Sushi Plate, Assorted: 6 pieces	420	3	36
Combination (Sushi & Sushi Rolls) 2 Sushi + 6 small & 3 medium rolls	400	7	72
Dipping Sauces: Average, 2 Tbsp	30	0	7
Ginger Vinegar Dressing, 2 Tbsp	20	0	5
Edamame: (young green soybeans):			
Boiled beans (no pods), 4 oz	160	7	12
Steamed (in pods), 4 oz	60	3	5
Katsu-don, Pork with Rice	1100	39	141
Miso Soup, with Tofu pieces, 1 cup	85	3	11
Sake Wine, (16% alcohol), 3 fl.oz	115	0	7
Seaweed Salad, 1.5 oz	20	2	0
Sukiyaki, (Beef/Tofu/Veggies), 8 oz	400	24	32
Tempura:			
3 large shrimp & veggies	320	18	25
1 shrimp only	60	4	3
Teppan Yaki, (Steak, Seafood & Veggies), 10 oz serving	470	30	15
Teriyaki: Beef, 4 oz	350	25	4
Chicken, 4 oz	260	9	7
Salmon, medium, 6 oz	270	8	3
Yakatori, 1 skewer, 2.5 oz	140	5	1

Kosher/Deli Foods

Item	C	F	Cb
Bagel/Bialy, 1 small, 2 oz	160	2	32
Beiglach, (Cheese Knish)	350	17	35
Blintzes: Average, 1 only	120	1	25
With Sour Cream & Preserves	370	10	30
Borscht, (Without Sour Cream): 1 cup	85	3	14
Diet/Reduced Calorie, 1 cup	30	1	7
Cabbage Roll, (meat/rice), 5 oz	170	6	21
Chicken Broth: 1 cup	80	8	0
With vegetables	100	8	5
With noodles	150	9	16
Lowfat, plain, 1 cup	25	1	0
Cholent, 1 medium serving, 1 cup	350	16	48
Chopped Liver: 1 serving, 3 oz	110	6	5
With Egg Salad, ¼ cup	100	7	3
Farfel, dry, ½ cup	90	0.5	21
Gefilte Fish Balls:			
Regular, 2 oz	55	2	4
With Jelled Broth	80	2	6
Cocktail size, 1 oz	30	1	2
Sweet: Medium, 2 oz	65	2	4
With Jelled Broth	95	2	9
Hallah, (Yeast Bread), 1 slice, 1 oz	85	2	14
Herring: Smoked, 2 oz	120	8	0
In Sour Cream, 2 oz	150	10	0
Kasha, cooked, ½ cup	100	0.5	20
Kipfel, (Vanilla/Almdond Cookie), 1 pce	60	2	7
Knaidlach ~ *See Matzo Balls*			
Knish: Kasha/Potato, 1 only	130	4	22
Cheese, 1 only	350	17	35
Kreplach, beef, 1 piece	40	1	6
Kugel, potato/noodle, 1 serving	300	20	25
Latkes, (Potato Pancake): 2 oz	200	11	22
3 Latkes w/ Sour Cran Apple Sauce	750	25	95
Lochshen: Plain, 1 cup	130	2	26
Pudding, 1 cup	380	13	48
Lox, (Smoked Salmon), 2 oz	65	2	0
Mandelbrot, (Almond Bread), 1 slice, ¼″ thick	45	2	5
Matzo, 1 oz board	110	0.5	21
Matzo Balls: 2 small, or 1 large, 2″	90	3	12
Extra large ball, 3″	180	6	24
Matzo Ball Soup:			
Cup w/ 2 small or 1 large ball	150	5	27
Bowl w/ Chkn & Noodles	325	13	34
Jerry's Deli, large bowl	560	17	56
NY Cheesecake, 4 oz	350	24	26
Pierogi, potato/cheese, 1 piece	90	4	11
Reuben S'wich, w/ ½ lb Corned Beef	920	60	28
Schmaltz, (Rend'd Chicken Fat), 1 T.	90	10	0

Korean Food

	C	F	Cb
Bibimbab, (Veg. & Beef on Rice), 1 cup	565	15	89
Bulgogi, (Barbeque Beef), 3.5 oz	325	12	15
Galbi (Short Ribs), 16 oz	975	61	16
Gujeolpan, (Pancake with Meat & Vegetables), 1 cup with 1 pancake	340	11	39
Japchae, (Noodle w/ Veggies & Meat), 1¼ cups	365	19	34
Sides:			
Kimchee, (Cabbage Relish), ½ cup	30	0	6
Namool, (Assorted Vegetables), 1 cup	125	6.5	9
Soups: *Per Serving*			
Muguk, (Radish & Chive Soup), 6 oz	105	7	6
Samgyetang, (Ginseng Chkn Soup):			
Without Chicken Skin, 1 cup	520	11	60
With Chicken Skin, 1 cup	725	35	60
Yuk Gae Jang, (Spicy Beef Soup), 1¼ cups	180	13	5

Lebanese/Middle East

	C	F	Cb
Baba Ghannouj, 2 Tbsp, 1 oz	70	6	2
Baklava, (Pastry, Nuts, Syrup), 1 pastry, 1¾ oz	245	18	18
Cabbage Rolls, (Cabb. Leaf, Meat, Rice), 1 roll, 3 oz	100	3	12
Cous Cous, (Semolina, Milk, Fruit, Nuts), 1 cup	400	21	43
Falafel, (Chick Pea Fritter), Fried, 1 medium, 1 oz	60	4	4
Hummus, ¼ cup, 2.2 oz	105	3	5
Fried Kibbi, (Wheat, Meat Pinenuts), 1 piece, 3 oz	180	8	15
Kafta, (Ground Lamb, Ssge on Skewer), 1 skewer, 1.5 oz	85	5	2
Kibbeh Naye, (raw Lamb, Bulgur & Spice) 1 cup, 9 oz	450	18	28
Lebanese Omelet, 1 serving, 4 oz (Egg, Spinach, Pinenuts, Onion)	200	12	13
Pilaf, (Rice, Onion, Raisins, Apr., Spice) 1 cup	400	11	60
Shawourma, (Spit-Roast Beef), 4 oz serving	280	15	2
Shish Kabob, 1 stick, 2.5 oz	130	7	2
Spinach Pie, 1 piece, 3.5 oz	290	21	20
Sweet Almond Sanbusak, (Pastry, Almonds, Spices), 1 piece	200	15	11
Tabouli, 1 serving, 4 oz	125	7	13
Tahini Sauce, average, 1 Tbsp	90	8	2

Mexican

	C	F	Cb
Burritos *(Taco Bell):* Bean	370	10	56
Supreme Beef	420	16	53
Chili, plain, ¼ cup	90	6	8
Chili con Carne: With Beans, 1 cup	310	17	15
Without Beans, 1 cup	370	28	10
Chimichangas, Beef, 5 oz	400	19	43
Chorizo Sausage, 2 oz	265	23	0
Churro, (1), 1.5 oz	150	8	18
Corn Chips, ½ cup, 1 oz	160	10	17
Enchilada, average	330	10	49
Fajitas, Chicken	200	7	20
Guacamole, average, 2 Tbsp, 1 oz	45	4	2
Horchata: *(Don Jose)*, 1 cup, 8 fl.oz	140	4	25
Cacique, 1 pint bottle, 16 fl.oz	320	7	62
Margarita, with 1.5 oz Tequila	160	0	6
Masa, (Pre-mixed for Tamales), 1 oz	80	5	9
Menudo:			
With Hominy, 1 cup	240	9	19
Without Hominy, 1 cup	170	9	2
Nachos: With cheese, peppers, 1 portion, 6-8 nachos, 7 oz	600	33	60
With cheese, beans, beef, peppers, 1 portion, 6-8 nachos, 9 oz	570	31	56
Del Taco: Regular, 4 oz	300	19	30
Macho Nachos, 17 oz	1000	56	94
Taco Bell, BellGrande®, 10.8 oz	780	40	84
Nopal Cactus Salad, 1 cup	130	9	11
Papas Fritas, (1), 6 oz	325	18	40
Piloncillo, (Brown Sugar):			
1 Tbsp, 0.5 oz	50	0	13
Cone, small, 3", 3 oz	325	0	81
Quesadilla, Cheese	490	28	39
Queso Fresco, ¼ cup	80	4.5	8
Refried Beans, ¾ cup, 6 oz	160	3	26
Rice Pudding, (Arroz Con Leche), 4 oz	140	3	24
Soup, Black Bean, 1 bowl	200	3	34
Tacos *(Taco Bell):*			
Crunchy: Regular	170	10	12
Supreme	200	12	15
Soft: Crispy Potato	270	13	31
Grilled Steak	250	14	19
Taco Salad with Salsa	840	52	85
Taco Sauce, average, ¼ cup	15	0	3
Taco Shell, regular	50	2	8
Tamales, Beef/Chicken, av. 4.5 oz	250	11	27
Taquitos, Beef & Cheese, 4.5 oz	330	15	36
Tostada (*Taco Bell*)	250	10	29
Tortilla, Corn, 6" diameter	70	1	14
Tortilla Chips, 1 oz	150	8	18
Soup, Black Bean, 1 bowl	200	3	34

Extra Food Listings ~ See Fast Food Section
(Examples: Del Taco, Taco Bell, Taco Cabana, Taco Time)

Mexican (Cont)

	C	F	Cb
Breads:			
Bolillos, 1 roll, 3.5 oz	240	4	42
Mexican Cornbread, 4" square	210	11	19
Pan de Leche, 1 roll, 1.3 oz	110	2.5	20
Telera, 2 oz	150	1.5	19
Cakes· Cookies· Pastries Pan Dulce:			
Banderilla, 1 piece	140	10	8
Bigotes, 7"	570	22	44
Capirotada, (Bread Pudding), 10 oz	810	38	107
Cinnamon Cookies, 2	125	8	13
Concha, av. all varieties:			
Small (3" diameter), 2.5 oz	250	8	38
Medium (4" diameter), 3.5 oz	350	11	53
Large (5" diameter), 5.5 oz	550	18	84
Cream Puff, with Custard, 4.3 oz	255	14	25
Cuernos, (Horns), 3 oz	340	17	41
Donut, large, 4", 3.5 oz	440	21	58
Elotes, 3.5 oz	450	24	51
Empanadas, average all varieties:			
Medium, 3 oz	300	14	42
Large, 4 oz	400	19	56
Fiesta Cookie, (1), 2.3 oz	280	8	47
Galletas Mixtas:			
Small, 1 oz	100	2.5	16
Medium, 2 oz	200	5	32
Large, 3 oz	300	7.5	48
Guayaba, 3.3 oz	360	14	53
Jelly Roll, (1), 3.3 oz	240	4	46
Mantecadites, 4.5 oz	670	42	64
Mini Cupcake, (1),1.8 oz	180	8	25
Muffins/Nino Enbuelto, large, 6 oz	465	11	48
Nuez, 3.3 oz	380	17	52
Ojo de Buey, 4 oz	360	15	55
Orejas, 1 medium, 3 oz	310	15	38
Pan Dulce, 1 bun	330	10	45
Panquecitos, 2.5 oz	260	11	36
Piedras, 4 oz	470	15	76
Polvorones: Small, 1.5 oz	180	9	24
1 large, 3 oz	370	18	48
Pound Cakes, mini, 3.5 oz	380	16	52
Puerquitos, 3.5 oz	350	12	55
Rebanadas, 3.5 oz	390	18	51
Roles De Canela, (Cinn. Roll), 4.5 oz	490	15	81
Roscas, 1 piece, 2.8 oz	360	18	44
Semitas (*Bimbo*), 1 piece, 2.2 oz	210	6	33
Sopapillas, (flaky pastry puffs): 1 piece	100	7	10
With Honey & Cream	200	14	18
Strawberry Crema Roll, 2.5 oz slice	240	5	45
Extra Food Listings ~ *See CalorieKing.com*			

Polish

	C	F	Cb
Cabbage Rolls, w/ Sour Cream, 2 small	220	10	30
Chicken Casserole, w/ Mshrms, 1 cup	520	27	5
Kielbasa, (Sausages, Onions, fried),			
2 large	350	28	2
Meatballs,			
in sour cream, 3 x 1$\frac{1}{2}$" balls	300	16	11
Pierogi, Fruit/Vegetables, 3" ball	80	2	15
Pork Goulash, (Pork/Vegetable Stew)	550	21	38
Pot Roast, with Vegetables	630	21	28

Soul Foods

	C	F	Cb
Breakfast Sausage, fried, 2 patties	250	17	0
Brunswick Stew, 1 cup, 8.5 oz	320	14	19
Cornbread, homemade, 3 oz	200	7.5	28
Fatback, 0.5 oz	110	11	0
Ham Hock, pickled, 3 oz	200	12	0
Hog Maw, 1 oz	70	4.5	0
Hominy, cooked, $\frac{3}{4}$ cup	110	0.5	25
Hush Puppies, 5 pieces	260	12	35
Kale, cooked, $\frac{1}{2}$ cup	20	0.5	4
Opossum, roasted, without bone, 3 oz	190	9	0
Oxtail, cooked, without bone, 2 oz	85	4.5	0
Pig's Ear, $\frac{1}{4}$ ear	50	3	0
Pig's Foot, $\frac{1}{2}$ foot	70	4.5	0
Pig's Tail, $\frac{1}{3}$ tail	115	10	0
Poke Salad, cooked, $\frac{1}{2}$ cup	16	0.5	3
Pork Brains, braised, 3 oz	115	8	0
Pork Chitterlings, simmered, 3 oz	260	25	0
Pork Cracklings, 0.5 oz	80	6	0
Pork Neck Bones, cooked, no bone, 2 oz	100	4.5	0
Pork Skin, 1 cup	70	4.5	0
Pork Tongue, $\frac{1}{3}$ tongue	75	5.5	0
Sousemeat, 1 oz	60	4.5	0
Succotash, $\frac{1}{2}$ cup	80	1	17
Sweet Potato Pie, $\frac{1}{8}$ of 9" pie	250	12	34
Tripe, 2 oz	55	2	0
Vienna Sausage:			
2 small, 1 oz	90	8	1
1 small, 0.5 oz	45	4	0.5

OLD McDONALDS FARM

128   FOR PEOPLE WHO WANT BETTER

Brooklyn

Spanish

	C	F	Cb
Arroz Abanda, (Fish with Rice)	340	8	31
Arroz Con Pollo, (Rice/Chkn Salad)	500	23	50
Clams Marinara, 8 clams	330	16	22
Cochifrito, (Lamb with Lemon/Garlic)	650	25	5
Cochinillo Asado,			
(Rst Suckling Pig), 2 slices	300	15	3
Cocido Madrileno,			
(Madrid-Style Boiled Dinner)	450	27	18
Flan de Leche, (Caramel Custard)	325	9	52
Fritadera de Ternera, (Sauteed Veal)	450	27	2
Gazpacho, 1 bowl	60	0	15
Mole Poblano, ½ cup	205	14	16
Paella a la Valenciana,			
(Chicken & Shellfish Rice)	900	42	70
Pollo a la Espanola, (Chicken)	475	30	4
Ternera al Jerez, (Veal with Sherry)	660	29	6
Zarzuela, (Fish & Shellfish Medley)	530	27	40

Thai Foods

	C	F	Cb
Appetizers: Satay Pork, 1 oz	100	4	2
Spring Roll, 1.3 oz	110	6	13
Soups, Tom Yam (Hot & Sour):			
Spicy Shrimp/Seafood:			
1 cup	100	4	6
1 bowl	160	7	10
Vegetarian, 1 cup	50	0	11
Curries: Chicken with Ginger, 1 cup	390	34	4
Thick Red Curry with Beef, 1 cup	600	50	7
Thai Chicken Curry, 1 cup	340	23	4
Massaman Curry, 1 cup	680	57	8
Green Curry with Pork, 1 cup	480	44	5
Pad Thai, large serving, 18 oz	990	38	125
Fish: Steamed with Spicy Thai Sce	450	8	46
Crispy Fried, 5 oz	290	15	9
Spicy Chicken, stir-fry	450	22	14
Spicy Garlic Tofu, stir-fry	340	18	18
Sticky Thai Rice: Plain 1 cup, 6 oz	170	0.5	36
With Coconut & Sesame Seeds, 1 cup	880	28	120
Stir-fried Rice Noodles, 1 cup 5.5 oz	270	9	40
Stir-fried Vegetables, 1 cup	100	3	18
Salads: Green Papaya Salad	160	0	40
Spicy Prawn, 9 shrimp	170	3	15
Thai Beef Salad, 1 serving	260	9	15
Thai Chicken, 1 serving	330	9	17
Thai Noodle, 1 serving	410	13	45
Satay Chicken & Peanut Sauce,			
1 satay stick	390	24	20
Sauce, Peanut Satay,			
½ cup, 4 oz	160	10	13

Vietnamese

	C	F	Cb
Banh Cuon, (Steam Rice w/ Pork), 1 roll	105	7	8
Bo Nuong, (Beef Satay), 2 sticks	265	9	4
Bo Xao Dau Phong,			
(Ginger Beef with Onion, Fish Sce)	750	30	10
Ca Chien Gung, (Whole Snapper/Ginger)	600	16	6
Canh Chay, (Vegetable/Tofu Soup)	80	3	13
Cari Chicken, 1 cup	475	29	16
Cari Chicken, with Rice Noodle,			
1 cup curry & 1 cup noodles	660	29	60
Cari Chicken, with Steamed Rice,			
1 cup curry & 1 cup rice	650	29	55
Cuu Xao Lan, (Curried Lamb and			
Veggies in Coconut)	900	40	80
Ga Chien, (Crisp Chick + Plum Sauce)	900	40	105
Ga Nuong, (Chicken Satay + Sauce)	240	10	4
Ga Xao Rau, (Marinated Chicken			
Braised with Vegetables)	800	26	100
Gio Lua, (Lean Pork Pie), ⅙ of pie	245	12	0
Goi Cuon, (Cold Spring Rolls), 1 roll	60	1	7
Rau Cai Xao Chay, (Stir Fried Veggies)	400	15	65
Thit Bo Vien, (Beef Balls), 6 balls	225	14	2
Thit Heo Goi Baup Cai,			
(Spicy Cabb. Rolls with Pork), 1 roll	200	7	11
Soup: *Per Bowl, ½ Cup*			
Bun Bo Hue, (Hot & Spicy Soup):			
Without Pork Feet	340	9	35
With Pork Feet	830	45	35
Chicken & Rice Noodle Soup	400	3	55
Pho Bo, (Beef Noodle Soup)	410	7	59
Pho Ga, (Chicken Noodle Soup)	460	6	58
Pho Tai, (Rare Beef & Noodle Soup)	440	7	73
Salad, Goi Du Du,			
(Green Papaya), ½ cup	155	3	29
Sauce, Nuoc Cham (Hot Sauce)	5	0	1

Gourmet & Miscellaneous

	C	F	Cb
Ants Eggs/Larvae, 1 Tbsp	20	0	0
Ants, chocolate coated, 3 Tbsp	140	7	2
Bee Maggots, canned, 3 Tbsp	65	2	0
Caviar, black/red, 1 Tbsp	40	3	0
Caterpillars, canned, 2 oz	60	2	0
Frog Legs, fried, 1 pair (large)	125	7	0
Haggis, boiled, 4 oz	350	24	22
Locusts, roasted, 1 oz	35	1	0
Silkworms, raw, 1 oz	60	2	0
Snails in garlic butter, 6 large	200	10	4
Snake, roasted, 4 oz	160	6	0

Fast - Foods & *Restaurants*

Nutritional data is based on U.S. outlets

For More Restaurants & Full Nutritional Data
~ See CalorieKing.com

Fast - Foods & Restaurants

A&W® (Sept '17)
California Restaurants Only

	C	F	Cb
Burgers: Cheeseburger	400	21	39
Double Cheeseburger	455	26	40
Hamburger	340	16	39
Original: Bacon Cheeseburger	440	25	41
Bacon Double Cheeseburger	645	41	42
Papa Burger	550	33	43
Sandwiches:			
Crispy Chicken	440	18	51
Grilled Chicken: 1 tender	400	15	40
2 Tenders	475	13	51
Chicken Tenders, breaded, 3 pcs	260	9	5
Corn Dog Nuggets: Kid's 5 pieces	180	8	20
10 pieces	350	17	40
Hot Dogs: Plain	310	19	23
Coney Chili Dog	340	20	26
Coney Cheese Dog	380	23	28
Fries/Sides: Cheese Curds, 5 oz	570	40	27
Chili Cheese Fries, 7 oz	410	17	52
French Fries:			
Small/Kids, 2.5 oz	200	8	29
Regular, 4 oz	310	13	45
Large, 5.5 oz	430	17	61
Onion Rings, 7-9 rings	350	16	45
Sauces: Per 1.25 oz			
BBQ	90	0	22
Honey Mustard	140	11	10
Papas, Regular/Spicy	170	15	8
Spicy Ketchup	60	0	15
A & W Root Beer: Small, 16 fl.oz	220	0	58
Regular, 20 fl.oz	270	0	72
Large, 32 fl.oz	440	0	116
Famous Floats:			
A&W Root Beer Float:			
16 oz Cup	330	5	70
20 oz Cup	350	6	77
32 oz Cup	640	10	136
Diet Root Beer, 16 oz	170	5	30
Orange Float, 16 oz	320	5	74
Freeze:			
A&W Root Beer: 16 oz	370	8	68
32 oz	820	18	150
Diet Root Beer, 16 oz	270	8	39
Orange, 16 oz	420	8	82
Polar Swirls: Oreo/M&M's, av. 12 oz	700	25	107
Reese's, 12 oz	740	31	97
Shakes: Strawberry, 16 oz	670	29	90
Chocolate/Vanilla, av. 16 oz	710	30	100
20 oz Cup	890	38	123
Soft Serve: Includes Cone			
Small, 4 oz	200	5	32
Large, 5.5 oz	260	7	41
Sundaes: Choc./Strawberry, av.	310	8	50
Caramel/Hot Fudge, av.	350	10	56

Applebees® (Sept '17)
Appetizers: As Served

	C	F	Cb
Boneless Wings, plain	680	35	52
Dressings: Bleu Cheese	240	25	1
Classic Buffalo; Ranch, av.	205	21	2
Sauces: Honey BBQ	230	0	55
Sweet Asian Chili	250	2	56
Brew Pub Pretzels & Beer Chse Dip	1050	44	130
Cheeseburger Eggrolls	990	61	77
Chicken Quesadillas	840	51	59
Chips & Salsa	630	27	89
Grilled Chicken Wonton Tacos	460	17	47
Mozzarella Sticks	910	50	79
Salsa Verde Beef Nachos	1750	117	107
Spinach & Artichoke Dip	960	58	91
Steak Quesadilla	870	52	59
Burgers: *Without Sides*			
Classic Burger: without cheese	630	33	44
with Cheddar; Monterey Jack, av.	715	40	44
with Swiss	790	45	44
Quesadilla Burger	1180	85	42
The All Day Brunch	1170	77	61
The American Standard	1010	68	48
Triple Bacon	1170	81	46
Chicken: *Includes Standard Sides*			
Bourbon Street Chicken & Shrimp	640	31	41
Chicken Tenders, Basket	1150	66	101
Crispy Brewhouse Chkn	1080	62	80
Fiesta Lime Chicken	1140	63	91
Handhelds: *Without Sides*			
BBQ Brisket Tacos	1220	70	101
Chicken Fajita Rollup	1060	65	60
Clubhouse Grille	1100	63	82
Nashville Hot Chicken Sandwich	1340	90	91
Lighter Fare: *Includes Standard Sides*			
Caprese Mozzarella Chicken	700	32	47
Cedar Grilled Lemon Chicken	580	26	48
Pepper-Crusted Sirloin & Wh. Grains	380	3	38
Shrimp Wonton Stir Fry	630	15	98
Pasta: *As Served*			
4-Cheese Mac & Cheese,			
w/ Honey Pepper Chkn Tenders	1460	64	155
Spin. & Artichoke Gr. Chkn Cavatappi	1040	44	110
Three-Cheese Chicken Cavatappi	1280	70	108
Seafood: *Includes Standard Sides*			
Double Crunch Shrimp	1230	58	145
Hand-Battered Fish & Chips	1520	102	105
Hand Breaded Fish & Chips	1570	98	121
New England Fish & Chips	1990	137	134

Updated Nutrition Data ~ www.CalorieKing.com
Persons with Diabetes ~ See Disclaimer (Page 22)

Applebees® cont... (Sept '17)

From-The Grill: Without Sides

	C	F	Cb
6 oz USDA Sirloin	230	9	2
8 oz USDA Sirloin	280	10	2
Butcher's Reserve 12 oz Top Sirloin	380	11	1
Cedar Grilled Salmon	340	22	2
Chef's Selection:			
Cedar Salmon w/ Maple Mustard	540	32	28
Grilled Shrimp Skewer	110	10	1
Shrimp 'N Parmesan Sirloin, 8 oz	580	37	6
Double Glazed Baby Back Ribs:			
Full Rack, without Sauce	790	50	4
Half Rack, without Sauce	390	25	2
Grilled Chicken Breast	190	4	2
Memphis Dry Rub, half rack	550	30	30
Sauce:			
Honey BBQ: Full rack	150	0	37
Half rack	80	0	18
Texas Style BBQ Sauce: Full rack	280	3	64
Half rack	170	2	38
Salads: Per Regular, with Dressing			
Crispy Chicken & Cornbread	1400	94	78
Grilled Chicken & Cornbread	1090	70	53
Oriental Grilled Chicken	1290	85	84
Pecan Crusted Chicken	1280	74	108
Southwestern Steak Salad	990	64	65
Fries & Sides: As Served			
4-Cheese Mac & Cheese	440	21	40
Baked Potato	390	24	41
Loaded	460	29	41
Classic Fries	430	20	57
Garlic Mashed Potatoes	260	14	30
Garlic Mashed Potatoes, loaded	490	34	34
Garlicky Green Beans	200	16	11
House Salad, w/out Dressing	190	12	11
Steamed Broccoli	90	8	6
Sweet Potato Fries	400	20	51
Wood-Fired Grilled Veggies	150	12	9
Soup:			
Chicken Tortilla Soup	180	8	20
Chili	340	18	14
French Onion	380	22	27
New England Clam Chowder	270	18	18
Souhwest Steak & Black Bean	180	6	18
Tomato Basil Soup	190	12	16
Desserts:			
Apple Chimi Cheesecake	1020	39	155
Blue Ribbon Brownie	1670	78	220
Chocolate Chip Cookie Sundae	1490	64	211
Hot Fudge Sundae	470	23	58
Triple Choc. Meltdown	980	52	125

Arby's® (Apr '18)

Sandwiches:

	C	F	Cb
Beef 'n Cheddar: Classic	450	20	45
Double	630	32	48
Half Pound	740	39	48
Roast Beef: Classic	360	14	37
Double	510	24	38
Half Pound	610	30	38
Buttermilk Chicken:			
Buffalo Chicken	550	26	52
Chicken Bacon & Swiss	660	33	55
Chicken Cordon Bleu	700	36	52
Crispy Chicken	560	27	52
Signature: Loaded Italian	680	40	49
Reuben	680	31	62
Roast Beef Gyro	550	29	48
Smokehouse Brisket	600	35	42
Turkey Gyro	470	20	48
Turkey:			
Grand Turkey Club	480	24	37
Roast Turkey & Swiss	710	28	79
Roast Turkey, Ranch & Bacon	800	34	79
Wraps: Roast Turkey & Swiss	520	29	39
Roast Turkey, Ranch & Bacon	620	34	39
Sliders: Buffalo Chicken	290	13	31
Chicken Tender 'n Cheese	290	12	30
Ham 'n Cheese	230	9	22
Jalapeno Roast Beef 'n Cheese	240	11	21
Roast Beef 'n Cheese	240	11	21
Chicken Tenders: 3 pieces	360	17	28
5 pieces	600	28	47
Dipping Sauces: Buffalo, 1 oz	10	1	2
Honey Mustard, 1 oz	140	13	5
Ranch, 1 oz	100	11	2
Curly Fries: Small, 4.5 oz	410	22	49
Medium, 6 oz	550	29	65
Large, 7 oz	650	35	77
Loaded Curly Fries, 8.2 oz	700	46	57
Snacks:			
Jalapeno Bites:			
5 pieces, no sauce	290	17	31
8 pieces, no sauce	470	27	50
Mozzarella Sticks: 4 pieces	440	23	37
6 pieces	650	35	56
Potato Cakes: 3 pcs	370	21	35
4 pieces	490	28	46
Steakhouse Onion Rings, 5 rings	420	21	52

continued next page...

Arby's® cont... (Jan '18)

Salads: Without Dressing

Chopped Farmhouse:	C	F	Cb
Crispy Chicken	430	24	26
Roast Turkey	230	13	8
Side Salad	70	5	4

Dressings: *Per 1.5 oz Packet*

	C	F	Cb
Balsamic Vinaigrette	130	12	4
Buttermilk Ranch	210	22	2
Dijon Honey Mustard	180	16	8
Light Italian	20	1	2
Kids Menu: Chicken Tenders (2)	240	11	19
Curly Fries, 2.75 oz	250	13	29
Roast Beef 'n Cheese Slider	240	11	21

Breakfast: *Per Serving*

Biscuits: Bacon, Egg & Cheese	480	29	38
Ham, Egg & Cheese	470	25	39
Sausage, Egg & Cheese	640	45	39
Croissants: Bacon, Egg & Cheese	440	27	29
Ham, Egg & Cheese	420	23	30
Sausage, Egg & Cheese	590	44	30
Sourdoughs:			
Bacon, Egg & Cheese	490	23	46
Ham, Egg & Cheese	470	19	47
Sausage, Egg & Cheese	640	39	47
Wraps: Bacon, Egg & Cheese	500	27	42
Ham, Egg & Cheese	440	22	42
Sausage, Egg & Cheese	630	41	42
Sauces: Arby's, 0.5 oz	15	0	3
Bronco Berry, 1 oz	60	0	15
Cheddar Cheese, 1.5 oz	50	3.5	4
Horsey, 0.5 oz	60	5	3
Marinara, 1 oz	20	0	4
Spicy Three Pepper, 0.5 oz	25	1	3
Tangy BBQ, 1 oz	40	0	9
Turnovers: Apple	430	18	65
Cherry	390	13	65
Iced Tea, Unsweetened	5	0	1
Juice, Capri Sun Fruit Juice, 6.5 oz	80	0	21

Shakes: Per Small

Chocolate; Jamocha	545	18	88
Vanilla	450	17	67

Sodas: Without Ice

Dr Pepper, Small	180	0	48
Mist Twist, Small	190	0	50
Mountain Dew, Small	200	0	54
Pepsi, Small	180	0	49

Atlanta Bread Co® (Nov '16)

Breakfast Sandwiches:

	C	F	Cb
Egg & Cheese	410	13	55
Egg, Cheese & Ham	460	15	56
Egg, Cheese & Turkey Sausage	520	20	56
Side, Breakfast Potatoes	170	9	20
Sandwiches: Chicken Salad	630	27	59
Honey Maple Ham	420	7	66
Roast Beef	400	6	57
Roasted Turkey	380	3	58
Veggie	460	17	59

Half Sandwich/Panini & Half Salad Options:
Without Salad Dressing or Sandwich Condiments

Hummus & Edamame S'wch & Greek Salad	370	24	24
Ital. Veggie Panini w/ Caesar Salad	330	22	23
Rst Beef S'wich w/ Mont Amore Salad	300	10	34
Tuna Salad S'wich w/ Bals. Blue Salad	520	25	56
Veggie Sandwich with Greek Salad	360	17	38

Salads: Without Dressing or Bread

Buffalo Chicken	280	12	14
Chardonnay Brie	260	16	18
Salsa Fresca Salmon	280	11	23
Sides: Edamame	150	4.5	14
Black Beans & Corn	190	9	24

Au Bon Pain® (Sept '17)

Bagels: Per Bagel

	C	F	Cb
Asiago Cheese, 3.9 oz	330	7	50
Cinnamon Crisp, 3.9 oz	370	6	71
Everything, 3.3 oz	260	2	52
Honey 9 Grain, 3.6 oz	280	2	56
Onion Dill, 3.6 oz	260	1	53
Plain Bagel, 3.2 oz	250	1	51
Whole Wheat Skinny, 1.6 oz	90	1	21

Breakfast Sandwiches:

2 Eggs on a Bagel	390	11	51
with Bacon	450	15	51
with Cheese	450	16	51
Egg Whites, Cheddar w/ Skinny Bagel	210	7	22
Smoked Salmon Wasabi, on Onion Dill Bagel	390	9	58
Fruit Cup, Large, 12 oz	140	0.5	36
Yogurt/Parfait:			
Blueb. Yogurt & Wild Blueb. 10.2 oz	380	10	68
Greek, Van. Yog. & Wild Blueb., 10.2 oz	340	8	47
Strawb. & Greek Nonfat Yog.,11.3 oz	340	8	48
Oatmeal, Classic Medium, 12 oz	260	5	47

Sandwiches: Whole

Cafe: BLT	470	22	52
Black Angus Roast Beef & Cheddar	570	21	61
Herb Chicken Salad	470	13	58
Tuna Salad	460	10	60
Turkey & Swiss	660	28	66
Signature: Turkey Club	600	25	53
Chipotle Turkey & Avocado	680	30	63

Updated Nutrition Data ~ www.CalorieKing.com
Persons with Diabetes ~ See Disclaimer (Page 22)

Au Bon Pain® cont... (Sept '17)

Harvest Hot Bowls:	C	F	Cb
Mayan Chicken	600	16	81
Mediterranean Chicken	760	6	75
Roasted Vegetarian	770	40	83
Teriyaki Steak	600	9	96
Macaroni & Cheese, medium, 12 oz	880	43	92
Meat Lasagna, 10.7 oz	470	24	41
Soups: Chicken Gumbo, 12 fl.oz	200	9	23
Chicken Noodle, 12 f.loz	120	2.5	15
Clam Chowder, 12 fl.oz	350	20	32
French Onion, 12 fl.oz	110	5	15
Harvest Pumpkin, 12 fl.oz	230	13	24
Lobster & Corn Bisque, 12 fl.oz	280	16	25
Minestrone, 12 fl.oz	180	6	24
Vegetarian Chili, 12 fl.oz	260	2	46
Salads: Without Dressing			
Chicken Caesar Asiago	280	10	20
Chicken Cobb, w/ Avocado	440	26	15
Harvest Turkey	390	15	35
Vegetarian Deluxe	270	13	28
Dressings: Bleu Cheese, 2 oz	310	33	2
Caesar, 2 oz	250	25	3
Lite Buttermilk Ranch, 2 oz	120	11	5
Cakes, Cookies, Croissants : Per Item			
Brownie Bites, 5 oz	600	25	82
Cakes: Red Velvet Cupcake, 3 oz	400	22	46
Pound Cakes: Iced Lemon, 4.5 oz	470	21	66
Marble, 4 oz	450	24	54
Cookies: Chocolate Chip	370	18	54
Oatmeal Raisin	290	11	46
Croissants: Almond, 4 oz	500	31	48
Apple & Cinn., 3.4 oz	220	8	35
Chocolate, 4 oz	470	25	55
Ham & Cheese Croissant	410	22	25
Danish: Peach, 5 oz	400	15	60
Sweet Cheese, 4.7 oz	440	21	56
Muffins: Blueberry, 4.9 oz	480	25	59
Double Choc. Chunk, 4.7 oz	580	30	66
Raisin Bran, 4.7 oz	430	12	75
Palmier, 2.6 oz	380	20	46
Pecan Roll, 6 oz	740	42	86
Beverages: Caffe Latte, 16 fl.oz	140	7	12
Caramel Macchiato, 16 fl.oz	270	7	43
Hot Chocolate, 16 fl.oz	350	12	51
Raspberry Iced Tea, 24 fl.oz	180	0	50
Strawberry Smoothie, 16 fl.oz	290	0	68

Extra Menu Items ~ See CalorieKing.com

Auntie Anne's® (Sept '17)

Pretzels: With Butter	C	F	Cb
Cinnamon Sugar	470	12	84
Jalapeno	330	5	63
Original	340	5	65
Original Stix, 6 sticks	340	5	65
Pepperoni	480	16	65
Sour Cream & Onion	360	5	68
Sweet Almond	390	6	74
Dipping Sauces:			
Caramel Dip, 1.7 oz	170	2	37
Cheese Dip, 1.4 oz	100	8	2
Hot Salsa Dip, 1.1 oz	90	7	4
Light Cream Cheese, 1.25 oz	80	6	1
Marinara, 2 oz	45	1	7
Melted Cheese, 2 oz	150	12	6
Sweet Glaze, 1.7 oz	150	0	38
Sweet Mustard, 1.5 oz	90	3	14
Pretzel Dogs: Original	360	20	33
Cheese	370	20	33
Jalapeno & Cheese	370	20	34
Jumbo	610	29	67
Mini Pretzel Dogs (10)	630	35	56
Beverages: Per 16 fl.oz			
Frozen Lemonade Mixer,			
Blue Raspberry; Strawberry, av.	260	0	66

Back Yard Burgers® (Sept '17)

Black Angus Burgers: W/ Whtie Bun	C	F	Cb
Back Yard: Classic Burger	570	28	46
Double Classic	850	47	46
Black Jack Burger	670	40	42
Black & Bleu Burger	770	48	44
Chipotle Burger	800	46	56
Mushroom Swiss Burger	670	38	42
Chicken Sandwiches: With White Bun			
Blackened Chicken	580	25	50
Black Jack Chicken Club	730	41	46
Grilled Chicken	440	12	45
Hawaiian Chicken	500	12	59
Specialties:			
Chicken Tenders Basket,			
without Toppings, Sce or Bread	540	36	27
Veggie Burger, without Cheese	390	8	67
Turkey Burgers: With White Bun, without Cheese			
Classic	520	29	41
Club	580	34	41
Wild	520	27	43

continued next page ...

Fast - Foods & Restaurants

Back Yard Burgers® cont... (Sept '17)

Fries:	C	F	Cb
Chili Cheese Fries, seasoned, reg.	790	59	52
Seasoned Fries: Regular, 4.5 oz	480	36	38
Large, 6 oz	640	47	50
Sweet Potato Fries, regular, 6 oz	600	39	54
Waffle Fries: Kid's, 4.5 oz	620	42	49
Regular, 6 oz	820	56	66
Sides: Back Yard Chili	310	18	15
Coleslaw	35	1.5	4.5
Loaded Baked Potato	540	21	70
Panko Onion Rings, regular, 4 oz	300	14	37
Salads: Without Dressing			
Back Yard Salad: w. Grilled Chicken	360	12	23
with Blackened Chicken	470	23	23
Cranberry Pecan Chicken	690	31	53
Side Salad	140	6	14
Dressings: Bleu Cheese	220	24	1
Gorgonzola Vinaigrette	170	15	6
Honey Mustard	240	23	7
Ranch, Homestyle	150	15	2
Dessert/Cobblers: Apple/Cherry	390	16	58
Apple/Cherry Cobbler A La Mode	540	24	78
Ice Cream, A La Carte	150	8	20
Milk Shakes: With Whole Milk & Whipped Topping			
Chocolate	710	33	94
Chocolate Oreo	840	39	113

Baja Fresh® (Sept '17)

Baja Bowls: With Black Beans	C	F	Cb
Carnitas	680	18	92
Chicken	700	22	82
Shrimp	660	20	83
Steak	690	22	82
Veggie	540	14	90
Burritos: With Standard Components			
Baja: with Carnitas	800	41	63
with Chicken	820	46	53
with Steak	810	45	53
Bean & Cheese: With Pinto Beans			
Carnitas	1060	40	113
Chicken	1080	44	103
Steak	1070	44	103
Mexicano: With Black Beans			
Chicken	800	27	94
Steak	790	26	94
Ultimo: Carnitas	950	45	88
Chicken	970	50	78
Steak	960	50	78
Nachos: Regular Size, with Black Beans			
Carnitas	1110	56	106
Chicken	1150	60	101
Steak	1140	60	101

Baja Fresh® cont... (Sept '17)

Fajitas: With Pinto Beans	C	F	Cb
Chicken: with Corn Tortillas	1060	39	121
with Flour Tortillas	1250	44	146
Shrimp: with Corn Tortillas	990	35	123
with Flour Tortilla	1180	41	148
Steak: with Corn Tortillas	1050	38	121
with Flour Tortilla	1240	45	149
Wahoo: with Corn Tortillas	990	35	121
with Flour Tortillas	1180	40	146
Tacos: With Standard Toppings			
Americano, Soft Taco: Carnitas	220	9	21
Chicken	230	11	19
Wahoo, Crispy Taco	250	15	24
Baja, meat varieties, average	160	6	17
Salads: Without Dressing			
Baja Ensalada: with Carnitas	300	9	28
with Chicken	260	11	18
with Shrimp	280	12	19
with Steak	250	11	17
Tostada: Carnitas & Pinto Beans	1010	48	99
Chicken & Black Beans	1020	53	86
Shrimp & Pinto Beans	1000	51	90
Steak & Black Beans	1020	52	86
Sides: Guacamole, 8 oz	310	27	19
Rice & Black Beans	550	11	90
Rice & Pinto Beans	570	11	95
Tortilla Chips, 5 oz	710	28	99
Tortilla Chips & Guacamole	1020	55	119

For Complete Nutritional Data ~ see CalorieKing.com

Baskin Robbins® (Apr '18)

Cones:	C	F	Cb
Cake	25	0	5
Fresh-Baked Waffle	160	3.5	29
Sugar	45	0.5	9
Ice Creams: Per 4 oz Scoop			
Classic Flavors: Cherries Jubilee	220	11	26
Chocolate Chip	250	16	23
Chocolate	240	14	26
Jamoca Almond Fudge	260	15	28
Mint Chocolate Chip	250	16	23
Old Fashioned Butter Pecan	260	18	20
Oreo Cookies 'n Cream	260	15	27
Peanut Butter 'n Chocolate	300	20	25
Pistachio Almond	270	19	21
Pralines 'n Cream	270	14	32
Reese's P'nut Butter Cup	300	17	32
Rocky Road	270	15	29
Rum Raisin	240	11	29
Vanilla	240	16	21
Very Berry Strawberry	200	11	24
Wild 'n Reckless Sherbet	130	2	25

180

Updated Nutrition Data ~ www.CalorieKing.com
Persons with Diabetes ~ See Disclaimer (Page 22)

Baskin Robbins® cont... (Apr '18)

Ice Creams (Cont): Per 4 oz Scoop	C	F	Cb
Seasonal Flavors: Black Walnut	270	18	21
Chocolate Fudge	240	15	27
Creole Cream Cheese	230	13	24
Strawberry Cheesecake	250	13	28

Grab-N-Go: Per 1.3 oz Cookie

	C	F	Cb
Dark Chocolate Chunk Cookie	170	7	26
Double Fudge Cookie	160	6	26
Peanut Butter 'n Chocolate Cookie	160	7	23
White Chunk Macadamia Cookie			

Ice Cream Quarts: Per ½ Cup

	C	F	Cb
Chocolate	170	9	21
Mint Chocolate Chip	170	10	18
Vanilla, 2.6 oz	170	10	17

Soft Serve:

	C	F	Cb
Cups: Vanilla: Kid's, 3 oz	110	4.5	14
Regular, 6 oz	230	9	29
Large, 9 oz	340	14	43
Parfaits: M&M's, Regular	820	32	119
Oreo, Regular	710	28	104
Snickers, Regular	730	24	114

31 Below' Mix-In: Per 16 oz Medium Cup

	C	F	Cb
Butterfinger	850	34	120
Choc. Chip Cookie Dough	870	32	129
Heath	910	46	111
M&M's	1000	40	139
Oreo	720	29	99
Reese's PB Cup	910	45	109

Sundaes:

	C	F	Cb
Banana Royale	680	33	90
Brownie	810	42	99
Chocolate Chip Cookie Dough	1100	47	160
Made with Snickers	1060	43	155
Two Scoop	570	33	63
Warm Brownie	810	42	99

Beverages: Per Medium, 24 fl.oz

	C	F	Cb
Blasts: Caramel Cappuccino	790	25	130
Mocha Cappuccino	610	22	97
Fruit Blast: Mango	500	1.5	123
Strawberry Citrus	350	0	89
Tropical	370	0.5	93
Milk Shakes: Chocolate Chip	1030	54	117
Mint Chocolate Chip	1030	55	117
Smoothie: Mango Banana	620	2	149
Strawberry Banana	520	1	126
Tropical Banana	540	1.5	130

Big Apple Bagels® (Sept '17)

Bagels:	C	F	Cb
Regular, average all flavors, 5 oz	340	2	70
Bab's Choice Bagels, av., 5 oz	380	8	65

Cream Cheese: Per 2 Tbsp, 1 oz

	C	F	Cb
Plain/Cheddar/Veg./Onion, av.	90	9	2
Plain, Lite	60	4.5	3
Strawberry	90	7	5

Muffins:

	C	F	Cb
Mini: Blueberry (2), 2 oz	170	8	22
Cinnamon Swirl Cheesecake (2)	215	11	28
Lemon Poppyseed (2), 2 oz	200	10	25
Jumbo: Blueberry, 6 oz	510	24	66
Chocolate Cheesecake, 6 oz	600	36	66

Sandwiches:

	C	F	Cb
Breakfast: BLT	705	31	83
Lox & Cream Cheese	600	21	78
Morning Classic	485	11	73
Gourmet: Classic Turkey	550	14	74
Kick-N Roast Beef	580	15	79

Specialty:

	C	F	Cb
Big Apple Club	795	37	75
Chicken Caesar	610	19	78
Overstuffed: Classic Reuben	960	43	57
Corned Beef/Pastrami	660	19	77
Manhattan Club	1120	40	120
Toasted: Chicken Melt	815	32	80
Spicy Italian Sub	770	34	77
Tuna Melt	640	23	75

Biggby Coffee® (Jan '18)

Hot Drinks: Per Tall, 16 fl.oz, without Whipped Cream & Sugar	C	F	Cb
Caffe au Lait: with 2% Milk	100	4	9
with Non-Fat Milk	65	0	9
with Soy	90	3	11
Caffe Latte: with 2% Milk	175	7.5	16
with Non-Fat Milk	115	0	16
with Soy	160	5	19
Cappuccino: with 2% Milk	105	4.5	10
with Non-Fat Milk	70	0	10
with Soy	95	3	11
Chai Latte: with 2% Milk	315	7.5	51
with Non-Fat Milk	255	0	51
Dark Hot Chocolate: w/ 2% Milk	320	9	50
with Non-Fat Milk	260	1.5	50

Frozen Creme Freeze: Per 20 fl.oz, with 2% Milk, Whipped Cream & Sugar, without Reduced Calorie

	C	F	Cb
Avalanche Latte	640	19	108
Banana Chip	750	20	135
Coconut Creme	640	19	110
Mellow Mocha	645	19	109

Fast - Foods & *Restaurants*

BJ's Restaurant® (Sept '17)

Shareable Appetizers: Full Order	C	F	Cb
Ahi Poke	320	10	24
Boneless Wings, Hot & Spicy Buffalo	890	41	62
Mozzarella Sticks	810	39	76
Root Beer Glazed Ribs	490	21	61
Sliders	880	32	97

Handcrafted Burgers: Includes Thin Fries
Bacon Cheeseburger	1420	85	99
BJ's Brewhouse Burger	1040	52	95
Black & Bleu-House Bgr	1200	65	97
Classic Burger	1250	71	98
Portobello Swiss Burger	1460	82	107

Brunch: Avocado Toast
Avocado Toast	410	20	47
BJ's B'milk Pancakes, short stack	910	32	136
BJ's California Scramble	1140	64	84
EnLIGHTened Veggie Omelette	270	9	24

Enlightened Entrees: Includes Menu Set Sides
Cherry Chipotle Glazed Salmon	590	26	40
Mediterranean Chicken Pita Tacos	670	20	79
North Beach Mahi-Mahi & Shrimp	560	18	42
Quinoa Bowls: Roasted Salmon	1040	56	77
Roasted Chicken & Spinach	890	41	73
Seared Ahi Salad	580	31	43

Pasta: Includes Garlic Knot
Deep Dish Ziti	1400	91	99
Gr. Chicken Alfredo	1380	69	129
Italiano Vegetable Penne	740	31	93
Jumbo Spaghetti & Meatballs	1450	66	162
Shrimp & Asparagus Penne	730	21	97

Pizza, Deep Dish: Per Slice, ⅛ Med. Pizza
BBQ/Buffalo Chicken, average	310	10	35
BJ's Classic Combo;Pepperoni, av.	335	17	32
BJ's Favorite	310	15	33
Spicy Hawaiian Chkn	350	15	36
Sweet Pig; Vegetarian, average	265	10	34

Pizza, Tavern-Cut: Per Slice (1/12 Pizza)
Brewhouse; Italian Market	110	6	9
Garlic Chicken Pesto	100	5	9
Spicy Pig/Old Country Tomato, av.	80	4	10

Sandwiches: Includes Crispy Thin Fries
Barbeque Pulled Pork	1460	54	174
Calif. Chicken Club/Rst Beef, av.	1315	68	96
Triple Decker Sandwich	1310	67	99

Ribs & Steaks: Without Sides
Baby Back Pork Ribs, Half Rack	710	34	75
BJ's Classic Rib-eye	1080	67	5
House Top Sirloin	500	32	2

Fries: Crispy-Thin Fries
Crispy-Thin Fries	390	23	42
Wedge-Cut Seasoned Fries	390	21	48

Soups: Chicken Tortilla, Bowl
Chicken Tortilla, Bowl	280	12	30
Clam Chowder: Bowl	430	26	33
Sourdough Loaf	1470	42	219

BJ's Restaurant® cont... (Sept '17)

Salads: With Dressing & Toppings	C	F	Cb
BBQ Chicken Chopped Salad	930	48	64
Caesar Salad	810	64	44
Derby-Style Chkn Cobb	1060	74	19
Honey-Crisp Chicken	1370	103	77
Santa Fe	980	57	55

Desserts: Baked Beignet
Baked Beignet	630	25	91
Monkey Bread Pizookie	1260	56	177
Salted Caramel Pizookie	1360	55	200
Soda Floats, average all flav.	510	19	82

Drinks: Cream Sodas, average
Cream Sodas, average	165	0	41
Handcrafted Root Beer	200	0	51
Lemonade	210	0	53

For Complete Nutritional Data ~ see CalorieKing.com

Blimpie® (Sept '17)

Cold Deli Subs:	C	F	Cb

Per Regular, 6" White Sub, with Standard Menu Board Toppings
Blimpie Best	470	17	54
Club; Ham & Swiss	430	14	54
Roast Beef & Provolone	460	14	53
Tuna	460	21	41
Turkey & Provolone	480	22	48

Wraps: Chicken Caesar
Chicken Caesar	570	28	50
Southwestern	580	31	53

Hot Deli Subs: Per Regular White Sub with Standard Menu Board Toppings Unless Indicated
BLT	510	27	48
Meatball Parmigiana	740	38	59
Philly Cheesesteak	570	28	49

Salads: Regular, without Dressing
Buffalo Chicken	180	8	9
Garden	40	0	8
Grilled Chicken	160	5	6
Ultimate Club	310	16	11

Dressings: Creamy Caesar, 1.5 oz
Creamy Caesar, 1.5 oz	210	23	2
Creamy Italian, 1.5 oz	180	18	4
Thousand Island	210	20	6

Soups: Per 8.6 oz
Chicken Noodle	210	4	29
Cream of Broccoli with Cheese	190	11	15
Cream of Potato with Bacon	190	9	24
New England Clam Chowder	170	3	28
Vegetable Beef with Barley	100	3	14

Breakfast:
Biscuits: Bacon, Egg & Cheese
Bacon, Egg & Cheese	410	22	37
Sausage, Egg & Cheese	560	36	37
Bluffin, Egg & Cheese	240	8	29

Burritos: Ham, Egg & Cheese
Ham, Egg & Cheese	580	30	50
Sausage, Egg & Cheese	710	43	50
Sandwich, Grilled Bacon	520	23	49

Updated Nutrition Data ~ www.CalorieKing.com
Persons with Diabetes ~ See Disclaimer (Page 22)

Bob Evans® (Sept '17)

	C	**F**	**Cb**
Appetizers: With Listed Sauces			
Onion Petals	860	45	105
Twisted Cheese Sticks	640	38	52
Burgers: Low Calorie			
Big Farm Burgers:			
Hamburger	1150	81	50
Bacon Cheeseburger	840	50	51
Three Cheese Burger	780	44	50
Sandwiches: Low Calorie, with Set Menu Items			
Bob Evans Farmboy	650	37	46
Farmhouse Gr. Chkn	820	40	56
Five Chse Gr. Chse	1020	64	72
Farmouse Fried Chicken	880	49	73
Slow Roasted:			
Ham & Cheese	910	42	76
Pot Roast	840	50	51
Turkey Bacon Melt	640	32	48
Dinners: Low Calorie Option with Set Menu Items			
Beef: Black Angus Chopped Steak	920	64	53
Blackened USDA Choice Sirloin	920	53	55
Country Fried Steak	920	52	86
USDA Choice Sirloin	1030	64	55
Chicken:			
Breasts: Farm, 1 breast	570	23	48
Wildfire, 1 breast	600	23	54
Chicken Pot Pie	1370	86	117
Chicken Tenders, Homestyle	1020	54	94
Seafood: Gr. Salmon Fillet	740	41	48
Biscuit Breaded Fried Shrimp	860	46	88
Potato Crusted Flounder	640	31	61
Wildfire Grilled Salmon Fillet	790	41	61
Slow Roasted Entrees: Pot Roast	920	55	65
Turkey & Dressing	1090	52	112
Sides: Baked Potato	330	12	51
Loaded	570	32	53
Bread & Celery Dressing	340	15	42
Broccoli, with Butter	110	10	5
Coleslaw	200	14	19
French Fries	330	14	47
Glazed Baby Carrots	90	4.5	13
Green Beans with Ham	30	1.5	4
Hash Browns	220	12	28
Golden Brown Home Fries	250	17	24
Mac & Cheese	250	12	25
Mashed Potatoes: w/ Chicken Gravy	210	14	19
with Country Gravy	170	10	17
Sauces: Per 1 oz Ramekin			
A.1.	25	0	5
Bob Evans Wildfire	50	0	13
Honey Mustard	120	11	5
Ranch	100	10	0.5
Sriracha-Avocado Mayo	160	18	0.5

Bob Evans® cont... (Sept '17)

	C	**F**	**Cb**
Soups: Per Bowl, with 2 Saltine Crackers			
Cheddar Baked Potato	390	21	32
Chicken N Noodles	290	15	26
Farm Festival Bean	300	4.5	48
Hearty Beef Vegetable	230	5	36
Sausage Chili	460	29	35
Salads: High Calorie, with Set Menu Items			
Farmhouse Garden, Colonial Dressing	250	18	17
Dressings: Per 2 oz Ramekin			
Blue Cheese	280	30	4
Buttermilk Ranch	210	21	2
Sweet Italian	230	22	10
Breakfast:			
Farm-Fresh Eggs: *High Calorie, with Set Menu Items*			
Big Egg Breakfast	1350	99	69
Country Fried Steak & Eggs	1500	102	105
Farmers Choice	1470	90	126
Homestead	1500	111	83
Rise & Shine	1280	94	68
Sirloin Steak & Eggs	1470	102	70
3 Egg Omelets: *Low Calorie, with Set Menu Items*			
Veggie	850	58	53
Western	740	43	52
French Toast: *High Calorie, with Set Menu Items*			
Brioche	830	25	134
Hotcakes: *With Whipped Crm & Powdered Sugar*			
Cinnamon Supreme	870	22	153
Double Blueberry	890	19	167
Double Chocolate	910	23	163
Sausage Selection: *Low Calorie, with Set Menu Items*			
Sausage Gravy Bowl	830	49	82
Sunshine Skillet	770	51	51
Breakfast Sides: Banana Nut Bread	420	22	37
B'Milk Biscuit (2), with Butter	520	31	53
Country Gravy, cup	20	0.5	3
English Muffin, with Butter	150	3	25
Fresh Fruit Dish	60	0	14
Golden-Brown Fries	250	17	24
Grits, bowl	390	32	25
Hardwood Smoked Bacon, 1.4 oz	190	14	0.5
Hickory Smoked Ham, 3.5 oz	100	2.5	2
Sausage Gravy, cup	230	16	14
Sausage Links (3)	190	16	0
Sausage Patties (2)	320	26	2
Shredded Hash Browns	220	12	28
Turkey Sausage Links (2)	140	7	2
Wheat Toast with Butter, 2 slices	170	6	24
Dessert: Coconut Cream Pie, 1 slice	590	36	63
French Silk Pie, 1 slice	650	43	59
Peanut Butter Brownie Bites (8)	880	40	120

Fast - Foods & *Restaurants*

Bojangles® (Sept '17)

Biscuit:	C	F	Cb
Plain	340	17	40
Bacon, Egg & Cheese	480	28	42
Cajun Filet	550	27	55
Cajun Gravy Biscuits	460	23	51
Country Ham	450	24	40
Sausage	540	35	40
Sausage, Egg & Cheese	580	38	40
Smoked Sausage	490	29	41
Steak	570	35	49
Chicken: Breast (1)	280	13	10
Leg (1)	100	5	5
Thigh (1)	240	17	9
Wing (1)	100	7	5
Homestyle Tenders, 4 pieces	500	24	41
Supremes, 4 pieces	390	19	29
Sandwiches:			
Cajun Filet: Regular	650	30	65
Club	740	40	70
Grilled Chicken: Regular	470	22	41
Club	570	30	42
Pulled Pork BBQ	460	21	48
Fixins': Per Individual Size, Unless Indicated			
Bo-Tato Rounds, medium	370	19	45
Cole Slaw	170	11	20
Green Beans	40	0	8
Macaroni & Cheese	260	13	29
Mashed Potatoes 'N Cajun Gravy	120	4.5	17
Seasoned Fries: Small	250	16	37
Medium	340	21	50
Picnic size	610	38	90
Salads: Without Dressing or Croutons			
Chicken Supreme	450	24	31
Garden	160	10	10
Grilled Chicken	290	14	11
Sweets: Bo-Berry Biscuit (1)	470	23	61
Cinnamon Twist (1)	370	21	41
Sweet Potato Pie	370	24	35

Boston Market® (Sept '17)

Sandwiches:	C	F	Cb
Per Whole with Set Menu Board Toppings			
All-White Chicken Salad	830	48	62
Meatloaf Carver	880	42	84
Roasted Turkey Carver	810	44	62
Rotisserie Chicken Carver	730	34	63
Individual Meals: Without Sides Or Bread			
Meatloaf, regular	450	26	23
Rotisserie Chicken, half	500	24	1
St Louis Style BBQ Ribs, ½ rack	990	75	22

Boston Market® cont...Mar '17)

Salads: Entree Size, with Dressing	C	F	Cb
Chicken Caesar, 10.8 oz	480	29	17
Mediterranean, 13.4 oz	510	34	17
Southwest Santa Fe, 13.7 oz	550	30	26
Sides: Without Gravy/Sauce			
Creamed Spinach	250	20	11
Fresh Steamed Veggies	60	3.5	7
Fresh Vegetable Stuffing	220	10	28
Green Beans	90	5	7
Macaroni & Cheese	270	9	36
Mashed Potatoes	240	10	32
Rotisserie Potatoes	120	2.5	22
Southwest Rice	260	9	39
Sweet Corn	130	4	21
Sweet Potato Casserole	460	13	83
Soups:			
Chicken Noodle	220	8	21
Chicken Tortilla, with Toppings	320	18	19
Desserts:			
Apple Pie, 1 slice	440	21	58
Chocolate Brownie (1)	310	12	49
Chocolate Cake, 1 slice	560	32	65
Pecan Pie, 1 slice	640	35	75

For Complete Nutritional Data ~ see CalorieKing.com

Boston Pizza® Canada (Sept '17)

Starters:	C	F	Cb
Oven Roasted Wings, 12.5 oz	780	50	9
Poutine, 14 oz	610	30	67
Spinach & Artichoke Dip, 14.7 oz	850	66	36
Burgers: Dble Bacon BBQ Burger	1110	78	60
Pepperoni & Bacon Pizzaburger	1160	75	68
Spicy Perogy Burger	1420	115	54
Gourmet Pastas: Full Order, without Garlic Toast			
Boston's Lasagna	790	23	107
Montréal Smoked Meat Pasta	890	16	142
Spicy Sausage Arrabiata Penne	1230	54	142
Gourmet Pizza: Per Individual Pizza			
Classic Crust: Boston Royal	780	26	97
Deluxe	770	27	92
Hawaiian	700	19	100
Pepperoni	750	28	89
Thin Crust:			
Bacon Double Cheeseburger	520	23	53
The Meateor	520	25	51

Boston Pizza® Canada cont... (Sept '17)

Sandwiches: Without Sides

	C	F	Cb
BBQ Pulled Pork	1070	57	92
Big Dipper	1320	72	117
Boston Brute	800	24	108
Buffalo Chicken	920	35	119
Chipotle Chicken Club	950	4	86
Smoked Meat	910	59	40

Salads: Full Order with Dressing

Crispy Chicken Pecan	1160	88	44
Market Spinach & Shrimp	790	57	36

Desssert:

NY Cheesecake	600	32	76
The Panookie, with ice cream	880	38	133

For Complete Nutritional Data ~ see CalorieKing.com

Braum's® ~ see CalorieKing.com

Bruegger's® (Sept '17)

Bagels:

	C	F	Cb
Blueberry, 4.1 oz	310	2	63
Jalapeno Cheddar, 5.5 oz	440	9	75
Plain, 4.1 oz	300	2	60
Sesame; Whole Wheat, av., 4 oz	310	3	60

Cream Cheese: Per 1.5 oz

Bacon Scallion, Jalapeno, av.	140	12	5
Honey Walnut	150	12	8
Light Herb Garlic/Plain	100	6	4
Plain	130	11	6
Smoked Salmon	150	13	3

Breakfast Bagel S'wiches: With Standard Toppings

Egg & Cheese	430	18	63
Egg White, Cheese & Bacon	460	12	64
Plain Bagel: Smoked Salmon	460	10	66
Sriracha Egg	650	30	70
Western	670	34	67

Deli Sandwiches: With Standard Toppings

BLT on Wheat Bread	610	44	38
Chicken Breast on Plain Bagel	550	6	81
Garden Veggie on Plain Bagel	360	2	72
Ham On Wheat Bread	470	10	67

Hot Paninis: On Ciabatta with Standard Toppings

Four Cheese & Tomato	570	26	59
Harvest Turkey	690	24	84
Primo Pesto Chicken	560	19	58
Roast Beef Cheddar Melt	630	26	72
Tuna Salad on Plain Bagel	520	14	61

Signature & Classic Sandwiches: With Standard Toppings

Herby Turkey/Sesame Bagel	570	15	75
Leon. da Veggie/Asiago Parm. Bgl	490	14	70
Sm. Salmon Egg Salad/Pumpnkl Bgl	580	11	91
Turkey Chipotle Club/Evrythng Bread	810	45	66

Bruegger's® cont... (Sept '17)

Café Salads: Without Dressing

	C	F	Cb
Blue Apple, 7 oz	360	18	30
Chicken Caesar, 7.7 oz	200	8	14
Pastrami Cobb, 10.3 oz	280	16	15

Dressings: Balsamic Vinaig., 1 oz

Balsamic Vinaig., 1 oz	60	6	3
Caesar, 1 oz	80	7	2
Ranch	90	10	1

Dessert Bars:

Chocolate Chunk Brownie, 3.3 oz	440	22	55
Cheesecake Brownie, 3.1 oz	340	18	43
New York Coffee Cake, 5.1 oz	590	29	77

For Complete Menu & Data ~ see CalorieKing.com

Burgerville® (Sept '17)

Burgers: With Standard Ingredients

	C	F	Cb
American Colossal	540	29	40
American ½ lb Colossal	800	47	40
Double Cheeseburger	480	28	31
Original: Hamburger	340	17	31
Cheeseburger	380	21	31
Pepper Bacon Cheeseburger	670	40	37
Tillamook Cheeseburger	600	34	38

Fish & Chips: With Lemon & Tartar Sce

Halibut, 3 pieces	1040	71	73
Halibut, 4 pieces	1130	75	80

Sandwiches: With Menu Set Ingredients

Deluxe Griled Chicken	550	25	42
Deluxe Crispy Chkn	780	43	67
Halibut Fish with Lettuce	460	27	40

French Fries: Small, 2.8 oz

French Fries: Small, 2.8 oz	220	11	28
Regular, 5 oz	400	19	50
Large, 6.5 oz	510	25	65

Salads: Full Size, Without Dressing

Grilled Chicken Club	170	9	4
Smoky Blue Cheese	150	6	17
Wild Smoked Salmon & Hazelnuts	170	11	5

Dressing: Blue Cheese

Dressing: Blue Cheese	180	18	2
Honey Mustard	200	19	8
Ranch	190	20	2

Breakfast:

B'fast Platter, Bacon, Engl. Muffin	760	45	63
Burger, w/ Pepp. Bacon, Chedd. Chse	470	27	25
Burrito, Ssg Patty & Chedd Cheese	690	45	40

Ice Cream Sundaes: With Whipped Cream

Caramel	390	19	50
Hot Fudge	390	19	51
Triple Berry	350	18	41

Burger King® (Apr '18)

Whopper Sandwiches:

	C	F	Cb
Whopper	660	40	49
without Mayo	500	22	49
with Cheese & Mayo	740	46	50
Bacon & Cheese Whopper	790	51	50
Double Whopper Sandwich	900	58	49
With Cheese	980	64	50
Whopper Jr	310	18	27

Flame Broiled Burgers:

	C	F	Cb
Bacon Cheeseburger	300	15	27
Bacon Double Cheeseburger	370	20	27
Bacon King Sandwich	1150	79	49
Cheeseburger	270	12	27
Double Cheeseburger	350	18	27
Extra Long Cheeseburger	590	34	45
Hamburger	220	8	26
Homestyle Cheeseburger	550	27	48

Grilled Dogs:

	C	F	Cb
Classic Dog	310	16	32
Chili Cheese Dog	330	19	28

Chicken Sandwiches:

	C	F	Cb
Crispy Chicken Jr.	450	30	34
Crispy Chicken Sandwich	670	41	54
Grilled Chicken Sandwich	470	19	39
Original Chicken Sandwich	660	40	48
Spicy Crispy Chicken Jr.	390	21	37

Chicken Nuggets:

	C	F	Cb
4 pieces	170	11	11
6 pieces	260	16	16
10 pieces	430	27	27
Chicken Fries, Regular, 9 pieces	280	17	20

Dipping Sauces:

	C	F	Cb
BBQ	40	0	11
Buffalo	80	8	2
Chicken Fry	140	13	6
Ranch; Zesty Onion Ring, av.	145	15	2
Big Fish S'wich	510	28	51
Veggie Burger: M'Star	390	15	42
Without Mayo	310	7	42

French Fries:

	C	F	Cb
Small, 4.3 oz	320	14	44
Medium, 5.8 oz	380	17	53
Large, 7 oz	430	19	60

Onion Rings:

	C	F	Cb
Small	320	16	41
Medium	410	21	53
Large	500	25	64

Garden Fresh Salads:

Bacon Cheddar Ranch Chicken:

	C	F	Cb
Crispy, w/ Dressing	710	50	34
Grilled, w/ Dressing	620	41	18

Garden Grilled Chicken:

	C	F	Cb
Crispy, without Dressing	440	25	31
Grilled, without Dressing	340	15	16
Garden Side Salad, w/o Dressing	60	4	3
Dressing, Ken's Ranch, 1.5 oz pkt	260	28	2

Burger King® cont... (Apr '18)

Breakfast:

	C	F	Cb
Biscuits: Bacon, Egg & Cheese	380	23	29
Ham, Egg & Cheese	370	21	30
Sausage	390	25	28
Sausage, Egg & Cheese	510	35	29
Burrito, Egg-Normous Burrito	910	55	73

Croissan'wich:

	C	F	Cb
Bacon, Egg & Cheese	340	18	30
Egg & Cheese	300	15	30
Fully Loaded	610	40	31
Ham, Egg & Cheese	330	16	31

King Croissan'wich:

	C	F	Cb
with Double Sausage	700	51	31
with Ham & Sausage	530	34	31
with Sausage & Bacon	580	39	31
French Toast Sticks: 5 pieces	380	18	49
with 1 oz Breakfast Syrup	500	18	79
Hash Browns: Small, 3 oz	250	16	24
Medium, 6 oz	500	33	48
Large, 8 oz	670	44	65
Oatmeal, Orig. Maple Flavored	170	3	32
Platters: Pancakes & Sausage	610	31	72
Ultimate Breakfast	1190	66	123

Sweets:

	C	F	Cb
Cinnamon Roll	280	11	41
Chocolate Chip Cookie (1)	165	8	24
Pies: Dutch Apple	340	14	51
Hershey's Sundae	310	19	32
Reese's P'nut Butter	310	19	31
Snickers	300	16	36
Sundaes: Caramel	290	6	53
Chocolate Fudge	280	7	47
Vanilla Soft Serve, in cone	190	4.5	32

Shakes:

	C	F	Cb
Chocolate	610	16	103
Chocolate Oreo	610	19	99
Oreo	730	21	121
Strawberry	640	15	113
Vanilla	580	15	98

Smoothies:

	C	F	Cb
Strawb. Ban.,16 fl.oz	310	1	71
Tropical Mango, 16 fl.oz	370	0	86
Beverages: Frappe, av., 16 fl.oz	405	16	62

Coca Cola/Sprite: *With 50% Ice*

	C	F	Cb
Value, 15 fl.oz	140	0	39
Small, 20 fl.oz	190	0	51
Medium, 30 fl.oz	290	0	77
Large, 40 fl.oz	380	0	102
Minute Maid Orange Juice, 10 fl.oz	140	0	33
Icee, Coke/Fanta Cherry, 16 oz	140	0	38
Iced Coffee: Regular, 16 oz	150	8	19
Vanilla, 16 oz	190	8	28
Sweet Tea, 20 oz	120	0	35

Updated Nutrition Data ~ www.CalorieKing.com
Persons with Diabetes ~ See Disclaimer (Page 22)

Captain D's Seafood® (Sept '17)

From The Grill: Without Sides	C	F	Cb
Blackened Tilapia	210	7	1
Grilled Salmon	220	10	1
Gr. Steak Tips, 1 kabob	110	4	2
Grilled Whitefish Fillet	180	8	2
Lemon Pepper Whitefish Fillet	180	8	1
Shrimp Scampi, 1 serving	980	67	70
Other Favorites:			
Cheese Sticks, 1order	500	32	35
Jalapeno Poppers, 1 order	510	36	40
Seafood:			
Butterfly Shrimp (6)	360	27	24
Popcon Shrimp	490	27	48
Stuffed Crab, 1 piece	140	10	11
Side Dishes:			
Baked Potato, plain, (1)	210	0	48
Coleslaw, 1 order	180	13	15
French Fries, 1 serving	330	22	28
Hushpuppy (1)	80	4	9
Dessert, Chocolate Cake, 1 order	300	11	49

Caribou Coffee® (Sept '17)

Without Whipped Cream Unless Indicated

Hot Coffees: Per Medium	C	F	Cb
Classic: Coffee Of The Day, 2% Milk	90	3.5	9
Cappuccino, with 2% Milk	110	4.5	10
Espresso, 4 oz	0	0	0
Latte, with 2% Milk	180	7	17
Macchiato, with 2% Milk	20	1	1
Hot Chocolate: Per Medium, with Whipped Cream			
Milk Chocolate, 2% Milk	600	36	50
Specialty, Mint Condition Mocha,			
Milk Choc., 2% Milk, medium	630	34	68
Cold Beverages: Per Medium, Without Whipped Cream			
Blended Fruit & Yogurt Smoothies:			
Mango Orange Key Lime	450	0	113
Strawberry Banana	380	0	88
Classics: Iced Americano	5	0	0
Iced Latte, with 2% Milk	90	3.5	8
Iced Mocha, Milk Choc., 2% Milk	280	7	39
Coolers: Chocolate, Milk Chocolate	660	24	93
Coffee	350	7	72
Vanilla	430	6	93
Specialty Blended Cooler:			
Caramel High Rise	540	12	107
Mint Condition, Milk Chocolate	590	9	114
Turtle Mocha, Milk Chocolate	700	15	127
Vanilla White Mocha, White Choc.	600	9	121

Carl's Jr.® (Apr '18)

California menu only. Please check instore for further nutritional information.

	C	F	Cb
Charbroiled Burgers:			
Famous Star with Cheese	670	37	57
Super Star with Cheese	920	56	59
Teriyaki Burger	660	29	71
The Big Carl	920	58	56
Western Bacon Cheeseburger	750	35	75
Double	1010	55	76
1/2 lb Thickburgers: Original $6	980	69	59
Guacamole Bacon	1200	89	51
Lettuce Wrapped	630	55	9
Chicken Sandwiches:			
Bacon Swiss Crispy Chicken Fillet	770	41	58
Big Chicken Fillet	650	33	55
Charbroiled: BBQ Chicken	370	5	49
Chicken Club	590	27	46
Santa Fe Chicken	550	25	45
Spicy Chicken Sandwich	490	29	43
Chicken Tenders, hand breaded,			
5 pieces, without Sauce	440	21	21
Chicken Stars,			
6 pieces, without Sauce	270	15	19
Breakfast:			
Bacon & Egg Burrito	570	35	32
Breakfast Burger, Single	730	43	47
Grilled Cheese & Sausage S'wich	660	43	43
Hash Brown Nuggets: Small, 3.8 oz	350	23	32
Medium, 4.2 oz	390	26	36
Large, 6 oz	560	37	52
Loaded B'fast Burrito	760	48	46
Steak & Egg Burrito	630	36	37
Fries: CrissCut Fries, 5 oz	450	29	42
Natural Cut: Small, 3.5 oz	300	15	39
Medium, 6 oz	430	21	55
Large, 6.5oz	460	22	59
Fried Zucchini, 5 oz	380	23	39
Onion Rings, 4.5 oz	530	28	61
Salads: Without Dressing			
Charbroiled Chicken Salad	280	9	19
Garden, Side	140	7	15
Dressings: Per 2 oz Package			
Blue Cheese	310	34	2
House	210	23	5
Low-Fat Balsamic	20	1	3
Dessert: Choc. Chip Cookie, 2.5 oz	330	17	43
Chocolate Cake, 3 oz	290	11	46
Strawberry Swirl Cheesecake, 3.5 oz	320	17	3
Malts: With Ice Cream			
Oreo Cookie	780	40	94
Other flavors, average	765	36	99
Shakes: With Ice Cream			
Oreo Cookie	710	39	79
Vanilla; Chocolate; Strawberry, av.	695	35	85

Carvel® (Sept '17)

Carvelanche:	C	F	Cb
Oreo/Reeses, av: Small, 12 oz	590	29	69
Regular, 16 oz	865	46	99
Large, 24 oz	1300	68	151
Classic Sundaes: Per Small, 12 oz			
Caramel	700	36	84
Hot Fudge	540	30	60
Strawberry	610	34	67
Sundae Dashers: Per Regular, 16 oz			
Banana's Foster	1020	31	176
Fudge Brownie	1170	60	147
Mint Chocolate Chip	1230	64	157
Peanut Butter Cup	1420	86	134
Strawberry Shortcake	730	38	91
Ice Cream:			
Chocolate/Vanilla, average:			
Junior Cup, 4.5 oz	260	14	28
with Carvelite	175	4	30
Small Cup, 7.5 oz	430	24	47
with Carvelite	285	6	52
Medium Cup, 9.5 oz	550	30	60
with Carvelite	360	8	65
Thick Shakes: Per 16 oz			
Chocolate; Vanilla, av.	650	29	90
Strawberry	600	31	70

Charley's Grilled Subs® (Sept '17)

Subs: Regular, Includes Standard Toppings, without Sauce or Dressings

	C	F	Cb
Bacon 3 Cheese Steak	720	31	56
Chicken Buffalo/Teriyaki, av.	610	18	60
Chicken California	690	28	52
Italian Deli Deluxe	750	36	58
Pepperoni Steak	780	37	55
Philly Cheesesteak	640	24	58
Philly Chicken	590	17	58
Turkey Cheddar Melt	670	21	62
Ultimate Club	710	27	61
Salads: Cheese or Dressings not included			
Grilled Chicken; Grilled Steak, av.	130	3	8
Fries: Original	400	22	46
Cheese Gourmet	550	31	62
Ultimate Gourmet	720	49	61
Breakfast: Hashbrowns	460	29	45
Omelet Platter: Bacon, Egg & Chse	1010	63	74
Sausage, Egg & Cheese	1110	70	73
Steak, Egg & Cheese	1050	62	74
Sandwiches: Bacon, Egg & Chse	490	26	36
Sausage, Egg & Cheese	590	33	36
Steak, Egg & Cheese	520	25	36
Toast, 2 slices	130	2	24

For Complete Menu & Data ~ see CalorieKing.com

Cheesecake Factory® (Sept '17)

Cheesecake: Per Slice	C	F	Cb
Original	800	n/a	62
Godiva Chocolate	1230	n/a	97
Reese's P.B. Chocolate Cake	1480	n/a	153
White Chocolate Raspb. Truffle	1120	n/a	88
Small Plates & Snacks: Ahi Tartare	260	n/a	19
Beets with Goat Cheese	360	n/a	31
Crispy Crab Bites	350	n/a	11
Crispy Cuban Roll	770	n/a	49
Dynamite Shrimp	570	n/a	40
Fried Zucchini	530	n/a	30
Loaded Baked Pot. Tots	950	n/a	56
Stuffed Mushrooms	470	n/a	15
Glamburgers & Sandwiches: Without Sides			
American Cheeseburger	1280	n/a	75
Bacon-Bacon Burger	1590	n/a	74
Classic Burger	1380	n/a	64
Crispy Shrimp S'wich	1330	n/a	102
Grilled Turkey Burger	1070	n/a	67
Kobe Burger	1380	n/a	83
Mushroom Burger	1400	n/a	69
Smokehouse BBQ Bgr	1380	n/a	97
Veggie Burger	1220	n/a	113
Glamburger Sides: French Fries	470	n/a	72
Green Salad	190	n/a	8
Sweet Potato Fries	470	n/a	72
Fish & Seafood:			
Fish & Chips	1550	n/a	118
Shrimp Scampi	1900	n/z	130
Sthrn Fried Catfish	1380	n/a	96
Pasta: Four Cheese	1210	n/a	106
with Chicken	1490	n/a	106
Fettuccine Alfredo with Chicken	2660	n/a	130
Louisiana Chicken Pasta	2510	n/a	162
Specialties: Baja Chicken Tacos	1500	n/a	165
Cajun Chicken "Littles"	2030	n/a	222
Chicken Bellagio	2010	n/a	153
Chicken Enchiladas	1380	n/a	106
Chicken with Lemon Couscous	1440	n/a	72
Crispy Chkn Costoletta	2590	n/a	102
Eggplant Parm.	1430	n/a	131
Factory Burrito Grande	1670	n/a	148
Famous Factory Meatloaf	1630	n/a	117
Grilled Fish Tacos	1500	n/a	165
Grilled Steak Tacos	1530	n/a	157
White Chicken Chili	570	n/a	36
Salads: Includes Dressing			
Caesar	1320	n/a	34
Santa Fe	1730	n/a	104
Seared Tuna Tataki	540	n/a	17

n/a = not available

Chick-fil-A® (Apr '18)

	C	F	Cb
Breakfast:			
Bagel, Chicken, Egg & Cheese	480	18	51
Biscuits: Plain, buttered	300	13	41
Bacon, Egg & Cheese	420	21	40
Chicken	450	21	50
Egg White Chicken Grill	300	7	31
Sausage, Egg & Cheese	600	40	41
Bowl, Hash Brown Scramble	450	28	19
Burrito, Hash Brown Scramble	450	22	34
Chick-n-Minis,			
4 pieces	350	14	39
Hash Browns, 2.7 oz	240	16	23
Parfait, Greek Yogurt, fruit topping	240	8	29
Chick-fil-A Sandwiches: *Without Sauce*			
Chicken	440	19	40
Deluxe	500	23	42
Grilled Chicken	310	6	36
Grilled Chicken Club	430	16	37
Spicy Deluxe	540	25	43
Cool Wrap, Grilled Chicken,			
without sauce	360	14	30
Chicken: *Without Dipping Sauce*			
Chick-n-Strips, breaded, 4 count	470	23	29
Nuggets: Breaded, 8 count	260	12	9
Grilled, 8 count	140	3.5	2
Salads: *Without Dressing*			
Cobb, with Breaded Ckn Nuggets	510	28	28
Grilled Market, with Chick-n-Strips	560	28	47
Spicy Southwest, w/- Grilled Filet	450	19	37
Dressings: Avocado Lime Ranch	310	32	3
Creamy Salsa	290	31	3
Garlic & Herb Ranch	280	29	2
Light Italian	25	1.5	3
Sauces: BBQ Sauce	45	0	11
Honey Mustard Sauce	45	0	11
Polynesian Sauce	110	6	13
Sweet & Spicy Sriracha Sauce	45	0	10
Sides: Fruit Cup, medium	50	0	12
Chicken Noodle Soup,			
small bowl	130	3.5	15
Side Salad, with toppings	160	11	12
Superfood Side Salad, with toppings:			
Small	150	9	18
Large	190	9	25
Waffle Potato Fries: Med.	360	18	43
Large	460	24	56
Dessert: Chocolate Chunk Cookie	350	16	50
Icedream Cone, large	260	6	45
Frosted Coffee, large	300	7	51
Milkshakes: Chocolate, large	720	26	108
Cookies & Cream, large	750	31	107
Vanilla, large	620	25	86

Chili's® (Sept '17)

	C	F	Cb
For The Table: *As Served*			
Bottomless Tostada Chips w/ Salsa	910	45	113
Classic Nachos: Beef	1640	108	57
Chicken	1470	93	58
Southwestern Eggrolls	800	41	82
Texas Cheese Fries, full order	1800	127	86
Triple Dipper: *Serving for One*			
Big Mouth Bites	800	55	47
Original Chicken Crispers	510	33	22
Burgers: *Without Side Fries*			
Classic Bacon Beef	880	56	46
Oldtimer, with Beef Burger	750	44	45
Southern Smokehouse w/ Beef	1130	69	75
Crispers & More: *As Served, with Set Sides*			
Cajun Pasta with Grilled Chicken	1200	53	112
Original Tempura	1320	6	121
Fresh Mex Bowls: *As Served*			
Bowls: Chipotle Chicken	900	38	79
Margarita Chicken	950	34	102
Prime Rib	860	41	86
Pairings: Beef Enchilada	300	17	20
Beef Taco	300	15	22
Cheese Enchilada	340	24	17
Chicken Quesadilla	710	51	34
Tostada Beef	360	20	27
Tostada Chicken	330	17	26
Lighter Choices: *As Served*			
Ancho Salmon	590	27	41
Grilled Chicken Salad	440	23	23
Mango Chile Chicken/Tilapia, av.	510	17	56
Margarita Grilled Chicken	610	14	65
Top Shelf Tacos: *Per Taco, without Sides*			
Pork Carnitas	330	19	16
Prime Rib	260	15	16
Ranchero Chkn	270	14	18
Spicy Shrimp	270	16	22
Baby Back Ribs: *Full Rack, without Sides*			
Original BBQ	950	56	34
House BBQ	960	58	33
Texas Dry Rub	1080	72	32
Steaks: *As Served*			
Classic Sirloin, 6 oz	680	37	41
Classic Ribeye	1050	64	40
Country-Fried Steak	1290	67	121
Sides: *As Served*			
Homestyle Fries	390	17	53
Loaded Mashed Potatoes	380	23	32
Southwestern Mac 'n' Cheese	480	30	36
Spiced Panko Onion Rings	400	19	48
Salads: *Includes Dressing*			
Boneless Buffalo Chicken	1020	72	45
Caribbean with Seared Shrimp	620	27	82
Quesadilla Explosion	1470	99	83
Sweet Stuff: *Per Slice*			
Cheesecake	730	43	76
Molten Chocolate Cake	1200	62	158

For Complete Menu & Data ~ see CalorieKing.com

Chipotle® (Sept '17)

Tortillas:	C	F	Cb
Burrito Size Flour Tortillas (1)	320	9	50
Taco Size: Crispy Corn Tortilla (3)	200	9	9
Soft Corn Tortillas (Taco), (3)	210	1.5	42
Soft Flour Tortillas (Taco), (3)	250	8	40
Meal Components: Barbacoa, 4 oz	170	7	2
Black/Pinto Beans, average, 4 oz	130	1.5	22
Brown Rice, 4 oz	210	6	36
Carnitas, 4 oz	210	12	0
Cheese, 1 oz	110	8	1
Chicken, 4 oz	180	7	0
Fajita Vegetables, 2.5 oz	20	0	5
Guacamole, 3.5 oz	230	22	8
Lettuce, 1 oz	5	0	1
Sofritas, 4 oz	150	10	9
Steak, 4 oz	150	6	1
Condiments:			
Salsa: Chili Corn, 3.5 oz	80	1.5	16
Green Tomatillo, 2 oz	15	0	4
Red Tomatillo, 2 oz	15	0	4
Tomato, 3.5 oz	25	0	5
Sour Cream, 2 oz	110	8	1
Extras, Chips, serving, 4 oz	540	25	73

Chuck E. Cheese® (Sept '17)

Appetizers:	C	F	Cb
Cheesy Breadsticks (1)	170	11	13
Parmesan Breadstick (1)	240	10	30
Tater Bites, Plain, 8 oz	590	33	71
Sandwiches & Wraps:			
BBQ Chicken Ciabatta	1080	58	100
Italian Sub Ciabatta	1120	76	70
Sandwiches & Wraps: Per Half Sandwich/Wrap			
BBQ Chicken Ciabatta	540	29	50
Italian Sub Ciabatta	560	38	35
Wraps: Chicken Caesar	400	20	29
Club	470	30	28
Specialty Pizzas: Per Medium Slice			
BBQ Chicken	210	9	24
Cali Alfredo; Meat Combo	200	10	19
Super Combo	190	9	19
Vegetarian	160	6	19
Traditional Wings:			
Small: with BBQ or Sweet Chili Sauce	450	27	17
with Blue Cheese	660	55	3
Desserts: Apple Pie Pizza, whole	440	9	86
Cinnamon Pizza, whole	830	28	134

Church's Chicken® (Sept '17)

Chicken: Per Serving	C	F	Cb
Original: Breast, 1 piece	250	14	9
Leg, 1 piece	150	8	6
Thigh, 1 piece	360	27	12
Wing, 1 piece	290	18	8
Spicy: Breast, 1 piece	280	17	12
Leg, 1 piece	160	9	9
Thigh, 1 piece	380	25	21
Wing, 1 piece	350	20	19
Tender Strips, average, 1 piece	100	5	5
Sides: Per Small Serving			
Baked Macaroni & Cheese, 4.7 oz	210	12	19
Cole Slaw, 4.2 oz	170	11	16
Dinner Roll (1), 1.7 oz	60	1	11
French Fries, 2.6 oz	210	9	29
Honey Butter Biscuits (1), 2.2 oz	230	15	25
Jalapeno Cheese Bombers (4)	220	11	24
Mashed Potatoes & Gravy, 4.5 oz	110	1	24
Okra, 3.4 oz	260	15	30
Sauces: BBQ, pkt	45	0	11
Creamy Jalapeno, pkt	120	13	2
Honey Mustard/Ranch, av., pkt	140	15	2
Dessert, Apple Pie	270	13	37

Cici's Pizza® (Sept '17)

	C	F	Cb
Adventurous Taste Pizzas: Per Slice			
BBQ Pork	200	7	27
Zesty Ham & Cheddar/Veggie, av.	170	6	23
Deep Dish Pizza, 1 slice	170	6	21
Flatbread, Spinach Alfredo, 1 slice	140	7	14
Traditional Pizzas: Per Slice			
Alfredo; Spin. Alf.; Zesty Ham & Ched	160	5	22
Beef; Pepperoni & Jalap; Ssg, av.	190	7	24
Wings: BBQ (5)	260	12	16
Buffalo (5), average	215	13	4
Garlic Parmesan (5)	270	18	5
Sides: Chicken & Pasta Soup, 8 oz	90	2.5	13
Pasta with Marinara Sauce, 7 oz	300	4	56
Dessert, Pizzas, average, 1 slice	130	3	23

Cinnabon® (Sept '17)

	C	F	Cb
Cinnabon Classic Roll (1)	880	37	127
MiniBon Roll (1), 3.4 oz	350	15	51
Bites: Cinnabon Classic (4)	440	17	64
Caramel Pecan Bites (4)	580	29	73
Centre of The Roll Classic (1)	750	34	105
Chillata: Chocolate Mocha, 16 fl.oz	370	14	61
Oreo	810	38	109
Strawberry/Strawb. Banana, av.	525	11	106

Claim Jumper® (Sept '17)

Appetizers: As Served

	C	F	Cb
Southwest Eggrolls	1190	53	114
Three Cheese Potatocakes (3)	1075	71	80

Burgers & Sandwiches: Without Sides

	C	F	Cb
Grilled Cobb Sandwich	1210	78	78
Widow Maker Burger	1370	87	84
Calzones: Specialty	1430	80	137
Traditional	1350	66	140

Meals: As Per Menu Description

	C	F	Cb
Favorites: Country Fried Steak	2030	107	189
Giant Stuffed Chicken Baker	990	34	118
Meatloaf & Mashed Potatoes	1300	75	117
Pasta: Black Tie Pasta	1535	84	126
Parmesan Crusted Chicken	975	47	83
Pizza: Calif. Works, Classic Crust	1295	64	127
Steakhouse, Flatbread	820	47	65
Specialties: BBQ Baby Back Pork Ribs,			
Full Rack	1745	111	111
Roasted Tri-Tip with Demi Glaze	800	47	19
Seafood: Atlantic Salmon, Blcknd	715	42	48
Tilapia Bianca, with Shrimp,			
Artichoke Hearts & Sauce	1165	80	56

Entree Salads: Without Dressing or Bread

	C	F	Cb
Calif. Citrus Chkn, Charbroiled	865	53	58
Seared Ahi Spinach	515	24	31

Soups: Per Bowl

	C	F	Cb
New England Clam Chowder	525	45	23
Potato Cheddar	710	61	31
Sweets: Choc. Motherlode Cake	2770	144	340
Italian Lemon Cake	1240	62	158

Coldstone Creamery® (Sept '17)

Ice Creams:

	C	F	Cb
Amaretto: Like it	330	20	33
Love it	530	31	53
Gotta have it	790	47	80
Chocolate: Like it	320	20	33
Love it	520	31	53
Gotta have it	780	48	79

Hot Stone:

	C	F	Cb
Brownie A La Cold Stone, 11 oz	810	55	99
Chocolate Lava Meltdown, 9 oz	730	36	97
Churro Caramel Crave, 8.6 oz	700	33	98

Sorbet:

Strawberry Mango:

	C	F	Cb
Like it	220	0	55
Love it	350	0	87
Gotta have it	520	0.5	13

Cosi® (Sept '17)

Bowls: W/ Set Menu Components

	C	F	Cb
Adobo Chicken with Avocado	680	21	99
Thai Curry Chicken	740	22	101
Thai Curry Tofu	740	26	103

Soups:

	C	F	Cb
Broccoli Cheddar: Bowl	770	66	28
Cup	510	44	19
Macaroni & Cheese: Bowl	990	56	82
Cup	680	39	56
Medit.Lentil: Bowl	370	17	45
Cup	250	11	30
Smart Fit Chicken Noodle: Bowl	190	4	19
Cup	120	2.5	12
Turkey Chili: Bowl	360	7	67
Cup	240	5	45

Salads: With Menu Set Dressing

	C	F	Cb
Cobb	740	56	20
Greek	535	47	20
Signature	620	45	40

Breakfast:

	C	F	Cb
Santa Fe Wrap, 8.8 oz	470	29	30
Spinach Florentine Wrap, 7.3 oz	380	22	28
Squagel (Plain) S'wich Cosi Club	560	21	64

Pastries:

	C	F	Cb
Banana Nut Muffin, 4 oz	500	31	47
Chocolate Croissant, 3 oz	360	16	46
Dessert: Blondie Brownie, 2.25 oz	280	14	36
Chocolate Chunk Brownie, 2.25 oz	300	16	39

Cousins Subs® (Sept '17)

Subs: Per 7.5", Standard Toppings

Grilled To Order:

	C	F	Cb
Chicken Bacon Cheddar	640	24	53
Chkn Bacon Mshrm	760	34	59
Chkn Cheese Steak	590	20	52

Classics:

	C	F	Cb
Club, with Mayo	680	39	50
Italian Special, with Oil	830	48	52
Tuna with Mayo	650	36	51

Deli Fresh:

	C	F	Cb
Ham & Provolone, with Mayo	670	32	53
Roast Beef & Cheddar, with Mayo	740	37	52
Turkey Breast w/ Mayo	535	31	53

Soup: Per Cup

	C	F	Cb
Beef Steak with Noodles	105	3.5	12
Cheddar Cauliflower	110	5	13
Chicken Noodle	110	3	16
Cream of Potato	170	8	21
New England Clam Chowder	150	2.5	25

For Complete Nutritional Data ~ see CalorieKing.com

Fast - Foods & Restaurants

Culver's® (Sept '17)

ButterBurgers:	C	F	Cb
Original: Single	390	17	39
Double	560	30	39
Triple	730	43	39
Cheddar with Bacon, Single	510	26	39
Cheddar:			
Single	470	24	39
Double	720	44	39
Culver's Bacon Deluxe:			
Single	610	36	42
Double	850	56	43
Culver's Deluxe:			
Single	570	34	42
Double	810	52	43
Mushroom & Swiss, Single	500	26	40
Sourdough Melt, Single	460	25	34

Sandwiches:	C	F	Cb
Beef Pot Roast	410	13	41
Crispy Chicken	460	14	58
Grilled Reuben Melt	660	38	43
North Atlantic Cod Filet	600	33	50
Pork Tenderloin	630	25	73

Sides:	C	F	Cb
Green Beans, reg.	130	9	9
Chili Cheddar Fries	670	32	78
Crinkle Cut Fries, reg.	360	14	53
Mashed Potatoes & Gravy, regular	130	1	25
Wisconsin Cheese Curds, 5.3 oz	510	25	51

Dinners: With Fries, Cole Slaw, Dinner Roll & Butter & Accompanying Sauce

	C	F	Cb
Butterfly Jumbo Shrimp, 6 pieces	1080	53	129
North Atlantic Cod, Fried, 2 pieces	1470	98	108

Soup:	C	F	Cb
Broccoli Cheese, 10.5 oz	220	12	17
Chicken Noodle, 10.5 oz	110	2	14
Potato au Gratin, 10.5 oz	330	20	28

Salads: Without Dressing

	C	F	Cb
Chicken Cashew w/ Grilled Chicken	460	24	16
Cranberry Bacon Bleu, with Grilled Chicken	360	14	14
Garden Fresco with Grilled Chicken	360	14	18
Side Salad	60	2	6

Kid's Meals:	C	F	Cb
Corn Dog, Kids	240	14	23
Chicken Tenders, Breaded, 2 pieces	270	12	21
Grilled Cheese Sourdough Sandwich	350	18	36

Dressings:	C	F	Cb
Chnky Bleu Chse, 1.8 oz	310	33	2
French Dressing, 1.8 oz	190	13	19
Ranch, 1.75 oz	180	19	2
Sesame Ginger, 2 oz	70	0	16

Culver's® cont... (Sept '17)

Concrete Mixers: No Toppings	C	F	Cb
Chocolate, regular	700	36	88
Cookie Dough, regular	1010	56	113

Sundaes: Per 2 Scoops	C	F	Cb
Banana Split	1060	60	121
Caramel Cashew	1000	51	121
Fudge Pecan	1040	64	107
Turtle	1040	62	112

Beverages:	C	F	Cb
Chocolate Malt, reg.	880	39	120
Chocolate Shake, reg.	820	38	108
Strawberry Malt, reg.	770	38	96
Strawberry Shake, reg.	730	38	86

D'Angelo's® (Sept '17)

Burgers: Without Condiments	C	F	Cb
Regular	450	18	45
Cheeseburger	510	23	45
Steak #9	710	3	55
Western Bacon Cheddar	780	42	51

Deli Sandwiches: Per Medium, with Standard Toppings on Italiab Sub

	C	F	Cb
Cranberry Pecan Chicken Salad	1005	58	78
Roast Beef & Cheese	780	38	76
Tuna Salad	990	68	61

Wraps: Per Medium, with Standard Toppings, on Tortilla Wrap

	C	F	Cb
Buffalo Chicken	1080	65	65
Chicken Caesar	1150	66	75
Cobb BLT	760	35	85

Fresh Entree Salads: With Dressing, without Pokket

Entree: Caesar	630	53	26
Greek	240	13	17

Grilled Topped:	C	F	Cb
Chicken Cobb	800	58	26
Steak Cobb	870	64	26
Steak Greek	780	62	20

Soup: Per Bowl	C	F	Cb
Beef Stew	330	12	34
Extreme Broccoli & Cheddar	370	28	18
Main Lobster Bisque	540	43	24
New England Clam Chowder	480	27	46

For Complete Menu & Data ~ see CalorieKing.com

Dairy Queen® (Jan '18)

Burgers:	C	F	Cb
Cheeseburger: Original	370	18	31
Deluxe	460	24	39
GrillBurgers: ¼ lb Bacon Cheese	630	36	42
½ lb Cheese	800	49	42
½ lb Flame Thrower	970	68	39
¼ lb Mushroom Swiss	590	36	37

Updated Nutrition Data ~ www.CalorieKing.com
Persons with Diabetes ~ See Disclaimer (Page 22)

Dairy Queen® cont... (Jan '18)

Sandwiches:

	C	F	Cb
Artisan Bakes!:			
Chicken Bacon Ranch	500	20	45
Kansas City BBQ PulledPork	430	15	69
Turkey BLT	550	26	45
Chicken Strip Baskets: Without Beverage			
4 pieces, with Country Gravy	1000	49	103
6 piece, with Country Gravy	1250	61	121
Hot Dogs: Regular	340	20	28
Chili Cheese	420	26	28
Snack Melts: Buffalo Chicken	290	16	21
Chicken Bacon BBQ	280	11	27
Salads: Without Dressing			
Chicken BLT:			
Crispy Chicken	400	21	28
Grilled Chicken	270	11	10
Side Salad	25	0	5
French Fries, regular, 4 oz	290	13	39
Onion Rings, 4 oz	360	16	48
Breakfast: Bacon Biscuit S'wich	420	26	19
Chicken & Gravy	420	21	29
Country Platter:			
with Bacon	1150	73	55
with Ham	850	42	60
Ham Biscuit Sandwich	350	18	19
Pancake Platter with Sausage	510	21	60
Desserts: Per Medium			
Blizzard Treats: Banana Split	580	16	97
Butterfinger	720	25	109
Cookie Dough	1040	41	151
Heath	870	37	119
Oreo Cookies	780	29	117
Reese's Peanut Butter Cups	750	32	102
Salted Caramel Truffle	1040	48	142
Turtle Pecan Cluster	900	48	105
DQ Dipped Cone, Chocolate, med.	460	22	59
DQ Sundaes: Caramel	430	11	73
Hot Fudge	430	15	66
Strawberry	330	10	53
Bakes, Hot:			
Fudge Stuffed Cookie	640	33	80
Triple Chocolate Brownie	540	25	74
Shakes: Caramel	750	25	115
Chocolate	710	3	110
Strawberry	620	23	87
Vanilla	660	23	97
Add Malt	90	1	17
Moo Latte: Per Medium, with Whipped Topping			
Caramel	570	17	96
Mocha	580	22	88
Vanilla	530	16	90

Daphne's Greek Cafe® (Sept '17)

Califonia Menu Only. Check Instore for Latest Information

Starters:

	C	F	Cb
Fire Feta & Warm Pita	340	7	39
Hummus & Warm Pita	320	12	47
Classic Pita Sandwiches: Without Tzatziki Sauce			
with Chicken	410	16	41
with Crispy Shrimp	410	17	48
with Falafel	640	17	96
with Gyro	680	45	49
Plates: Without Pita or Tzatziki Sauce			
Cali-Greek Bowls:			
with Crispy Shrimp	930	37	109
with Falafel	1160	39	165
with Grilled Chicken	930	37	109
with Grilled Shrimp	1060	46	91
Mediterranean Veggie,			
with Rice & Greek Salad	1050	60	110
Classic Greek Salads: W/ Dressing, w/o Pita & Sauce			
Crispy Shrimp	440	31	25
Falafel	670	31	74
Grilled Chicken	440	30	18
Add, Pita & Tzatziki	130	3	21
Sides: Cucumber-Tomato Salad	120	11	5
Fire Roasted Vegetables	70	3	12
French Fries	440	22	55
Greek Salad, small	140	12	7
Moroccan Carrot-Walnut Salad	180	13	15
Pita Chips	220	6	36
Pita Bread	190	3	36
Seasoned Rice	360	8	68
Tabouli Salad	220	15	20
Tzatziki	40	1	3

Davanni's® (Sept '17)

Half Hoagies: With 6" White Bun & Standard Toppings

	C	F	Cb
Assorted	490	30	39
Cheese	500	31	39
Chicken & Bacon w/ Honey Mustard	505	22	46
Chicken Parmigiana	445	16	40
Club	495	27	40
Pastrami	470	27	40
Roast Beef	470	25	39
Southwestern Chicken	535	26	43
Tuna Melt	645	44	42
Turkey Bacon Chipotle	565	33	39
Pasta: As Served, with Garlic Toast			
Chicken Florentine, half portion	570	23	56
Lasagna, half portion	625	43	37

continued next page...

Davanni's® cont... (Sept '17)

Pizzas: Per ⅛ of Medium Pizza

	C	F	Cb
Five Meat: Thin Crust	255	13	19
Traditional Crust	305	13	30
Solo, Thin Crust	655	36	44
Veggie: Thin Crust	220	10	19
Traditional Crust	275	10	30
Works: Thin Crust	265	14	19
Traditional Crust	315	15	30

Del Taco® (Sept '17)

Breakfast:

	C	F	Cb
Burritos: Breakfast	430	21	38
Half Pounders: Bacon	640	36	38
½ lb Chorizo/Steak, av.	510	26	39
Hash Brown Sticks, 5 pieces	230	17	18
Tacos: Bacon	230	14	15
Chorizo	520	28	39
Carne Asada Steak	240	13	16
Egg & Cheese	190	11	15
Burgers:			
Bacon Dble Del Cheeseburger	740	51	35
Del Cheeseburger	470	28	34
Double Del Chseburger	690	47	35
Crinkle Cut Fries: Kids, 3 oz	160	10	17
Small, 4 oz	210	13	22
Medium, 6 oz	320	19	34
Macho, 8.8 oz	470	28	49
Chili Cheddar Fries, 10.5 oz	570	35	42
Burritos: ½ lb Bean & Cheese	470	10	69
Classic Gr. Chicken	530	33	40
Del Beef	500	24	40
Del Combo	540	17	64
Epic: Bacon Ranch Chkn Avocado	980	52	90
Carne Asada	750	24	90
Grilled Chicken Avocado	840	36	90
Macho Combo	950	37	100
Macho Nachos,			
Beef/Chicken/Steak, av.	950	48	98
Platos: Per Plate			
2 Street Tacos:			
Beer Battered Fish	1060	45	139
Carne Asada Steak	960	35	127
Grilled Chicken	940	35	127
Carne Asada Wet Burrito	1300	48	150
Chicken Verde, Wet Burrito	1220	48	154
Quesadillas: Mini Bacon	170	9	14
Cheddar; Spicy Jack, average	460	27	32
Chicken Cheddar/Spicy Jack, av.	550	31	35

Del Taco® cont... (Sept '17)

Tacos:

	C	F	Cb
Beer Battered Fish	230	12	26
Chicken Street	170	7	20
Del Taco: Crunchy Beef	310	20	14
Soft Beef	300	18	17
Grilled Chicken	210	12	16
Salads: Without Dressing			
Chicken, Bacon Avocado	590	46	23
Mexican Chopped Chicken	510	23	39
Signature Taco	550	29	38
Sides:			
Bean & Cheese, 7.8 oz	320	3.5	52
Hashborn Sticks (5)	230	17	18

Denny's® (Jan '18)

Breakfast:

	C	F	Cb
Favorites: *With Hash Browns, without Bread*			
Country Fried Steak & Eggs, 11 oz	520	33	38
Grand Slamwich, 19 oz	1260	79	87
Moons Over My Hammy, 17 oz	970	62	57
Omelettes:			
Ham & Cheese Omelette, 13 oz	780	54	20
Loaded Veggie	620	44	24
Philly Cheesesteak	880	64	25
Ultimate	820	65	20
Skillets: *Without Eggs*			
Bourbon Chicken, 20 oz	870	39	67
Santa Fe, 9 oz	530	37	33
Supreme, 10 oz	560	42	34
Slams:			
All American, w/ Hash Browns, 15 oz	930	74	19
French Toast, 11 oz	860	53	65
Honey Jalapeno Bacon, 15 oz	800	35	95
Lumberjack, w/out bread, 23 oz	970	49	96
Pancakes: *Without Hash Brown, Egg & Meat*			
Blueberry	460	11	80
Cranberry Orange	710	10	144
Peanut Butter Cream	1000	49	124
Salted Caramel & Banana	920	24	164
Sticky Bun	680	16	124
Sides: Bacon Strips (4)	210	16	2
Buttermilk Biscuit (2)	470	26	54
Cheddar Cheese Hash Browns,5 oz	250	18	15
English Muffin, w/out Margarine	110	0.5	22
Grilled Ham, 3 oz slice	90	3	1
Hash Browns, 1 serve	170	12	15
Hearty Breakfast Sausage (1)	350	31	5
Oatmeal, w/ Milk & Br. Sugar, 10 oz	240	2	45
Red Skinned Potatoes, 4 oz	200	9	27
Wheat Toast, with Margarine	230	33	29

Updated Nutrition Data ~ www.CalorieKing.com
Persons with Diabetes ~ See Disclaimer (Page 22)

Denny's® cont... (Jan '18)

Appetizers:	C	F	Cb
Bacon Cheddar Tots,			
with Sour Cream (10)	580	34	54
Chkn & Ssg Quesadilla, w/ Ranch	1140	82	58
Chicken Strips: with Buffalo Sauce	700	30	68
with Sweet & Tangy BBQ Sauce	760	21	106
Loaded Bacon Cheddar Tots (10)	850	55	59
Mozzarella Cheese Sticks, w/o Sce	560	22	60
Zesty Nachos: Half Size	960	59	83
Full size	1840	113	160

Lunch Burgers & Sandwiches:

Burgers: Without Sides	C	F	Cb
Bacon, Avocado Cheeseburger	1010	68	50
Bacon Gouda	1100	71	55
Bourbon Bacon	940	53	65
Honey Jalapeno Bacon Sriracha	1010	63	53
Slamburger	860	51	52

Sandwiches: Without Sides	C	F	Cb
Cali Club	820	48	55
Club	830	39	74
The Grand Slamwich	1090	68	72
The Super Bird	620	31	43

Dinners: Without Sides or Bread	C	F	Cb
Brooklyn Spag. & M'balls, 20 oz	990	48	86
Chicken Strips, 7 oz	490	17	53
Country Fried Steak, w/ Gravy, 10 oz	560	3	35

Melts: Without Sides	C	F	Cb
Chicken Philly	760	40	57
Pot Roast Melt	900	48	54
Prime Rib Philly	910	52	62
Sirloin Steak, 8 oz	330	14	2
T-Bone Steak, 13 oz	540	34	0
with Shrimp, 18 oz	800	43	32
Tilapia Ranchero, 9 oz	320	13	7

Soups: Without Bread	C	F	Cb
Broccoli & Cheddar: Cup	160	11	11
Bowl	240	16	16
Chicken Noodle: Cup	150	5	18
Bowl	230	8	27
Clam Chowder: Cup	210	12	21
Bowl	310	18	31
Loaded Baked Potato: Cup	360	24	25
Bowl	470	31	36
Vegetable Beef: Cup	200	11	27
Bowl	310	16	40

Sides, Lunch/Dinner:	C	F	Cb
Bacon & Cheddar Tots,			
w/ Sour Crm (6)	300	15	31
Bacon Strips (2)	100	8	1
Broccoli, 3 oz	25	0	4

Denny's® cont... (Jan '18)

Sides, Lunch/Dinner (Contd)	C	F	Cb
Caesar Salad, 6 oz	280	22	15
Cheddar Mashed Potatoes	200	11	179
French Fries, 4 oz	400	22	46
Fresh Sauteed Zucc. & Squash, 3 oz	70	6	3
Fresh Steamed Zucc. & Squash	15	0	3
Fried Chicken Strip Cobb Salad,			
without Dressing, 15 oz	790	42	57
Garden Salad, w/out Dressing, 7 oz	170	9	16
Garlic Toast/Dinner Bread, 2 pieces	190	7	25
Golden-Fried Shrimp, 6 pieces	220	9	22
Hash Browns, 1 serving	170	12	15
Honey Jalapeno Bacon, 2 slices	190	13	0
Mashed Potatoes, 1 serving	120	5	17
Onion Rings (6)	390	22	44
Prime Rib Cobb Salad,			
without Dressing	560	38	20
Red Skinned Mashed Potatoes	200	9	27
Sweet Petite Corn, 5 oz	210	13	20
Veggies for Dipping, with Ranch	220	21	7
Whole Grain Rice, 5 oz	240	2.5	48

Salads: Without Bread	C	F	Cb
Avocado Chicken Caesar,			
with Caesar Drssng	730	59	10
Cranb. Apple Chicken			
with Balsamic Dressing	570	21	66
Prime Rib Cobb, without Dressing	560	38	20

Dressings: Per 1.5oz	C	F	Cb
Blue Cheese	160	16	2
Caesar	250	26	1
French	130	8	2
Honey Mustard	180	15	12
Ranch	200	21	1
Thousand Island	160	16	7

Sauces: Per 1.5 oz	C	F	Cb
Bourbon	100	0	25
Buffalo	70	7	1
Sweet & Tangy BBQ	110	0	30

Desserts: As Served	C	F	Cb
Banana Split, 21 oz	1160	51	169
Caramel Apple Pie Crisp, 13 oz	760	26	126
Chocolate Lava Cake	700	34	85

Beverages:	C	F	Cb
Iced Cappuccino, 9 oz	200	5	31
Lemonade Iced Tea, 12 oz	80	0	21
Strawb. Lemonade, 12 oz	210	0	55
Milk Shake, Vanilla, 16 oz	800	43	97

For Complete Nutritional Data ~ see CalorieKing.com

Dippin' Dots® (Sept '17)

Flavored Ices: Per ½ Cup, 3 oz

	C	F	Cb
Rockin' Cherry with Popping Candy	130	0.5	30
Other varieties	100	0	26

Frozen Yogurt: Per ½ Cup

Strawberry Cheesecake	100	0	21
YoDots: Cookies 'N Cream	140	3	27
Chocolate & Vanilla	110	1.5	24
Cookie Dough	150	3	29

Ice Cream: Per ½ Cup

Banana Split	160	8	20
Choc. Chip Cookie Dough	230	11	32
Mint Chocolate	170	8	21
Strawberry	160	8	18

Donatos Pizza® (Sept '17)

Pizzas: Per Slice

	C	F	Cb
Hand Tossed Signature Pizzas: Per Slice of 14" Pizza			
Chicken Spinach Mozzarella	290	11	30
Founder's Favorite	320	13	4
Mariachi Beef	300	12	35
Mariachi Chicken	230	6	20
Sriracha Jack	360	16	40
The Works	270	12	30
Thick Crust Signature Pizzas: Per Slice of 12" Pizza			
Bourbon BBQ Bacon	150	6	16
Chicken Spinach Mozzarella	140	6	13
Double Bacon Pepperoni	170	9	14
Founders Favorite	160	7	14
Margherita	140	7	13
Serious Meat	160	8	14
Sriracha Jack	140	7	14

Oven Baked Subs:

Big Don: Italian Sub, Marinara	600	25	62
Chicken Bacon Cheddar	770	38	61
Fresh Vegy	490	19	62
Ham & Smoked Prov.	560	21	61
Hot Chicken	830	42	72
Meatball	800	36	70
Stromboli: Deluxe	860	33	95
Pepperoni	980	45	94
Three Meat	970	42	94

Salad: Entree Size, with Menu Set Dressing

Chicken Caprese	390	25	17
Chicken Harvest	600	37	42
Italian Chef	500	43	11

Wings: Without Dipping Sauce

Boneless Chkn: Mild/Hot Sce, av.	395	22	25
Asian Sauce	450	17	51
BBQ	410	16	43

For Complete Nutritional Data ~ see CalorieKing.com

Domino's® (Sept '17)

12" Hand Tossed: Per Slice, ⅛ Pizza

	C	F	Cb
Bacon, Beef & Sausage	280	14	27
Beef, Green Pepp., On. & Mshrm	210	7	27
Black Olives, Green Peppers,			
Onions, Mushrooms, Tomatoes	200	7	27
Ham & Pineapple	200	6	28
Pepperoni	220	9	26
Pepperoni & Sausage	250	11	26
Sausage	240	11	26
Sausage, Beef & Pepperoni	270	14	26

14" Thin Crust: Per Slice, ⅙ Pizza

Bacon, Beef & Sausage	300	19	19
Beef, Green Pepp., On. & Mshrm	220	12	19
Black Olives, Green Peppers,			
Onions, Mushrooms & Tomatoes	190	9	19
Ham & Pineapple	200	9	20
Pepperoni	210	12	18
Pepperoni & Sausage	250	16	18
Sausage	240	15	18

14" Brooklyn: Per Slice, ⅙ Pizza

Beef, Green Pepp., On. & Mshrm	270	11	29
Black Olives, Green Peppers,			
Onions, Mushrooms, Tomatoes	260	10	30
Ham & Pineapple	270	10	31
Pepperoni	290	14	28
Pepperoni & Sausage	340	19	28
Sausage	330	18	28

12" Hand-Tossed: Per Slice, ⅛ Pizza

Buffalo Chicken	260	2	26
Deluxe	230	10	27
ExtravaganZZa	280	13	28
MeatZZa	270	13	27
Ultimate Pepperoni	270	13	26

12" Handmade Pan: Per Slice, ⅛ Pizza

Cali Chicken Bacon Ranch	370	21	30
Deluxe	310	16	30
Memphis BBQ Chicken	330	16	33
Spinach & Feta	300	15	29

14" Thin Crust: Per Slice, ⅛ Pizza

Buffalo Chicken	260	15	17
Cali Chicken Bacon Ranch	320	21	18
Honolulu Hawaiian	250	13	20
Memphis BBQ Chicken	260	14	22
Wisconsin 6 Cheese	250	14	18

Domino's® cont... (Sept '17)

Chicken Wings: W/out Sauce

	C	F	Cb
Barbecue, 4 wings	240	13	18
Hot, 4 wings	200	13	8

Chicken Dipping Cups: Per 1.5 oz Container

	C	F	Cb
Blue Cheese	200	21	2
Kicker Hot	45	4	2
Ranch	200	21	2
Sweet Mango Habanero	60	0	17

BreadBowl Pasta: Per ½ Bowl

	C	F	Cb
Chicken Alfredo, 10.5 oz	690	25	91
Chicken Carbonara, 11.6 oz	730	28	92
Italian Sausage Marinara, 11.85 oz	730	27	96
Pasta Primavera, 11 oz	660	24	91

Oven Baked Sandwiches: Per Sandwich

	C	F	Cb
Buffalo Chicken with Blue Cheese	840	42	74
Chicken Bacon Ranch	880	44	72
Chicken Parmesan	760	30	74
Italian	820	40	72
Mediterranean Veggie	700	28	76
Philly Cheese Steak	740	31	76
Sweet & Spicy Chicken Habanero	810	30	89

Salads: Per Serving without Dressing

	C	F	Cb
Chicken Caesar	210	7	15
Classic Garden	200	9	17

Salad Dressings: Per 1.5 oz Package

	C	F	Cb
Caesar Dressing	210	23	2
Italian	160	17	4
Light Balsamic Dressing	90	9	5
Ranch Dressing	200	21	2

Bread Side Items:

	C	F	Cb
Breadsticks, 2 pieces	190	9	23
Jalap. Bacon Stuffed Cheesy Bread	150	6	17
Parmesan Bread Bites, 5 pieces	150	4	23
Spin. & Fetta Stuffed Cheesy Bread, 1 piece	150	6	17
Stuffed Cheesy Bread, 1 piece	140	5	17

Bread Dipping Sauces: Per Container

	C	F	Cb
Garlic, 1 oz cup	250	28	0
Marinara, 2 oz	30	0	6

Cinna Stix:

	C	F	Cb
2 sticks	200	9	26
8 sticks	1600	72	208

Sweet Icing, Dipping Cup

	C	F	Cb
Sweet Icing, Dipping Cup	250	2.5	57

Dessert: Choc. Lava Crunch Cake

	C	F	Cb
Choc. Lava Crunch Cake	350	17	47
Dipped Choc. Chunk Cookie	380	18	55
Marbled Cookie Brownie	190	9	25

Dunkin' Donuts® (Jan '18)

Bagels: Per Bagel

	C	F	Cb
Plain; Onion, average	310	1	64
Cinnamon Raisin	320	1	66
Everything	340	3	67
Sesame Seed	350	5	65
Sour Cream & Onion	330	1.5	66
Whole Wheat	320	2	61

Danish: Apple Cheese

	C	F	Cb
Apple Cheese	400	19	53
Cheese	420	21	52
Strawberry Cheese	400	19	52

Donuts: Apple 'n Spice

	C	F	Cb
Apple 'n Spice	260	14	29
Bavarian Kreme	270	15	31
Boston Kreme	300	16	37
Bowtie Donut	320	16	40
Chocolate Frosted Cake	350	19	40
Double Chocolate	350	20	39
French Cruller	260	18	21
Jelly	270	14	32
Old Fashioned Cake	290	19	28
Powdered	320	19	33
Strawberry Frosted	280	15	32
Sugar Raised	230	14	22
Vanilla Creme	330	20	35

Muffins: Blueberry, Regular

	C	F	Cb
Blueberry, Regular	460	15	76
Reduced Fat	410	10	75
Chocolate Chip	550	21	83
Coffee Cake	590	24	87
Corn; Honey Bran Raisin, av.	450	15	71

Munchkins: Cinnamon

	C	F	Cb
Cinnamon	60	3.5	6
Glazed	70	4	7
Jelly	70	4	8
Sugared Raised	60	4	5
Toasted Coconut	90	5	10

Other Bakery Items: Brownie (1)

	C	F	Cb
Brownie (1)	440	23	58
Blueberry Coffee Cake, ⅛ cake	190	6	31
Chocolate Chip Coffee Cake, ⅛ cake	230	9	34
Original Coffee Cake, ⅛ cake	230	9	33

Bakery Sandwiches:

	C	F	Cb
Chicken Bacon Ciabatta	580	22	63
Chicken Salad Croissant	580	39	42
Deluxe Grilled Cheese: w Bacon	510	29	40
with Ham	480	25	40
Grilled Cheese	450	24	40
Ham & Cheddar Ciabatta	390	12	50
Snack 'n Go: Chicken Wrap	300	17	21
Steak Wrap	250	15	15
Tuna Melt on Croissant	700	50	43
Tuna Salad on Plain Bagel	580	25	68
Turkey Cheddar Bacon Ciabatta	440	17	47

continued next page...

Dunkin' Donuts® cont... (Jan '18)

Breakfast:

	C	F	Cb
Hash Browns, 6 pieces	140	8	17
Oatmeal,			
Brown Sugar Flavored Oatmeal,			
with Dried Fruit Topping	310	2	66
Plain Bagels:			
Bacon, Egg & Cheese	520	18	67
Egg & Cheese	470	14	67
Ham, Egg & Cheese	500	15	67
Sausage, Egg & Cheese	680	33	67
Big N' Toasted, with Toast	630	38	43
Biscuits: Bacon, Egg & Cheese	530	34	38
Sausage, Egg & Cheese	680	49	38
Croissants: Bacon, Egg & Cheese	560	36	41
Egg & Cheese	500	31	40
Ham, Egg & Cheese	520	32	40
Sausage, Egg & Cheese	700	50	41
English Muffins:			
Bacon, Egg & Cheese	350	18	32
Ham, Egg & Cheese	320	14	32
Sausage, Egg & Cheese	500	33	33
Multigrain Flatbread,			
Turkey Sausage	480	28	32
Wake-Up Wraps:			
Bacon, Egg & Cheese	210	13	14
Egg & Cheese	180	11	13
Ham, Egg & Cheese	200	11	14
Turkey Sausage	280	18	13

Hot Beverages: Per Medium Size

	C	F	Cb
Chocolate: Original	330	10	59
Mint	300	10	52
Dunkaccino	350	15	52

Cold Beverages: Per Medium, 24 fl.oz

	C	F	Cb
Coolatta:			
Strawberry Fruit	370	0	88
Vanilla Bean	630	9	138

Iced Latte: Per Medium, 24 fl.oz, with Whole Milk without sugar

	C	F	Cb
Brown Sugar Cinnamon Swirl	350	9	55
Maple Pecan Swirl	350	9	56
Mocha Swirl	350	10	54
Peppermint Mocha Swirl	360	10	60
Pumpkin Swirl	340	9	53

Iced Macchiato: Per Medium, 24 fl.oz, with Whole Milk

	C	F	Cb
Caramel Swirl	290	6	49
French Vanilla Swirl	280	6	49
Maple Pecan Swirl	290	6	50
Peppermint Mocha Swirl	290	7	53

Eat 'N Park® (Sept '17)

Breakfast:

	C	F	Cb
Bananas Foster French Toast,			
2 slices	440	6	88
Omelettes: Ham & Cheese	665	47	6
Meat Lover's	760	58	6
Pancakes:			
Buttermilk (2)	325	3	65
Blueberry (2)	335	3	68
Scramblers:			
All-American with Bacon	605	27	58
Waffles: Belgian (1)	275	11	37
Strawberry (1)	370	17	48

Appetizers:

	C	F	Cb
Chicken Quesadilla	1030	62	62
Fried Cheese Sticks	590	35	41
Fried Ravioli	895	59	66
Mac 'n Cheese Bites	950	74	55

Burgers:

	C	F	Cb
Black Angus:			
American Grill	705	45	32
Mushroom & Onion	750	43	41
Superburger	1040	69	28
Classic: Black Angus	670	41	38
Black Angus Bacon Cheeseburger	755	46	37
Black Angus Cheeseburger	710	41	39
Garden Burger	420	15	60
Original, Superburger	680	42	38

Sandwiches: With Menu Board Standard Add-Ins

	C	F	Cb
BLT	505	14	68
Buffalo Chicken Wrap, with Ranch	825	47	60
Chargrilled Chicken	475	16	41
Classic Grilled Cheese	720	37	70
Hot Turkey	500	7	74
Reuben	1020	72	45
Shredded Pot Roast	540	31	28
Turkey Club	850	46	48
Whale of a Cod Fish	930	35	96

Dinners: Without Sides

	C	F	Cb
Baked Chicken Parmigiana:			
with Marinara Sauce	955	39	97
with Meat Sauce	1105	50	93
Baked Lemon Sole, 2 fillets	305	21	1
Chicken Fillets, 5 pieces	545	27	29
Classic Liver & Onions	290	13	11
Nantucket Cod	390	27	8
Smothered Ground Sirloin Steak	445	27	8
Spaghetti with Marinara Sauce	665	9	124
Spaghetti with Meat Sauce	835	22	120
Whale of a Cod	625	30	39

Continued Next Page....

Updated Nutrition Data ~ www.CalorieKing.com
Persons with Diabetes ~ See Disclaimer (Page 22)

Eat 'N Park® cont... (Sept '17)

Salads: *Without Dressing*	C	F	Cb
Buffalo Chicken	635	35	46
Greek Chicken	315	9	24
Grilled Chicken	485	20	33
Steak	750	45	34
Dressings: Per 2 oz			
Balsamic Vinaigrette	120	10	8
Bleu Cheese	320	32	2
Greek Vinaigrette	180	18	2
Italian	250	27	2
Ranch	200	20	4
Thousand Island	190	19	4
White Balsamic	160	16	4
Desserts:			
Ice Cream, 2 scoops	295	16	33
Pies: Apple Pie, 1 slice	395	14	65
Blackberry Pie, 1 slice	430	14	72
Coconut Cream Pie, 1 slice	475	23	59
Dutch Apple Pie, 1 slice	405	16	65
Sundaes: Caramel, 2 scoops	475	19	73
Oreo	560	24	80

Edo Japan® (Sept '17)

	C	F	Cb
Bento Box: Without Teriyaki Sauce			
Beef Yakisoba, 20.3 oz	840	29	102
Chicken Yakisoba, 20.5 oz	790	24	102
Sizzling Shrimp, 22 oz	790	15	122
Sukiyaki Beef, 20.3 oz	880	27	120
Teriyaki: Without Teriyaki Sauce			
Beef & Shrimp, 17 oz	660	18	82
Sukiyaki Beef, 14.8 oz	580	15	80
Soup: Per 33 oz Bowl			
Beef Udon	580	17	72
Chicken Udon	550	13	72
Maki Sushi: Per 6 Pieces			
California Roll, 7.6 oz	430	17	61
Spicy Tuna Roll, 6.5 oz	300	2.5	54
Nigiri Sushi: Per 1 Piece			
Ebi (Steamed Prawn), 1.7 oz	70	0.5	12
Salmon Sashimi, 0.7 oz	30	1.5	1

Einstein Bros® (Sept '17)

Bagels:	C	F	Cb
Bagels: Asiago Cheese	300	4	54
Blueberry	290	1	60
Chocolate Chip	300	3.5	58
Cinnamon Sugar	320	6	59
Garlic	280	2	57
Honey Whole Wheat	260	3	49
Onion	270	1.5	55
Potato	280	4	52
Sesame	290	2.5	56
Gourmet Bagels:			
Apple Cinnamon	450	9	83
Green Chile	330	8	53
Power Protein	350	6	64
Six-Cheese	370	10	53
Spinach Florentine	360	11	53
Bagel Dogs:			
Original	530	26	57
Asiago	580	29	57
Egg Sandwiches: 1 Egg Classic on Plain Bagel			
Applewood Bacon & Spinach	490	18	55
Cheddar Cheese	420	13	57
Ham & Swiss	530	18	58
Turkey Sausage & Cheddar	570	22	58
Signature Sandwiches: 1 Egg on Plain Bagel			
Bacon & Spin. on Spin. Florentine	720	42	56
Chorizo Sunrise	790	47	60
Farmhouse	730	34	64
French Toast Egg	720	32	78
Santa Fe	560	22	60
Salads: Without Dressing			
Chicken Caesar	210	6	18
Strawberry Chicken	220	6	24
Tostinis: BBQ Chicken	540	13	66
Buffalo Chicken & Bacon	630	23	58
Italian Chicken	690	32	60
Roasted Veggie	510	21	62
Turkey Club	690	33	60
Wraps: Santa Fe	710	39	60
Turkey Club Mex	740	42	57
Cream Cheese: Per 1.2 oz Schmear			
Reduced Fat:			
Garlic Herb/Garden Veggie	110	9	5
Honey Almond; Strawberry, av.	120	8	10
Plain	120	12	2
Onion and Chive	120	10	4
Sweets: Blueberry Muffin, 4 oz	420	20	57
Cinnamon Twist, 3.4 oz	360	16	50
Snickerdoodle Cookie, 2.9 oz	420	20	59

El Pollo Loco® (Sept '17)

Starters: Per Small Serving	C	F	Cb
Chicken Tortilla w/ Tortilla Strips	210	9	19
without Tortilla Strips	140	5	10
Bowl: Original Pollo, 18.1 oz	610	10	87
Ultimate Double Chicken, 24.7 oz	930	30	93
Burritos:			
Chicken Avocado, 17.9 oz	950	53	74
Chicken Fajita, 17.1oz	870	38	84
Chipotle Chicken Avocado	920	41	89
Ranchero Chicken	930	45	86
Flame-Grilled Chicken: Skin On			
Breast; Thigh, av.	220	12	0
Leg; Wing, av.	90	4.5	0
Stuffed Quesadillas:			
Chicken Avocado	960	61	59
Chicken Fajita Avocado	910	54	63
Salads: Without Dressing			
Classic Chicken	240	8	19
Mexican Cobb	520	25	38
Tacos:			
Crunchy Chicken, 4.6 oz	230	11	19
Grande: Avocado & Chicken, 6.4 oz	340	20	20
Avocado Shrimp, 6.2 oz	320	18	20
Taco al Carbon: Chicken, 3.2 oz	160	6	18
Shrimp, 3 oz	160	7	17
Tostada Salads: With Shell, without Dressing			
Chicken,17.3 oz	860	42	77
Double Chicken, 21.6 oz	1030	50	82
Under 500 Calories: Without Dressing			
Black Bean Bowl, Shrimp, 18.5 oz	480	12	57
Chicken Avocado Tortilla Wrap	480	20	46
Double Chicken Avocado Salad	380	15	15
Dressings: Creamy Cilantro: 3 oz	320	35	2
Light Creamy Cilantro, 1.5 oz	70	5	5
Ranch, 1.5 oz	230	24	2
Sides: Black Beans, 6 oz	140	1	24
Cole Slaw, 4 oz	130	10	9
Cut Corn with Red Peppers, 5 oz	160	5	24
Gravy, 1 oz	10	0	2
Macaroni & Cheese, 6 oz	310	19	24
Mashed Potatoes, 5 oz	110	1.5	23
Pinto Beans, 6 oz	200	4	29
Condiments:			
Pico de Gallo, 1.5 oz	15	1	2
Salsa: Avocado, 1.5 oz	30	2.5	2
House; Roja, av.,1.5 oz	10	0	2
Sour Cream, 1.3 oz	80	7	1
Dessert, Two Cinnamon Churros	320	22	30

Fatburger® (Sept '17)

Burgers: Without Extras	C	F	Cb
Burgers: Small	400	21	37
Medium	590	31	46
Large	850	41	69
Turkeyburger	480	21	50
Veggieburger	510	20	60
Hot Dogs: Without Extras			
Chili Cheese	480	27	35
Regular Hot Dog	320	15	32
Sandwiches: Without Extras			
Chicken: Crispy	560	27	53
Grilled	430	14	42
Fish	560	31	55
Fries: Fat Fries	380	18	47
with Chili	480	24	52
with Chili & Cheese	590	33	53
Skinny Fries	390	15	58
with Chili Cheese	600	30	64
Add-Ons: American Cheese, 1 slice	70	5	1
Cheddar Cheese, 1 slice	110	9	1
Mayonnaise, 1 serving	90	10	1
Relish, 1 serving	20	0	5
Sides: Chili Cup	200	11	10
with Cheese & Onions	320	20	12
Onion Rings	540	29	64
Shakes: Chocolate	910	45	115
Cookies & Ice Cream	1180	59	163
Maui-Banana	940	44	126
Peanut Butter	950	53	114
Strawberry; Vanilla, average	885	44	112

For Complete Nutritional Data ~ see CalorieKing.com

Fazoli's® (Sept '17)

Oven-Baked Pasta: Per Serving	C	F	Cb
Baked Ziti	590	20	73
Chicken Broccoli Penne	810	34	73
Chicken Parmigano	750	20	97
Penne Romano	800	37	76
Penne with Creamy Basil Chicken	830	38	69
Twice-Baked Lasagna	690	29	74
Top It Options:			
Bacon	90	8	0
Broccoli	70	5	4
Italian Meatballs	230	18	5
Italian Sausage	200	16	3
Roasted Chicken	120	4	3

Continued Next Page....

Updated Nutrition Data ~ www.CalorieKing.com
Persons with Diabetes ~ See Disclaimer (Page 22)

Fazoli's® cont... (Sept '17)

Samplers: Per Serving	C	F	Cb
Classic Sampler	940	29	129
Spicy Sampler	1110	42	129
Ultimate Sampler Platter	1060	25	160

Signature Pastas:			
Chicken Carbonara	890	30	100
Ultimate Fettuccine	930	34	101
Ultimate Spaghetti	920	36	105

Submarinos:			
Meatball da Vinci	920	56	65
Primo Italiano	840	45	60
Turkey Club Classico	710	35	55

For Complete Nutritional Data ~ see CalorieKing.com

Firehouse Subs® (Sept '17)

Hot Subs: Per Medium White Sub, with Standard Toppings and Dressings	C	F	Cb
Ham	760	38	69
Roast Beef	740	37	53
Turkey	680	35	58
Veggie	720	45	60
Specialty: Club on a Sub	770	40	63
Engineer	690	35	59
Hero	800	38	63
Hook & Ladder	720	36	62
Italian	940	58	65
Meatball	840	50	61
Sides, Chili, Bowl	300	16	26

Under 500 Calorie Salads: Without Dressing

Canadian Chopped:			
Hook & Ladder (Smoked Turkey)	340	16	21
House Chopped, without Meat	190	14	11

Firehouse Chopped:			
with Grilled Chicken	260	8	15
with Ham	310	10	27
with Turkey	220	7	15
Italian, with Grilled Chicken	485	32	18

Five Guys® (Sept '17)

Burgers:	C	F	Cb
Bacon Burger	780	50	39
Bacon Cheeseburger	920	62	40
Cheeseburger	840	55	40
Hamburger	700	43	39
Little Burgers: Bacon Burger	560	33	39
Bacon Cheeseburger	630	39	40
Cheeseburger	550	32	40
Hamburger	480	26	39

Five Guys® cont... (Sept '17)

Dogs:	C	F	Cb
Bacon Dog; Cheese Dog	620	42	40
Bacon Cheese Dog	695	48	41
Hot Dog	545	35	40

Fries:			
Cajun Style, 14.5 oz	955	41	131
Five Guys Style, 14.5 oz	955	41	131

Flame Broiler® (Sept '17)

Bowls: With White Rice	C	F	Cb
Beef	620	11	74
Chicken	600	14	68
Chicken & Veggie	510	14	49
Half & Half	610	13	71
The Works	520	13	52

Plates: With White Rice			
Beef	840	18	94
Rib	1100	44	95
The Works	700	19	63

Freshens® (Sept '17)

Smoothies: 100% Juice	C	F	Cb
Blended Fruit Classics: Per 20 fl.oz			
Bangin' Berry	370	0	90
Caribbean Craze; Maui Mango	330	0	81
Jamaican Jammer; Or. Sunrise	320	2	70
Peach On The Beach	280	3	61
Purple Rein	320	0	79
Tropical Therapy	480	6	109
Wild Strawberry	340	0	87
Protein, Peanut Butter	500	12	76

Crepes:			
Buffalo Chicken	410	22	25
Chicken Caesar	600	44	25
Chipotle Ranch Turkey Melt	520	31	25
Denver, with Bacon	520	29	27
Honey Mustard Chicken	460	22	36
Pesto Chicken	490	29	27
Southwest Chicken	580	33	36

Rice Bowls: Buffalo Chicken			
Buffalo Chicken	600	22	69
Florence	450	12	62
KC BBQ	590	11	90
Mexican	710	29	83
Power Protein	670	27	70
Spicy Korean	520	8	89

Salad: Buffalo Chicken			
Buffalo Chicken	480	27	29
Grilled Chicken Caesar	520	37	26
Roadhouse BBQ Chicken	420	17	42
Strawberry & Kale	490	15	56

Godfather's Pizza® (Sept '17)

Golden Crust Pizza: Per Slice	C	F	Cb
Cheese: Medium, 1/8 pizza	210	8	25
Large, 1/10 pizza	230	10	27
Combo: Med., 1/8	280	13	27
Large, 1/10 pizza	310	15	29
Super Combo: Medium, 1/8 pizza	310	15	28
Large, 1/10 pizza	360	18	30
Mozza-Loaded:			
All Meat Combo: Medium, 1/8 pizza	360	19	28
Large, 1/10 pizza	390	21	30
Original Crust Pizza:			
BLT: Mini, 1/4 pizza	220	11	19
Medium, 1/8 pizza	370	18	32
Jumbo, 1/12 pizza	500	25	42
Buffalo Chicken: Mini, 1/4 pizza	170	7	18
Medium, 1/8 pizza	270	9	32
Jumbo, 1/12 pizza	380	14	41
Super Taco Pie: Mini, 1/4 pizza	220	9	22
Medium, 1/8 pizza	370	17	36
Jumbo, 1/12 pizza	450	20	46
Thin Crust Pizza:			
BBQ Chicken: Medium, 1/8 pizza	190	8	18
Large, 1/10 pizza	220	10	21
Pepperoni: Medium, 1/8 pizza	210	10	21
Large, 1/10 pizza	270	16	18
The Don: Medium, 1/8 pizza	280	17	16
Large, 1/10 pizza	350	19	25
Sides:			
Breadstick, Golden, av., 1 oz	80	3	11
Cheesestick, average, 1.2 oz	100	5	11
Chicken Wings: Bone-In, Buff., 3 oz	190	14	2
Breaded Hot Wing, full order, 8 oz	920	54	38
Garlic Bread: 1 piece	160	9	17
with Cheese, 1 piece	200	12	17
Potato Wedges, 4 oz	140	7	18

Gold Star Chili® (Sept '17)

Burritos & Burrito Bowls:	C	F	Cb
Gold Star Chili Burrito	970	33	126
Grilled Chicken Bowl	905	29	111
Coneys: Cheese	310	19	21
Coney	225	12	21
Sriracha Coney	315	19	22
Ways, Regular:			
2-Way	395	10	54
3-Way	680	34	55
4-Way, Bean	825	34	81
5-Way	840	33	87
Super 5-Way	1180	48	122
Chili By The Bowl:			
Gold Star	205	10	10
Veggie	200	3	34

Gold Star Chili® cont...(Sept '17)

Double Deckers:	C	F	Cb
Ham & Bacon	515	29	40
Ham & Turkey	620	26	48
Turkey & Bacon	590	30	44
Sandwich, Crispy Chicken	355	20	24
Salads: Without Dressing			
Cafe	305	13	34
Chili	685	36	62
Spring Harvest	185	5	29
Fries: French	400	16	58
Cheese	575	30	59
Chili Cheese	680	36	63
Sriracha	425	16	64

Golden Corral® (Sept '17)

Breakfast:	C	F	Cb
Corned Beef Hash, 1/2 cup	230	15	14
Biscuit	230	15	20
Potato Hash Brown Casserole, 1/2 c.	100	3.5	14
Sausage & Egg Burrito	320	19	22
Scrambled Eggs, 1/2 cup	180	14	2
Hot Buffet: Without Sides			
Beef: Pot Roast, 1/2 cup	150	7	8
Roast, carved, 3 oz	110	3	0
Salisbury Steak (1), 3 oz	70	3	7
Steak, Smothered Chopped, 5.9 oz	290	18	4
Chicken: Breast, Grilled, 3.4 oz	70	1.5	0
Fried Chicken, 5 oz	270	14	14
Piccata, 5 oz	220	13	6
Pot Pie, Mini, 7.9 oz	400	24	34
Fish: Baked, 3 oz	150	8	1
Florentine Fish, 1 piece	180	12	1
Pork: Chops, Southern Style, 3 oz	230	16	8
Steaks (1), 4.6 oz	250	13	17
Sides: Baby Carrots, steamed, 1/2 c.	90	7	8
BBQ Baked Beans, 1/2 cup	160	1	35
Breaded Okra (10)	110	7	10
Creamed Spinach, 1/2 cup	170	12	10
Fried Cubed Potatoes, 1/2 cup	160	9	19
Vegetables, Medley Campfire, 1/2 c.	90	5	9
Salad Buffet: Per 1/2 Cup Unless Indicated			
Caesar, without dressing, 1 cup	110	8	8
Chicken	250	22	3
Coleslaw	110	9	6
Potato Steakhouse	150	5	26
Seafood	140	10	9
Spinach Bacon, 1 cup	120	9	4
Tuna	190	11	4
Dressings: Balsamic Vinaig., 2 Tbsp	20	0	5
Caesar, 2 Tbsp	150	15	2
Ranch, 2 Tbsp	110	12	2

Updated Nutrition Data ~ www.CalorieKing.com
Persons with Diabetes ~ See Disclaimer (Page 22)

Great American Bagel Co® (Apr '16)

Bagels:	C	F	Cb
Asiago Cheese	520	16	72
Cheddar Herb	390	8	66
Cinnamon Raisin	380	3.5	76
Jalapeno Cheddar	370	7	63
Plain	360	4	71
Spinach Tomazzo	640	20	86
Tomazzo	520	13	77
Paninis: On Regular Baguette			
Chicken Pesto	770	35	70
Ham & Swiss	600	26	58
Philly Beef	920	40	92
Turkey Club	680	29	67
Sandwiches: Asiago Omelet	720	29	80
BLT	550	17	72
Chicken Parmigiana	740	22	81
Ham	460	9	71
Roast Beef	465	9	71
Turkey	435	5	72
Cream Cheese Filling: Per 1 oz			
Plain	100	10	1
Strawberry; Vegetable, average	90	8	4
Pastries:			
Cookies: Chocolate Chunk, 4 oz	110	3.5	19
Oatmeal Raisin, 4 oz	120	5	18
Muffins: Banana Nut, 4.25 oz	430	18	61
Blueberry, 4.25 oz	430	16	64

Green Burrito® (Sept '17)

Burritos:	C	F	Cb
Bean & Cheese	660	25	76
Green: Chicken	930	38	96
Steak	940	38	96
Grilled, Beef; Chicken; Steak, av.	840	33	89
Specialties:			
Quesadillas: Cheese	640	34	53
Chicken	780	40	56
Steak	790	39	56
Rice, Bean & Chips Platter	340	10	51
Super Nachos, average	735	44	53
Taco Salad, Chicken; Steak	875	53	60
Tacos:			
Crunchy Beef Taco	210	12	16
Soft Chicken Taco	250	12	18
Sides: Chips, 2 oz	300	17	35
Cilantro lim Rice, 3.4 oz	90	5	21
Guacamole, 2.7 oz	100	8	5
Pinto Beans, 3.7 oz	90	1.5	13

(The) Great Steak® (Sept '17)

Breakfast Sandwiches:	C	F	Cb
Bacon, Egg & Cheese	550	31	38
Sausage, Egg & Cheese	660	42	38
Steak, Egg & Chse	540	27	38
Burgers:			
Bacon Cheeseburger	1050	72	45
Cheeseburger	840	54	45
Hamburger	730	46	44
Philly Cheeseburger	780	48	44
Sandwiches: 7"			
Bacon Cheddar Cheesesteak	590	23	55
Buffalo Chicken Philly	750	38	61
Chicagoland Cheesesteak	610	24	59
Chicken Bacon Ranch	820	44	60
Great Steak Cheesesteak	790	45	55
Ham Delight	780	44	64
Orig. Philly Cheesesteak	510	17	55
Pastrami Philly	800	46	57
Reuben Philly	710	37	56
Super Steak Cheesesteak	800	45	57
Turkey Philly	750	42	57
Ultimate Chicken Philly	800	44	60
Veggie Delight	490	19	61
Wisconsin Inside-Out	530	26	50
Baked Potatoes:			
Bacon & Cheese	440	23	36
Broccoli & Cheese	250	6	45
The Great Potato: Chicken	460	19	49
Ham	450	19	52
Steak	470	20	46
Turkey	430	17	48
The King	540	32	38
Fries:			
Bacon Ranch: Regular	650	42	51
Large	1520	91	139
Great Fry: Kids	270	13	36
Regular	370	18	48
Large	930	40	132
King Fry, regular	480	27	52
Salads: Without Dressing			
Great Salad: Chicken	370	22	16
Ham	360	22	19
Steak	390	23	17
Turkey	350	20	19
Salad Dressings: Mayo, reg., 1 oz	200	22	0
Ranch, 1 oz	150	16	2
Thousand Island, 1 oz	130	12	4
Sauce: BBQ, 1 oz	50	0	12
Buffalo, 1 oz	10	0	1
Honey Mustard, 1 oz	40	1	7
Teriyaki, 1 oz	25	0	3

Haagen-Dazs® (Sept '17)

Classic Flavors: Per ¹/₂ Cup

	C	F	Cb
Belgian Chocolate	330	21	30
Brownies a La Mode	280	16	28
Butter Pecan	300	22	20
Caramel Cone	320	20	28
Cherry Vanilla	290	17	29
Choc. Chip Cookie Dough	290	17	30
Chocolate Chocolate Chip	300	19	26
Chocolate Peanut Butter	330	22	25
Coffee; Green Tea	250	17	20
Cookies and Cream	250	16	22
Dulce de Leche	270	16	28
Espresso Chocolate Cookie Crumble	310	21	25
Mint Chip	280	18	25
Pineapple Coconut	230	13	25
Rocky Road	290	17	29
Rum Raisin	250	16	22
Sea Salt Caramel Truffle	300	17	32
Strawberry	240	15	22
Vanilla Bean	270	17	25
Vanilla Swiss Almond	290	19	24
Vanilla Tangerine & Shortbread	290	18	26
White Chocolate Raspberry Truffle	280	16	31

Gelato,

	C	F	Cb
Sea Salt Caramel, ½ cup	250	17	20

Sorbet: Per ¹/₂ Cup

	C	F	Cb
Mango	150	0	38
Orchard Peach	140	0	34
Raspberry; Zesty Lemon, average	115	0	29

Ice Cream Bars/Cones ~ See Page 109

Hardee's® (Jan '18)

Burgers:

	C	F	Cb
All Natural Grass Fed, 11 oz	780	49	56
Cheeseburgers: ¹/₄ lb	440	23	37
¹/₃ lb	640	33	56
²/₃ lb	970	59	57
Double, 5.7 oz	380	19	33
Small, 4.5 oz	300	13	33
Hamburger, Small, 4.2 oz	250	9	32
Thickburgers: ¹/₄ lb	530	35	34
Original: ¹/₃ lb	780	48	56
²/₃ lb	1100	73	57
Bacon Cheese: ¹/₃ lb	850	54	54
²/₃ lb	1170	79	55
Double, ²/₃ lb	1130	77	58
Frisco: ¹/₃ lb	840	55	46
²/₃ lb	1150	80	47
Mushroom 'N' Swiss:			
¹/₃ lb	680	38	53
²/₃ lb	1000	63	54

Hardee's® cont... (Jan '18)

Sandwiches:

	C	F	Cb
Chicken: Big Chicken Fillet, 11 oz	710	36	64
Charbroiled: BBQ, 7.8 oz	350	6	46
Chicken Club	560	28	38
Spicy Chicken	440	23	44
Hot Ham 'N' Cheese: Regular	290	11	29
Big	530	20	51
Roast Beef: Regular	310	14	28
Big	500	23	48

Chicken Tenders: Without Sauce

Hand Breaded:

	C	F	Cb
3 pieces, 4.5 oz	260	13	13
5 pieces, 7.5 oz	440	21	21
Chili Dog, Jumbo	390	26	23

Fried Chicken Pieces:

	C	F	Cb
Breast, 5.2 oz	370	15	29
Leg, 2.4 oz	170	7	15
Thigh, 4.3 oz	330	15	30
Wing, 2.3 oz	200	8	23

Sides:

	C	F	Cb
Coleslaw, 4 oz	270	22	17
Crispy Curls:			
Small, 4.1 oz	360	18	46
Medium, 5.36 oz	470	23	60
Large, 6.5 oz	570	28	72
Green Beans, 4.7 oz	40	1.5	5
Mashed Potatoes & Gravy, 5 oz	90	1	17
Side Salad, w/out Dressing, 6.7 oz	120	7	7

Fries & Onion Rings:

	C	F	Cb
Beer Battered Onion Rings, 4.5 oz	410	24	45
Natural Cut Fries:			
Kid's, 3 oz	240	12	31
Small, 3.7 oz	300	15	47
Medium, 5.9 oz	490	24	63
Large, 6.5 oz	530	26	69

Kids Meals: Includes Kid's Fries, w/out Drink

	C	F	Cb
Cheeseburger	520	23	62
Chicken Tenders	400	19	37
Hamburger	470	20	61
Hotdog	570	34	50

Updated Nutrition Data ~ www.CalorieKing.com
Persons with Diabetes ~ See Disclaimer (Page 22)

Hardee's® cont... (Jan '18)

Better For You:	C	F	Cb
Low Carb It: 1/3 lb Thickburger	440	35	9
Breakfast Bowl	660	52	10
Charbroiled Chicken Club S'wich	340	22	13
Trim It, Charbr. BBQ Chkn S'wich	190	3.5	24
Breakfast:			
Low Carb Bowl	680	59	2
Breakfast Burritos:			
Loaded	580	30	46
Made From Scratch Biscuits:			
Bacon, Egg & Cheese	610	38	46
Bacon, Swiss, Cheese & Egg	840	54	56
Biscuit 'N' Gravy	620	39	57
Chicken Fillet	650	41	53
Cinnamon 'N' Raisin	320	14	46
Country Ham	500	30	44
Country Steak	640	42	52
Jelly	460	26	52
Loaded Omelet	620	39	57
Made From Scratch, Buttermilk	430	26	43
Monster	880	61	48
Sausage	620	43	44
Sausage and Egg	690	48	46
Smoked Sausage, Egg & Cheese	790	57	48
Platter: with Bacon	900	57	64
with Ham	880	43	75
with Sausage	1070	72	76
Sandwich, Frisco Breakfast	450	19	45
Breakfast Sides: Grits, 5 oz	110	4.5	17
Hash Rounds: Small, 2.9 oz	260	15	23
Medium, 4.2 oz	370	22	33
Large, 5.8 oz	510	30	45
Desserts:			
Apple Turnover, w/out Cinnamon Sugar	270	13	35
Chocolate Chip Cookie (2), 2 oz	240	10	36
Freshed Baked (1), 2 oz	290	15	35
Single Scoop Ice Cream:			
Vanilla: Bowl, 4 oz	240	13	27
Sugar Cone, 4.4 oz	300	14	37
Ice Cream Shakes:			
Choc.; Strawb., av., 14 oz	705	34	86
Vanilla, 14 oz	700	33	86

Hissho Sushi® (Sept '17)

Starters: With White Rice	C	F	Cb
Chicken Gyoza, 4 oz	180	6	20
Pork Gyoza, 4 oz	230	11	23
Spring Rolls: Regular	185	4	30
Ocean	180	2	29
Squid Salad, 4 oz	95	2	7
Maki Rolls: With White Rice			
Rolls: Blazing California, 7 oz	405	12	65
California, 7 oz	295	3	59
Dynamaite Roll, 7 oz	470	13	66
Eel, 7 oz	375	1	69
Hissho Healthy, 6 oz	210	1	46
Nippon Favorite, 6 oz	300	4	45
Philadelphia, 7 oz	385	12	60
Snow Crab, 7 oz	295	3	55
Spicy, 7 oz	430	11	62
Sushicado, 7 oz	290	3	54
Veggie Roll, 7 oz	275	2	57
Specialty Rolls: Per 7 oz Roll Unless Indicated			
Caterpillar	480	5	84
Living Color	370	5	51
Mango Tango	420	10	58
Salmon Lover	720	32	63
Sriracha Party	540	14	77
Tempura Shrimp, 9 oz	665	19	108
TNT	545	14	71
Wasabi Crunch	550	19	76

Hot Dog on a Stick® (Sept '17)

Menu Items:	C	F	Cb
American Cheese on a Stick	260	16	21
Beef Hot Dog on a Bun	340	23	22
Turkey Hot Dog on a Stick	240	13	23
Veggie Dog on a Stick	220	8	24
Pepperjack Cheese on a Stick	240	14	19
Sides, French Fries, 4.5 oz	410	22	49
Dessert, Funnel Cake Sticks, with Powdered Sugar, (10)	210	8	31
Beverages: Per Regular Size, 16 fl.oz			
Lemonade: Original	150	0	38
Cherry	210	0	52
Lime	230	0	57

Hungry Howie's Pizza® (Sept '17)

Counts may vary in Florida.

	C	**F**	**Cb**
Specialty Pizza: 12" Pizza, Per ⅛ Slice			
BBQ Chicken, Butter Crust	240	8	30
Buffalo Chicken, Ranch Crust	210	8	25
Works, Cajun Crust	310	16	26
Veggie, Ranch Crust	200	6	27
Subs: Per Large 8" Sub, with Set Menu Toppings			
Italian	660	23	81
Ham & Cheese	590	15	68
Steak, Cheese & Mushroom	610	18	81
Turkey Club	660	18	80
Veggie	610	19	83
Wings, Boneless, Buffalo, 3 pieces	280	11	21
Salads: Half of Regular Size, without Dressing			
Antipasto	170	10	10
Chef	140	8	9
Garden	70	2	12
Greek	140	7	15
Dressings: Per 1 oz			
Creamy Italian	120	12	2
Greek	110	11	2
Ranch	140	14	1
Thousand Island	140	14	4

In-N-Out Burger® (Sept '17)

	C	**F**	**Cb**
Burgers:			
Hamburger: with Onion	390	19	39
w/ Mstrd & Ketchup, w/o Spread	310	10	41
Protein Style w/ Lettuce Wrap, without Bun	240	17	11
Cheeseburger: with Onion	480	27	39
w/ Mstrd & Ketchup, w/o Spread	400	18	41
Protein Style w/ Lettuce Wrap, without Bun	330	25	11
Double Double: with Onion	670	41	39
w/ Mstrd & Ketchup, w/o Spread	590	32	41
Protein Style w/ Lettuce Wrap, without Bun	520	39	11
French Fries, 4.5 oz	395	18	54
Drinks: Milk, 10 fl.oz	180	6	18
Coca-Cola, 16 fl.oz	195	0	54
Dr Pepper; 7-Up, av., 16 fl.oz	200	0	53
Lemonade, 16 fl.oz	180	0	40
Root Beer, 16 fl.oz	220	0	60
Shakes:			
Chocolate, 15 fl.oz	590	29	72
Strawberry, 15 fl.oz	590	27	81
Vanilla, 15 fl.oz	580	31	67

IHOP® (Sept '17)

	C	**F**	**Cb**
Made To Stack Pancakes:			
Chocolate Chocolate Chip:			
Buttermilk version (2)	305	10	47
Chocolate version (2)	315	11	48
Double Blueberry (2)	300	7.5	51
NY Cheesecake (2)	470	18	68
Orig. Buttermilk (3)	430	17	57
Strawberry Banana (2)	335	7.5	61
Syrups: Per 1 fl.oz			
Blueb.; Butter Pecan; Old Fashioned	110	0	27
Boysenberry; Strawberry	100	0	26
Sugar-Free Syrup	15	0	6
Made To Top Griddle Faves: With Set Toppings			
French Toast: Original	750	36	85
Bananas Foster Brioche	1010	49	123
Brioche, Plain	720	35	82
Strawberry Banana	880	31	131
Waffle, Belgian	520	27	60
Crepes: With Set Toppings			
Banana with Nutella	960	45	121
Chicken Florentine	900	53	48
German Crepes	680	34	76
Strawberries & Cream	800	30	117
Swedish	660	30	81
Made To Order Omelettes: Without Pancakes or Sides			
Big Steak	1150	78	47
Chicken Fajita	960	63	24
Garden Omelette	830	66	16
Spinach & Mushroom	890	70	20
Made to Build Combos:			
Biscuits & Gravy Combo,			
2 Fried Eggs, with Country Gravy	1330	83	107
Breakfast Sampler, w/out Eggs	920	56	69
Chicken Fried Chicken,			
2 Fried Eggs, with Country Gravy	1060	60	85
Pork Chops, 4 oz, 2 Poached Eggs	1040	60	67
T-Bone Steak, 10 oz, & 3 Fried Eggs	970	50	59
Sandwiches: Without Sides			
Chicken Clubhouse Super Stacker	1090	68	62
Double BLT	660	42	43
Ham & Egg Melt	1080	53	78
Patty Melt	1030	65	64
Sandwich Sides: French Fries	320	15	41
Hash Browns	280	18	28
Onion Rings	500	28	57
Entrees: With Menu Set Sides, without Garlic Bread, Soup or Salad			
Chicken Cordon Bleu	1070	71	57
Pot Roast	820	43	64
Roast Turkey & Fixings	1000	40	106
T-Bone Steak, with Pancakes, 12 oz	750	40	41

For Complete Menu & Data ~ see CalorieKing.com

Jack in the Box® (Jan '18)

	C	F	Cb
Sandwiches & Burgers:			
Bacon Swiss Buttery Jack	885	59	48
Bacon Ultimate Cheeseburger	930	65	32
Classic Buttery Jack	815	52	50
Double Jack	830	58	34
Jumbo Jack: with Cheese	600	40	33
without Cheese	520	33	32
Junior Bacon Chseburger	480	31	32
Sourdough Jack	700	45	39
Spicy Sriracha Burger	680	45	38
Ultimate Cheeseburger	840	59	31
Chicken & Fish:			
Chicken Fajita Pita	345	12	36
Chicken Sandwich	510	31	42
Chicken Teriyaki Bowl	690	6	134
Crispy Chicken Strips, 4 pieces	565	24	53
Homestyle Ranch Chicken Club	710	33	66
Jack's Spicy Chkn S'wich	550	29	48
with Cheese	630	35	49
Sourdough Grilled Chicken Club	580	30	38
Brunchfast: Brunch Burger	770	55	32
Bacon & Egg Chicken Sandwich	650	39	37
Southwest Scrambler Plate,			
with Bacon	500	28	38
Breakfast:			
Biscuit: Bacon, Egg & Cheese	410	25	26
Sausage, Egg & Cheese	535	38	27
Breakfast Jack: Reg.	350	18	30
with Sausage	485	33	29
Burrito: Meat Lovers, with salsa	790	50	50
Grand Sausage, with salsa	1045	70	68
Croissants: Sausage	555	39	32
Supreme	450	27	32
Hash Browns	185	13	17
Sandwiches: Extreme Sausage	650	49	29
Loaded	705	47	36
Ultimate	520	31	30
Snacks & Sides:			
Bacon Cheddar Potato Wedges	680	41	58
Chiquita Apple Bites,2 oz	30	0	7
Egg Rolls (3), without sauce	440	22	46
French Fries: Small	300	14	40
Medium	430	20	58
Large	550	25	75
Panko Onion Rings (8), 4.3 oz	445	24	52
Seasoned Curly Fries: Small	280	16	30
Medium	430	25	46
Large	480	28	52
Stuffed Jalapenos: 3 Pieces	220	12	21
7 Pieces	510	29	49

Jack in the Box® cont... (Jan '18)

Salads: W/out Dressing or Toppings	C	F	Cb
Chicken Club: with Crispy Chicken	515	28	36
with Grilled Chicken	370	20	11
Side Salad	20	0	4
Southwest Chicken,			
with Grilled Chicken Strips	350	15	27
Dressings: Creamy Southwest	190	19	3
Ranch	250	25	5
Low Fat Balsamic Vinaigrette	25	1.5	3
Dipping Sauce: Barbecue, 1 oz	40	0	10
Buttermilk, 1 oz	110	11	2
Frank's Red Hot Buffalo, 1 oz	10	0	1
Sweet & Sour, 1 oz	40	0	10
Teriyaki	50	1	11
Sandwich Sauce:			
Creamy Bacon Mayo, 0.7 fl.oz	120	13	1
Creamy Sriracha Sauce, 0.8fl.oz	120	13	1
Mayo-Onion, 0.5 fl.oz	90	10	0
Tartar Sauce, 0.5 fl.oz	50	4.5	2
Desserts:			
Chocolate Overload Cake	300	7	57
Churros, Mini (5)	345	18	42
New York Style Cheesecake	310	17	32
Ice Cream Shakes: 16 fl.oz, with Whipped Topping			
Chocolate	780	28	103
Oreo Cookie	795	42	92
Strawberry	760	38	97
Vanilla	685	38	78

For Complete Nutritional Data ~ see CalorieKing.com

Jack's® (Sept '17)

Burgers & Sandwiches:	C	F	Cb
Big Bacon	800	57	36
Big Jack Burger	720	47	43
Cheeseburger	440	23	38
Chicken Fillet Sandwich	560	29	46
Double Cheeseburger	680	43	38
Grilled Chicken S'wich	410	17	35
Hamburger	400	19	38
Chicken: Breast	480	29	20
Fingers & Fries, 4 piece	720	32	60
Fries, regular	310	13	42
Breakfast: Double Gravy Biscuit	950	58	90
Sausage, Egg & Cheese Biscuit	630	46	34
Steak Biscuit	580	41	42

Jamba Juice® (Sept '17)

Freshly Squeezed Juice: 16 fl.oz

	C	F	Cb
Orange Berry Antioxidant	200	1	48
Purely Carrot	130	0.5	30
Purely Orange	220	1	52
Tropical Kick-Start	210	1	50

Smoothies: Per Small

	C	F	Cb
Classic: Banana Berry	280	1	67
Mango-A-Go-Go	300	1.5	69
Peach Pleasure	280	1	65
Razzamatazz	290	1	67
Strawberry Surf Rider	320	1	78
Strawberries Wild	260	0	62
Fruit & Veggie: Apple 'n Greens	250	1	60
Berry UpBEET	240	1	52
Greens 'n Ginger	330	1	83
Protein: Chocolate	370	6	53
Cookies 'n Crème	480	15	59
PB & Banana	490	22	44
Super Blend:			
Apples 'N Charge	410	15	52
Green Up 'N Go	250	10	30
PB 'N Jealous	380	14	47

Tasty Bites:

	C	F	Cb
Artisan Flat Bread: *Per Flatbread*			
Four Cheese	330	13	37
Sweet 'n Spicy	330	11	38
Baked Goods: *Per Item*			
Apple Cinnamon Pretzel	380	4	76
Cheddar Tomato Twist	240	4.5	41
Sourdough Parmesan Pretzel	410	10	67
Sweet Belgian Waffle	320	15	42
Breakfast Wraps: Spinach 'n Chse	240	8	30
Turkey Sausage 'n Cheese	320	16	29
Steel-Cut Oatmeal: *With Soymilk*			
Plain	180	2.5	35
Add: Apple Cinnamon	70	0	16
Banana	50	0	13
Blueberries	10	0	2
Brown Sugar Crumble	40	1	8
Clover Honey	30	0	9
Strawberries	5	0	1
Toasted Bistro Sandwiches:			
Ham, Jarlsberg & Dijon	290	8	33
Roast Chicken, Cheddar & Honey Dijon	290	7	34
Three Cheeses	330	14	32

Energy Bowls: Per 16 fl.oz

	C	F	Cb
Acai Primo	490	10	99
Chunky Strawberry	590	17	96
Fruit & Greek Yogurt	390	4	62
Island Pitaya	470	8	100

Jersey Mike's Subs® (Sept '17)

Cold Subs: Per Regular, on White, without Vinegar, Oil or Mayo Unless Indicated

	C	F	Cb
#1 BLT, with Mayo	780	48	67
#2 Jersey Shore Favorite	550	14	69
#3 American Classic	540	14	68
#5 Super Sub	570	15	70
#6 Roast Beef & Provolone	700	23	66
#7 Turkey Breast & Provolone	530	12	66
#8 Club Sub with Mayonnaise	860	45	69
#9 Club Supreme w/ Mayonnaise	930	48	68
#10 Albacore Tuna	800	43	70
#13 Original Italian	680	25	71
#14 Veggie	660	28	68

Hot Subs: Per Regular on White Roll

	C	F	Cb
#15 Meatball & Cheese	800	41	71
#17: Chicken Philly	700	23	69
Steak Philly	640	22	69
#18 Grilled Chicken Parmesan	620	18	64
#19 BBQ Beef	780	18	96
#20 Reuben	670	24	75
#42: Chipotle Chicken, with Mayo	990	53	72
#43: Chipotle Steak, with Mayo	920	52	71
#55: Big Kahuna Chkn	760	27	70
#56: Big Kahuna Steak	690	26	70

Signature Wraps: Flour/Spinach/Tomato Tortilla

	C	F	Cb
Baja	680	26	63
Buffalo Chicken	840	43	64
Caesar	650	28	57
Turkey Honey Mustard	560	20	63

Salads: Without Dressing

	C	F	Cb
Chef, 16 oz	250	10	16
Feta with Chicken, 16.7 oz	340	9	17
Gorgonzola, with Chicken, 17.8 oz	580	26	36
Mike's, 10.26 oz	60	0	13
Soup: Boston Clam Chowder, bowl	190	9	22
Cream of Broccoli, bowl	140	9	13
Vegetable, Beef & Barley, bowl	140	4.5	17
Wisconsin Cheese, bowl	340	24	24

Dressings: Per 2 Tbsp, 1 oz

	C	F	Cb
Caesar	150	15	2
Chipotle Mayo	180	20	0
Golden Italian	110	11	3
Ranch	120	12	2
Russian	160	16	4
Desserts: Choc Chip Cookie, 1.5 oz	190	9	26
Blondie Brownie, 4 oz	520	30	59
Drinks: Mountain Dew, 22 oz	310	0	84
Mug Root Beer, 22 oz	300	0	79
Tropicana Fruit Punch, 22 oz	310	0	77

Updated Nutrition Data ~ www.CalorieKing.com
Persons with Diabetes ~ See Disclaimer (Page 22)

Jimmy John's® (Sept '17)

Subs: (8") Figures Based on French Bread w/ Standard Toppings & Mayo, Unless Indicated

	C	F	Cb
#1 Pepe	625	30	59
#2 Big John	535	22	56
#3 Totally Tuna, without mayo	710	34	62
#4 Turkey Tom	505	20	57
#5 Vito with Italian Vinaigrette	655	31	60
#6 Vegetarian	695	40	61
JJBLT	615	31	56

Giant Club Sandwiches: Figures Based on 8-Grain Bread w/ Standard Toppings & Mayo, Unless Indicated

#7 Gourmet Smoked Ham	775	37	65
#8 Billy Club	800	39	63
#9 Italian Night w/ Mayo & Vinaig.	955	56	66
#10 Hunter's Club	815	40	61
#11 Country Club	765	36	64
#12 Beach Club	835	46	66
#13 Gourmet Veggie Club	995	64	67
#14 Bootlegger	675	29	61
#15 Club Tuna w/o drssng	1010	58	68
#16 Club Lulu	755	38	61
#17 Ultimate Porker	765	39	62

Plain Slims: Figures Based on French Bread without Toppings, Dressing or Mayo

Slim 1 Ham & Provolone Cheese	570	13	76
Slim 2 Roast Beef	480	5.5	73
Slim 3 Tuna Salad	800	35	78
Slim 4 Turkey Breast	450	3	74
Slim 5 Salami Capicola & Cheese	660	23	75
Slim 6 Double Provolone	610	21	75

Sides:

Jimmy Chips: Average	150	9	16
Thinny, 1 oz	130	5	20
Cookies: Chocolate Chunk, 3 oz	410	19	56
Raisin Oatmeal, 3 oz	370	13	57
Jumbo Kosher Dill Pickle, 6.9 oz	20	0	4

Johnny Rockets® (Sept '17)

Starters & Shareables:

	C	F	Cb
Chili Bowl	490	38	16
Fries: American	480	19	69
Bacon Cheese	830	44	82
Cheese	740	37	82
Chili Cheese	1000	56	93
Sweet Potato	590	31	75
Onion Rings	790	36	80
Rocket Wings, traditional	600	43	19

Johnny Rockets® ...cont (Sept '17)

Original Hamburgers:

	C	F	Cb
Hamburger #12	950	60	57
Original Burger	900	59	54
Rocket: Single	930	59	52
Double	1400	96	52
Route 66	980	67	49
Smoke House: Single	1080	65	67
Double	1640	109	67
Streamliner	400	10	56

Chicken Tenders, (6), w/o sauce 880 56 42

	880	56	42

Chicken Philly Cheese Steak,

with American Cheese	660	24	58
Hot Dogs: Rocket Dog	610	26	77
Rocket Chili Dog	830	53	56

Philly Cheese Steaks: Without Substitutions

Beef	810	41	55
Chicken	660	24	58

Rocket Melts: Standard, without substitutions

BBQ Chicken Bacon Melt	1090	40	89
Patty Melt	880	54	53
Tuna Melt	730	47	47

Sandwiches: Without Substitutions

BLT, on White Bread	520	31	47
Chicken Club, on White Bread	930	36	77
Grilled Chicken, on Hamburger Bun	610	30	47
Tuna Salad, on White Bread	800	59	48

Salads: Without Dressing

Crispy Chicken	660	45	21
Grilled Chicken Club	510	28	10
Garden Salad	280	19	7

Breakfast: Standard, without Subsititutions

French Toast & Bacon	330	11	49
Pancakes & Bacon	570	19	85
Patty n' Eggs	1370	89	90
S'wiches: Egg, Bacon, Wh. Bread	810	60	46
Egg, Bacon Rye	850	61	50
Egg, Ham, English Muffin	820	54	55
The Works	1000	70	55

Desserts: Apple Pie 620 34 74

Apple Pie	620	34	74
Super Sundae: with Hot Fudge	660	41	65
with Hershey's Chocolate Syrup	610	36	62
with Strawberry Syrup	580	36	55

Shakes:

Banana; Strawberry, average	810	43	90
Butterfinger	960	52	107
Chocolate	900	44	112
P'nut Butter Banana	1170	71	107
Strawb. Oreo Crumble	970	50	114

For Complete Menu & Data – see CalorieKing.com

Fast - Foods & *Restaurants*

KFC® (Jan '18)

Chicken On The Bone: Per Piece

	C	F	Cb
Original Recipe: Breast, 6 oz	390	21	11
Drumstick, 1.87 oz	130	8	4
Thigh, 3.7 oz	280	19	8
Whole Wing, 1.5 oz	130	8	3
Extra Crispy: Breast, 6.3 oz	530	35	18
Drumstick, 1.9 oz	170	12	5
Tenders, 1 order	140	7	8
Thigh, 3.5 oz	330	23	9
Whole Wing, 1.7 oz	170	113	5
Kentucky Grilled: Breast, 4.6 oz	210	7	0
Drumstick, 1.4 oz	80	4	0
Thigh, 2.5 oz	150	9	0
Whole Wing, 1 oz	70	3	0
Spicy Crispy: Breast, 5.2 oz	350	20	
Drumstick, 1.6 oz	130	8	5
Thigh, 2.8 oz	270	20	10
Whole Wing, 1.2 oz	120	8	5

Go Cups:

	C	F	Cb
Chicken Littles	570	28	60
Exta Crispy Tenders	540	27	50
Fiery Buff. Hot Wings	480	25	49
HBBQ Hot Wings	540	25	61
Hot Wings	480	25	43
Popcorn Nuggets	570	32	53
Popcorn Nuggets: Kids	290	19	19
Large	620	39	39

Wings: Without Dipping Sauce

	C	F	Cb
Fiery Buffalo, Hot	70	4	5
Honey BBQ, Hot	90	4	9
Hot	70	4	3

Dipping Sauces & Condiments: Per 0.9 oz Container

	C	F	Cb
Buttermilk Ranch Sauce	100	10	2
Colonel's Buttery Spread	35	4	0
Creamy Buffalo Sauce	70	7	2
Finger Linkin' Good; Honey Mstrd, av.	125	11	6
Honey Sauce	30	0	8
Ketcup	30	0	8
Lemon Juice	5	0	1
Strawberry Jam	35	0	9
Summertime BBQ Sauce	40	0	9
Sweet & Tangy Sauce	45	0	12

KFC Famous Bowls & Pot Pie:

	C	F	Cb
Chicken Pot Pie, 14 oz	790	46	66
Famous Bowl:			
Snack Size, 7 oz	270	13	28
Large	710	34	81

Sandwiches: Includes Mayo

	C	F	Cb
Chicken Littles	300	15	26
Crispy Twister	630	34	53
Double Crunch	520	26	46
Zinger	480	24	39

KFC® cont... (Jan '18)

Salads: W/out Dressing or Croutons

	C	F	Cb
Caesar, Side	40	2	2
House Side Salad	15	0	3

Dressings & Add-Ins:

	C	F	Cb
Creamy Parmesan Caesar, 2 oz	260	26	4
Light Italian, 1 oz	15	0.5	2
Original Ranch Fat Free, 1.5 oz	35	0	8
Croutons, Parm. Garlic, 1 pouch	60	3	8

Homestyle Sides: Per Single Portion

	C	F	Cb
BBQ Baked Beans, 4.5 oz	240	1.5	43
Biscuit, 2 oz	180	9	22
Coleslaw, 4.2 oz	170	12	14
Corn on the Cob, 2.5 oz	70	0.5	17
Macaroni & Cheese, 4.8 oz	170	6	22
Mashed Potatoes, with Gravy, 5 oz	120	4	19
Potato Wedges, 3.8 oz	270	13	34
Sweet Kernel Corn	80	0.5	20

Desserts:

	C	F	Cb
Apple Turnover, 2.9 oz	230	10	32
Cafe Valley Choc. Chip cake, 1 slice	300	15	39
Cafe Valley Lemon Cake, 1 slice	210	11	28
Cafe Valley Mini Choc. Chip Cake (1)	300	12	49
Chocolate Chip Cookie (1)	160	8	22
Oatmeal Raisin Cookie (1)	150	6	22
Oreo Cookies & Creme Pie	270	13	35
Reese's Peanut Butter Pie, 2.6 oz	300	17	33

Beverages:

	C	F	Cb
7-Up; Dr Pepper; Mug Root Beer, average			
12 fl.oz	140	0	35
16 fl.oz	190	0	46
20 fl.oz	240	0	58
Code Red Mountain Dew: 12 fl.oz	170	0	46
16 fl.oz	230	0	62
20 fl.oz	290	0	77
30 fl.oz	430	0	116
Dole: Classic Lemonade, 20 fl.oz	150	0	39
Strawberry Lemonade, 20 fl.oz	170	0	45
Mountain Dew: 12 fl.oz	160	0	44
16 fl.oz	220	0	59
20 fl.oz	270	0	73
30 fl.oz	410	0	110
Tropicana Fruit Punch: 12 fl.oz	170	0	45
16 fl.oz	230	0	60
20 fl.oz	280	0	75

Kilwins® ~ *see CalorieKing.com*

Kolache® ~ *see CalorieKing.com*

210

Updated Nutrition Data ~ www.CalorieKing.com
Persons with Diabetes ~ See Disclaimer (Page 22)

Krispy Kreme® (Sept '17)

Doughnuts:	C	F	Cb
Original Glazed:			
Regular	190	11	22
Mini size (3)	250	12	30
Apple Fritter	350	19	42
Chocolate Iced: Cake	280	13	37
Custard Filled	300	15	37
Glazed	240	11	33
with Sprinkles	250	11	36
Kreme Filling	350	19	41
Cinnamon Apple Filled	270	14	31
Cinnamon Bun	270	15	29
Cinnamon Sugar	190	10	21
Cruller: Glazed	210	10	29
Chocolate Iced Glazed	260	10	40
Double Chocolate Éclair	400	21	50
Double Dark Chocolate	370	19	45
Dulche De Leche	300	16	35
Glazed: with Kreme Filling	340	19	40
Lemon Filled	290	14	36
Maple Iced	240	11	34
Powdered Cake	240	12	29
Powdered Strawberry Filled	270	14	30
Strawberry Iced	240	11	33
Strawb. Shortcake Éclair	360	17	50
Sugar Doughnut	190	10	21
White Iced w/ Chocolate Drizzle	250	11	37
Doughnut Holes: Glazed Cake (4)	190	8	28
Glazed Blueberry Cake (4)	190	7	28
Original Glazed (5)	220	11	25
Hot: Chocolate, w/ 2% Milk, 12 oz	390	14	57
Mocha Latte, w/ Skim Milk, 12 oz	260	4.5	41
Kool Kreme:			
Cone, Chocolate	310	9	52
Doughnut Sundae, Orig. Glazed	450	17	69
Frozen Coffees: With Whipped Cream			
Caramel, 12 fl.oz	350	11	58
Mocha, 12 fl.oz	330	11	52
Vanilla Latte, 12 fl.oz	330	10	54
Frozen Lemonade, 12 fl.oz	200	0	52
Iced Lattes: Per 12 fl.oz with 2% Milk			
Caramel Latte, with Wh. Cream	310	7	50
Hazelnut	190	3.5	32
Iced Mocha, 2% Milk, 12 fl.oz	280	10	38
Skinny Iced Lattes: With 2% Skim Milk			
Caramel, 12 fl.oz	160	1.5	29
Vanilla, 12 fl.oz	70	0	12

For Complete Menu & Data ~ See CalorieKing.com

Krystal® (Sept '17)

Krystals:	C	F	Cb
Original	130	6	15
Angus Bacon & Cheese	450	23	40
Bacon Cheese; Double	190	10	16
Cheese	150	8	15
Triple	240	15	16
Chik, regular	280	16	23
Pups: Chili Cheese Pup	230	14	16
Corn	250	17	18
Regular	160	9	21
Fries:			
French Fries: Small	140	9	14
Medium	240	15	24
Large	300	19	30
Loaded: Chili Cheese Fries	670	47	40
Junk Yard	800	59	42
Wings: Bone in (12)	1170	90	36
Boneless: with Buffalo Sauce (12)	970	49	70
with BBQ Sauce (12)	1080	47	103
Breakfast:			
Plates: *With Three Eggs*			
Bacon & Biscuit	480	30	29
Bacon & Toast	330	19	16
Sausage & Biscuit	520	36	28
Sausage & Toast	370	24	16
Sandwiches: Bacon on Toast	300	13	30
Krystal Sunrisers (2)	420	32	15
Sausage on Toast	340	19	29
Sausage Gravy Biscuit	370	21	41
Scramblers:			
Original: with Bacon	300	19	16
with Sausage	340	24	15
Low-Carb Scrambler,			
with Sausage	370	33	1
Sides: Grits, bowl	210	5	36
Kryspers (5)	240	18	21
Dessert, Apple Turnover	290	18	31
Coca-Cola:			
Small	190	0	52
Medium	230	0	65
Large	350	0	98
Hand-Spun Shakes: Regular			
Chocolate	650	18	114
Strawberry	560	17	92
Vanilla	510	17	80
Sundaes: Choc.; Strawb., av.	310	8	57
Oreo	350	13	54

For Complete Menu & Data ~ see CalorieKing.com

LaRosa's Pizzeria® (Sept '17)

Classic Pizzas:	C	F	Cb
Hand Tossed: *Per Slice, 1/8 of 14" Large Pizza*			
Chicken Bacon Ranch	340	18	30
Double Pepperoni	430	19	45
Garlic Chicken	415	18	46
Hawaiian	435	17	49
Zesty BBQ Chicken	435	16	52
Traditional: *Per Slice, 1/12 of 14" Large Pizza*			
Chicken Bacon Ranch	290	17	20
Double Pepperoni	235	13	19
Hawaiian	240	12	22
Zesty BBQ Chicken	240	11	24
Deluxe Pizzas:			
Hand Tossed: *Per Slice, 1/8 of 14" Large Pizza*			
Buddy Deluxe	510	25	47
Meat Deluxe	575	40	47
Original Deluxe	495	23	47
Veggie Deluxe	360	11	49
Pan: *Per Slice, 1/8 of 14" Large Pizza*			
Buddy Deluxe	520	27	47
Meat Deluxe	590	32	47
Original Deluxe	505	25	47
Veggie Deluxe	375	13	49
Calzones: Standard Toppings, w/out Dipping Sauce			
Philly Chicken with 4 Cheese	820	26	107
Philly Cheese Steak with 4 Cheese	870	33	105
Three Meat with 4 Cheese	1070	52	106
Pasta Dinner: Without Bread, Soup or Salad			
Lasagna, with Meat Sauce	1100	66	72
Ravioli: Cheese, with Pasta Sauce	750	29	89
Meat, with Pasta Sauce	730	26	89
Meat & Cheese, w/ Pasta Sauce	740	27	89
Ziti: Chicken Alfredo	1180	57	121
Sausage Pelucci w/ Spag. Sce	1040	42	136
Fresh Salad: Regular, w/out Dressing or Breadstick			
Antipasto For One	500	38	15
Crispy Chicken	500	27	37
Grilled Chicken	300	12	16
JoJo's BLT	160	9	12
Tossed Garden Salad	160	9	12
Salad Dressings: Per 2 oz Cup			
Bleu Cheese	280	30	2
Honey French	250	19	18
Italian	320	34	4
Soup: Baked Onion, w/ crackers	230	10	27
Minestrone, with crackers	140	4	24

LaRosa's Pizzeria cont... (Sept '17)

Appetizers: *Without Sauce*	C	F	Cb
Cheesy Flatbread	1470	92	109
Garlic Fries	630	33	75
Fried Mozzarella Cheese Stick (5)	550	35	40
Garlic Bread (6)	900	42	114
Rondo: Pepperoni (6)	1360	80	106
Spinach/Cheese, average, 4.5 oz	1215	67	107
Wings, Boneless: BBQ (5)	380	17	36
Diablo (5)	440	25	33
Garlic-Romano (5)	560	42	27

La Salsa Fresh Mexican® (Sept '17)

Breakfast:	C	F	Cb
Burritos: Chicken	660	30	56
Steak	700	36	55
Huevos Ranchero Platter: Chicken	500	14	59
Chorizo	610	27	61
Steak	550	20	58
Taco	200	10	114
Burritos: Without Chips			
Black Beans & Cheese:	720	37	62
with Carnitas	820	41	62
with Grilled Chicken	810	40	63
California Steak, w/ Black Beans	830	39	81
Grande, Black Beans,			
with Carnitas/Chicken/Steak, av.	760	30	79
Pinto Beans & Cheese: Plain	810	37	79
with Chicken	910	40	80
with Steak	970	49	80
Overstuffed Burrito:			
with Carnitas	860	35	56
with Grilled Chicken	860	32	59
with Steak	980	49	58
Platters:			
Enchiladas:			
Pinto Beans: Carnitas; Chicken, av.	985	53	59
Cheese	850	49	58
Steak	1070	63	59
Three Pepper Fajita Flour Tortilla:			
Black Beans: Carnitas	700	29	55
Chicken	690	27	58
Steak	820	44	57
Taquitos & Quesadillas:			
Pinto Beans: Carnitas; Chicken, av.	1600	76	134
Cheese	1470	72	129
Steak	1660	84	134
Tacos: Without Chips			
Baja Grilled Fish	260	12	23
Baja Shrimp	250	9	23
Guadalajara Carnitas	300	17	22

Updated Nutrition Data ~ www.CalorieKing.com
Persons with Diabetes ~ See Disclaimer (Page 22)

La Salsa® cont... (Sept '17)

Favorites: Without Chips

	C	F	Cb
Classic Quesadillas: Carnitas	980	58	59
Cheese	880	54	59
Chicken	980	57	60
Steak	1040	65	60
Fire Roasted Bowls:			
Black Beans: Carnitas	510	18	54
Chicken	500	16	55
Steak	570	25	55
Nachos:			
Black Beans: with Carnitas	1150	56	93
with Chicken	1150	54	95
with Steak	1210	63	94
Pinto Beans:			
with Carnitas	1190	56	101
with Chicken	1170	54	98
with Steak	1230	63	98
Stuffed Fajitas: Carnitas	930	49	59
Cheese	830	45	59
Chicken	930	48	60
Steak	990	57	60

Little Caesars® (Sept '17)

14" Pizza: Per Slice, 1/8 Pizza

	C	F	Cb
Specialty Classic Round:			
3 Meat Treat	330	16	31
Hula Hawaiian, ham/bacon, av.	275	9	35
Italian Sausage	270	11	31
Ultimate Supreme	300	13	32
Veggie	270	10	32
Hot-N-Ready:			
Classic Pizza:			
Cheese	250	8	31
Pepperoni	280	11	31
Deep Deep Dish: Cheese	320	11	39
Pepperoni	350	14	40
***Caesar Wings:** Per 8 Wing*			
BBQ	640	40	32
Buffalo, Mild	560	40	0
Garlic Parmesan	720	56	8
Oven Roasted	560	40	0
***Caesar Dips:** Per 1.5 oz Container*			
Buffalo Ranch	230	24	3
Buttery Garlic, 0.5 oz	380	42	0
Cheezy Jalapeno	210	22	3
Ranch	250	26	3
***Bread:** Crazy Bread, 1 stick*	100	3	15
Ital; Pepp. Chse Bread	135	6	15
***Crazy Sauce,** for Bread*	45	0	10

Lone Star Steakhouse® (Oct '13)

Appetizers: Per Serving

	C	F	Cb
Lone Star Wings, mild, 3.5 oz	305	20	5
Spin. & Artichoke Dip, 3.5 oz	160	13	4.5
Texas Rose, 3.5 oz	285	19	25
***Meals:** Without Sides, Toppings & Sauce*			
Chopped Steak, 9.6 oz	710	52	0
NY Strip, 9.6 oz	525	28	0
Texas Ribeye, 12.5 oz	710	40	5.5
Ribs Combo:			
Baby Back Ribs, with Chicken	740	30	46
Seafood:			
Fried Shrimp Entree, 11.7 oz	865	40	97
Grilled Shrimp: 3.5 oz	60	2	5.5
11 oz	190	7	17
Sweet Bourbon Salmon: 6oz	240	11	0
9 oz	360	16	0
Burgers:			
Bubba, 15.7 oz	1085	57	67
Swiss & Mushroom, 15.2 oz	845	38	53
***Salads:** Per Serving, Includes Dressing*			
Dinner, Caesar, 6.3 oz	145	11	8
Grilled Chicken Caesar	480	24	19
Lettuce Wedge	395	34	10
***Sides:** Per Serving*			
Garlic Mashed Potatoes, ½ cup	130	5	19
Steak Fries, 8 oz	610	26	86
Texas Seasoned Rice, 8 oz	100	3.5	14

Long John Silver's® (Sept '17)

Chicken,

	C	F	Cb
Chicken Tenders, 1 piece 2.1 oz	150	7	11
Sandwiches & Tacos:			
Baja Fish Taco	410	21	40
Crispy Fish Sandwich	400	16	44
Seafood:			
Baked Cod, 1 piece, 6 oz	160	1	1
Battered: Alaskan Pollock,			
1 piece, 3.2 oz	200	10	16
Cod, 1 piece, 3 oz	190	11	9
Shrimp, 3 pieces, 1.5 oz	100	7	5
Crab Cake, 1 cake, 2.2 oz	280	15	26
Snack Box: Breaded Clam Strips	340	20	35
Popcorn Shrimp, 3 oz	210	9	24

Continued Next Page....

Long John's® cont... (Sept '17)

Sauces & Condiments:

	C	F	Cb
Dipping Sauces: BBQ, 1 oz	40	0	10
Cocktail, 0.9 oz	20	0	4
Honey Mustard, 1packet	60	6	2
Ketchup, 1 pouch	30	0	8
Louisiana Hot Sauce, 1 tsp	0	0	0
Malt Vinegar, 0.5 oz	0	0	0
Marinara, 1 oz	15	0	4
Sweet Thai Chili, 1 oz	60	0	14
Tartar, 0.5 oz packet	40	4	3
Sides: Baked Potato, 12 oz	295	0	67
Breaded Mozzarella Sticks (3)	370	23	24
Brocc. Cheese Soup, 1 bowl, 7.4 oz	220	18	8
Clam Chowder, 1 bowl, 8 oz	230	16	16
Cole Slaw, 4 oz	170	11	18
Corn	160	8	9
Crumblies, 1 oz	170	12	13
Fries, 3.7oz	350	17	44
Hushpuppy, 2 pups, 1.5 oz	150	7	19
Jalapeno Cheddar Bites (5), 1 oz	240	16	18
Rice, 5 oz	180	1	37

For Complete Menu & Data ~ see CalorieKing.com

Macaroni Grill® (Sept '17)

Tappas & Antipasti:

Per Whole Appetizer as Served

	C	F	Cb
Calamari Fritti	760	55	33
Goat Cheese Peppadew Peppers	350	11	56
Loaded Fries	1020	74	68
Mac & Cheese Bites w/ Truffle Dip	920	70	44
Spicy Ricotta Meatballs	530	39	14
Meals: with Menu Set Sides			
Carne: Fig Marsala Pork Chop	1000	66	35
Grilled Lamb Chops	790	63	19
Rosemary Ribeye	1430	120	18
Chicken: Caprese	560	22	40
Marsala	790	32	61
Scalopine	1110	74	51
Under a Brick	1590	145	20
Classics: Eggplant Parmesan	1340	90	103
Fettuccine Alfredo	1040	59	86
Lasagna Bolognese	1110	67	69
Mom's Ricotta Meatballs:			
with Bolognese	1260	73	88
with Pomodoro	1100	62	84

Macaroni Grill® cont... (Sept '17)

Meals (Cont): Per Whole Entree

	C	F	Cb
Classics (Ctnd):			
Mushroom Ravioli	930	66	53
Penne Rustica	1060	52	82
Truffle Mac &Cheese	1060	89	24
Pesce: Lobster Ravioli	920	74	36
Parmesan-Crusted Sole	1330	94	94
Artisan Pizzas: Per Whole Meal, as Served			
Cheese	1170	41	146
Farmhouse	1330	56	146
Margherita	1140	41	146
Pepperoni	1360	57	146
Kids: Chkn Tenders w/ Broccolini	860	45	67
Macaroni & Cheese	540	31	44
Pepperoni Pizza	630	25	72
Spaghetti & Meatballs, with Pomodoro Sauce	660	37	48
Salads: Includes Dressing			
Bibb & Blue, entrée	520	42	17
Caesar, with Chicken, entrée	650	41	16
Steak & Greens	950	71	32
Side: Florentine	300	22	22
Fresh Green	190	16	11
Dessert: Gelato, Vanilla	310	13	42
Homemade Choc. Cake	940	58	101
Lemon Passion	740	45	77
New York Style Cheesecake	690	41	70
Tiramisu	600	39	54

Manhattan Bagel® (Sept '17)

Bagels: Per Bagel

	C	F	Cb
Californian: Blueberry, 3.8 oz	300	1	65
Chocolate Chip, 3.8 oz	290	2.5	58
Cinnamon Raisin, 4 oz	290	1	63
Egg, 3.6 oz	300	5	54
Everything; Poppy, av., 3.7 oz	275	2.5	56
Pumpernickel, 3.6 oz	240	1.5	53
Gourmet: Asiago, 4.4 oz	340	4	64
Blueberry Glaze, 4.6 oz	370	1	79
Super Cinnamon, 4.6 oz	360	1	77
Signature Flavors: Cheddar, 4 oz	320	1.5	67
Multigrain, 4.3 oz	350	2	70
Poppy, 4.2 oz	330	3	64
Rye, 4 oz	310	1.5	66
Cream Cheese: Plain, 1.3 oz	120	12	2
Lox, 1.25 oz	110	11	4
Scallion, 1.3 oz	140	12	5

Manhattan Bagel® cont... (Sept '17)

Breakfast: On Plain Bagel

	C	F	Cb
Egg & Cheese	530	19	64
Egg Bacon & Cheese	580	23	64
Egg, Pork Roll & Cheese	770	37	66
Omelet Wrap, Egg, Cheese & Ham	650	30	55

Deli Sandwich:

Chicken Salad Croissant, 8.9 oz	680	44	60
Rst Beef on Cheddar Roll, 10.5 oz	510	12	68
White Albacore Tuna Wrap, 8.6 oz	540	28	53
Signature Lunch: Bronx Bomber	580	27	54
Chelsea Chicken, 11.5 oz	750	37	59
Village Veggie Wrap, 10.7 oz	580	33	62

Salad: Without Dressing

Garden Market, 9.3 oz	140	5	21
NY Deli Chef, 13.2 oz	410	22	21

Marie Callender's® (Sept '17)

Appetizers:

	C	F	Cb
Crispy Chicken Tenders, 12.9 oz	870	47	72
Crispy Green Beans, 10.5 oz	810	52	75
Mozzarella Sticks, 8.6 oz	690	42	46

Burgers and Sandwiches: With Fries, w/out Cheese

Original Burger	1290	87	84
Frisco Chicken Breast	1290	81	95
Meatloaf on Cheese Sourdough	1250	78	96
Roasted Turkey Croissant Club	1450	97	95

Main Meals: As Per Menu

Comfort Classics:

Double Shrimp Pasta	1210	65	100
Home-Style Meatloaf Dinner	650	38	33

Delightful Dishes:

Avocado Shrimp Stack	590	33	53
Chicken Street Taco	440	13	51
Mahi Mahi Cabo Taco	570	23	53

From The Grill:

Cajun Salmon & Jumbo Shrimp	1280	63	115
St. Louis BBQ Ribs & Shrimp Skewer	800	47	39
Pies, Chicken Pot Pie, w/out sides	1140	79	70

Salads: Includes Dressing

Calif. Waldorf Chicken with Mango	740	40	73
Crunchy BBQ Chicken	1060	56	90
Traditional Caesar, with Chicken	700	43	28
Sides: Cornbread, w/ Honey Butter	340	21	33
French Fries, 4 oz	380	20	45
Loaded Mashed Potatoes, 6.2 oz	340	23	23
Macaroni & Cheese, 6.4 oz	230	9	26

Soups: Per Bowl

Chicken Tortilla	230	10	26
Clam Chowder	270	13	22
Hearty Vegetable	90	3	13
Split Pea & Ham	220	13	17

Marie Callender's® cont... (Sept '17)

Breakfast: As Per Menu

	C	F	Cb
Classics: Croissant Sandwich	1100	70	76
Eggs Benedict: California	1210	67	126
Traditional	1060	54	110
Hearty Man's Combo	1540	80	155
Tremendous Ten with Bacon	1350	61	155
Griddle Greats: Belgian Waffles	600	19	99
Buttermilk Pancakes (3)	670	28	92
Old Fashioned French Toast	830	31	123
Platters: Belg. Waffle, w/ Bacon	820	34	101
French Toast, with Bacon	770	25	105
Pancake, with Sausage	1060	59	96
Omelettes: BTA	1610	84	161
Oh My	1710	87	156
Spanish	1550	78	166
Quiche: Bacon, 1 slice	990	79	45
Ham, 1 slice	1030	83	39

Desserts: Per Slice Unless Indicated

Pies: Apple	630	39	66
Banana Cream, with Meringue	510	24	66
Chocolate Cream, with Meringue	570	25	77
Coconut Cream with Meringue	590	29	75
Razzleberry	650	39	71

For Complete Nutritiona Data ~ see CalorieKing.com

Max & Erma's® (Sept '17)

Shareables: As Served

	C	F	Cb
Baja Fish Taco: Crispy	1120	43	134
Grilled	760	28	84
Chicken Fajita Quesadilla	820	54	51
Potato Skins	1990	91	232
Spinach Dip	660	49	28
Wings with Blue Cheese Dressing:			
Cherry Cola BBQ	2090	120	118
Sweet Chili	1840	120	54

Burgers: Without Fries

Cola BBQ Bacon	1320	80	93
Garbage, 6 oz	1650	118	60
Sauteed Mushroom & Swiss	1200	85	53
Tortilla	1260	84	61

Salads: Entrée Size, w/ Dressing, w/out Breadstick

3rd Street	1190	97	41
Grilled Chicken Santa Fe	1090	83	46
Village	430	37	14
Sides: Baked Potato	220	0	51
Creamy Coleslaw	160	12	14
Fresh Fruit Salad	90	0	23
Mashed Potatoes	290	11	43
Seasoned Fries	290	9	49

Dessert:

Banana Cream Pie	820	38	111
Chocolate Cake a la Mode	1650	83	216

For Complete Menu & Data ~ See CalorieKing.com

Fast - Foods & Restaurants

McAlister's Deli® (Sept '17)

Sandwiches:

	C	F	Cb
Black Angus Club	840	43	73
California Turkey Reuben	950	46	81
Four Cheese Griller	760	38	66
French Dip	520	15	43
Grilled Chicken Club	830	37	78
Harvest Chicken Salad	730	48	55
Horseradish Roast Beef	680	30	70
McAlister's Club	810	39	78
Reuben	900	41	76
Smoky Pepper Jack Turkey	780	36	72
Sweet Chipotle Chicken	630	15	77
The Italian	760	39	49
The Veggie	570	39	46

Mellow Mushroom® (Sept '17)

Burger:

	C	F	Cb
Carnie Burger	1270	87	56
Calzones:			
Chicken & Cheese	1300	34	163
Steak & Cheese	1280	40	151
Hoagies, Whole: Chicken &Chse	860	47	54
Italian	1120	79	54
Meatball	540	19	56
Mushroom Club	1090	71	57
Spiked Sausage	1010	63	49
Steak & Cheese	970	61	51
Tofu	740	48	54
Munchies: Garlic Bread	510	25	55
Magic Mushroom Soup	350	24	15
Meatball Trio	440	29	15
Roasted Red Potatoes	150	3	27
Spin. & Artichoke Dip, w/o bread	870	65	42
Stuffed Portobello	250	10	27
Wings: BBQ (10)	670	36	29
Sweet Thai Chili (10)	740	33	51
Pizzas: Per Medium Slice			
Buffalo Chkn; Holy Shitake Pie, av.	460	24	43
Funky Q Chicken; House Special, av.	445	17	47
Kosmic Karma; Mega-Veggie, av.	385	15	48
Salads: Per Regular Size			
Caesar, with Caesar Dressing	890	78	27
Greek, with Feta, without Dressing	250	15	17
Dressings: 1000 Island, 1 oz	130	12	4
Balsamic Vinaigrette, 1 oz	90	8	5
Caesar, 1 oz	160	17	0.5
Desserts: Choc Chunk Cookie	600	29	83
Oatmeal Raisin Cookie	480	17	75
Peanut Butter Cookie	580	32	65

Extra Menu Items ~ See CalorieKing.com

McDonald's® (May '18)

Beef Burgers/Sandwiches::

	C	F	Cb
Big Mac Burger	540	28	46
Cheeseburger	300	12	33
Double Cheeseburger	430	21	35
Hamburger	250	8	31
McDouble	380	18	34
Pico Guacamole, 1/4 lb	580	33	41
Sweet BBQ Bacon, 1/4 lb	700	38	52
Quarter Pounder: with Cheese	530	27	41
Double, with Cheese	770	45	42
Chicken Sandwiches: *On Artisan Roll*			
Artisan Grilled Chicken	380	7	44
Buttermilk Crispy Chicken	570	23	64
Garlic White Cheddar:			
Artisan Grilled Chicken	530	20	48
Buttermilk Crispy Chkn	700	34	67
Pico Guacamole:			
Artisan Grilled Chicken	550	20	50
Buttermilk Crispy Chicken	720	34	69
Sweet BBQ Bacon:			
Artisan Grilled Chicken	670	25	61
Buttermilk Crispy Chicken	830	39	80
McChicken, on regular bun	350	15	40
Filet-O-Fish Sandwich, regular bun	410	20	39
Chicken McNuggets: 4 pieces	180	11	11
6 pieces	270	16	16
10 pieces	440	27	26
20 pieces	890	53	53
Sauces: Per Packet			
Creamy Ranch	110	12	1
Siganture	100	9	3
Spicy Buffalo	30	3	1
Sweet 'N Sour; Tangy BBQ	50	0	11
French Fries: Kids, 1.3 oz	110	5	15
Small, 2.6 oz	230	11	29
Medium, 3.9 oz	340	16	44
Large, 5.9 oz	510	24	66
Ketchup, packet	10	0	2
Breakfast:			
Big Breakfast: with Reg. Biscuit	750	49	53
with Hotcakes	1350	65	155
Biscuits: *Regular*			
Bacon, Egg & Cheese	450	24	40
Sausage	460	30	36
Sausage with Egg	530	34	38
Steak, Egg & Cheese	530	30	40
Burrito, Sausage	300	16	26
Fruit 'N Yogurt Parfait	150	2	30

Fast - Foods & *Restaurants*

McDonald's® cont... (May '18)

Breakfast (Cont):

	C	F	Cb
Fruit & Maple Oatmeal:			
with brown sugar	310	4	62
w/out brown sugar	260	4	49
Hash Browns, (1), 2 oz	150	9	16
Hotcakes: Plain (3)	330	8	56
with Syrup and Whipped Butter	600	16	102
McGriddles:			
Bacon, Egg & Cheese	420	18	45
Sausage	430	24	42
Sausage, Egg & Cheese	550	32	45
McMuffins: Egg	300	12	30
Egg White Delight	280	10	29
Sausage	400	25	29
Sausage with Egg	470	30	30

Happy Meals:

Chicken McNuggets (4):			
+Apple Slices + 1% Low Fat Milk	295	13	27
+Apple Slices + Fat Free Choc Milk	325	11	38
+ Go-Gurt Strawb Yog. & Apple Jce	310	12	30
Hamburger:			
+Apple Slices + 1% Low Fat Milk	365	11	47
+Apple Slices +Fat Free Choc Milk	395	8	58
+ Go-Gurt Strawb Yog. & Apple Jce	380	9	60
Cheeseburger:			
+Apple Slices + 1% Low Fat Milk	415	15	49
+ Apple Slices & Fat-Free Choc Milk	445	12	60
+ Go-Gurt Strawb Yog. & Apple Jce	430	13	62

Mighty Kid's Meal:

Chicken McNuggets (6):			
+ Apple Slices+ Fat Free Choc Milk	415	16	43
+ Go-Gurt Strawb Yog. + Apple Jce	400	17	45

Salads: Without Dressing

Bacon Ranch: Grilled Chicken	320	14	9
Buttermilk Crispy Chicken	490	28	28
Southwest: Grilled Chkn, w/ glaze	350	11	27
B'milk Crispy Chicken, wih glaze	520	25	46
Side Salad	15	0	3

Salad Dressings: Per Package

Newman's Own: Ranch, 2 fl.oz	200	17	11
Low-Fat: Balsamic Vinaig., 1.5 fl.oz	35	1.5	3
Family Recipe Italian, 1.5 fl.oz	50	1.5	8
Snacks: Apple Slices	15	0	4
Yoplait Go-Gurt, Strawberry, 1 tube	50	0.5	8

Desserts & Shakes:

Baked Apple Pie, 2.6 oz	230	10	33
Cookies: Choc. Chip, (1)	170	7	23
Oatmeal Raisin (1), 1 oz	140	5	22

McDonald's® cont... (May '18)

Desserts & Shakes (Cont):

	C	F	Cb
Pie, Strawberry & Creme	290	15	34
McFlurry: M&M Candies, regular	630	22	96
Oreo Cookies, 12 fl.oz	510	17	80
Soft Serve: Kiddie Cone	45	1	5
Vanilla Cone	200	5	32
Sundaes:			
Hot Caramel, 6.4 oz	380	12	61
Hot Fudge, 6.3 oz	380	14	53
Strawberry, 6.3 oz	310	10	50
Milk: 1% Low-Fat, 8 fl.oz	100	2.5	12
Fat-Free Chocolate Milk, 8 fl.oz	130	0	23
Juice, Apple, box	35	0	9

Soda: With Ice, approximately 30%

Coca-Cola or Sprite, average:			
Extra Small, 12 fl.oz cup	110	0	30
Small, 16 fl.oz cup	150	0	40
Medium, 21 fl.oz cup	215	0	56
Large, 30 fl.oz cup	290	0	75
Dr Pepper:			
Extra Small, 12 fl.oz cup	120	0	32
Small, 16 fl.oz cup	170	0	46
Medium, 21 fl.oz cup	210	0	58
Large, 30 fl.oz cup	290	0	79
Powerade, Mountain Berry Blast:			
Extra Small, 12 fl.oz cup	70	0	16
Small, 16 fl.oz cup	90	0	22
Medium, 21 fl.oz cup	120	0	31
Large, 30 fl.oz cup	170	0	42
Sweet Tea, medium	110	0	28

McCafe:

Frappes: With Whipped Topping			
Caramel; Mocha, average:			
Small	420	17	60
Medium	510	21	72
Large	670	27	96
Shakes:			
Chocolate: 12 fl.oz cup	530	15	87
16 fl.oz cup	630	18	103
22 fl.oz cup	850	23	141
Vanilla: 12 fl.oz cup	490	14	79
16 fl.oz cup	590	17	95
22 fl.oz cup	800	22	131
Smoothies, all flavors:			
Small, 12 fl oz cup	200	0.5	45
Medium, 16 fl oz cup	245	1	56
Large, 22 fl oz cup	340	1	77

...McCafe cont next page

Fast - Foods & *Restaurants*

McDonald's® cont... (May '18)

McCafe:

Hot Chocolate: *With Whipped Cream & Toppings*

	C	F	Cb
Whole Milk: Small, 12 fl oz	370	14	51
Medium, 16 fl oz	440	16	61
Nonfat Milk: Small, 12 fl oz	290	4	52
Medium, 16 fl oz	340	4	62

Iced Coffee: *With Liquid Sugar & Light Cream*

Regular: Small, 16 fl.oz	140	5	24
Medium, 22 fl.oz	170	5	30
Large, 30 fl.oz	240	7	44
Caramel: Small, 16 fl.oz	140	5	23
Medium, 22 fl.oz	190	7	31

Iced Mocha: *W/ Whole Milk, Syrup, Whipped Cream & Toppings*

Small, 16 fl.oz	290	11	40

Mimi's Cafe® (Sept '17)

Breakfast:

Benedicts: *With Roasted Potatoes*

	C	F	Cb
Original	880	56	51
Smoked Salmon	810	52	52

Omelets: *With Roasted Potatoes Unless Indicated*

Bacon Avocado	930	67	28
Hickory-Smoked Ham & Cheese	680	47	25
Mushroom Bacon & Brie	780	57	26
Smoked Salmon	570	37	22

Griddle: *With Roasted Potatoes*

Brioche French Toast	500	17	66
Cinnamon Roll French Toast	730	31	94
Orange Crème French Toast	1090	42	145

Appetizers:

Baked Brie To Share	440	17	56
Calamari	350	9	32
Warm Spinach Artich. Dip, 15 oz	700	40	64

Lunch & Dinner: *Without Side Choices*

Burgers:

Bacon Avoc. Sourdough	1240	87	41
Brioche Cheeseburger	820	45	51
Hickory Bacon Cheddar	1250	67	90

Craft Sandwiches:

Chicken Cordon Bleu	1100	49	92
West Coast Reuben	1190	70	76

Entrees:

Chicken Pot Pie	860	56	60
French Pot Roast	510	32	22
Quiche Lorraine	420	28	16
Roasted Chicken Crepes	360	27	12

Sides:

Broccoli	110	9	5
Golden Buttermilk Onion Strings	190	3	36
Idaho Russet Fries	150	4	27
Mashed Potatoes	130	4	21
Roasted Potatoes	290	19	26
Sauteed Spinach	70	4	5

Mr. Goodcents® (Sept '17)

Cold Subs: *Per 8" Wheat Bread Sub with Standard Toppings*

	C	F	Cb
Centsable	590	29	62
Garden Veggie	510	17	48
Goodcents Original	660	36	61
Oven Roasted Chicken Breast	490	18	60
Penny Club	500	19	61
Pepperoni	840	56	58
Tuna Salad	630	33	65

Toasted Sub: *Per 8" Wheat Bread Sub with Standard Toppings*

Chicken Bacon Ranch, w/ Cheddar	710	31	57
Meatball	720	28	69

Pasta:

With Alfredo Sauce	840	40	103
With Marinara Sauce & Meatballs	910	33	119
Chicken Alfredo	970	43	104
Chicken Parmesan	810	23	109

Garlic Bread, 1 piece, 2 4 oz | 290 | 12 | 44

Soup: *Per 16 oz Bowl*

Broccoli Cheese	360	28	16
Chicken Homestyle Noodle	140	4	20
Potato with Bacon	420	28	36

Mr. Hero® (Sept '17)

7" Subs & Burgers:

Burgers:

	C	F	Cb
Cheeseburger	720	50	44
Hamburger	640	44	44
Romanburger	810	57	45

Chicken Subs:

Chicken Bacon Ranch	550	23	48
Chicken Philly	500	21	44

Deli Subs: *Per 7" Sub with Menu Board Toppings*

Italiano	570	27	54
Original Italian	530	27	50
Tuna 'N Cheese	670	53	45
Turkey	330	2.5	49

Steak Subs:

Hot Buttered Cheesesteak Deluxe	660	42	41
Sicilian Parm	570	31	41
Zesty Bacon & Swiss	510	25	43

Pitas:

Chicken	450	13	45
Gyro	580	31	50

Sides: *Per Regular Size*

Mozzarella Sticks	525	34	36
Onion Petals	545	36	52
Potato Waffer Fries	360	27	29

Desserts:

Oreo Cheesecake	270	18	24
Snickers Cheesecake	270	18	23
Strawb. Swirl Cheesecake	250	17	21

Updated Nutrition Data ~ www.CalorieKing.com
Persons with Diabetes ~ See Disclaimer (Page 22)

Mrs Fields Cookies® (Sept '17)

Brownies: Per 2.15 oz Brownie	C	F	Cb
Butterscotch Blondie	260	10	38
Double Fudge; Pecan Fudge, av.	265	14	33
Special Walnut Fudge & Blondie	260	13	35
Toffee/Walnut Fudge, average	265	14	33
Brownie Bites:			
Butterscotch Blondie (3)	200	8	29
Double/Toffee Fudge (3)	200	10	27
Coffee Cake,			
Chocolate Chip, small, 2.35 oz	240	11	30
Bite Size Nibblers Cookies:			
Cinn. Sug. (3)	180	8	25
Peanut Butter (3)	170	9	19
Semi-Sweet Chocolate (3)	170	8	23
Triple Chocolate (3)	160	8	22
White Chunk Macadamia (3)	180	9	22
Cookies: Butter; Debra's Special (1), av.	200	8	28
Cut Out (1)	280	11	44
Oatmeal, Raisins and Walnuts (1)	200	9	27
Peanut Butter (1)	200	12	24
Semi-Sweet: Chocolate (1)	210	10	29
with Walnuts (1)	220	11	28
Triple Chocolate (1)	210	10	28
White Chunk Macadamia (1)	230	12	28
Muffins: Per 1.9 oz			
Blueberry	190	9	24
Chocolate Chip	200	10	26

For Complete Nutritional Data ~ see CalorieKing.com

My Favorite Muffin® (Sept '17)

Muffins: Per Large Muffin	C	F	Cb
Large: Blueberry	590	36	60
Boston Cream Pie	740	33	105
Choc. Chip	790	39	100
Carrot Cake	850	42	112
Deep Dish Apple Pie	560	22	85
Lemon Poppy Seed	670	32	90
Pumpkin Spice	600	26	86
Strawberry Cheesecake	580	31	67

Nathan's Famous® (Sept '17)

Burgers:	C	F	Cb
Super Cheeseburger, 5 oz	960	67	48
Cheesesteak, Original Philly, 10.5 oz	680	33	52
Chicken:			
Sandwiches: Grilled Chicken, 8.2 oz	470	21	43
Krispy Chicken, 8.5 oz	660	37	58
Tenders, Krispy, 3 pieces, 6.3 oz	520	31	32
Wings, Original Buffalo, 10.5 oz	690	49	34

Nathan's Famous® cont... (Sept '17)

Hot Dogs: With Natural Casings	C	F	Cb
Original, 3.5 oz	280	18	24
Chili, 5.5 oz	400	27	30
Chili Cheese, 6.5 oz	460	31	33
Hot Dog Nuggets, 3.5 oz	350	28	20
Corn Dog, on a stick, 3.2 oz	380	21	39
Fries::			
Bacon Cheese, regular, 10 oz	710	51	46
Crinkle Cut: Cheese, regular, 9 oz	570	38	46
French, regular, 7.5 oz	510	34	42

New York Fries® ~ See CalorieKing.com

Ninety Nine® (Sept '17)

Standout Starters: As Served	C	F	Cb
Boneless Wings & Skins Sampler	1890	125	107
Mozzarella Moons	870	52	63
Outrageous Pot. Skins	1470	101	84
Burgers: Without Sides			
Bacon & Cheese Burger	900	58	48
Sweet Heat Burger	1320	93	67
Vermont Cheddar Bgr	1100	76	54
West Coast Turkey Bgr	800	48	42
Sandwiches & Wraps: Without Sides			
Honey BBQ Chicken Wrap	850	33	100
Triple Decker Turkey Club S'wich	700	31	58
Meals: Served with Set Sides Unless Indicated			
Fish & Chips	1570	105	107
Macadamia Crusted Chicken	1240	82	92
New England Shoreline Combo	1890	126	132
Original Crispy Chicken Tenders	1750	112	128
Prime Rib: 12 oz, without sides	670	39	3
18 oz, without sides	940	53	3
Smthrd Sirloin Tips, w/o sides, 24 oz	1050	62	18
Salads: As Served			
Chicken Caesar	730	42	52
Gr. Chicken Kabob	770	48	44
Fire Grilled Cobb, w/out Dressing	660	41	25
Sides:			
Baked Potato with Sour Cream	310	8	52
Double Bleu Iceberg Wedge	460	42	11
French Fries	1040	64	107
Honey Butter Bisc., w/ Honey Butter	230	11	29
Pasta: with Butter	740	28	104
with Marinara	660	10	124
Perfect Coleslaw	150	12	10
Russet Mashed Potatoes	260	11	36
Dessert,			
Towering Midnight Fudge Cake	790	40	96

Noodles & Company® (Sept '17)

Noodles & Pasta: Regular Size

	C	F	Cb
Alfredo MontAmore	1320	79	104
Buttered Noodles	720	34	90
Japanese Pan Noodles	690	18	112
Mushroom Stroganoff	850	43	99
Pad Thai	1330	75	139
Penne Rosa, w/ Parmesan/Feta, av.	695	26	96
Pesto Cavatappi, w/ Feta	740	33	91
Spaghetti	610	18	91
Spaghetti & Meatballs	970	49	95
Spicy Korean Beef Noodles	910	21	141
Steak Stroganoff	940	46	100
Thai Green Curry, with Shrimp	970	27	142
Wisconsin Mac & Cheese	1050	46	117

Salads: Per Regular Size

	C	F	Cb
Grilled Chicken Caesar	400	26	18
Napa Market, with Chkn	600	45	24
The Med, with Chicken	370	15	33

Soups: Per Regular Size

	C	F	Cb
Thai Chicken	370	22	31
Tomato Basil Bisque	430	28	37

Extras:

	C	F	Cb
Cheesy Garlic Bread (3)	320	17	30
Potsticker (6), with sauce	380	10	54
Side Caesar Salad	90	6	6
Wisconsin Mac & Cheese, side	340	16	36

Dessert:

	C	F	Cb
Chocolate Chunk Cookie	490	22	69
Rice Crispy	540	18	94
Snoodledoodle Cookie	460	13	88

O'Charley's® (Sept '17)

Appetizers: As Served

	C	F	Cb
Chicken Tenders, Chipotle	1160	40	107
Nashville Deviled Eggs	720	61	24
Spicy Jack Cheese Wedges (7)	720	48	44
Top Shelf Combo Platter	1880	132	74

Burgers: Without Sides

	C	F	Cb
Better Cheddar Bacon	1000	68	49
Classic Cheeseburger	930	61	47
Prime Rib Steakhouse Burger	1060	65	72
Southwest Blackbean	760	38	77
Wild West Burger	1290	94	64

Chicken & Pasta: With Sides Unless Indicated

	C	F	Cb
Chicken Tenders & Fries	1410	85	74
New Orleans Cajun Chicken Pasta	1170	61	99
Peach Chutney Chkn, w/out Sides	470	8	69
Shrimp Scampi Pasta	950	43	104

O'Charley's® cont... (Sept '17)

Classic Combos: Without Sides

	C	F	Cb
Steak & Chicken Tenders, 9 oz	1160	76	26
Steak & Garlic Shrimp	870	68	28
Steak & Half Rack Baby Back Ribs	890	49	48
Steak & Savannah Crab Cake	910	67	26

Ribs: Without Sides

	C	F	Cb
Prime Rib Blackened: 8 oz	850	71	6
12 oz	1160	96	6
16 oz	1470	121	6
Prime Rib Grilled: 8 oz	840	70	3
12 oz	1150	95	3
16 oz	1460	121	3
Slow Roasted Prime Rib: 8oz	830	70	3
16 oz	1460	120	4

Sandwiches: Without Sides Unless Indicated

	C	F	Cb
BLTC	720	4	56
Cajun BBQ Prime Rib	770	48	48
Chicken, Carolina BBQ	650	22	74
Classic French Dip	1020	44	79
Nashville Hot Chicken, with Fries	1600	101	119
Open Faced Prime Rib	700	47	31
Southern Fried Chicken	1300	75	94

Seafoodl Favorites: Without Sides Unless Indicated

	C	F	Cb
Grilled Blackened Atl. Salmon, 9 oz	510	31	3
Hand Battered Fish & Chips	1420	92	85
Hand Breaded Catfish, w/ Fries & Slaw	1720	124	103
Savannah Crab Cake Dinner	980	73	49

Steaks: Without Sides

	C	F	Cb
Bacon & Bourbon Glazed Filet	640	42	28
Barrel House Pork Chops	920	45	62
Grilled Top Sirloin, 12 oz	530	36	1
Rib-Eye Steak	840	71	1
Slow Roasted Prime Rib, 8 oz	830	70	3

Sides:

	C	F	Cb
Baked Potato (1)	200	1	50
Broccoli, 5 oz	110	8	6
French Fries, 6 oz	400	24	40
Loaded Baked Potato, 1 portion	490	27	53
Sweet Potato Fries, 1 portion	280	19	27

Salads: Per Full Salad, with Dressing

	C	F	Cb
California Chicken	1020	67	71
Classic Cobb	1140	92	36
Sthrn Fried Chicken	1550	110	48
Sthrn Pecan Chicken Tender	1550	106	95

Signature Soup: Per Bowl

	C	F	Cb
Chicken Harvest	210	13	20
Chicken Tortilla	190	7	20

Desserts:

	C	F	Cb
Country Apple Pie, 1 slice	630	35	77
Double-Crust Cherry Pie, 1 slice	600	35	69
French Silk Pie, 1 slice	580	43	49
Goo Goo Crunch	1450	93	155
Ooey Gooey Caramel Pie, 1 slice	640	39	76
Southern Pecan Pie, 1 slice	730	45	78

For Complete Menu & Data ~ see CalorieKing.com

Old Spaghetti Factory® (Sept '17)

Appetizers: As Served

	C	F	Cb
Shrimp, Spinach & Artichoke Dip	590	40	39
Sicilian Garlic Cheese Bread	1220	78	97

Entrées, Lunch/Dinner:

Classics:

	C	F	Cb
Spaghetti: w/ Clam Sauce, 15 oz	810	31	107
with Marina Sauce, 15 oz	560	5	108
with Meat Sauce, 15 oz	650	11	108
with Sicilian Meatballs, 21 oz	1040	36	115

Factory Favorites:

Chicken Parmigiana, 18 oz	750	29	70
Spinach & Cheese Ravioli, 11 oz	470	16	63
Spinach Tortellini, w/ Alfredo Sce	940	56	86

Managers Favorites:

Marinara: Clam, 15 oz	690	18	107
Meat, 15 oz	600	8	108
Mushroom, 16.5 oz	610	10	109

Signature Selection:

Chicken Picatta	1150	76	63
Crab Ravioli, 11 oz	810	45	73
Spaghetti Vesuvius, 17.2 oz	850	29	110

Olive Garden® (Jan '18)

Appetizers:

Calamari	870	56	67
Sauce: Marinara	45	2.5	6
Ranch	210	21	3
Spicy Calabrian Tenders	900	67	19
Spicy Shrimp Scampi Fritta	560	37	34

Entrées:

Lunch:

Fettuccine Alfredo Mini Pasta Bowl	650	45	47
Grilled Vegetable & Chees Piadina	630	37	52
Lasagna Classico	640	36	39
Spag. & Meat Sce Mini Pasta Bowl	360	12	51

Dinner:

Eggplant Parmig.	1060	54	113
Fettuccini Alfredo	1010	56	97
Five Cheese Ziti al Forno	1220	71	103
Grilled Chicken Parmigiana	760	29	54
Lasagna Classico	930	53	56
Ravioli di Portobello	820	46	73
Tour of Italy	1520	96	92

Desserts:

Black tie Mousse Cake	750	50	76
Tiramisu	470	27	54
Warm Apple Crostata	630	29	83
Zeppoli, without sauce	810	28	119

On the Border® (Sept '17)

Appetizers: As Served

	C	F	Cb
Border Sampler	2180	147	116
Fajita Quesadillas:			
Chicken	1190	82	59
Steak	1280	97	56

Burritos: Witout Bean & Rice

Classic Chicken Tinga	670	34	44
Classic Ground Beef	990	62	49

Chimichangas: W/out Rice, Beans & Sauce

Chicken Tinga	840	46	57
Ground Beef	990	58	66

Enchiladas: W/out Bean and Rice

Ranchiladas	1180	73	43
Suizas	760	43	52

Salads: W/out Dressing

Fajita: Chicken	410	19	24
Steak	490	27	27
Grande Taco Salad: Chkn Tinga	710	46	49
with Ground Beef	830	57	51

Tacos: Without Beans and Rice

Brisket Tacos (2)	850	42	44
Grilled Fish Tacos Del Mar (2)	850	62	31
Southwest Chicken Taco (3)	1510	105	30
Soup: Chicken Tortilla, 1 cup	310	18	22
1 Bowl	510	26	44
Sides: Black Beans	220	2	38
Cilantro Lime Rice	180	2	37
Corn Tortillas (3)	130	2.5	33
Mexican Rice	220	6	37
Refried Beans	240	8	30

Dressings: Per Serving

Ranch Dressing	230	24	2
Smoked Jalapeno Vinaigrette	250	24	8

For Complete Nutritional Data ~ see CalorieKing.com

Orange Julius® (Sept '17)

Julius Originals: Per Medium Size

	C	F	Cb
Berry Pomegranate	430	0	108
Mango Pineapple	450	0	114
OrangeBerry	330	0	82
Strawberry Banana	530	8	114

Premium Fruit Smoothies: Per Medium Size

Berry Pomegranate	380	0	91
Pina Colada	340	0	80
Strawberry	300	0.5	71

Light Smoothies: Per Medium Size

Orange	170	0	41
Strawberry	200	0	50
Tripleberry	210	0	55
Boost, Banana, Small drink	30	0	7

Outback Steakhouse® (Sept '17)

Aussie-Tizers: Per Whole Dish, with Selected Dressing/Sauce	C	F	Cb
Alice Springs Chicken Quesadillas	1610	96	91
Aussie Cheese Fries: Small	1160	83	70
Large	1770	117	124
Bloomin' Onion	1950	155	123
Crab Cakes	790	66	22
Kookaburra Wings, medium/hot	1445	127	14
Seared Peppered Ahi, large	390	22	18
Steakhouse Quesadilla, regular	1590	107	78
Volcano Shrimp	960	73	55

Forkless Features: *Without Sides*

	C	F	Cb
Cripsy Chicken Sandwich	880	52	69
Outback Burger, without Cheese	710	43	42
Steakhouse Philly S'wich	1030	61	140
The Bloomin' Burger	1160	83	58

Chicken, Ribs, Chops:

	C	F	Cb
Alice Springs Chicken & Fries, 8 oz	920	50	73
Baby Back Ribs & Fries, full order	1280	75	78
Grilled Chkn On The Barbie, 8 oz, with Seasonal Mixed Veggies	490	16	28
Parmesan-Herb Crusted Chicken, with Mixed Veggies	670	32	30
Queensland Chicken & Shrimp Pasta	1140	48	100

Signature Steaks: *Without Sides*

	C	F	Cb
Outback Centre Cut Sirloin: 6 oz	210	7	0
9 oz Sirloin	320	10	0.5
Ribeye, 10 oz	540	35	0
Sirloin, 12 oz, & Grilled Shrimp	580	22	5
Victoria's Filet Mignon, 6 oz	240	9	0

Straight From The Sea: *W/ Seasonal Mixed Veggies*

	C	F	Cb
Bacon Bourbon Salmon, 10 oz	810	52	23
Perfectly Grilled Salmon, 10 oz	710	46	20
Tilapia, w/ Pure Lump Crab Meat	690	37	25

Entree Salads: *With Dressing*

	C	F	Cb
Aussie Cobb Salad: w/ Crispy Chkn	840	52	47
with Grilled Chicken	530	27	19
Brisbane Caesar:			
w/ Grilled Chkn	560	37	20
with Grilled Shrimp	560	38	22
Steakhouse	940	5	50

Side Salads: *With Dressing*

	C	F	Cb
Premium: Blue Cheese Pecan Chopped	530	40	31
Blue Cheese Wedge	440	34	27
Regular: Caesar	270	24	11
House: with Blue Cheese Vinaig.	370	29	20
with Caesar Dressing	300	25	14
with Creamy Blue Cheese	370	33	13
with Honey Mustard	340	26	24
with Thousand Island	360	31	18

Outback Steakhouse® cont... (Sept '17)

Soups:	C	F	Cb
Baked Potato: Cup	280	17	23
Bowl	520	32	47
Chicken Tortilla Soup: Cup	170	9	13
Bowl	260	4	21
Clam Chowder: Cup	360	22	23
Bowl	710	44	47
French Onion	420	29	21

Sides:

	C	F	Cb
Aussie Fries	410	17	57
Broccoli & Cheese	390	30	16
Fresh Seasonal Mixed Veggies	160	10	17
Grilled Asparagus	70	4.5	5
Homestyle Mashed Potatoes	240	15	21
Loaded Mashed Potatoes	300	20	22
Steakhouse Mac & Cheese	830	49	64
Sweet Potato, with all toppings	410	11	72

Kid's Menu: *Without Sides or Drink*

Entrees:	C	F	Cb
Boomerang Cheeseburger	600	36	40
Chicken Fingers	470	29	28
Grilled Cheese-A-Roo	580	21	77
Grilled Chicken on the Barbie	160	3.5	0
Junior Ribs, BBQ Sauce	300	21	2
Mac-A-Roo 'N Cheese	510	19	65

Desserts: *Per Whole Dish*

	C	F	Cb
Chocolate Thunder	1540	106	137
Double chocolate Mini Parfait	710	49	60
NY Style Cheesecake, w/ Choc. Sce	1100	75	92
Triple Layer Carrot Cake	1290	68	174

For Complete Menu & Data ~ see CalorieKing.com

Panda Express® (Jan '18)

Appetizers:	C	F	Cb
Chicken Egg Roll (1), 2.75 oz	200	10	20
Chicken Potsticker (3), 3.3 oz	160	6	20
Cream Cheese Rangoon (3), 2.4 oz	190	8	24
Crispy Shrimp (3), 1.8 oz	130	6	13
Veggie Spring Rolls (2), 3.4 oz	190	8	27

Entrées:

	C	F	Cb
Beef: Beijing Beef, 5.6 oz	470	26	46
Broccoli Beef, 5.4 oz	150	7	13
Shanghai Angus Beef: with Asparagus, 5.4 oz	310	19	16
with String Beans, 5.4 oz	320	19	17
Chicken Breast:			
String Bean, 5.6 oz	190	9	13
Sweet & Sour, 5.8 oz	300	12	40
SweetFire, 5.8 oz	380	15	47

Panda Express® cont... (Jan '18)

Entrees (Cont):

	C	F	Cb
Shrimp: Crispy Shrimp (6), 3.5 oz	260	13	26
Honey Walnut Shrimp, 3.7 oz	360	23	35
Vegetables: Eggplant Tofu, 6.1 oz	340	24	23
Country Style Bean Curd, 5.7 oz	190	12	14
Hot Szechuan Tofu, 5.5 oz	140	8	10
Mixed Vegetables, 4.3 oz	35	0	8
Sides: Chow Mein, 9.4 oz	510	20	80
Fried Rice, 9.3 oz	520	16	85
Steamed White Rice, 8.1 oz	380	0	87
Soup, Hot & Sour: Cup, 12.2 oz	120	5	14
Bowl, 17.4 oz	170	6	20
Dessert, Choc Chip Chunk Cookie	160	7	25

Panera Bread® (Sept '17)

Bagels:

	C	F	Cb
Asiago Cheese	330	6	55
Cinnamon Crunch	430	7	82

Breakfast Sandwiches, Grilled:

	C	F	Cb
Bacon, Egg & Cheese on Asiago Chse	590	30	45
Sausage, Egg & Cheese on Ciabatta	560	29	45
Steak & Egg on Everthing Bagel	540	18	59
Bowls, S'west Chkn Tortilla Broth	480	16	51

Sandwiches: *Per Full Sandwich*

	C	F	Cb
Bacon Turkey Bravo on Tomato Basil	630	25	57
Mediterranean Veggie on Tomato Basil	420	12	62
Napa Almond Chicken Salad, on Sesame Semolina	700	26	90
Roasted Turkey & Avocado BLT, on Sourdough	600	28	49
Tuna Salad, on Black Pepper Foccacia	660	35	57
Flatbread: BBQ Chicken (1)	380	6	41
Tomato Mozzarella (1)	350	18	35
Panini, Frontega Chicken on Focaccia	750	24	85

Pasta:

	C	F	Cb
Chicken Tortellini Alfredo, 2 cups	750	39	68

Mac & Cheese:

	C	F	Cb
Small	470	30	36
Bread Bowl	1140	35	166

Salads: *Full Size, with Dressing, without Bread*

	C	F	Cb
Asian Sesame w/ Chkn	410	20	27
Chicken Caesar	450	27	17
Chinese Cashew & Chkn	540	27	45
Greek	400	36	13
Strawberry Poppyseed with Chkn	340	13	31

Panera Bread® cont... (Sept '17)

Soups: *Per Cup, without Bread*

	C	F	Cb
Baked Potato	220	13	22
Broccoli Cheddar	230	13	19
Crm of Chkn & Wild Rice	180	10	18
New England Clam Chowder	370	25	27
Vegetarian Creamy Tomato	200	9	25

Cakes & Brownies:

	C	F	Cb
Cinnamon Crumb Coffee Cake, 1 slice	470	25	53
Double Fudge Brownie (1)	520	22	80
Cookies: Chocolate Chipper (1)	380	19	51
Oatmeal Raisin with Berries (1)	340	13	54

Pastries & Sweets:

	C	F	Cb
Bear Claw (1)	540	31	59
Cobblestone (1)	560	12	102
Pecan Roll (1)	720	46	69
Muffin: Apple Crunch	450	12	80
Pumpkin Muffin	580	22	90
Muffie, Chocolate Chip	320	14	46

Papa Gino's® (Sept '17)

Appetizers:

	C	F	Cb
BBQ Chicken Tender (2), 5.2 oz	360	18	33
Buffalo Chicken Tender (2), 5.4 oz	390	25	22
Cheddar Breadsticks (10)	560	19	72
Chicken Tender (2), 4.4 oz	350	20	24
Burgers: Cheeseburger, 6.7 oz	570	32	37
Classic Double, 12.8 oz	1040	67	43
Hamburger, 6.3 oz	520	28	35
French Fries, small, 5 oz	470	24	66

Pasta:

	C	F	Cb
Mac & Cheese, 17.8 oz	1040	60	87
Ravioli, 12.4 oz	560	21	67
Spaghetti & Meatballs, 19.8 oz	780	28	109

Pizzas:

Thin Crust: *Per Slice, 1/8 Large Pizza*

	C	F	Cb
Boss BBQ Chicken	320	12	38
Cheese	230	7	32
Colossal Meat Pulled Pork	390	19	34
PapRoni	280	16	23
Pepperoni	250	12	22
Super Veggie	230	10	24
Works	260	13	23

Subs: *Per Small Sub*

	C	F	Cb
BLT	690	35	67
Italian	590	24	64
Meatball Parmesan	790	38	79
Steak & Cheese	710	33	63
Super Steak	750	33	72
Tuna	730	39	64
Turkey Club	600	22	67

Fast - Foods & *Restaurants*

Papa John's® (Sept '17)

Pizzas:

	C	F	Cb
Original Crust (14"): *Per 1/8 of Large 14" Pizza*			
BBQ Chicken & Bacon	340	11	45
Buffalo Chicken	380	17	40
Cheese	290	10	38
Grilled Chicken & Bacon	270	7	37
John's Favorite	390	20	36
Pepperoni	320	13	38
Pepperoni & Sausage	360	17	38
Thin Crust (14"): *Per 1/8 of Large 14" Pizza*			
BBQ Chicken & Bacon	270	12	27
Buffalo Chicken	300	18	22
Cheese	210	11	20
Grilled Chicken & Bacon	190	8	19
John's Favorite	320	22	18
Pepperoni	250	14	20
Pepperoni & Sausage	310	20	20
Wings: *With Dipping Sauce*			
BBQ, 8 wing	880	57	20
Buffalo, 8 wings	840	58	8
Honey Chipotle, 8 wings	900	57	27
Chicken Poppers: 5 Poppers	180	7	15
10 Poppers	370	14	29
15 Poppers	550	22	44
Sides:			
Breadsticks (2)	300	4	54
Garlic Parm (2)	340	10	54
Wisconsin Stuffed Cheesesticks (1)	240	12	24
Desserts: Brookie	190	9	26
Double Chocolate Chip Brownie	240	12	34

Papa Murphy's® (Sept '17)

Pizzas:

	C	F	Cb
Original Crust: *Per 1/12 of Family Size Pizza*			
BBQ Chicken	340	13	37
Chicken Garlic	330	15	30
Cowboy	370	19	32
Gourmet Vegetarian	320	16	32
Hawaiian	270	10	33
Murphy's Combo	350	18	33
Papa's Favorite	350	17	33
Pepperoni	300	14	31
Rancher	320	14	32
Spicy Fennel Sausage	350	16	35
Thai Chicken	340	12	40
Stuffed Pizzas: *Per 1/16 of Family Size Pizza*			
5 Meat	460	18	52
Big Murphy	450	18	53
Chicago Style	450	18	52
Chicken and Bacon	440	17	51

Papa Murphy's® cont... (Sept '17)

Pizzas (Cont):

	C	F	Cb
Thin Crust: *Per Slice, 1/8 of Large Pizza*			
Cowboy	250	15	18
Hawaiian	180	8	19
Murphy's Combo	240	14	18
Pepperoni	200	11	16
Rancher	210	11	17
Salads: *Per Whole Salad, w/out Dressing or Croutons*			
Club, 13 oz	270	16	12
Garden, 14.5 oz	190	11	13
Italian, 13 oz	270	19	11

Pei Wei Asian Diner® (Sept '17)

	C	F	Cb
Shareables: *Without Sauce*			
Crab Wontons (4)	340	20	26
Korean BBQ Tacos (2)	520	23	51
Traditional Edamame	320	13	20
Vegetable Spring Rolls (4)	460	20	52
Sauces: Soy	15	0	2
Sweet Chile, 2 oz	140	0	34
Thai Peanut Dipping Sauce, 2 oz	230	15	20
Sushi Rolls: *Per 4 Rolls*			
Classic California	200	7	26
Kung Pao Shrimp	450	21	49
Salmon Avocado Roll	190	8	21
Spicy Tuna Roll	120	1.5	19
Rice Bowls: *Without Side Choices*			
Honey Seared:			
Chicken: Small	850	44	83
Regular	1160	59	112
Steak: Small	860	46	83
Regular	1150	60	111
Pei Wei Spicy with Shrimp:			
Small	570	26	76
Regular	790	33	107
Sweet & Sour, regular:			
with Chicken	950	48	96
with Shrimp	910	50	93
with Steak	950	49	95
Salad Bowls: *With Dressing*			
Ahi Aavocado	740	41	72
Asian Chopped Chicken	750	44	47
Thai Steak & Mango	940	59	67
Vietnamese Rice Noodle	1000	48	87
Soup: Hot & Sour	540	18	45
Thai Wonton	480	14	66

Pepe's Mexican® ~ *see CalorieKing.com*

Perkins® (Sept '17)

Breakfast: Without Side Choices	C	F	Cb
Classic: Eggs Benedict	690	45	42
Country Fried Steak & Eggs	740	45	47
Hearty Man's Combo	800	69	11
Steak Medallions & Eggs	530	28	8
Perfect Platters: *Without Extras*			
Belgian Waffle	560	26	63
Brioche French Toast	770	40	65
Cinn. Roll French Toast	800	45	71
French Toast, plain	620	32	53
Lemon Blueberry	850	35	114
Syrups & Toppings:			
Apricot Syrup, 2 oz	120	0	30
Glazed Blueberries, 6 oz	200	0	51
Glazed Strawberries, 6 oz	140	0	36
Pancake/Twinberry Syrup, 2 oz, av.	130	0	33
Sugar Free, 2 oz	10	0	3
Omelets: *Without Optional Sides*			
Everything	550	40	14
Farmers	660	54	8
Granny's Country	970	47	98
B'fast Side Choices: Bacon, 4 slices	140	12	0
Biscuits (2), Jumbo, with butter	650	36	68
Blueberry Muffin with butter	650	33	81
Breakfast Potatoes, 5 oz	250	12	32
Eggs (2)	170	13	2
English Muffin, with butter	230	11	28
Fresh Cut Fruit, 4 oz	70	0	19
Ham, grilled, 5.6 oz	160	4.5	6
Hash Browns, 4 oz	490	13	87
Oatmeal, w/ 2% Milk & Brown Sugar	330	6	60
Potato Pancakes (2), w/out extras	440	18	59
Sausage Links (2)	240	24	1
Smoked Sausage, 4.1 oz	380	34	8
Sticky Bun, with butter	790	41	98
White Toast (2), with butter	310	16	34
Whole Wheat Toast (2), w/ butter	310	13	38
Burgers: *Without Side Choices*			
BBQ Beef Bacon Supreme	1070	62	76
Classic Burger	710	42	44
Classic Cheeseburger	700	42	44
The Beef Tangler	1090	72	57

Perkins® (cont... Mar '17)

Sandwiches: W/out Side Choices	C	F	Cb
Chicken Strips Melt, on S'dough	1290	80	88
Grilled Chicken Breast	510	20	44
Reuben Melt	1090	61	79
Roast Beef & Swiss	730	50	33
Turkey & Avocado BLT	700	39	47
Lunch & Dinners: Without Sides			
Fork Worthy Entrées:			
Chicken Strips Dinner	800	43	59
Country Fried Steak Dinner	570	32	45
Fish 'n Chips, with Tartar Sauce	1370	87	107
Grilled Garlic Tilapia & Shrimp	550	20	57
Grilled Salmon	430	29	2
Steak Medallions & Mushrooms	480	29	6
Turkey & Dressing, w/- Cranb. Sce	510	20	39
Sides: Apple Sauce, 3 oz	40	0	9
Baked Potato, with Sour Cream	300	12	42
Buttered Corn	150	8	17
French Fries, 7 oz	570	36	56
Green Beans & Bacon, 4 oz	45	2.5	4
Herb Rice Pilaf, 6.5 oz	270	6	50
Macaroni & Five Cheese, 5.2 oz	300	16	26
Mashed Potatoes & Gravy, 8.6 oz	240	9	34
Sauteed Spinach, 4 oz	70	3.5	4
Side Salad with Croutons, witout Dressing	110	4.5	13
Tater Tots	470	28	47
Soups: *Per Bowl, Includes Crackers*			
Chicken Noodle	260	6	37
Tomato Basil	460	26	46
Salads: *Includes Set Dressing*			
Chopped Cobb	510	30	18
Honey Mstrd Chkn Crunch	980	63	63
Southwest Avocado	820	50	61
Dessert:			
Muffins: *Includes Whipped Butter Blend*			
Apple Cinnamon	630	33	76
Banana Nut	790	46	85
Blueberry	650	33	81
Pies: *Per Slice*			
Caramel Apple, 7.2 oz	500	22	68
Cherry	580	27	75
Lem. Meringue, 7 oz	500	17	80
Southern Pecan, 5.5 oz	670	33	86
Wildberry, no sugar added, 7 oz	470	27	50

Peter Piper Pizza® (Sept'17)

Appetizers:	C	F	Cb
Boneless Wings: *Per 10 oz Serving*			
Mild Buffalo	1010	67	56
Sweet BBQ	1130	58	110
Cheddar Bacon Roll (1)	350	18	34
Garlic Cheese Bread, 3.25 oz	390	17	45
Handmade Breadsticks, with Marinara Sauce (6)	1190	31	199

Dipping Sauces:			
BBQ	240	0	60
Buffalo	120	9	6
Ranch	320	36	2
Sweet Chili	200	0	46
Xtra Hot Buffalo	90	6	5

Signature Pizzas:			
Original Crust: *Per 1/8 of Large 14" Pizza*			
5 Meat Supreme	360	15	39
California Veggie	290	9	41
Cheese	320	11	39
Chicago Classic	330	13	40
Hearty Hawaiian	310	9	41
New York 3 Cheese w/ Pepperoni	390	18	39
Pizza Mexicana	390	18	39
Spinach Alfredo	350	15	37
The Werx	310	11	40
Veggie Harvest	300	9	42
Original Crust: *Per 1/12 of Extra Large 16" Pizza*			
5 Meat Supreme	350	16	34
California Veggie	250	8	35
Cheese	280	10	34
Chicago Classic	300	12	35
Hearty Hawaiian	270	8	36
New York 3 Cheese w/ Pepperoni	350	16	34
Pizza Mexicana	340	15	34
Spinach Alfredo	310	14	32
The Werx	290	11	34
Veggie Harvest	260	8	36

Salads: *Small Size, without Dressing*			
Caesar, with Croutons	320	14	35
Mandarin Cranberry	150	6	26

Dessert:			
Cinnamon Crunch, small slice	380	9	69
Vanilla Soft Serve: Cone	200	6	35
Cup	180	6	31

P.F. Chang's® (Sept'17)

Street Fare:	C	F	Cb
Cauliflower Tempura	550	36	57
Chang's BBQ Spare Ribs	1210	64	62
Chang's Chicken Lettuce Wraps	580	29	48
Chang's Vegetarian Lettuce Wraps	470	21	39
Crispy Green Beans	1040	81	71
Dynamite Shrimp	490	39	26
Edamame with Kosher Salt	400	17	25
Northern Style Spare Ribs	1130	63	41
Salt & Pepper Calamari	750	40	72

Entrées:			
Beef: *Per Whole Meal, without Rice*			
A La Sichuan	810	35	77
Beef with Broccoli	710	37	45
Mongolian	790	42	43
Wok Fired Filet Mignon	1070	63	68
Chicken: *Per Whole Dish, without Rice*			
Chang's Spicy	960	35	102
Crispy Honey Chkn	1200	48	130
Korean BBQ Chicken Stir-Fry	910	46	73
Kung Pao	1090	64	58
Orange Peel Chkn	980	39	92
Sesame Chicken	990	36	102
Seafood: *Per Whole Meal, without Rice*			
Chang's Lobster & Shrimp Rice	1090	50	113
Crispy Honey Shrimp	1040	41	131
Kung Pao Shrimp	840	55	47
Oolong Chilean Sea Bass	630	37	42
Orange Peel Shrimp	660	29	78
Salt & Pepper Prawns	650	32	45
Walnut Shrimp with Melon	1420	113	69

Vegetarian: *Without Rice*			
Buddha's Feast, steamed	250	4	32
Coconut Curry Vegetables	1270	90	73
Ma Po Tofu	950	62	61
Stir-Fried Eggplant	480	23	65

Noodles & Rice:			
Fried Rice: Combo	1250	40	162
with Beef	1100	32	156
with Chicken	1080	28	159
with Pork	1140	36	161
with Shrimp	990	24	157
Long Life Noodles & Prawns	970	40	109

Updated Nutrition Data ~ www.CalorieKing.com
Persons with Diabetes ~ See Disclaimer (Page 22)

P.F. Chang's® cont... (Sept '17)

Noodles & Rice (Cont):

	C	F	Cb
Lo Mein: Beef	860	28	106
Chicken	830	21	110
Combo	920	29	111
Pork	920	32	112
Shrimp	760	18	109
Vegetables	630	10	114
Hokkien Street Noodles	970	26	131

Market Sides: Per Serving

	C	F	Cb
Brown Rice	190	0	40
Chili Garlic Green Beans	320	16	40
Sichuan-Style Asparagus	300	16	33
White Rice, 6 oz	220	0	49
Wok-Charred Brussels Sprouts	210	13	22
Wok'd Spinach w/ Garlic	60	9	15
Salad: Asian Caesar	570	45	24
Mandarin Crunch	880	58	78
Vietnamese Noodle	640	11	113
Dessert: Banana Spring Rolls	1030	42	152
Berries & Cream Shortcake, small	500	38	37
New York Style Cheese Cake	890	57	82
The Great Wall of Chocolate	1730	72	264

Pita Pit® ~ See CalorieKing.com

Pizza Hut® (Jan '18)

Hand-Tossed Style: Per 1/8 of Medium 12" Pizza

	C	F	Cb
Cheese	210	8	26
Chicken-Bacon Parmesan	230	9	25
Meat Lover's	280	15	25
Pepperoni	220	10	25
Pepperoni Lover's	270	13	26
Primo Meats	280	15	25
Supreme	240	11	26
Ultimate Cheese Lover's	230	10	25
Veggie Lover's	200	7	26

Original Pan: Per 1/8 of Medium 12" Pizza

	C	F	Cb
Cheese	240	10	28
Meat Lover's	310	17	28
Pepperoni	250	12	27
Pepperoni Lover's	300	15	28
Premium Garden Veggie	240	10	29
Supreme	270	13	28
Ultimate Cheese Lover's	260	13	27
Veggie Lover's	220	9	29

Rectangle Slices: Per Slice, 1/8 of Pizza

	C	F	Cb
BBQ Bacon Cheeseburger	290	13	34
Bacon Spinach Alfredo	260	12	28
Cheese	240	10	29

Pizza Hut® cont... (Jan '18)

Personal Pan: Per 1/4 of 6" Pizza

	C	F	Cb
BBQ Bacon Cheeseburger	210	9	25
Meat Lover's	210	12	17
Pepperoni	150	7	17
Pepperoni Lover's	180	9	17
Primo Meats	200	12	17
Supreme	170	9	17
Ultimate Cheese Lover's	170	8	17
Veggie Lover's	140	5	18

Skinny Slice: Per 1/8 of Medium 12" Pizza

	C	F	Cb
BBQ Bacon Cheeseburger	270	11	33
Bacon Spinach Alfredo	230	11	25
Italian Meatball	220	8	27
Supreme	240	11	27

Thin 'n Crispy: Per 1/8 of Medium 12" Pizza

	C	F	Cb
Cheese	180	7	22
Chicken-Bacon Parmesan	220	10	21
Four Pepper Pepperoni	180	7	23
Meat Lover's	260	14	22
Pepperoni	200	9	22
Pepperoni Lover's	250	13	22
Supreme	210	9	23
Ultimate Cheese Lover's	210	10	21
Veggie Lover's	170	6	24

Pastas, Tuscani: Per Whole Pan

	C	F	Cb
Creamy Chicken Alfredo	890	49	74
Meaty Marinara	720	31	78
Sides: Bone Out Baked Wings (1)	60	2	4
Breadstick (1), without sauce	140	4.5	19
Buffalo Chicken Nachos	1110	50	132
Fried Chicken Tender (1)	240	14	14
Fried Curly Fries	370	20	42
Fried Onion Rings, with Ketchup	860	50	93
Garlic Bread, 1 piece	140	8	15
Spin. Dip, w/ Chips	850	60	53
Stuffed Garlic Knot	80	2.5	10

Salad: Entree Size, without Dressing

	C	F	Cb
Asian	330	15	24
BLT	400	26	26
Chicken Caesar	470	25	27
Harvest	470	19	48
Zesty Italian	370	22	30
Dressing: Blue Cheese, 1.5 oz	200	21	2
Buttermilk Ranch, 1.5 oz	200	22	2
Honey French, 1.5 oz	190	15	13
Desserts: Hot Cinnamon Apple Pie	170	9	22
Hershey's: Hot Choc. Brownie	290	11	45
Toasted S'mores Cookie (1)	240	10	33

Pizza Ranch® (Sept '17)

Figures based on West Coast Outlets **C** **F** **Cb**

Pizza:

Original Crust: *Per Slice, 1/10 of Medium Pizza*

	C	F	Cb
Bacon Cheeseburger	200	8	20
BLT	250	14	21
Bronco	210	9	21
Buffalo Chicken	200	9	20
California Chicken	220	10	20
Chicken Bacon Ranch	240	12	20
Chicken Broccoli Alfredo	190	8	20
Macaroni & Cheese	210	8	25
Pepperoni	210	10	19
Prairie (Veggie)	180	7	21
Roundup	200	8	21
Stampede	210	9	22
Sweet Swine	180	6	22
Texan Taco	230	9	27

Thin Crust: *Per 1/10 Slice of Medium Pizza*

	C	F	Cb
BBQ Chicken	140	5	13
BLT	200	13	11
California Chicken	170	10	10

For Complete Menu & Data ~ see CalorieKing.com

Pollo Tropical® ~ See CalorieKing.com

Popeye's® (Sept '17) **C** **F** **Cb**

Chicken Pieces: Mild & Spicy with Skin

	C	F	Cb
Breast, average	430	27	14
Leg, average	165	10	5
Thigh, average	270	20	8
Wing	210	14	8
Nuggets: 4 pieces, 1.8 oz	150	9	10
6 Pieces 2.7 oz	230	14	14
Tenders: Mild, 3 pieces, 4.5 oz	340	14	26
Spicy, 3 pieces, 4.5 oz	310	15	16
Sandwiches & Wraps: Each			
Blackened BBQ Chicken Po'Boy	340	7	49
Chicken & Sausage Jambalaya	220	11	20
Chicken Po'Boy	660	34	61
Loaded Chicken Wrap	310	13	33
Shrimp Po' Boy	690	42	66
Seafood: Catfish Fillets, 5 oz	460	29	27
Butterfly Shrimp (8)	290	17	21
Popcorn Shrimp, 3 oz	330	9	28

Popeye's® cont... (Sept '17)

Sides:

	C	F	Cb
Biscuit, 2 oz	260	15	26
Cajun Fries, regular, 3 oz	260	14	30
Cajun Rice, regular, 4.3 oz	170	5	25
Cole Slaw, regular, 4.9 oz	220	15	19
Corn on the Cob (1), 7.8 oz	190	2	37
Mashed Potatoes, regular, 5 oz	110	4	18
Onion Rings (12)	560	38	50
Red Beans & Rice, regular, 5.2 oz	230	14	23

Breakfast:

	C	F	Cb
Biscuits: Bacon	400	25	37
Chicken	490	26	47
Egg	510	29	41
Egg & Sausage	690	45	43
Sausage	540	36	41
Sausage & Gravy	510	33	42
Grits	370	5	80
Hash Rounds	360	20	41

Desserts:

	C	F	Cb
Hot Sweet Potato Pie 3.4 oz	350	19	41
Mardi Gras Cheesecake, 3 oz	310	19	32
Mississippi Mud Pie, 3 oz	280	7	51
Sliced Pecan Pie, 3.4 oz	410	21	52

Port of Subs® (Sept '17)

Figures Based on West Coast Outlets **C** **F** **Cb**

Cold Submarine S'wiches: Per 5" Sub with Cheese, Lettuce, Tomato Vinegar, Oil, Salt & Oregano

	C	F	Cb
#1 Ham, Salami, Capicolla Pepperoni, Provolone	475	22	43
#2 Ham & Turkey, Provolone	400	13	42
#3 Salami & Turkey, Provolone	440	18	43
#4 Ham, Salami, Provolone	425	18	42
#5 Smoked Ham, Turkey, Cheddar	405	14	43
#6 Vegetarian, 3 Chse	430	20	44
#7 Roast Beef, Prov.	400	14	42
#8 Turkey, Provolone	415	13	45
#10 Rstd Chicken Breast, Provolone	390	12	42
#11 Ham, American Cheese	470	22	44
#12 Salami, Provolone	435	20	42
#13 Pepprd Pastrami Turkey, Swiss	410	15	43
#15 Salami, Pepperoni, Provolone	445	22	42
#16 Chkn, Pepperoni, Pepper Jack	350	14	41
#17 Tuna, Provolone	490	25	43
#18 Roast Beef, Turkey, Provolone	410	14	43

continued next page...

Port of Subs® cont... (Sept '17)

Figures Based on West Coast Outlets **C F Cb**

Wraps: With 12" Flour Tortilla, Cheese, Lettuce, Tomato, Onion, Vinegar, Oil, Salt & Oregano

	C	F	Cb
#2 Ham, Turkey, Provolone	590	24	57
# 8 Turkey Provolone	610	24	60
#11 Ham, with American Cheese	740	38	60

Fresh Salads: W/ Lettuce, Tomato & Onion, w/o Dressing

	C	F	Cb
Caesar, with Parmesan, 6 oz	35	0	7
Garden, 10 oz	65	2	10
Grilled Chkn, 10 oz	235	4	11

Salad Dressings:

Blue Cheese, 1.5 oz	220	23	2
Caesar, 1.5 oz	240	23	2
Ranch, 1.5 oz	260	28	2
Croutons, 1 package	30	1	5

Sides: Per Regular, 8 oz

Caesar Bow Tie Pasta Salad	355	18	37
Cucumber Salad	125	11	4
Macaroni Salad	515	41	44
Potato Salad	325	13	52

Desserts:

Brownie, 2.3 oz	280	6	50
Chocolate Chunk Cookie, 4 oz	500	22	70
Oatmeal Raisin Cookie, 4 oz	460	20	68
White Choc.Macadamia Nut Cookie	520	26	66

Fountain Beverages: Without Ice

Coca Cola: 22 oz	270	0	74
32 oz	395	0	108
Barq's Root Beer: 22 oz	305	0	83
32 oz	445	0	120
Cherry Coke: 22 oz	285	0	77
32 oz	415	0	112
Smoothies: Strawb. Bomb, 8 oz	250	0	63
Mand. Orange Passion Fruit, 8 oz	240	1	59
Average other flavors, 8 oz	220	1	53

Pret A Manger® (Sept '17)

Baguettes:

	C	F	Cb
Chicken Mozzarella	550	20	57
Tuna & Cucumber	560	29	52
Roast Beef, Arugula & Parmesan	530	19	53

Hot Food: Per Pack

Baguette, Chipotle Chicken	630	20	70
Burrito, Pret's Chicken	650	25	70
Spinach & Tomato Mac & Chse	460	23	44
Wrap, Falafel & Red Pepper	700	28	87

Pret A Manger® cont (Sept '17)

Pots:

	C	F	Cb
Asian Greens Veggie, 5.4 oz	200	13	16
Banana & Honey, 8.7 oz	400	14	53
Blueberry & Pinenut, 2.7 oz	130	9	5
Egg & Quinoa, 4.9 oz	240	16	15
Seasonal Berries Yogurt, 7.3 oz	240	10	25

Sandwiches:

Balsamic Chicken & Avocado, 8.5 oz	480	25	40
California Club, 9.4 oz	390	17	39
Chicken & Bacon, 7.9 oz	480	27	35
Classic Cheddar & Tomato, 7 oz	430	25	35
Tuna Salad, 8.7 oz	460	29	32
Veggie Club, 11.8 oz	630	40	46

Soups:

Green Chicken Pozole, 15.6 oz	240	7	27
Miso, 12 oz	50	1.5	6
Moroccan Lentil, 12 oz	380	17	45
Tomato Feta, 12 oz	230	14	23

Salads: Without Dressing

Chef, 8.9 oz	290	15	14
Chicken Avoc., 7.7 oz	400	23	25
Kale Chicken Caesar, 7.5 oz	280	10	11
Souvlaki Chicken,15.5 oz	380	18	23
Veggie Fiesta, 17.3 oz	470	27	38

Bakery: Per Pack

Croissants: Almond	370	21	39
Pain au Chocolate	300	15	34
Pain au Raisin	395	20	46
Cookies: Carrot Cake, 2.5 oz	270	14	35
Chocolate Chunk, 2.5 oz	320	15	41
Harvest, 2.5 oz	280	12	40
Muffin, Blueberry, 4.5 oz	420	16	63

Pretzelmaker® (Sept '17)

Pretzels: Per Small Serving **C F Cb**

	C	F	Cb
Bites: Salted, 6 oz	500	14	85
Cinn. Sugar, 6 oz	530	14	90
Whole: Plain, 4 oz	310	3	66
Cinnamon Sugar, 5 oz	450	12	79
Garlic, 5 oz	430	12	74
Parmesan, 5 oz	450	15	66
Ranch, 5 oz	440	12	72
Pretzel Dogs: Mini (8)	430	29	33
Jalapeno (1), 6 oz	450	24	34

continued next page...

229

Fast - Foods & *Restaurants*

Pretzelmaker® cont... (Sept '17)

Sauces: Per 2 oz	C	F	Cb
Caramel	100	1	22
Cheddar Cheese	80	6	6
Cream Cheese	200	20	2
Nacho Cheese	80	6	4
Pizza Sauce	30	1	6
Vanilla Glaze	170	0	42

Beverages: *Per 20 oz Unless Indicated*

Blended Drinks:

	C	F	Cb
Cool Cappuccino	430	22	58
Mango Madness	500	16	90
Mocha Mania	580	22	94
Power Pomegranate	490	16	86
Strawberry Bananza	500	16	85
Fresh Lemonade: Original, 20 oz	140	0	38
Strawberry; Raspberry, 20 oz, av.	210	0	52

Qdoba® (Apr '18)

Please Note: Nutritional Information is based on a single serving of each menu ingredient listed.

Burritos: *Each with 12.5" Flour Tortilla, Cilantro-Lime Rice, Black Beans, Salsa Verde, Lite Sour Cream, Lettuce and Shredded Cheese*

	C	F	Cb
Marinated Grilled Chkn	1035	37	124
Pulled Pork	1005	33	129
Seasoned Ground Beef	1055	40	124

Burritos: *With 12.5" Flour Tortilla, 3-Cheese Queso Pinto Beans, Roasted Chili Corn Salsa, Guacamole & Lite Sour Cream*

	C	F	Cb
Marinated Grilled Chicken	1020	47	104
Marinated Gr. Steak	1030	47	102
Pulled Pork	990	43	109
Seasoned Ground Beef	1040	50	104

Grilled Quesadillas: *With 12.5" Flour Tortilla, Shredded Cheese, Pico de Gallo and Fajita Vegetables*

	C	F	Cb
Grilled Chicken	685	30	64
Pulled Pork	655	26	60

3-Cheese Nachos: *Per Serving, with Tortilla Chips, 3-Cheese Queso, Salsa Roja, Guacamole & Sour Cream*

	C	F	Cb
Grilled Chicken	1120	64	98
Pulled Pork	1090	60	103

Qdoba® cont... (Apr '18)

Knock Out Tacos: Set Ingredients	C	F	Cb
Bohemian Veg	230	9	28
Drunken Yardbird	220	8	25
Mad Rancher	230	10	21
Two Timer	290	13	28
Triple Threat	250	12	17
The Gladiator	280	17	16

Taco Salads: *With Crunchy Flour Tortilla Bowl, Black Beans, Lettuce, Shredded Cheese, Brown Rice, Lite Sour Cream, Guacamole & Cilantro Lime Dressing*

	C	F	Cb
Grilled Chicken	1270	66	116
Pulled Pork	1240	62	121
Seasoned Ground Beef	1290	69	116

Chips & Dip: *Includes Tortilla Chips*

	C	F	Cb
3- Cheese Queso	750	41	81
3-Cheese Queso, Guac. & Salsa Roja	900	51	92

Breakfast Burritos: *With 12" Flour Tortilla*

Chorizo & Seasoned Potato:

	C	F	Cb
with 3-Cheese Queso Sauce	820	40	80
with Shred. Cheese & Salsa Roja	820	38	79

Quiznos Subs® (Jan '18)

Subs: *Per 8" Regular Japaleno Cheddar Sub, with Standard Menu Toppings Unless Indicated*

All Natural Chicken:	C	F	Cb
Baja	780	31	76
Carbonara	860	40	73
Honey Mustard	830	34	80
Mesquite	780	32	73
Southwest Chicken	860	45	73
Steak:			
Black Angus Steak,			
On Rosemary Parmesan	780	27	88
Chipotle Steak & Cheddar	840	44	73
French Dip	760	30	79
Peppercorn Steak	840	42	76
Deli Classic:			
Classic Italian	930	51	78
Spicy Monterey	630	17	83
Tuna Melt	660	22	76
Turkey Ranch & Swiss	700	6	75
Veggie Guacamole	810	44	81

Grilled Flatbreads: *Per Menu Board Toppings*

	C	F	Cb
Classic Italian	470	29	33
Honey Bacon Club	450	22	41
Turkey Bacon Guacamole	450	24	33

continued next page...

Quiznos Subs® cont... (Jan '18)

	C	F	Cb
Salads: Per Full, without Dressing			
Apple Harvest Chicken	400	17	42
BBQ Chicken Ranch	270	10	15
Honey Mustard Chicken	260	13	8
Savory Soups: Per Regular Bowl, with 2 Crackers			
Broccoli Cheese	245	15	22
Chicken Noodle	145	4.5	18
Breakfast:			
Subs: Bacon, Egg & Cheddar	470	24	38
Ham, Egg & Cheddar	360	13	39
Sausage, Egg & Cheddar	490	28	39
Desserts:			
Chocolate Chunk Cookie	390	19	54
Chocolate Brownie	310	16	40
Cinnamon Sugar Cookie	400	17	58
Oatmeal Raisin Cookie	360	12	58

Rally's/Checkers® (Sept '17)

	C	F	Cb
Burgers/Sandwiches:			
Baconzilla	810	52	40
Big Buford	660	39	39
Cheese Champ	430	21	39
Cheese Double	480	25	38
Roadhouse	670	40	49
Classic Wings: Buffalo, 5 pieces	360	23	3
Honey BBQ, 5 pieces	430	23	19
Garlic Parmesan, 5 pieces	510	40	3
Fries:			
Fries, medium	500	24	63
Chili Cheese	590	30	72
Fully Loaded	870	56	72

Ranch One® (Sept '17)

	C	F	Cb
Sandwiches:			
Chicken & Cheese	390	12	40
Chkn Philly, 9.3 oz	410	13	40
Grilled Classic Chicken, 9.4 oz	680	47	37
Original Crispy Chicken, 11.5 oz	640	31	60
Other Favorites:			
Chicken Fajitas, 10 oz	540	24	53
Chicken Platter, with Rice, 11.9 oz	270	6	28
Popcorn Chkn:			
Small, 5.5 oz	310	10	30
Large, 7.5 oz	420	14	40
Salads: Completed			
Grilled Chicken Caesar, 13.3 oz	430	30	14
Southwest Chicken, 17.5 oz	680	43	44
Fries:			
Medium, 5.8 oz	380	19	43
Large, 10.9 oz	530	27	58
Cheese Fries: Medium, 7.3 oz	490	27	46
Large, 11 oz	760	44	66

Red Hot & Blue® (Sept '17)

	C	F	Cb
Starters:			
Catfish Fingers	590	19	75
Nachos, with Chili	1005	51	103
Shakin' Bacon Cheese Fries	2440	60	106
Burgers:			
ALL IN	915	52	46
Classic Blues	665	32	44
Ribs, Full Slab:			
Dry	1870	144	28
Sweet	1895	142	44
Favorite Entrees: Delta Catfish	835	42	57
Delta Surf & Turf	1025	68	38
Southern Fried Chicken Crispers	760	35	50
Rib & Crispers Platter	1060	68	39
BBQ Platters: Five Meat	935	63	15
Delta Double with Memphis Chkn	900	54	12
Pulled Pork	325	21	7
Smoked Sausage	965	68	36
Sandwiches:			
Fried Delta Catfish	655	25	71
Grilled Chicken	360	6	40
Pulled Pork	370	15	37
Sides: BBQ Beans	255	2	48
Collard Greens	50	2	7
Fried Ocra	190	8	29
Mashed Potatoes, with Gravy	310	14	44
Memphis Fries, 6 oz	345	19	38
Potato Salad	405	28	33
Sweet Potato	495	0	114
Sweet Potato Fries	375	19	49
Salads: Grilled Chicken Caesar	770	46	47
Southern Fried Chicken	710	31	60

Red Lobster® (Sept '17)

	C	F	Cb
Seaside Starters: Menu Set Sides			
Crispy Calamari & Vegetables	1770	122	138
Crispy Shrimp Lettuce Wraps	620	18	93
Lobster, Artichoke & Seafood Dip	1050	56	106
Lobster & Langostino Pizza	690	34	53
Mozzarella Cheesesticks	810	44	67
Parrot Isle Jumbo Cocktail Shrimp	610	39	52
Signature Shrimp Cocktail	130	0	11
Sweet Chili Shrimp	1100	76	77
Lunch Entrees: With Menu Set Sides & Dipping Sauce			
Classic Caesar Salad with Chicken	640	48	19
Crab Linguini Alfredo, half portion	650	32	59
Crunchy Popcorn Shrimp	420	18	49
Maple Glazed Chicken	340	5	46
Shrimp Linguine Alfredo, half	620	32	55

Red Lobster® cont... (Sept '17)

Dinner Entrées: Includes Menu Set Sides, Condiments and Dipping Sauce

	C	F	Cb
Fish: Hand Battered Fish & Chips	900	48	74
Parmesan-Crusted Tilapia	550	31	18
Lighthouse/Fresh Fish Menu:			
Garlic-Grilled Shrimp	390	16	34
Maple-Glazed Chicken	500	8	54
Wood-Gr. Peppercorn Sirloin & Shrimp	530	19	37
Seafood Bakes: Bar Harbor Lobster	1680	93	117
Roasted Maine Lobster	1220	66	112
Shrimp: Coconut Shrimp Bites	400	22	38
Seaside Shrimp Trio	1300	66	101
Shrimp Linguini Alfredo, full	1340	59	118
Walt's Favorite Shrimp	620	28	68
Wood-Grilled:			
Cheeseburger	1380	86	99
Shrimp Skewers	300	10	33
Tacos, with Lobster Meat	660	30	73
Side Dishes:			
Baked Potato, Plain	210	2	45
Cheddar Bay Biscuit	160	10	16
Coleslaw	260	20	17
Creamy Lobster Mashed Potatoes	330	18	31
French Fries	290	12	42
Garden Salad, without dressing	70	1.5	12
Grilled Zucchini & Squash	150	12	8
Tomato Mozz. Caprese	120	8	7
Wild Rice Pilaf	140	3	25
Salads:			
Caesar Salad: *With Dressing*			
with Gr. Chicken	640	48	19
with Gr. Shrimp	600	48	19
With Salmon	830	65	18
Sauces: 100% Pure Melted Butter	300	33	0
Blue Cheese Dressing	230	24	2
Caesar Dressing	300	32	0
Cocktail Sauce	45	0	11
Honey Mustard Dressing	200	18	9
Marinara Sauce	35	2	4
Desserts:			
Chocolate Wave	1130	63	136
Key Lime Pie	400	14	59
Triple Choc. Brownie a la Mode	470	25	58
Warm Apple Crostada	610	31	76
Warm Chocolate Chip Lava Cookie	920	42	126

For Complete Nutritional Data ~ see CalorieKing.com

Red Robin® (Sept '17)

Nutritional Information varies between restaurants. Please refer to Red Robin's website for further information.

Appetizers:	C	F	Cb
Creamy Artichoke & Spinach Dip	780	43	66
Fried Pickle Nickels	790	51	70
Guacamole, Salsa & Chips	810	39	81
Nachos, OMG	1490	83	105
Pretzel Bites	650	20	97
The O-Ring Shorty	1120	78	84
Towering Onion Rings	1890	121	171
Wings'n'Yukon Chips, Buzz Sce, large	1230	72	51
Jump Starters: *Without Dressing*			
Cheese Sticks	600	32	53
Clamstrips	690	53	44
Fresh Fried Mshrms	410	23	48
Sweet Potato Fries	380	15	62
Wisconsin Cheese Curds	710	57	23
Entrées: *With Menu Set Sides*			
Arctic Cod Fish & Chips	1560	92	136
Clucks & Fries	1350	82	102
Ensenada Chicken Platter, 1 piece	220	7	11
Prime Rib Dip	680	24	64
Sear-ious Salmon	450	35	7
Shrimp & Cod Duo	1060	64	86
Finest Burgers: Black & Bleu	980	58	59
Citrus Harissa Salmon	870	58	49
The Marco Pollo	740	32	49
The Southern Charm	1150	59	94
Fire Grilled Burgers: A.1.	1110	69	71
Bleu Ribbon	1130	70	73
Burnin' Love	920	58	60
Chili Chili Chseburger	870	48	57
Grilled Turkey	680	39	53
Guacamole Bacon	950	59	50
Keep It Simple, Beef	750	33	78
Prime Chophouse	1110	66	81
Red Robin Gourmet Cheeseburger	820	47	55
Royal Red Robin	1160	81	48
Sauteed 'Shroom	840	48	52
Whiskey River BBQ	1180	76	71
Sandwiches & Wraps:			
BLTA Croissant	800	38	83
Caesars Chkn Wrap	760	43	55
Nacho Chicken Bacon Wrap	1480	81	127
Philly Cheesesteak Sandwich	930	62	54
Whiskey River BBQ Chicken Wrap	1040	58	71
Wrappin' California Club	1050	58	92

Red Robin® cont... (Sept'17)

Soups:	C	F	Cb
Chicken Tortilla: *Includes Tortilla Strips*			
1 Cup	210	10	18
1 Bowl	380	18	31
Clam Chowder: *Includes Croutons*			
1 Cup	240	15	18
1 Bowl	390	25	28
French Onion: *Includes Baguette, Au Jus & Croutons*			
1 Cup	180	12	14
1 Bowl	410	23	41
Salads: Without Dressing Unless Indicated			
Banzai, with Dressing	570	17	68
Crispy Chicken Tender	900	50	60
Mighty Caesar, with Caesar Dressing	680	50	24
Simply Grilled Chicken	310	8	25
Southwest Sombrero	790	48	46
Sides: Chili Chili Cheese Fries	840	54	60
Coleslaw	80	5	7
Mac & CHeese	320	22	21
Onion Rings	550	31	62
Steamed Broccoli	30	0	6
Steak Fries	370	17	49
Tavern Menu Burgers:			
Big Ghost	820	46	58
Big Pig Out	990	63	50
Four Cheese Melt	700	40	49
Red's Big Tavern	870	54	50
The Big Smoky Jack	860	49	59
Desserts:			
Gooey Chocolate Brownie Cake	795	28	132
Mountain High Mudd Pie	1390	59	194
Milkshakes, Banana; Choc., av.	545	21	78
Smoothie: Coconut Pineapple	505	14	93
Hawaiian Heart Throb	325	2	79

Roly Poly® (Sept'17)

Wraps:	C	F	Cb
Per 6" White Tortilla Unless Indicated			
Chicken: Basil Cashew Chicken	300	10	30
Catalina Chicken	315	11	28
Chicken Caesar	310	11	30
Chicken Fajita	315	9	28
Cobb Salad	255	12	27
Oriental Chicken	230	4	29
Santa Fe Chicken	305	11	28
Ham & Smoked Pork: Ital. Classic	335	12	32
Key West Cuban Mix	330	9	44
Peachtree/Pork Melt	310	11	27
Southside Club	365	17	30
Tuna: Classic Tuna Melt	340	17	26
Popeyes Tuna on Wheat	305	10	31
Texas/Thai Hot Tuna, average	300	11	30
Turkey: California	330	12	30
Tuscan	220	2	31

Round Table Pizza® (Sept'17)

Appetizers:	C	F	Cb
Boneless Wings:			
with BBQ Sauce, 8 pcs	565	14	73
with Buffalo Sauce, av., 8 pcs	440	14	41
Garlic Bread: 1 piece	70	3.5	9
with Cheese, 1 piece	100	6	9
Garlic Parmesan Twists, 1 twist	170	5	26
Pizzas: Per 1/12 of Large 14" Pizza			
Original Crust: Cheese	230	9	25
Chicken & Garlic Gourmet	250	11	25
Gourmet Veggie	240	10	27
Guinevere's Garden Delight	220	8	26
Hawaiian	220	8	27
Italian Garlic Supreme	270	14	25
King Arthur Supreme	270	13	26
Maui Zaui, with Polynesian Sce	260	10	29
Montague's All Meat Marvel	290	15	25
Smokehouse Combo	290	14	26
Triple Play Pepperoni	250	12	24
Pan Crust: Cheese	300	11	38
Chicken & Garlic Gourmet	340	13	39
Gourmet Veggie	320	12	41
Guinevere's Garden Delight	300	10	39
Hawaiian	300	10	40
Italian Garlic Supreme	360	16	39
King Arthur Supreme	340	14	39
Maui Zaui w/ Polynesian Sauce	340	12	43
Montague's All Meat Marvel	350	15	37
Smokehouse Combo, Chicken	370	16	40
Triple Play Pepperoni	330	14	36
Skinny Crust: Cheese	190	9	18
Chicken & Garlic Gourmet	220	11	18
Gourmet Veggie	200	10	20
Guinevere's Garden Delight	180	8	19
Hawaiian	190	8	20
Italian Garlic Supreme	240	14	18
King Arthur Supreme	240	13	19
Maui Zaui w/ Polynesian Sauce	220	10	22
Montague's All Meat Marvel	260	15	18
Smokehouse Combo, Chicken	250	14	20
Triple Play Pepperoni	220	12	17
Sandwiches: Chicken Club	800	43	59
Ham Club	740	40	60
RT Veggie	630	32	65
Turkey Club	720	38	59
Tukey Pesto	710	37	56
Turkey Sante-Fe	730	40	57

For Complete Nutritional Data ~ see CalorieKing.com

Fast - Foods & *Restaurants*

Rubio's Mexican Grill® (Sept '17)

Burritos: Each with Flour Tortilla, with Chips

Beef:	C	F	Cb
Baja Grilled, with Steak	890	34	99
Especial, with Steak	1120	39	149
Chicken:			
Baja Grilled, with Chicken	850	31	100
Especial, with Chicken	1080	36	150
Seafood: Beer Battered Fish	1170	69	109
Classic Grilled Shrimp	980	47	106
Grilled Wild Mahi Mahi	950	37	120
Shrimp & Bacon	1150	63	106
Veggies & More: Bean & Cheese	950	36	120
Especial with Veggies	1050	37	159

Enchiladas: With Black Beans & Mexican Rice

Two Cheese, w/ Fire-Rstd Sauce	850	37	82
Two Chicken, w/ Fire-Rstd Sauce	830	30	83
Two Shrimp, with Verde Sauce	830	33	91

Tacos: Each, with Corn Tortilla

Grilled Gourmet: Chicken/Steak	335	19	21
Fish Taco Especial (1)	390	25	29
Seafood, Blackened:			
Wild Alaskan Salmon	250	10	26
Wild Mahi Mahi	240	10	24
Seafood, Grilled:			
Wild Alaskan Salmon	230	10	23
Wild Mahi Mahi	230	9	22

Sides:

Black Beans: Reg., 4 oz	120	2	19
Large, 9.4 oz	280	3	46
Citrus Rice: Reg., 2.3 oz	100	2	21
Large, 6 oz	270	4	53
Mexican Rice: Regular, 2.3 oz	100	2	20
Large, 6 oz	270	4	53
Pinto Beans (Not Fried): Reg., 4 oz	120	1	19
Large, 10.9 oz	300	2	51
Tortilla Chips: Regular, 1.8 oz	210	3	43
Large, 4 oz	460	5	96
Salsas, average all types	10	0	2

Salad & Bowls: *Entrée Size, Includes Dressing*

Calif. Bowl, w/ Chkn/Salsa verde	660	23	81
Chipotle Orange Salad, w/ Shrimp	430	26	36
Chipotle Ranch Salad:			
with Blackened Ono	590	38	39
with Grilled Chicken	490	35	20
with Pan Seared Shrimp	450	36	19

Ruby Tuesday® (Sept '17)

Shareables: Per Whole Dish

	C	F	Cb
Crispy Buffalo Chicken Bites, honey	605	21	62
Crispy Thai Chicken Bites	555	21	48
Philly Cheesesteak Potstickers	255	8	30
Queso & Chips	1125	68	108
Shrimp Fondu, with Chips	1245	74	97
Spinach Artichoke Dip, with Chips	1050	62	97
Thai Spring Rolls	570	25	67

Burgers/Sandwiches: With Fries

Avocado Grilled Chicken S'wich	1095	48	104
Avocado Turkey Burger	1255	67	104
Grilled Chicken Sandwich	1000	41	100

Burger Baskets: With Fries

Bacon Cheeseburger	1225	63	100
Classic Cheeseburger	1130	56	100
Colossal Burger	1680	90	123
Ruby's Classic Bgr	1075	52	100
Smokehouse Burger	1385	68	125
Triple Prime Burger	1075	52	100
Triple Prime Cheeseburger	1130	56	100

Lunch/Dinner Entrees: Without Sides

Chicken: Chicken Bella	350	16	8
Chicken Fresco	360	21	3
Hickory Bourbon	250	5	18
Smoky Mountain	495	23	15
Pasta & More:			
California Primavera	960	62	74
with Grilled Chicken	1140	66	75
with Grilled Shrimp	1020	63	74
Chicken & Broccoli Penne	1395	89	87
Crispy Chicken Mac 'N Cheese	1575	84	119
Parmesan Shrimp Pasta	1080	52	87
Ribs & Chops:			
Hickory Boubon Glazed Pork Chop	930	42	60
Classic BBQ Ribs: Half Rack	470	22	21
Full Rack	940	46	42
Texas Dusted Ribs: Half Rack	590	33	24
Full Rack	1100	68	30
Seafood:			
Grilled Salmon	490	30	0
Blackened Tilapia	200	6	1
Hickory Bourbon Salmon	415	20	18
New Orleans Seafood	350	15	3
Steak: New York Strip, 10 oz	565	40	0
Petite Sirloin, 6 oz	305	17	1
Ribeye, 12 oz	750	56	0
Top Sirloin, 8 oz	420	22	2

Updated Nutrition Data ~ www.CalorieKing.com
Persons with Diabetes ~ See Disclaimer (Page 22)

Ruby Tuesday® cont... (Sept '17)

Sides:	C	F	Cb
Baked White Chedd. Bacon Mac 'N Chse	535	28	39
Caesar Salad, with Caesar Dressing	325	27	12
French Fries	510	25	64
Fresh Baked Potato	250	3	51
Garden Salad	230	15	11
Green Beans	65	4	5
Grilled Asparagus	70	2	7
Grilled Zucchini	15	0	2
Garlic Cheese Biscuit	100	6	12
Loaded Baked Potato	560	27	51
Mashed Potatoes	295	16	32
Onion Rings	350	19	37
Rice Pilaf	190	1	40
Steamed Broccoli	45	2	5
Sweet Potato Fries	445	23	55

Salads: *With Standard Components & Dressing*

	C	F	Cb
Chopped: BBQ Chicken Salad	1090	60	72
Crispy Chicken Cobb	1055	62	65
Kale Caesar:			
with Grilled Chicken	982	65	43
with Grilled Salmon	1015	71	43
Mediterranean Chicken	965	59	48
Traditional: BBQ Chicken	1270	77	77
Crispy chicken Cobb	1230	80	68
Kale Caesar, with Grilled Chicken	980	65	43

Dressings: *Per 1 Serving*

	C	F	Cb
Buttermilk Blue Cheese	180	19	1
Creamy Caesar	170	19	1
Honey Mustard	100	8	5
Italian Herb Vinaigrette	130	14	2
Lite Ranch	70	5	6
Soups: Broccoli & Cheese	290	20	19
Garden Vegetable	110	1	18
Roasted Tomato	340	18	33

Desserts:

	C	F	Cb
Apple Crumble Skillet	875	46	103
Cake: Blueberry Lemon	560	27	72
Caramel Crunch	760	37	99
Chocolate Fall	1375	59	180
Cookies & Cream	725	32	95
Key Lime	765	44	86
New York Cheesecake	975	61	90

For Complete Menu ~ see CalorieKing.com

Runza® (Sept '17)

Burgers:	C	F	Cb
¼ LB: BBQ Bacon & Swiss	530	32	26
Bacon Cheeseburger	510	31	26
Cheeseburger	420	22	28
French Onion	490	29	26
Hamburger	370	18	26
Spicy Jack	570	38	23
Swiss Mushroom	480	29	24

Chicken Sandwiches:

	C	F	Cb
BBQ Grilled	400	11	40
Buffalo/Deluxe, av.	360	11	37
Spicy Jack Grilled	530	27	35
Wraps: uffalo Mini Chicken	320	16	31
Ranch Mini Chicken	310	16	31
Chicken Strips, 2 pieces	220	12	14
Runza Sandwiches: Original	530	20	67
BBQ Bacon Runza	730	34	72
BLT Runza	745	40	68
Cheese Runza	580	24	69
Cheesesburger Runza	590	24	72
Spicy Jack Runza	750	41	69
Southwest Runza	650	28	75
Swiss Cheese Mushroom Runza	620	28	68

Sides:

	C	F	Cb
French Fries: Small	210	9	28
Medium	300	13	40
Large	440	19	59
French Onion Dip	70	5	3
Frings, Medium	320	17	39
Homemade Chili	290	11	26
Onion Rings: Medium	320	19	35
Large	550	31	58

Salads: *Without Dressing Unless Indicated*

	C	F	Cb
Asian Chicken, with Dressing	360	7	48
Southwest Chicken Salad, w/ Salsa	310	15	26
Side Salad	20	0	4
Sweet Berry Chicken	370	19	21
Dressings: Honey Mustard	200	18	9
Ranch	180	18	3

Soups: *Per Bowl*

	C	F	Cb
Boston Clam Chowder	280	15	29
Broccoli Cheese	240	16	20
Chicken Tortilla	150	6	16

Kids:

	C	F	Cb
Junior: Cheeseburger, plain	250	13	18
Hamburger, plain	200	9	16
Swiss Cheese Mushroom Burger	300	17	17

Desserts:

	C	F	Cb
Choc. Chip Cookie	370	18	53
Ice Cream Cones, all flavors	260	7	40
Shake, Cappuccino, regular	490	12	82
Sundaes: Caramel; Chocolate	300	7	51
Turtle	360	13	53

235

Fast - Foods & *Restaurants*

7-Eleven® (May '18)

Breakfast Sandwiches:	C	F	Cb
Biscuits:			
Sausage, 3.3 oz	330	22	28
Spicy Chicken, 4.5 oz	270	14	30
Croissants:			
Sausage, Egg & Cheese, 4.7 oz	450	32	23
English Muffin:			
Egg, Bacon & Chse, 4.5 oz	300	14	28
Egg, Cheese & Sausage, 5 oz	390	25	24
Salads: *Per Container*			
Balsamic Garden Salad, with Chicken, 6.5 oz	170	9	18
BLT, 8 oz	270	18	12
Caprese Salad, 4.5 oz	150	11	7
Chicken Caesar, 7.5 oz	390	28	17
Chicken Caesar Pasta Salad, 9 oz	540	24	61
Kale & Quinoa Salad, 6 oz	300	18	30
Mediterranean Pasta Salad, 8.5 oz	490	29	49
Side, 5 oz	30	0	7
Sandwiches/Melts:			
Chicken, Bacon Ranch Melt, 7.4 oz	560	22	56
Chicken Salad Sandwich, 6.6 oz	470	21	49
Double Cheeseburger, with American Cheese, 9.6 oz	800	54	35
Egg Salad Sandwich, 6.8 oz	480	24	50
Go!Smart Turkey Sandwich	300	2.5	48
Grilled Chicken Sandwich, with Honey Mustard BBQ Sauce, 6 oz	340	10	39
Italian Melt, 7.8 oz	610	39	38
Southwest Turkey Sandwich, 8 oz	560	28	48
Steak & Cheese Melt, 7.8 oz	680	35	57
Sides:			
Hash Browns (1), 2 oz	100	5	12
Potato Wedges (6), 0.7 oz	240	4.5	27
Taquitos:			
Chicken & Monterey Jack, (2), 5.3 oz	330	12	44
Drinks: Cappuccino, 8 fl.oz	180	4	36
Caramel Macchiato, 8 fl.oz	190	5	34
Cuban Coffee, with milk, 8 fl.oz	200	7	34
French Vanilla Cappuccino, 8 fl.oz	190	6	34
Skinny, 8 fl.oz	140	4.5	30
Hot Chocolate, 8 fl.oz	170	2.5	37
Peppermint Mocha, 8 fl.oz	180	4	36
Pumpkin Spice Late, 8 fl.oz	190	6	35
Slurpees, average all flavors:			
12 oz cup	95	0	26
22 oz cup	175	0	44
28 oz cup	220	0	56
Sugar Free, 12 oz cup	30	0	9

Saladworks® (Sept '17)

Salads: W/out Dressing or Bread	C	F	Cb
Bently	290	15	11
Buffalo Bleu	350	12	29
Chicken Caesar	370	15	29
Cobb	370	23	19
Farmhouse	270	12	28
Fire Roasted Cabo	350	17	25
Greek	200	11	17
Mandarin Chicken	185	4	25
Mediterranean	330	23	16
Nuevo Nicoise	360	13	40
Sophie's Salad	310	13	35
Thai Chicken	200	6	20
Tivoli	470	21	41
Turkey Club	290	7	38
Paninis: Buffalo Chicken	870	36	85
Caprese	940	47	94
Chicken Mozzarella	620	25	63
Turkey Melt	1020	49	90
Sandwiches: Avocado BLT	830	55	60
Loaded Chicken	370	9	28
Tuna Salad	410	8	57
West Coast Turkey	580	30	51
Wraps: Bentley	550	21	63
Buffalo Bleu	660	20	82
Chicken Caesar	610	20	81
Cobb	690	33	71
Farmhouse	590	20	82
Fire Roasted Cabo	670	25	78
Greek	500	19	69
Madarin Chicken	530	12	83
Mediterranean	650	34	92
Nicoise	490	18	63
Sophie's Salad	550	17	81
Thai Chicken	410	9	70
Tivoli	610	27	63
Turkey Club	460	14	61
Soups: Per Medium Serve, without Bread Roll			
Baked Potato	345	23	28
Chicken Dumpling	180	5.5	21
Chicken Noodle	180	5	18
Chicken Tortilla	260	14	19
Homestyle Tomato	300	21	25
Lasagna, with Turkey Sausage	235	11	21
Maine Lobster Bisque	470	39	21
New England Clam Chowder	370	26	22

Sandella's® (Sept '17)

Grilled Flatbread:

	C	F	Cb
Buffalo Chicken	420	10	47
Brazilian Bacon	560	17	79
Brazilian Chicken	510	10	73
El Paso	710	19	97
Hawaiian	610	17	89
Meatball	630	29	56
Pesto Chicken	610	28	56
Spinach & Bacon	660	39	52

Without Meat:

	C	F	Cb
Artichoke	570	23	65
Bianco	530	27	52
Brazillian	440	9	71
Healthy Veggie	360	7	54
Italian Veggie	400	10	59
Margherita	360	9	51
Pesto & Peppers	530	27	52

Paninis: With Standard Toppings

	C	F	Cb
Americana	580	25	54
Arizona Chicken	660	23	78
Basilico	530	20	50
BBQ Chicken	490	2.5	92
Beef Fajita	640	28	59
Bistro Ham & Brie	560	19	70
Brazilian Beef, without cheese	500	6	86
Buffalo	600	25	48
Napoli Chicken	440	17	50
Holiday Ham	770	21	110
Pastrami Melt	500	15	52
Philly Cheese	590	25	55
Spinach, Ham & Swiss	550	20	61
Tuscan Chicken	540	21	55

Quesadillas: With Standard Toppings

	C	F	Cb
California	500	23	53
Mediterranean	400	16	53

Salads: Includes ½ Flatbread

	C	F	Cb
Fiesta, with Light Bals. Vinaigrette	360	8	54
Greek, with Light Bals. Vinaigrette	310	15	37

Rice Bowls: Includes Flatbread & Standard Toppings

	C	F	Cb
Black Bean & Rice	840	20	130
Chicken Fajita	750	20	104

Wraps: With Standard Toppings

	C	F	Cb
California Turkey	410	10	55
Chipotle Chicken	350	7	55
Pesto Turkey	460	15	54
Sweet & Spicy Chicken	400	7	64

Sarku Japan® (Sept '17)

Bento Box:

	C	F	Cb
Fried Rice: Beef	830	32	98
Chicken	1020	49	98
Shrimp	750	27	96

D'Lite Meals:

Vegetarian:

	C	F	Cb
Fried Rice	430	10	79
Noodles	640	14	109
Steamed Rice	410	6	83

Combos: With Steamed Rice

	C	F	Cb
Teriyaki: Beef	580	16	80
Beef & Shrimp	690	21	85
Chicken	640	24	79
Chicken & Shrimp	750	29	85
Shrimp	530	12	80

Sushi Hand Rolls:

	C	F	Cb
Salmon Skin (1)	210	7	27
Seafood (1)	170	1.5	29
Spicy Tuna (1)	180	3.5	27
Sauce, Teriyaki, 1.5 oz	45	0	9
Sides: Chicken Egg Roll	160	6	21
Dumplings (6)	260	12	29
Edamame	170	7	11
Miso Soup	50	2	6
Seaweed Salad	70	2	13
Shrimp Tempura (3)	390	30	23
Vegetarian Spring Roll	190	9	15

Schlotzsky's® (Sept '17)

Sandwiches: Per Medium Size

Angus: *With Standard Bun & Toppings*

	C	F	Cb
Corned Beef Reuben	890	38	81
Pastrami & Swiss	830	33	79
Pastrami Reuben	900	40	84
Chipotle Chicken	530	9	78
Deluxe Original	980	47	81
Fiesta Chicken	810	31	78
Fresh Veggie	500	14	74
Ham & Cheese, Original	730	25	81
Roast Beef & Cheese	780	30	81
Smoked Turkey Breast	500	6	80
The Original	780	34	78
The Sicilian	730	44	42
The Tuscan	700	42	48
Turkey Bacon Club	770	30	81
Turkey Original	820	33	81
Turkey & Guacamole	520	11	78
Turkey Bacon Club	770	30	81

Large Size Sandwiches ~ Double above Medium figures

continued next page...

Schlotzsky's® cont... (Sept '17)

10" Pizzas: Per Pizza	C	F	Cb
BBQ Chicken & Jalapeno	920	21	148
Combination Special	960	38	119
Double Cheese	840	27	115
Fresh Veggie	920	35	118
Grilled Chicken & Pesto	910	29	114
Pepperoni & Double Cheese	980	42	115
Oven Baked Pasta:			
Bayou Chicken	800	41	66
Chicken Pesto Carbonara	930	45	79
Tomato-Basil Canestrelli	550	19	70
Salads: Without Dressing or Breadsticks			
Chicken Caesar	680	17	29
Cranberry, Apple, Pecan & Chicken	640	27	68
Southwest Chicken	600	29	44
Turkey Avocado Cobb	610	33	42
Dressings: Per 3 oz			
Butttermilk Ranch	320	33	4
Chunky Blue Cheese	460	49	3
Red Wine Vinaigrette	280	28	3
Robusto Italian	430	43	9
Tuscan Caesar	430	45	2
Soup: Per Bowl			
Broccoli Cheddar	185	12	14
Chicken & Wild Rice	280	14	25
Chicken Tortilla	315	16	27
Loaded Baked Potato	385	31	29
Timberline Chili	380	21	27
Tomato Basil	320	26	21
Chips:			
Baked: Regular; BBQ	130	3	25
Other varieties, average	230	14	24
Kidz Meals: Without Cookie or Drink			
Cheese Pizza	540	17	78
Ham Sandwich	220	2	40
Pepperoni Pizza	590	22	78
Turkey Sandwich	220	2	40
Desserts:			
Brownie (1)	370	19	49
Cookies: Chocolate Chip (1)	160	7	24
Oatmeal Raisin; Sugar, (1), av.	155	5	24

Second Cup® ~ *see CalorieKing.com*

Shakey's® (Sept '17)

Pizzas: Per Slice, ½ Large Pizza	C	F	Cb
Cheese:			
Pan Crust	185	6	26
Thin Crust	150	5.5	18
Firehouse: Pan Crust	255	12	27
Thin Crust	220	12	19
Garden Veggie: Pan Crust	185	5.5	27
Thin Crust	150	5.5	19
Margherita:			
Pan Crust	175	5	26
Thin Crust	135	4.5	18
Rustic Garlic Chicken: Pan Crust	190	5.5	26
Thin Crust	155	5.5	18
Shakey's Special: Pan Crust	210	6.5	31
Thin Crust	195	10	18
Texas BBQ Chicken: Pan Crust	205	5	29
Thin Crust	170	5	21
Ultimate Meat: Pan Crust	280	14	26
Thin Crust	245	13	18
Additional Toppings: Beef	35	3	0
Cheese	15	1	1
Chicken	15	0.5	0
Pepperoni	25	2.5	0
Sausage	45	4	1
Shareables: Per Serving, Unless Indicated			
Chicken Strips (5)	620	31	48
Mojo Potatoes (5)	215	11	25
Mojo Supreme, serves 4-6	1950	120	160
Shakey's Spicy Wings (6)	495	29	27
Shakey's Famous Chicken: Per Piece			
Fried Chicken: Breast	475	26	16
Leg	170	9	6
Thigh	350	24	10
Wing	130	9	4

Shari's® (Sept '17)

Breakfast: As Served	C	F	Cb
Bacon & Eggs without extras	290	22	2
BMP Frittata	920	70	22
Bone-In Hickory Ham & Potato P'cakes	890	38	76
Breakfast Cannoli	740	34	92
Country Omelette without extras	680	52	8
Denver Omelette without extras	660	51	10
Eggs Benedict with Hashbrowns	810	46	61
French Toast	790	51	69
Fresh Caramel Pecan Cinn. Roll	1190	41	182
Meat Lover's Frittata	1120	84	35
Panini	970	61	70
Quiche Lorraine	690	39	62
Sausage & Eggs without extras	630	57	2

Shari's® cont... (Sept '17)

Breakfast (Cont):

	C	F	Cb
Shari's Potato Pancakes	570	17	96
The Shari's Sampler	1080	76	55
Ultimate Country Fried Steak	1200	85	66
USDA Top Sirloin Steak	790	51	30
Waffle without extras	260	4	49
Extras: Apple Topping	230	4.5	45
Biscuits & Gravy (1)	320	18	34
Butter & Syrup	680	10	146
Hashbrowns & White Bread	510	27	59
Pancake (1)	280	7	49
Strawberry Topping	220	4.5	42

Lunch: Without Side Choices

	C	F	Cb
Burgers: Bavarian	970	43	60
Bleu Cheeseburger	650	33	46
Cheddar Cheesebuger	680	35	46
Hamburger	600	29	46
Pepperjack Cheese	700	38	46
Ranch Hand BBQ Bacon Chsebgr	1110	72	65
Swiss Cheeseburger	640	32	46
Flatbread Paninis, Pastrami	700	28	58
Quiche: BMP Trio	390	27	23
Ham & Cheese Trio	380	25	22
Salads: Entrée Size, with Dressing			
Northwest Steak/ Raspb Vinaig.	710	31	67
Rustic Tuscan Chkn/Ital. Dressing	510	32	21
Spinach Cobb/ Bleu Chse Vinaig.	760	44	46
Sandwiches: Per Whole Sandwich			
Crispy Chicken BLT	910	56	65
Cuban, on Ciabatta	540	23	47
Prime Rib Dip	540	21	52

Dinner: With Menu Set Sides & Bread

	C	F	Cb
Beer Battered Fish & Chips	1740	134	118
Cedar Plank Salmon	750	44	48
Chicken Mushroom Alfredo	1080	54	94
Country Fried Steak Dinner	1310	80	112
Gr. Chkn Mozzarella Bruschetta	610	28	48
Prime Rib Stroganoff	1280	79	95
Slow Cooked Pot Roast	1440	78	91

Sides, Lunch Dinner:

	C	F	Cb
Baked Potato, Plain	160	0	37
French Fries	390	25	40
Garlic Parmesan Tater Tots	570	42	35
Golden Fried Shrimp	420	17	43
Key West Vegetables	130	9	9
Loaded Mashed Potatoes	410	21	42
Onion Rings (6)	390	24	39
Red Skin Mshd Potato	260	8	40
Rice Pilaf	90	4.5	10
Sauteed Mushrooms	150	14	4

Shari's® cont... (Sept '17)

Sides, Lunch/Dinner (Cont):

	C	F	Cb
Shrimp Scampi	360	30	2
Shrimp Skewers (2)	190	11	1
Steakhouse Mac 'n Cheese	510	27	45
Tater Tots, Plain	370	26	33
Desserts:			
Cheesecake, 1 slice	350	22	34
Chocolate Lava Cake 1 slice	710	30	104
Classic Pies: Per Slice, as Served			
Banana Cream Dream	460	24	53
Chocolate Cream Supreme	540	30	62
Gourmet Pies: Per Slice, as Served			
Caramel Pecan Crunch	770	49	76
Peanut Butter Chocolate Silk	660	45	60
S'mores Galore	560	31	68
Velvet Chocolate Silk	580	38	56

Sheetz® (Sept '17)

Breakfast Sandwiches:

	C	F	Cb
Dreamy Bacon Croissant	400	22	33
Twisted BLT	740	42	62
Walker Breakfast Ranger	550	23	58
Burgerz: Big Mozz Burger	600	27	48
Boss Bacon Burger	710	50	26
Cowboy Burger	650	33	46
El Gringo Burger	640	33	55
Twisted Swiss Burger	760	41	59
Hot Dogs: BLT	450	28	33
Firehouse	390	22	35
Junkyard	340	16	38
Philly	340	17	35
Shmokehouse	370	18	37
Mac & Cheese Platter:			
Boom Chicka	910	34	113
Meatball	1010	43	109
Morning	870	34	108
Szechuan Fire	770	21	110
Sandwichez:			
Deli: Boom Boom BLT	820	46	52
Ciabatta Bing	620	34	53
Garden of Eatin	440	16	54
Grilled Chicken: Big Mozz	560	18	51
Carolina Slaw	440	16	37
Twisted Brunch	810	41	59
Subz: Per 6" Standard Menu Sub/Flatbread			
Big Philly Sub	640	25	66
Cali Turkey Flatbread	720	43	44
Protein Parm Sub	460	15	47
Southwest Veggie Sub	440	18	56
Spring Chicken Sub	450	19	39

continued next page...

Fast - Foods & *Restaurants*

Sheetz® cont... (Sept '17)

Sidez:

	C	F	Cb
Coleslaw	80	3.5	12
Crispy Chicken Stripz: 3 pieces	330	11	39
5 pieces	550	18	65
Fryz, no sauce, 1 cup	390	13	64
Hard Cooked Egg (1)	70	4.5	0
Jalapeno Poppers, w/o Sce	330	18	35
Loaded Fryz, plain	600	20	97
Mac & Cheese, plain, 1 order	590	13	98
Onion Rings, no sauce, 1 cup	470	27	52
Popcorn Chicken, without Sauce:			
Regular	300	14	28
Large	610	28	55

Sizzler® (Sept '17)

Burgers & Sandwiches:

	C	F	Cb
⅓ lb Burgers: Bacon Cheeseburger	950	67	44
Classic: Burger	830	57	44
Cheese Burger	920	64	45
Double Mega Bacon	1250	91	44
Malibu Melt	1840	155	69
Turkey Patty	510	30	39
Sandwiches: Double Hibachi Chkn	440	4	14
Grilled Chicken Club	580	19	39
Malibu Chicken	870	63	52

Hot Entrées: Small, without Sides, Condiments, Dipping Sauce or Optional Accompaniments

Chicken: Grilled Hibachi Chicken	220	2	7
Italian-Herb Chicken, 7 oz	230	6	1
Malibu Chicken, Single	680	60	14
Pasta: Fettuccine Alfredo	960	51	85
Cajun Penne	1030	71	108
Ribs:			
BBQ: 6 bones	1870	145	32
9 Bones	2820	213	61
Seafood: Fish & Chips, 2 pieces	1410	102	93
Grilled Salmon, 6 oz	370	23	3
Ultimate Shrimp Trio	1230	62	85
Steaks:			
Burgundy Mushroom Sirloin Tips	480	16	38
Combos: Steak & Hibachi Chicken	500	14	20
Steak & Lobster Tail	720	51	2
Steak & Malibu Chicken	920	62	30
Porterhouse, 20 oz	1430	108	2
Tri Tip: Slow Roast BBQ, 5 oz	680	39	52
6 oz	790	44	54
Tri Tip Sirloin: 8 oz	340	16	0.5
10 oz	440	20	3
12 oz	530	24	3

Sizzler® cont... (Sept '17)

Sides:

	C	F	Cb
Baked Potato: Foil	350	13	54
Loaded Foil	530	32	54
Salted	510	30	55
Loaded	760	57	55
Baked Yam with Maple Topping	410	11	75
Balsamic Brussels Sprouts	150	7	20
Broccoli, steamed	40	0	7
with Butter	70	4.5	7
Button Mushroom Saute	180	17	5
Cilantro Lime Rice	150	7	20
Garlic Mashed Potatoes	150	2.5	9
Green Beans	80	5	8
Grilled Onions	80	6	7
Roasted Corn with Herb Butter	80	2.5	13
Roasted Red Potatoes	130	0	8
Spinach Saute	70	1.5	5
Street Fries, 5 oz	350	22	37
Sweet Potato Fries	610	48	39
Vegetable Medley	80	45	8
Zucchini Planks	20	0	3

For Complete Menu & Data ~ see CalorieKing.com

Skyline Chili® (Sept '17)

Burritos:

	C	F	Cb
Chili Deluxe	610	33	38
Original	610	31	54
Coneys/Sandwiches:			
Coneys: Cheese, w/ onions & mstrd	350	23	25
Coney, plain	220	13	22
Sandwiches: Chili Cheese,			
with onions & mustard	290	17	24
Plain; With onions & mustard, av.	175	8	22
Ways: Per Regular Serving			
Chili Spaghetti with Cheese:			
3 Way; 4 Way Onion, average	810	44	52
4 Way Bean	890	44	66
5 Way	900	44	70
Bowls: Chili	200	12	0
Loaded Chili	480	28	20
Vegetarian Black Beans & Rice	400	14	48
Steamed Potatoes: 3-Way Potato	620	26	65
Cheddar Potato	630	33	65
Sour Cream Potato	460	19	65
Salads: Without Dressing			
Buffalo Chicken	220	11	12
Greek	210	12	17
Wraps:			
BLT: Small	530	34	36
Large	850	55	58
South Western Chicken	680	29	70
Fries: Chili Cheese	840	53	61
Regular	430	24	51

Updated Nutrition Data ~ www.CalorieKing.com
Persons with Diabetes ~ See Disclaimer (Page 22)

Smoothie King® (Sept'17)

Fruit Smoothies: Per 20 oz Cup

Figures Include Turbinado. Without Turbinado, deduct 100 calories and 23 carbs.

	C	F	Cb
Fitness Blends:			
Orig. High Protein: Banana	350	9	37
Chocolate	420	9	49
Pineapple	320	9	30
Peanut Power Plus:			
Chocolate	700	26	98
Strawberry	680	21	112
The Activator:			
Blueberry Strawberry	300	1.5	49
Chocolate	220	3	24
Strawberry Banana	270	1.5	42
The Hulk: Chocolate	800	32	105
Strawberry	965	32	145
Vanilla	800	32	105
Slim Blends:			
Slim-N-Trim: Chocolate	250	3	41
Strawberry	240	2	52
Vanilla	210	2.5	40
Take A Break Blends:			
Banana Boat	475	4	101
Caribbean Way	395	0	97
Muscle Punch	360	1	84
Pineapple Surf	460	1	104
Yogurt D-Lite	275	4	46
Wellness Blends: Acai Adventure	435	5	92
Mangosteen Madness	380	0	94

32 fl.oz Cup: Multiply 20 fl.oz figures by 1.5
40 fl.oz Cup: Multiply 20 fl.oz figures by 2

Kids Cup Smoothies: *Per 12 fl.oz Cup*

	C	F	Cb
Apple Kiwi Bunga	155	0	37
Choc-A-Laka	210	4	32
Lil' Angel	210	0	52
Strawberry Bluegurt Blitz	160	0	35

Snappy Tomato® (Sept'17)

Pizza: Per Slice, ⅛ of Large Pizza

	C	F	Cb
Buffalo Grilled Chicken	250	5	32
Cheese	220	7	30
Hawaiian	370	18	33
Pepperoni	340	17	31
Ranch	370	21	31
Snapperoni	390	22	31
Supreme	340	17	32
Ultimate	460	26	33
Veggie	240	8	33
Wings, Plain, no sauce (3), 2.6 oz	160	11	0

Sonic Drive-In® (Sept'17)

	C	F	Cb
Burgers:			
Bacon Cheeseburger	870	54	54
Bacon Double Cheeseburger	1280	87	54
Cheeseburger: w/ Mayo	780	46	54
with Ketchup	750	41	57
Double Cheeseburger with Mayo	1280	87	54
Jr. Burger	320	16	32
Jr. Dble Cheeseburger	560	34	33
Jr. Deluxe Cheeseburger	410	24	33
Toaster, Bacon Cheeseburger	910	52	67
Chicken:			
Sandwiches: Chicken Strip	460	21	49
Classic Crispy Chicken	530	26	54
Classic Grilled Chicken	460	17	44
Ultimate Chicken	780	39	67
Strips, Super Crunch (5)	580	28	44
Breakfast:			
Breakfast Bacon Toaster	620	32	52
Breakfast Burrito: Bacon	490	27	36
Ham	460	22	37
Sausage	500	29	36
CroiSonic Sandwich: with Bacon	580	38	32
with Sausage	640	46	32
Cinnasnacks, (3) with Frosting	640	32	81
French Toast Sticks, (4) w/out Syrup	590	31	71
Coneys & 6" Hot Dogs:			
All American Dog	410	20	45
Chicago Dog	420	19	49
Chili Cheese Coney	490	30	36
New York Dog	400	23	36
Original Pretzel Dog	390	18	41
Wraps: Crispy Chicken	530	22	57
Grilled Chicken	440	15	41
Natural Cut Fries: Small	250	12	33
Medium	290	13	38
Large	470	22	63
Sides: Per Medium Serving			
Ched 'R' Peppers	280	48	56
Chili Cheese Fries	450	26	43
Handmade Onion Rings	590	29	74
Mozzarella Sticks	540	27	52
Tater Tots	360	19	43

continued next page…

Sonic Drive-In® cont... (Sept '17)

Custard Concretes: Per Medium

	C	F	Cb
Banana, w/ Reeses P'nut Butter Cup	1420	62	99
Caramel, with Snickers Bars	1320	55	184
Dark Choc., w/ Oreo Cookie Pieces	1250	55	173
Vanilla, with Heath Toffee Pieces	1240	63	154
Ice Cream Cone, Vanilla	250	12	30

Ice Cream Sundaes:

	C	F	Cb
Caramel; Hot Fudge, av.	515	25	67
Pineapple	460	21	61
Strawberry	440	21	55
Waffle Cone, Vanilla	380	14	55

Waffle Cone Sundaes:

	C	F	Cb
Caramel & Snickers Bars	510	19	75
Other Flavors, average	525	21	78

Ice Cream Slushes, average:

	C	F	Cb
Small	560	21	90
Medium	760	28	125

Shakes: Per Medium

	C	F	Cb
Banana (fresh)	870	41	115
Caramel	870	42	113
Chocolate	850	40	113
Hot Fudge	950	48	117
Peanut Butter	1060	72	92
Strawberry	750	39	90

Sonic Blast: Per Medium

	C	F	Cb
Butterfingers	1030	53	126
Reese's Peanut Butter Cup	1060	60	116
Snickers	960	52	108

Sonic Master Blast: Per Medium

	C	F	Cb
Banana Split	1300	60	188
Caramel Brownie	1160	56	149
Malted Brownie Bliss	1070	49	143
Triple Chocolate	1210	59	161
Turtle Pecan	1260	72	144
Waffleberry Brownie	1010	49	130
Limeade: Small	110	0	28
Medium	180	0	47

Iced Coffee: Per Medium

	C	F	Cb
Chocolate	260	6	49
French Vanilla	150	6	24
Praline Pecan	150	6	233

For Complete Nutritional Data ~ see CalorieKing.com

Souplantation® (Sept '17)

Soups: Per 8 fl.oz Cup

	C	F	Cb
Big Chunk Chicken Noodle	105	2.5	11
Deep Kettle Chili	215	6.5	21
Shrimp Bisque	240	13	16
Yankee Clipper Clam Chowder	265	19	19

Souplantation® cont... (Sept '17)

Prepared Salads: Per ½ Cup

	C	F	Cb
Joan's Broccoli Madness	160	12	10
Quinoa & Feta	130	5	19
Red, White & Blue Potato, w/ Bacon	120	7	10
Texas Slaw	70	4.5	5
Tuna Tarragon	220	12	21

Hot Pasta: Per 1 Cup

	C	F	Cb
Beef & Sausage Bol., w/ Rigatoni	340	11	47
Macaroni & Cheese	330	14	40
Tomato & Spinach, with Penne	200	6	29

Bakery:

	C	F	Cb
Bread: Multigrain, East Coast, vegan	80	2	12
Sourdough: Californian, vegetarian	70	0	13
West Coast, vegan	110	0	22
Squaw Bread: Californian, vegan	110	0	23
West Coast, vegetarian	230	2.5	46
Focaccia: Cheesy Garlic,	60	2	9
Quattro Formaggio	70	2	9
Muffins: Brownie Bite (1)	170	11	18
Lemon (1), gluten free	210	8	29
Peach Poppyseed (1)	170	7	23

Desserts: Per ½ Cup

	C	F	Cb
Creamy Almond Rice Pudding	140	2.5	25
Dessert Ice Cream Bars,			
Chocolate/Vanilla, average	100	2.5	20
Lava Cake: Carrot & Cream Cheese	340	14	49
Chocolate	320	8	60
Vanilla Soft Serve: Cappuccino	140	4.5	28
Chocolate/Vanilla, av.	100	2	20
Creamy Lemon	160	4	34

For Complete Nutritional Data ~ see CalorieKing.com

Southern Tsunami® (Sept '17)

Rolls: With White Rice

Hybrid:

	C	F	Cb
Berry: Eel, 6 oz	240	6	43
Immitation Crab	230	5	44
Blueberry: Salmon, 8 oz	360	16	45
Smoked Steelhead, 8 oz	340	13	45
Tuna, 8 oz	340	15	45
Crunchy Dragon Roll: Salmon, 8 oz	560	31	59
Steelhead, 8 oz	530	28	59
Done Deal, Tuna, 7 oz	330	12	41
Happy Mango, 8 oz	410	19	51
Jalapeno, Tuna, 8 oz	290	10	48
Mango Shrimp, 6 oz	360	19	42
Red Rock, 7 oz	360	14	44
Spicy Mango, Tuna, 8 oz	380	20	45
Ultimate Chili, Salmon, 6 oz	290	11	39

Updated Nutrition Data ~ www.CalorieKing.com
Persons with Diabetes ~ See Disclaimer (Page 22)

Southern Tsunami® cont... (Sept '17)

Rolls (Cont): With White Rice

	C	F	Cb
Chef Samplers:			
A, 5.5 oz	240	7	37
Premium, 5.5 oz	260	9	35
Plus Rolls: *Per 12 oz*			
California	450	8	88
Cream Cheese Plus: Eel	620	25	82
Salmon/Smoked	590	23	76
Seaside Plus: Eel	670	21	103
Salmon	620	18	91
Spicy Plus: Salmon	640	28	78
Yellowtail	670	29	78
Vegetable Plus Combo	430	8	89
Wraps: Berry, 4.6 oz	200	9	28
California, 6.6 oz	270	15	26
Cream Cheese & Tuna, 6.6 oz	230	14	39
Mango, 6.6 oz	130	4.5	22
Spicy Crm Chse & Salmon, 6.6 oz	320	23	15
Salads: Without Dressing			
Edamame, 8 oz	300	6	30
Hawaiian Poke, w/ Steelhead, 14 oz	790	38	94
Sea Breeze, 4 oz	90	2.5	17
Tropical Mango, 7.5 oz	290	25	14
Dressings/Sauces:			
Ginger Dressing, 2 Tbsp	50	1.5	8
Peanut Sauce, 1.4 oz	60	0	12
Sweet Chili Sauce, 1.4 oz	100	0	24
Wasabe Dressing, 2 Tbsp	35	2	2

Starbucks® (Jan '18)

Brewed Coffee: Per16 fl.oz Grande without Whipped Cream

Caffe Misto (Au Lait):	C	F	Cb
with Coconut Milk	70	4.5	7
with Nonfat Milk	70	0	10
with Soy Milk	100	3	13
with Whole Milk	130	7	10
Chocolate: *Per 16 fl.oz Grande without Whipped Cream*			
Hot Chocolate:			
with 2% Milk	320	9	47
with Coconut Milk	270	10	42
with Soy Milk	320	8	51
with Whole Milk	360	13	47
Peppermint Hot Chocolate:			
with 2% Milk	390	9	65
with Nonfat Milk	340	2.5	65
with Soy Milk	390	7	69
with Whole Milk	420	13	65

Starbucks® cont... (Jan '18)

Hot Espresso Beverages:
Per 16 fl.oz Grande without Whipped Cream

	C	F	Cb
Caffe Latte: with Coconut Milk	140	8	15
with Nonfat Milk	130	0	20
with Soy Milk	190	6	24
with Whole Milk	230	12	19
Cappuccino: with Coconut Milk	140	8	14
with Nonfat Milk	80	0	12
with Soy Milk	120	3.5	16
with Whole Milk	140	7	12
Caramel Macchiato: Coconut Milk	200	8	32
with Nonfat Milk	200	1.5	36
with Soy Milk	250	6	39
with Whole Milk	280	11	35
Cinn. Dolce Latte: Coconut Milk	220	7	37
with Nonfat Milk	220	0	42
with Whole Milk	310	11	41
Espresso: 1 Doppio, 2 fl.oz	10	0	2
1 Solo, 1 fl.oz	5	0	1
Espresso Con Panna, 1 Solo, 1 fl.oz	30	2.5	2
Latte Macchiato: with 2% Milk	190	7	19
with Soy Milk	180	5	23
with Whole Milk	220	11	19
Iced Espresso: Per 16 fl.oz Grande w/out Whipped Cream			
Caffe Latte: with Coconut Milk	90	5	10
with Nonfat Milk	90	0	13
with Soy Milk	130	3.5	17
with Whole Milk	150	7	13
Vanilla Latte: with 2% Milk	190	4	30
with Coconut Milk	160	4.5	28
with Nonfat Milk	160	0	31
with Whole Milk	210	6	30
Coconutmilk Mocha Macchiato	210	9	30
Fizzios, Ginger Ale; Lemon Ale,			
Orange Cream,16 fl oz Grande, av.	100	0	26
Frappuccino Blended: Cold, Per 16 fl.oz Grande with			
Whole Milk without Whipped Cream			
Caffe Vanilla	310	3	68
Caramel	280	3.5	60
Coffee	240	3	50
Java Chip	350	7	68
Mocha	300	4	51
White Chocolate Mocha	300	5	61

continued next page... ...

243

Starbucks® cont... (Jan '18)

Frappuccino Blended Creme: | C | F | Cb

Per 16 fl.oz Grande with Whole Milk and Whipped Cream

	C	F	Cb
Double Chocolaty Chip	420	20	57
Green Tea, sweetened	430	16	68
Java Chip	470	18	72
Vanilla Bean Creme	400	16	60
Refreshers: Cool Lime, 16 oz	60	0	15
Valencia Orange, 16 oz	90	0	23
Very Berry Hibiscus, 16 oz	70	0	18

Smoothies: *Per 16 fl.oz Grande with 2% Milk, without Whipped Cream*

	C	F	Cb
Chocolate	320	5	53
Strawberry	300	2	60

Teas: *Per 16 fl.oz Grande, with Whole Milk*

Hot Tea Latte:

	C	F	Cb
Classic Chai Tea	270	7	45
Green Tea, sweetened	280	11	34

Iced Tea Latte:

	C	F	Cb
Chai	270	7	44
Green Tea, sweetened	250	10	31

Drink Extras:

	C	F	Cb
Caramel Drizzle, 1 teaspoon	15	0.5	2
Flavored Syrup: 1 Pump	20	0	5
Sugar-Free, 1 Pump	0	0	0
Mocha Syrup, 1 Pump	25	0.5	6

Sweetened Whipped Cream:

	C	F	Cb
Grande/Venti, cold drinks, av.	110	11	3
Grande/Venti, hot drinks	75	7	3

Breakfast, Hot:

	C	F	Cb
Bacon, Gouda & Egg B'fast S'wich	370	19	32
Sausage, Cheddar & Egg Sandwich	500	28	41

Bistro Protein Boxes: *As Prepared*

	C	F	Cb
BBQ Chicken	420	16	49
Cheese & Fruit	450	27	34
PB & J	520	26	53
Smoked Turkey	360	12	42

Paninis:

	C	F	Cb
Roasted Tomato & Mozzarella	350	13	42
Turkey Pesto	540	21	55

Sandwiches:

	C	F	Cb
Chicken Artichoke Flatbread	510	27	37
Chicken BLT Salad	470	25	35
Egg Salad	480	27	42
Turkey & Havarti	460	21	31

Starbucks® cont... (Jan '18)

Bakery: *Each*

	C	F	Cb
Almond Croissant, 3.5 oz	410	22	45
Apple Fritter, 4.2 oz	460	23	56
Banana Nut Bread, 4.4 oz	420	22	52
Blueberry Muffin, w/ Yogurt & Honey, 4 oz	380	16	53
Blueberry Scone, 3.5 oz	420	17	61
Butter Croissant, 2.2 oz	240	12	28
Cheese Danish, 2.8 oz	320	16	36
Chewy Chocolate Cookie, 1.6 oz	170	5	30
Chocolate Chip Cookie, 2.47 oz	310	15	42
Cinnamon Morning Bun, 3.9 oz	390	15	56
Classic Coffee Cake, 3.5 oz	390	16	57
Dble Choc. Chunk Brownie	490	28	55
Iced Lemon Pound Cake, 4.4 oz	470	20	68
Old-Fashioned Glazed D'nut, 4 oz	480	27	56
Greek Parfait, w/ Berries & Granola	220	3	36

Bottled Drinks ~ See Page 37

Steak Escape® (Sept '17)

Sandwiches: *With Set Menu Board Components*

Regular:

	C	F	Cb
Buffalo Chicken	820	33	97
Cajun Chicken	660	23	68
French Onion	830	33	75
Grand Escape	660	19	68
Turkey Club	550	14	65
Wild West BBQ	700	20	75

Wraps: *With Set Menu Board Components*

	C	F	Cb
Cajun Chicken	470	17	50
Grand: Chicken	490	18	51
Escape	520	18	50
Turkey Club	440	15	49
Wild West BBQ	550	19	56

Salads:

	C	F	Cb
Grilled: Chicken	410	25	14
Steak	440	24	15
Turkey	360	21	15
Without Meat	280	20	13
Loaded Potatoes: Bacon & Ranch	670	46	51
Cheddar & Bacon	430	17	56

For Complete Nutritional Data ~ see CalorieKing.com

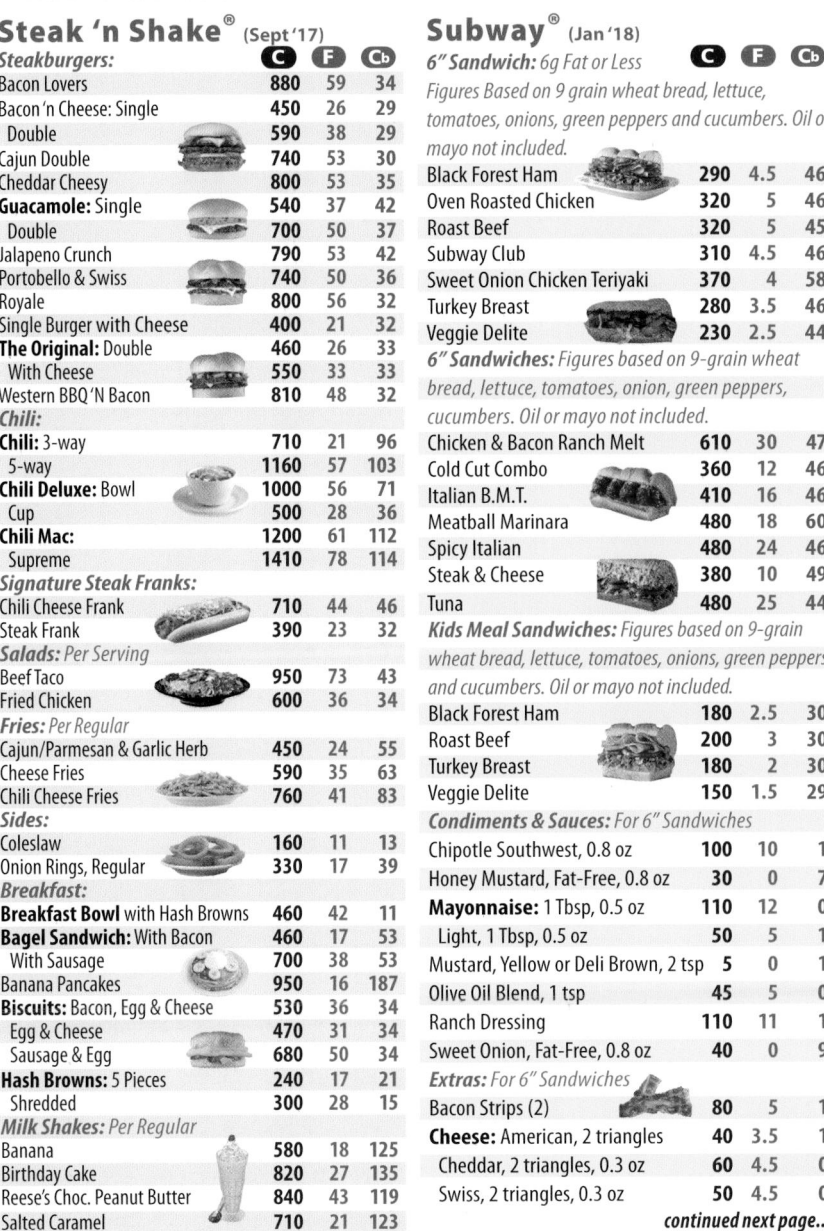

Steak 'n Shake® (Sept '17)

Steakburgers:	C	F	Cb
Bacon Lovers	880	59	34
Bacon 'n Cheese: Single	450	26	29
Double	590	38	29
Cajun Double	740	53	30
Cheddar Cheesy	800	53	35
Guacamole: Single	540	37	42
Double	700	50	37
Jalapeno Crunch	790	53	42
Portobello & Swiss	740	50	36
Royale	800	56	32
Single Burger with Cheese	400	21	32
The Original: Double	460	26	33
With Cheese	550	33	33
Western BBQ 'N Bacon	810	48	32
Chili:			
Chili: 3-way	710	21	96
5-way	1160	57	103
Chili Deluxe: Bowl	1000	56	71
Cup	500	28	36
Chili Mac:	1200	61	112
Supreme	1410	78	114
Signature Steak Franks:			
Chili Cheese Frank	710	44	46
Steak Frank	390	23	32
Salads: Per Serving			
Beef Taco	950	73	43
Fried Chicken	600	36	34
Fries: Per Regular			
Cajun/Parmesan & Garlic Herb	450	24	55
Cheese Fries	590	35	63
Chili Cheese Fries	760	41	83
Sides:			
Coleslaw	160	11	13
Onion Rings, Regular	330	17	39
Breakfast:			
Breakfast Bowl with Hash Browns	460	42	11
Bagel Sandwich: With Bacon	460	17	53
With Sausage	700	38	53
Banana Pancakes	950	16	187
Biscuits: Bacon, Egg & Cheese	530	36	34
Egg & Cheese	470	31	34
Sausage & Egg	680	50	34
Hash Browns: 5 Pieces	240	17	21
Shredded	300	28	15
Milk Shakes: Per Regular			
Banana	580	18	125
Birthday Cake	820	27	135
Reese's Choc. Peanut Butter	840	43	119
Salted Caramel	710	21	123

Subway® (Jan '18)

6" Sandwich: 6g Fat or Less

Figures Based on 9 grain wheat bread, lettuce, tomatoes, onions, green peppers and cucumbers. Oil or mayo not included.

	C	F	Cb
Black Forest Ham	290	4.5	46
Oven Roasted Chicken	320	5	46
Roast Beef	320	5	45
Subway Club	310	4.5	46
Sweet Onion Chicken Teriyaki	370	4	58
Turkey Breast	280	3.5	46
Veggie Delite	230	2.5	44

6" Sandwiches: *Figures based on 9-grain wheat bread, lettuce, tomatoes, onion, green peppers, cucumbers. Oil or mayo not included.*

Chicken & Bacon Ranch Melt	610	30	47
Cold Cut Combo	360	12	46
Italian B.M.T.	410	16	46
Meatball Marinara	480	18	60
Spicy Italian	480	24	46
Steak & Cheese	380	10	49
Tuna	480	25	44

Kids Meal Sandwiches: *Figures based on 9-grain wheat bread, lettuce, tomatoes, onions, green peppers and cucumbers. Oil or mayo not included.*

Black Forest Ham	180	2.5	30
Roast Beef	200	3	30
Turkey Breast	180	2	30
Veggie Delite	150	1.5	29

Condiments & Sauces: *For 6" Sandwiches*

Chipotle Southwest, 0.8 oz	100	10	1
Honey Mustard, Fat-Free, 0.8 oz	30	0	7
Mayonnaise: 1 Tbsp, 0.5 oz	110	12	0
Light, 1 Tbsp, 0.5 oz	50	5	1
Mustard, Yellow or Deli Brown, 2 tsp	5	0	1
Olive Oil Blend, 1 tsp	45	5	0
Ranch Dressing	110	11	1
Sweet Onion, Fat-Free, 0.8 oz	40	0	9

Extras: *For 6" Sandwiches*

Bacon Strips (2)	80	5	1
Cheese: American, 2 triangles	40	3.5	1
Cheddar, 2 triangles, 0.3 oz	60	4.5	0
Swiss, 2 triangles, 0.3 oz	50	4.5	0

continued next page....

Fast - Foods & *Restaurants*

Subway® cont... (Jan '18)

Breakfast:

	C	F	Cb
6" Egg White Omelet S'wich: *Includes 9 Grain Wheat Bread*			
Bacon, Egg White & Cheese	410	13	45
Egg White & Cheese	330	8	44
Egg White & Cheese with Ham	360	9	45
Steak, Egg White & Cheese	400	10	46
6" Regular Egg Omelet S'wich: *Includes 9 Grain Wheat Bread*			
Bacon, Egg & Cheese	450	18	44
Egg & Cheese	370	13	44
Egg & Cheese with Ham	400	14	45
Steak, Egg & Cheese	440	15	46
6" Regular Egg Omelet Flatbread: *Includes Flatbread*			
Bacon, Egg & Cheese	460	21	43
BMT	520	25	46
Egg & Cheese	380	15	42
Mega Melt	600	31	44
Sausage, Egg & Cheese	520	26	44
Sunrise Subway Melt	530	22	47
8" Pizza: Bacon	840	31	98
Cheese	720	23	97
Meatball	860	33	100
Pepperoni	840	33	97
Sausage	860	35	98
Flatizza: *Includes 9 Grain Wheat Bread*			
Cheese	400	16	43
Pepperoni	500	26	44
Spicy Italian	500	25	44
Veggie	410	17	45
Side of Hash Browns, 3.6 oz	220	10	30

Salads (6g Fat or Less): *Figures based on lettuce, tomatoes, spinach, onions, green peppers, olives & cucumbers. Dressing or croutons not included.*

	C	F	Cb
Black Forest Ham	110	3	13
Oven Roasted Chicken	150	3.5	13
Roast Beef; Subway Club, average	140	3.5	12
Sweet Onion Chkn Teriyaki, w/ Sce	230	3	34
Turkey Breast	110	2	13
Veggie Delite	60	1	11

Soup: *Per 8 oz Bowl*

	C	F	Cb
Beef Chili, with Beans	360	22	20
Black Bean	210	1	39
Broccoli & Cheddar	170	9	18
Creamy Chicken & Dumpling	150	4.5	20
Creamy Chicken & Wild Rice	190	11	16
Homestyle Chicken Noodle	110	3	14
Loaded Baked Potato	210	13	15
Tomato Basil	130	6	15

Subway® cont... (Jan '18)

Cookies & Desserts:

	C	F	Cb
Apple Slices, 1 package, 2.5 oz	35	0	9
Brownie, 3 oz	370	17	51
Chocolate Chip Cookie, 1.5 oz	200	10	30
Oatmeal Raisin Cookie, 1.5 oz	200	8	30
Raspberry Cheesecake, 1.6 oz	200	9	29

Sweet Tomatoes®

Same Menu & Data as Souplantation ~ See Page 242

Swiss Chalet® (Sept '17)

Canadian Outlets

	C	F	Cb
Starters: Chicken Spring Rolls (4)	340	16	31
Caesar Salad, without Dressing	90	3	13
Chalet Wings (10), w/out Sauce	560	34	13
Cheese Perogies (7)	420	10	69
Poutine, 12.2 oz	910	50	94
Burgers: *Without Sides or Accompanying Sauce*			
Classic Hamburger, with Mayo	520	21	50
Ultimate Bacon Cheeseburger	730	42	46
Veggie Burger with Mayo	440	15	50
Ribs: *With Sauce, without Sides*			
BBQ Side Ribs: ⅓ Rack	480	33	1
½ Rack	720	50	1
Full Rack	1440	100	2
BBQ Back Ribs: ½ Rack	460	30	0
Full Rack	920	61	1
Rotisserie Chicken: *Without Sides, Sauces or Bread*			
Chicken & Shrimp	940	35	88
Chicken Pot Pie, 1 pie	610	35	43
Double Leg: with skin	490	31	0
without skin	320	16	0
Half Chicken: with skin	530	27	0
without skin	380	14	0
Quarter Chicken:			
Dark Meat: with skin	240	16	0
without skin	160	8	0
White Meat: with skin	290	11	0
without skin	220	6	0
Sandwiches: *Without Sides or Accompanying Sauce*			
Chicken Club Kaiser: Dark Meat	740	36	45
White Meat	660	26	45
Rotisserie Chicken Kaiser:			
Dark Meat	570	18	47
White Meat	480	8	47
Entree Salads: *Without Dressing*			
Rotisserie Chicken Caesar	420	11	38
Spinach & Mandarin Chicken	400	16	28
Sweet Heat Salad with Chicken	340	9	30

Updated Nutrition Data ~ www.CalorieKing.com
Persons with Diabetes ~ See Disclaimer (Page 22)

Swiss Chalet® cont...(Sept '17)

Sides:

	C	F	Cb
Caesar Salad without Dressing	50	1.5	8
Creamy Coleslaw	200	14	15
Gravy	45	1.5	7
Mashed Potatoes	150	4	27
Medit. Tomato & Cucumber Salad	110	7	8
Sauteed Mushrooms	140	1	30
Seasoned Rice	240	3.5	48
Multigrain Roll	110	1	22
White Roll	110	0	22
Dip, Blue Cheese, 1 oz	140	14	2
Dressings: Chalet, 1 oz	160	14	6
Caesar, 1 oz	180	18	2
Ranch, 1 oz	140	14	2
Sauce: Chalet Dipping, 1 oz	25	0.5	5
Cajun; Sweet Chili 1 oz	50	0	12
Plum, 1 oz	100	0	26

Desserts/Pies:

Apple Pie	440	19	65
Classic Vanilla Cheesecake	380	25	32
Coconut Cream Pie	540	33	57
Lemon Meringue Pie	400	11	73
Pecan Pie	590	29	79

Taco Bell® (Jan '18)

Burritos: W/ Standard Components

	C	F	Cb
½ lb Cheesy Potato, w/ Beef	490	22	54
½ lb Seasoned Beef Combo	450	18	51
7-Layer, no meat	440	16	59
Beefy 5-Layer	500	19	64
Cheesy Potato Griller, no meat	340	13	50
Chili Cheese, no meat	370	17	40
Shredded Chicken	420	20	47
Smothered Beef	700	33	71
Supreme, with Seasoned Beef	410	15	51
XXL Grilled Stuft: Beef	870	40	96
Marinated Steak	840	35	93
Shredded Chicken	850	38	93
Nachos, Triple Layer, with Beef	400	19	43

Power Menu: With Standard Menu Component

Power Bowls: Chicken, shredded	520	23	54
Seasoned Beef	550	26	57
Steak	510	21	55

Specialties:

Chalupa Supreme: *With Standard Menu Components*			
Seasoned Beef	350	19	33
Shredded Chicken	340	18	32
Crunchwrap Supreme: *W/ Standard Menu Components*			
Seasoned Beef	530	21	71
Shredded Chicken	520	20	69

Taco Bell® cont... (Jan '18)

Specialties (Cont):

	C	F	Cb
Gordita Supreme: *With Standard Menu Component*			
Seasoned Beef	280	12	31
Shredded Chicken	270	11	30
Steak	270	9	30
MexiMelt, Beef	250	13	19
Meximelt Supreme, Shr. Chicken	270	14	19
Nachos BellGrande:			
Seasoned Beef	760	38	84
Shredded Chicken	740	37	83
Quesadillas: Fire Grilled Chicken	510	28	38
Steak	510	28	38

Tacos: With Standard Menu Components

Crunchy: Seasoned Beef	170	9	13
Supreme. S'nd Beef	190	11	15
Double Decker:			
Regular, Seasoned Beef	320	13	36
Supreme, Fire Grilled Chicken	320	12	36
Soft: Seasoned Beef	180	9	17
Supreme, Seasoned Beef	210	10	20
Shredded Chicken	200	9	18

Taco Salads: With Standard Menu Components

Express Fiesta, Seasoned Beef	580	25	65
Fiesta: Seasoned Beef	760	39	77
Shredded Chicken	740	37	75
Steak	730	34	75
Sides: Black Beans & Rice	190	3.5	35
Cheesy Fiesta Potato	230	12	28
Chips & Guacamole	230	14	23
Pintos 'n Cheese	190	7	22
Seasoned Rice	120	2	23

Breakfast: With Standard Menu Components

Crunchwrap: Bacon & Eggs	670	42	51
Sausage Patty & Eggs	700	46	51
Grande Scrambler Burrito:			
Bacon & Eggs	650	34	64
Sausage Patty & Eggs	680	38	64
Quesadillas: Bacon	460	24	37
Sausage Crumbles	450	24	37
Steak	440	21	37
Sweets: Caramel Apple Empanada	280	13	38
Cinnabon Delights:			
4 Pack	310	18	35
12 Pack (serves 4)	930	53	104
Cinnamon Twist	170	6	7

Note: Nutritional data in New York outlets may vary slightly.
Please check Taco Bell website

Fast - Foods & *Restaurants*

Taco Cabana® (Sept '17)

Cabana Burritos: | C | F | Cb
Includes Flour Tortilla, Rice, Refried Beans, Romaine, Meat, Shredded Cheese, Pico de Gallo & Sour Cream

	C	F	Cb
Beef	1030	48	106
Chicken Fajita	950	37	105
Chicken, Shredded	1010	43	108
Steak Fajita	990	44	107

Enchiladas:

	C	F	Cb
Beef (1)	220	14	14
Cheese (1)	320	23	13
Chicken (1)	280	14	20

Quesadillas: Personal, with Guacamole & Sour Cream

	C	F	Cb
Chicken Breast Fajita	740	42	51
Shredded Beef	710	41	51
Shredded Chicken	700	39	52
Steak Fajita	760	45	52

Sizzling Skillets: Includes Flour Tortilla, Grilled Onion, Bell Pepper, Rice, Shredded Cheese, Sour Cream, Guacamole, Lettuce & Pico de Gallo

2lb: Serves 2

	C	F	Cb
Chicken Fajita	1680	62	195
Shredded Beef	1760	78	195
Steak Fajita	1770	79	200

Tacos:

	C	F	Cb
Crispy: Beef	200	11	15
Shredded Chicken	190	9	16
Soft: Bean & Cheese	300	14	31
Beef	240	11	22
Black Bean	210	4	37
Carne Guisada	230	9	23
Chicken Breast Fajita	180	5	21
Shredded Beef	240	11	22
Shredded Chicken	230	9	23
Steak Fajita	210	8	22
Street, Beef (3)	410	17	48

Salads: Includes Shell, Lettuce Meat, Shredded Cheese, Guacamole, Pico de Gallo & Sour Cream

	C	F	Cb
Beef Cabana	770	53	43
Chicken Cabana	l750	48	45
Chicken Fajita Cabana	690	43	42
Steak Fajita Cabana	720	49	44

Sides & Add-Ons: Per Serving

	C	F	Cb
Borracho Beans, 4 oz	140	3	20
Guacamole, 3 oz	110	9	7
Queso, 3 oz	110	8	5
Refried Beans with Cheese, 4 oz	260	14	25
Rice, 4 oz	120	1	25
Salsa: Fuego; Roja, 1 oz	5	0	1
Verde, 1 oz	10	0	1
Sour Cream, 3 oz	160	15	3

Taco Del Mar® (Sept '17)

Baja Bowls: Per Regular Bowl, | C | F | Cb
with Rice, Refried Beans, Meat, Cheese & Pico de Gallo

Mondo:	C	F	Cb
Beef Steak Asada	500	14	63
Chicken; Shredded Beef	520	17	62
Ground Beef	570	23	62
Pork	500	15	61

Mondito:	C	F	Cb
Beef Steak Asada	370	10	51
Chicken	370	10	51
Ground Beef	390	13	51
Pork	360	10	50
Shredded Beef	370	10	51

Burritos: Includes Flour Tortilla, Rice, Refried Beans Meat, Cheese & Pico de Gallo

Mondito:	C	F	Cb
Beef Steak Asada	460	12	67
Chicken; Shredded Beef, av.	475	14	67
Ground Beef	500	17	67
Pork	470	13	66

Mondo:	C	F	Cb
Beef Steak Asada	810	21	115
Chicken; Shredded Beef	840	24	113
Ground Beef	880	30	114
Pork	830	24	113

Nachos: Includes Chips , Refried Beans, Meat, Cheese, Pico de Gallo, Guacamole & Sour Cream

Mondito:	C	F	Cb
Cheese	620	29	72
Beef Steak Asada; Beef; Chkn, av.	675	31	72
Ground Beef; Fish, average	700	35	75

Mondo:	C	F	Cb
Cheese	1050	62	95
Beef Steak Asada	1150	64	98
Chicken; Shredded Beef, av.	1180	68	97
Ground Beef	1220	74	97
Pork	1170	67	96

Platters: Includes Meat, Cheese, Rice, Refried Beans, Lettuce, Pico, Guacamole, Sour Cream & Enchilada Sauce

Enchilada: Per 2 Soft Corn Tortillas

	C	F	Cb
Beef Steak Asada (2)	810	27	107
Cheese (2)	810	32	105
Chicken; Shredded Beef, av., (2)	845	31	106
Ground Beef (2)	890	37	106
Pork (2)	830	30	104

Quesadillas: Includes Flour Tortilla, Meat, Cheese, Pico

Mondito:	C	F	Cb
Beef Steak Asada	390	17	40
Chicken; Shredded Beef, average	415	19	39
Ground Beef	430	22	40
Pork	410	19	39
Vegan	290	5	52

Taco Del Mar® cont... (Sept '17)

Taco Salads: Includes Shell, Cheese
Refried Beans, Lettuce, Cabbage, Meat & Pico de Gallo

	C	F	Cb
Mondito: Beef Steak Asada	480	23	51
Chicken	500	25	50
Ground Beef	520	28	50
Pork	500	24	50
Shredded Beef	500	24	50
Mondo: Beef Steak Asada	600	28	58
Chicken	640	32	56
Ground Beef	680	38	57
Pork	620	31	56
Shredded Beef	630	31	57
Veggie	720	29	96

Note: Nutritional Information varies from state to state.
Please refer to Taco Del Mar Website

Taco John's® (Sept '17)

Burritos:	C	F	Cb
Bean Burrito	370	11	53
Beef Grilled Burrito	590	32	53
Chicken Grilled Burrito	590	30	50
Meat & Potato: Beef Burrito	520	25	57
Chicken Burrito	480	21	56
Crunchy Chkn Burrito	580	27	67
Chips:			
& Queso, 6.7 oz	430	25	43
& Nacho Cheese, 5 oz	380	23	39
Mexi Rolls: *Without Nacho Cheese*			
4 Pieces, 8 oz	550	21	61
6 Pieces, 10 oz	710	27	77
Nachos:			
Super Nachos:			
Small, 6.7 oz	420	25	37
Regular, 12.6 oz	790	47	72
Potato Oles: *Per Serving*			
Small, 5 oz	480	27	52
Medium, 7 oz	670	38	73
Large, 9 oz	860	49	94
Super Potato Oles:			
Small, 9.7 oz	650	40	59
Regular, 16.8 oz	1090	67	98
Quesadilla Melt:			
Beef, 8.6 oz	550	29	46
Cheesy, 5.5 oz	450	24	40
Chicken, 8.6 oz	520	25	45
Tacos:			
Crispy Taco	170	10	11
Softshell Taco: Beef	220	10	23
Chicken	190	6	21
Stuffed Grilled Taco	540	27	58
Taco Bravo	330	13	38

Taco John's® (Sept '17)

Salads: *Without Dressing*	C	F	Cb
Beef Taco Salad	540	33	40
Chicken Taco Salad	500	27	39
Crunchy Chicken Taco	630	36	53
Crunchy Chicken Salad	370	18	29
Sides: *Per Serving*			
Refried Beans, 9.5 oz	320	17	46
Desserts:			
Churro, 2 oz	200	9	29
Mexican Donut Bites, 3.2 oz	290	12	47
Condiments:			
Bacon Ranch, 1.5 oz	120	9	10
House Dressing, 1.5 oz	70	7	2
Nacho Cheese, 3 oz	110	9	5
Salsa, 2 oz	10	0	2
Sour Cream, 2 oz	120	10	3
Breakfast:			
Burritos: Bacon & Potato, 7.7 oz	550	27	56
Potato & Bacon Oles Scrambler	1080	68	86
Spicy Chorizo, 8.2 oz	510	28	44
Sausage Scrambler, 8.7 oz	650	33	60

Taco Mayo® (Sept '17)

Burritos:	C	F	Cb
Bean	450	14	63
Beef	515	22	46
Double, Smothered Double Queso			
Chicken Platter	850	38	84
Fajita: Grilled Chicken	485	25	43
Grilled Steak	525	28	43
Super: Beef	525	21	56
Chicken	420	18	41
Quesadilla Platter:			
Chicken	675	37	46
Fajita Chicken	700	39	47
Fajita Steak	725	40	47
Tacos:			
Crispy Taco, Beef	160	9	10
Soft Taco: Beef	230	11	17
Chicken	185	6	16
Taco Burger	300	13	28
Salads: *As Per Menu Description*			
Acapulco Chicken	680	50	35
SalsaLita: Chicken	280	6	33
Steak, 12 oz	305	8	33
Taco: Beef	705	38	57
Steak, 11.3 oz	445	25	30
Sides:			
Mexicali Rice	160	1	36
Refried Beans	295	9	43
Potato Locos, Small	380	24	36

Fast - Foods & *Restaurants*

Taco Time® (Sept '17)

Burritos:	C	F	Cb
5 Alarm	420	15	58
Chicken B.L.T.	600	31	46
Sweet Pork	550	18	72
Big Juan: Chicken	590	16	79
Seasoned Beef Beef	650	22	83
Casita: Chicken	450	16	44
Seasoned Beef	510	22	48
Crisp Burrito:			
Chicken	380	17	39
Meat	390	17	43
Pinto Bean	380	13	53
Soft Burrito: Pinto Bean	380	10	56
Seasoned Beef	420	16	46
Veggie	440	17	60
Chimichangas:			
Green Chili Pork: Carnitas	590	21	65
Enchiladas	340	12	26
Nachos:			
Original	900	39	91
Chicken	970	39	92
Seasoned Beef	1020	45	96
Tacos:			
Soft Tacos: Chicken	360	10	42
Junior	300	13	29
Pork	440	16	43
Seasoned Beef	410	16	45
Super Soft Tacos: Chicken	500	16	61
Pork	590	21	62
Seasoned Beef	560	21	65
Fries:			
Mexi: Small, 3.2 oz	190	12	19
Regular, 4.7 oz	300	19	29
Stuffed: Small, 4.5 oz	320	20	29
Regular, 6.6 oz	460	28	42
Salads:			
Fiesta, Chicken,12.3 oz	340	11	37
Taco: Chicken, 8 oz	310	14	26
Seasn'd Beef , 7.5 oz	360	19	28
Soup, Enchilada, 8 oz	130	0.5	20
Breakfast:			
Burritos: *Regular Size*			
Bacon & Egg	450	20	48
Country	700	42	50
Sausage & Egg	560	30	48
Quesadilla	300	17	18
Taters & Gravy, regular	410	27	36
Desserts:			
Churro: Plain	210	16	15
Bavarian Cream	320	8	54
Cinnamon Crustos	320	5	64

TCBY® (Sept '17)

Soft Serve Frozen Yogurt: 4 fl.oz	C	F	Cb
Super Fro Yo: Bananas Foster	90	0	23
Cake Batter; Golden Vanilla	105	2	22
Cheesecake	105	2	22
Chocolate	110	1.5	23
Dutch Chocolate	95	0	23
Greek Honey Vanilla	100	0	20
Old Fashioned Vanilla	90	0	23
White Chocolate Macadamia	70	0	18
White Chocolate Mousse	120	1.5	24
Dairy Free/Sorbet:			
Chocoalte Almond	100	1	28
Kiwi Strawberry Sorbet	90	0	22
Limeade Sorbet	110	0	28
Mango Sorbet	95	0	24
Watermelon Sorbet	100	0	25
Vanilla Almond	100	1	28
No Sugar Added: Chocolate	65	0	18
Mountain Blackberry	65	0	18
Salted Caramel	70	0	18
Hand-Scooped Frozen Yogurt:			
Butter Pecan: Kid's, 4 fl.oz	220	10	27
Small, 6.4 fl.oz	350	16	43
Regular, 12.8 fl.oz	705	32	86
Chunky Choc. Cookie Dough:			
Kid's, 4 fl.oz	220	7	33
Small, 6.4 fl.oz	350	11	53
Regular,12.8 fl.oz	705	22	106
Cookies & Cream:			
Kid's, 4 fl.oz	200	6	32
Small, 6.4 fl.oz	320	10	51
Regular, 12.8 fl.oz	640	19	102
Peanut Butter Delight:			
Kid's, 4 fl.oz	250	13	30
Small, 6.4 fl.oz	400	21	48
Regular, 12.8 fl.oz	800	42	96
Pralines & Cream: Kid's 4 fl.oz	210	6	27
Small, 6.4 fl.oz	335	10	43
Regular, 12.8 fl oz	670	19	86
Vanilla Bean: Kid's,4 fl.oz	170	4.5	27
Small, 6.4 fl.oz	270	7	43
Regular, 12.8 fl.oz	545	14	86

Updated Nutrition Data ~ www.CalorieKing.com
Persons with Diabetes ~ See Disclaimer (Page 22)

TGI Friday's® (Sept '17)

Appetizers/Snacks:	C	F	Cb
Chicken Quesadilla	1060	67	54
Loaded Potato Skins, with Ranch Sour Cream	1620	91	167
Mozzarella Sticks, w/ Marinara	820	50	54
Pan Seared P'stickers, w/ Szech. Sce	590	25	72
Sesame Jack Chicken Strips	1090	35	159
Spinach & Queso Dip	770	54	66
Warm Pretzels, w/ Beer-Cheese Sauce	1190	60	125

Burgers: *Without Sides*			
Bacon Cheeseburger	840	54	47
BBQ'n	1160	74	77
Black Bean & Avocado	830	49	74
Jack Daniel's Burger	1110	55	110
Turkey Burger	520	22	48

Chicken & Seafood:			
Crispy Chkn Fngrs, fries & Hon Msrd	1030	59	87
Gr. Salmon, Jasmine Rice Pilaf & Spin.	980	57	55

Pasta,			
Bruschetta Chicken, full portion	860	35	93

Ribs: *With Coleslaw & Seasoned Fries*			
BBQ: Half Rack	870	48	75
Full Rack	1260	72	89
Jack Daniel's: Half Rack	1070	49	124
Full Rack	1600	73	173

Sandwiches: *W/out Sides*			
French Dip	800	48	51
Jack Daniel's Chicken	1110	57	100
Mediterranean Mahi Mahi Naan	480	15	55
Southern Fried Chicken	930	57	67

Steaks: *With Mashed Potatoes & Lemon Butter Broccoli*			
Flat Iron: with Parmesan Butter	780	52	33
with Jack Daniel's Glaze	900	42	87
Ribeye: with Parmesan Butter	960	58	33
with Jack Daniel's Glaze	1090	48	89
Sirloin: with Parmesan Butter	990	70	33
with Jack Daniel's Glaze	1120	60	89

Salads: *Includes Menu Set Dressing*			
Caesar, with 4 oz Flat Iron Steak	730	60	28
Pecan-Crusted Chicken	1220	84	82
Strawberry Fields Salad	610	47	40

TGI Friday's® cont... (Sept '17)

Salad Dressing: *Per 1.25 oz*	C	F	Cb
Balsamic Vinaigrette	190	19	4
Bleu Cheese	200	21	1
Honey Mustard	200	18	8
Ranch	130	14	1

Signature Sides:			
Coleslaw	100	8	5
Jasmine Rice Pilaf	420	11	72
Mashed Potatoes	250	15	19
Seasoned Fries	320	16	40
Sweet Potato Fries	390	20	50

Soups: *Per 10 oz Bowl*			
French Onion	310	17	25
White Chedd. Brocc. Chse	280	20	18
Soup Of The Day:			
New England Clam Chowder	500	30	45
Tomato Basil	300	24	20

Desserts: *Per Whole Dish*			
Brownie Obsession	1200	60	153
Oreo Madness	500	21	76
Vanilla Bean Cheesecake	920	57	88

Signature Slushes:			
Blue Raspberry	250	0	64
Mango Peach Lemonade	160	0	44
Red Bull Passion	210	0	54
Strawberry Lemonade	210	0	55

Thundercloud Subs® (Sept '17)

Subs: *Small, with Standard Toppings*	C	F	Cb
Classic: BLT	365	17	35
Smoked Chicken	265	4	35
Turkey	255	4	36
Low Fat: Genoa Salami	265	6	35
Roast Beef	290	4	35
Signature Subs:			
Club	445	19	38
California Club	475	23	40
NY Italian	540	30	37
Office Favorite	790	39	71
Texas Tuna	675	44	39
Veggie Delite, with Hummus	385	19	52

T.J. Cinnamons® (Sept '17)

Bakery:	C	F	Cb
Orig. Gourmet Cinn. Roll, 7.8 oz	840	42	106
Pecan Stick Bun, 8.3 oz	940	49	111

Tim Hortons® (Sept '17)

Breakfast:

	C	F	Cb
Biscuit Sandwich:			
Sausage, Egg & Cheese	530	35	34
Turkey Sausage, Egg & Cheese	430	23	35
English Muffin Sandwich:			
Bacon, Egg & Cheese	350	17	29
Steak, Egg White & Cheese	270	8	29
Grilled B'Fast Wraps:			
Farmer's Breakfast	650	38	55
Steak & Cheddar	440	21	40
Oatmeal, with Mixed Berries, reg.	210	3	44
Hash Brown, regular	130	7	16
Hot Bowls: Chili, 10 oz	300	16	18
Mac & Cheese, 10 oz	490	27	48
Soup: Chicken Noodle, 10 oz	120	1.5	21
Clam Chowder, 10 oz	190	7	23
Potato Bacon Cheddar, 10 oz	260	15	22
Paninis: Grilled Cheese	460	29	39
Steak & Cheese	400	17	35
Tuscan Chicken	420	15	42
Sandwiches:			
Italiano Grilled Bagel	640	27	64
Turkey Bacon Club	510	27	36
Wraps: Chicken/Steak Fajita, av.	430	20	40
Donuts: Apple Fritter	290	8	48
Boston Creme Filled	220	6	35
Chocolate, Glazed	280	14	37
Chocolate Dip	190	7	29
Double Chocolate	270	15	32
Honey Cruller	310	18	37
Old Fashioned, Plain	210	10	25
Timbits: Chocolate, Glazed	70	3	10
Apple Fritter; Honey Dip, average	50	1.5	9
Old Fashion, Plain	50	2.5	7
Bagels: 12 Grain	350	9	55
Other varieties, av., 4 oz	300	3	59
Cream Cheese Spread, Light, 1.5 oz	90	7	3
Cinnamon Roll, Frosted	400	14	60
Cookies, average, 1.84 oz	230	10	34
Croissants, Cheese	310	17	30
Danish, Maple Pecan	390	21	48
Greek Yogurt, with Berries, av.	250	5	29
Muffins: Choc. Chip, 4 oz	420	16	66
Cran Apple Walnut Bran, 4 oz	350	14	54
Lemon Poppyseed, 4 oz	370	14	56
Wild Blueberry, 4 oz	340	11	57
Beverages: Cappuccino, 10 oz	70	0	11
Hot Chocolate, 10 oz	240	6	45
Latte, 10 oz	80	0	12
Mocha Latte, 10 oz	190	6	26
Cold: Frozen Lemonade, Orig., 12 oz	140	0	34
Iced Capp®, w/ Milk, 12 oz	180	1.5	39
Iced Coffee, with Milk, 16 oz	45	0	9

Togo's® (Sept '17)

California Outlet ~ Please check

	C	F	Cb
local outlet for menu items and nutritional information			
Cold Sandwiches: Per Regular 6", with Menu Set			
Components on White Bread			
Albacore Tuna	670	27	72
Avocado & Provolone	720	38	74
California Club	740	34	71
Chicken Salad	620	22	70
Ham & Cheese	690	28	70
Hummus	670	26	93
Salami & Provolone	910	52	68
The Italian	880	47	70
Turkey & Avocado	700	32	74
Turkey & Cranberry	650	18	86
Viva Veggie	820	37	99
Hot Sandwiches: Per Regular 6", with Menu Set			
Components on White Bread			
Meatball	890	40	81
Pastrami	740	34	73
Pepperjack Pastrami Melt	1010	59	73
Roast Beef	710	21	67
Sandwich Dressings: Mayo, reg.	150	16	0.5
Boom Boom Sauce, regular	160	16	3
Sweet Baby Ray's BBQ, regular	35	0	9
Wraps: Per Whole 12" Spinach Tortilla Wrap, with Menu			
Set Components			
Asian Chicken	590	24	70
Chicken Caesar	540	20	65
Santa Fe Chicken	660	31	70
Salads: Per Full Salad, with Dressing			
Asian chicken	570	40	37
Chicken Caesar	390	24	21
Santa Fe Chicken	880	68	46
Salad Dressings: Caesar, 2.5 oz	150	12	8
Buttermilk Ranch, 2.5 oz	330	35	3
Italian Vinaigrette, 2.5 oz	310	33	2
Thousand Island, 2.5 oz	310	28	12
Soups: Broccoli Cheddar, 10 oz	380	24	31
Chicken Noodle, 10 oz	125	3	23
Chicken Tortilla, 10 oz	155	6	21
Garden Vegetable	90	0.5	18
Brownie, Choc. Chunk, 3 oz	430	22	57
Cookies: Dark Choc. Chunk, 3 oz	410	21	53
Oatmeal Raisin, 3 oz	360	13	57
Peanut Butter Chip, 3 oz	410	23	48

Tropical Smoothie Cafe® (Sept '17)

Menu & Nutrition Differ from Outlets to Outlet. Please Check Instore. Figures below Based On Irvine, CA

C F Cb

Breakfast:

	C	F	Cb
All American Omelet Wrap	420	20	37
Peanut Butter Crunch Flatbread	590	24	77
Southwest Omelet Wrap	480	26	38

Toasted Sandwiches: *Per Whole Ciabatta Sandwich*

Turkey Apple Dijon	780	9	69
Turkey Bacon Ranch	560	20	59
Tropical Chicken Salad	630	30	64

Toasted Wraps: *In Flour Tortilla*

Baja Chicken	640	25	66
Caribbean Jerk Chicken	590	17	74
Hummus Veggie	730	39	78
Island Buffalo Chicken	530	21	45
Supergreen Caesar Chicken	530	26	41
Thai Chicken	520	15	64

Classic Smoothies: *Per 24 oz with Turbinado*

Blimey Limey	440	0	111
Blueberry Bliss	340	5	86
Jetty Punch	370	0	94
Peaches 'N Silk	360	0	91
Sunny Day	460	0	116
Sunrise Sunset	360	0	89

Indulgent Smoothies: *24 oz with Turbinado*

Bahama Mama	500	4.5	117
Beach Bum	550	5	129
Mocha Madness	660	5	152
Peanut Butter Cup	710	20	127

Supercharged: *Per 24 oz with Turbinado*

Health Nut, with Soy	530	4.5	101
Lean Machine	490	0	124
Muscle Blaster, with Whey	470	2	96
Peanut Paradise, with Whey	690	17	105

Tubby's® (Sept '17)

Subs: *Per Regular 8" Tubby Sub, w/out Dressing or Sauce*

Deli-Subs:

	C	F	Cb
Ham & Cheese	540	11	78
Turkey Breast & Cheese	550	11	77

Grilled Burger Subs: Big Tub

	790	35	78
Cheeseburger Italiano	790	35	78
Loaded Burger	820	36	83
Pizza Burger	810	36	81

Tubby's® cont... (Sept '17)

Subs (Cont): *Per Regular 8" Tubby Sub, without Dressing or Sauce*

C F Cb

Grilled Chicken Subs: Gr. Chicken

	C	F	Cb
	450	4.5	75
Chicken & Broccoli	550	11	78
Chicken & Cheddar	540	11	75
Chicken Fajita	550	11	79

Grilled Steak Subs:

Loaded Steak	540	13	77
Pepper Steak & Cheese	540	13	77
Portabella Mushroom Steak	580	13	77
Steak & Cheese	540	13	75

Specialty Subs: BLT

	570	21	72
Cold Veggie	490	10	86
Italian Sausage	600	2	78
Meatball	790	33	83
Tuna	570	11	76

Uno Pizzeria & Grill® (Sept '17)

Appetizers: *Per Whole Dish*

	C	F	Cb
Mozzarella Sticks	1100	57	108
Muchos Nacos	1520	72	176
Shrimp & Crab Dip	1120	81	64

Burgers: *Without Sides*

BBQ, with Bacon & Cheddar	1430	103	40
Bacon Cheddar Burger	1410	103	35
Uno Burger	1050	29	35

Entrees:

Chicken: *Without Sides or Breadstick*

Baked Stuffed Spinoccoli	330	15	6
Stir Fry Chicken	520	10	83
Romano Crusted Chicken Parm.	1090	40	124

Deep Dish Pizza: *Per Individual Pizza*

Chicago Classic	2220	157	112
Numero Uno	1820	125	118
Prima Pepperoni	1720	118	110

Pasta: *Without Breadstick*

Chicken Spinoccoli	1260	62	106
Deep Dish Mac & Cheese	870	51	70
Shrimp Scampi	1190	54	128

Steak & Seafood: *Without Sides or Breadstick*

Grilled Shrimp & Sirloin	760	52	1
Sirloin: 6 oz	330	22	0
10 oz	560	37	0
Stockyard Strip Steak	400	10	1

Sides: Breadstick

	160	8	18
French Fries, 7.5 oz	450	33	35
Onion Rings, 7.5 oz	370	7	68
Red Bliss Mashed Potatoes	270	14	36
Roasted Seasonal Veggies, 7.2 oz	70	4	8

Dessert: All American

	640	28	90
Brownie Bowl	1130	53	152

253

Villa Fresh Italian® (Sept '17)

Pizzas: Per Slice

	C	F	Cb
Neapolitan: Buffalo	770	46	52
Deluxe	530	22	55
Sausage & Pepperoni	550	25	53
Stuffed: Baked Ziti	845	33	97
Spinach & Mushroom	735	33	79

Entrees:

Chicken Pasta Primavera, 16 oz	505	20	58
Fettuccini Alfredo, 14 oz	765	38	85
Mac & Cheese, 14 oz	725	54	39
Pasta Primavera, 16 oz	495	21	66
Spaghetti & Meatballs, 18 oz	840	28	112

Sides: Caesar Salad, 4 oz | 90 | 5 | 9

Garlic Roll,	260	10	34
Garden Salad, 3 oz	15	1	3
Greek Salad, 6 oz	125	10	7
Roasted Potatoes, 6 oz	210	12	24
Sauteed Vegetables, 6oz	85	6	6

Vocelli Pizza® (Sept '17)

Pizzas:

Artisan: *Per 1/8 of Medium Pizza, with Menu Set Cpomponents*

	C	F	Cb
Buffalo Chicken	240	9	26
Chicken Carbonara	260	11	27
Chicken Pesto	260	10	27
Chicken Spinaci	240	9	27
Deluxe	260	10	29
Hawaiian	280	11	30
Meat Magnifico	290	12	28
Philly Steak	270	13	25
Quattro Cheese	260	11	27

Pasta: *Single Serving*

Chicken Alfredo	1200	54	129
Chicken Parmesan	960	26	144
Chicken Pesto	1230	57	128

House Baked Subs: *On Italian Bread*

Buffalo Chicken	950	39	86
Chkn Parmesan	990	39	105
Meatball	1170	55	103

Salads: *Per Regular Size, without Dressing*

Chicken Caesar	180	4	14
Mediterranean	230	11	22
Tuscan Grilled Chicken	320	13	22

Stromboli: *With Menu Set Components, & Marinara Sauce*

Pepperoni	1410	62	149
Spicy Italian	1440	57	156
Steak	1230	37	158

Wahoo's Fish Taco® (Sept '17)

Bowls: W/ White Rice & Black Beans

	C	F	Cb
#7 Blackened/Charbroiled Chkn, av.	860	15	127
# 8 Charbroiled/Teriyaki Fish, av.	930	22	126
#9 Veggie	760	11	141
#10 Carnitas/Kahlua Pig, average	1025	25	131

Burritos: *With Brown Rice & White Beans*

Banzai Blackened or Charbroiled:

Chicken	575	16	77
Fish, average	620	21	77
Mushroom	490	14	81
Carne Asada	565	17	79
Carnitas	685	23	79
Shrimp	475	14	77
Vegetarian	485	14	82

Side Kicks, *Corn Tortillas, each* | 145 | 2 | 29

Wahoo's Sandwiches:

Blackened or Charbroiled:

Chicken, average	550	22	51
Fish, average	510	18	51
Carne Asada	500	19	52

Salads:

Banzai Veggie	295	18	24

Blackened or Charbroiled:

Chicken, average	415	22	14
Fish, average	485	29	14
Carne Asada	400	23	16

Soup, *Chicken Tortilla* | 55 | 1 | 5

For Complete Nutritional Data ~ see CalorieKing.com

WAWA® (Sept '17)

Breakfast Sizzlis:

	C	F	Cb
Bagels:			
Bacon, Egg & Cheese	410	18	43
Pork Roll, Egg & Cheese	420	19	43
Sausage, Egg & Cheese	500	28	43
Turkey Ssg, Egg White & Cheese	360	12	43
Biscuit, Sausage, Egg & Cheese	630	43	47
Croissants:			
Bacon, Egg & Cheese	420	27	26
Chorizo	570	39	39
Sausage, Egg & Cheese	510	38	26
Muffin, Ham, Egg White & Cheese	240	7	29

Cold Hoagies: *On 6" Shorti Roll w/out Toppings*

Egg Salad	650	37	61
Italian	450	13	57
Roast Beef	410	5	57
Tuna Salad	690	39	63
Veggie	290	3	55

WAWA® cont... (Sept '17)

	C	F	Cb
Hot Dogs: *Without Toppings, Sauce or Mustard*			
All Beef: ¼ Pound	420	28	21
Big Bacon Cheese Dog	810	47	57
Hot Hoagies: *On 6" Shorti Roll without Toppings*			
Beef Steak & Cheddar Cheese	550	19	59
Chicken Steak & Cheddar Cheese	550	17	59
Meatball & Cheddar Cheese	790	40	71
Soups: *Per Medium Serving*			
Baked Potato w/ Cheddar & Bacon	450	32	28
Broccoli Cheddar Soup	280	23	14
Chicken Noodle	190	7	20
New Eng. Clam Chowder	330	21	24
Tomato Soup	320	22	27
Quesadillas: *Without Toppings*			
Beef & Cheddar Cheese	480	22	39
Cheddar Cheese	400	20	38
Chicken & Cheddar Cheese	480	20	39
Sides: *Per Medium without Toppings*			
Chili	350	16	35
Macaroni & Cheese	500	25	49
Mashed Potatoes	470	28	50
Meatballs in a Cup	380	28	14
Rice	270	0	59
Bakery:			
Apple Fritter	510	19	79
Brownie	490	22	72
Muffins: Banana Walnut	610	33	74
Blueberry	570	28	72
Chocolate Chip	680	34	86
Hot Beverages: *Per 16 oz, without Extras*			
Hot Cappuccino, with 2% milk	130	5	13
Mocha Latte, with 2% milk	330	7	59
Smoothie, Strawberry Banana, without whipped cream, 24 oz	670	0	120

Wendy's® (Jan '18)

	C	F	Cb
Breakfast:			
Artisan Egg Sandwich	360	19	29
Honey Butter Chicken Biscuit	500	26	48
Morning Melt Panini	520	33	33
Oatmeal Bar	290	10	47
Sausage & Egg Burrito	390	29	14
Seasoned Home-Style Potatoes	230	8	35

Wendy's® cont... (Jan '18)

	C	F	Cb
Cheeseburgers:			
Dave's: Single	570	34	39
Double	810	51	39
Triple	1090	72	40
Baconator	950	62	38
Double Stack	390	21	25
Jr. Bacon Cheeseburger	380	22	26
Jr. Cheeseburger	280	13	25
Jr. Cheeseburger Deluxe	330	19	27
Jr. Hamburger	240	10	25
Son of Baconator	630	39	37
Sandwiches: *With Standard Toppings*			
Crispy Chicken	330	16	33
Grilled Chicken	360	8	38
H/Style Asiago Ranch Chicken Club	670	34	54
Homestyle Chicken	520	22	52
Spicy Chicken	510	21	51
Wraps: Grilled Chicken	270	10	24
Spicy Chicken	370	20	30
Chicken Nuggets:			
4 pieces	170	11	10
6 pieces	250	16	14
10 pieces	420	27	24
Dipping Sauces: *Per 1 oz*			
Barbecue	45	0	11
Buttermilk Ranch	120	12	2
Creamy Sriracha	120	12	3
Honey Mustard	90	7	7
Sweet & Sour	45	0	12
Fresh-Made Salads: *Full Size w/ Menu Set Dressing*			
Apple Pecan Grilled Chicken	560	24	52
BBQ Ranch Grilled Chicken	590	30	42
Spicy Chkn Caesar	720	43	41
Sides:			
Baconator Fries	490	28	46
Baked Potatoes:			
Bacon & Cheddar	480	17	66
Broccoli Cheese	430	11	70
Sour Cream & Chives	310	2.5	63
Natural Cut Fries: Kids/Value	230	10	30
Small, 4 oz	320	15	43
Medium, 5 oz	420	19	56
Large, 6.5 oz	530	24	70
Rich Meaty Chili: Small	170	5	16
Large	250	7	23
Frosty:			
Chocolate; Vanilla, average:			
Small	340	9	56
Medium	460	12	77
Large	575	15	96

Whataburger® (Sept '17)

Burgers & Sandwiches: **C** **F** **Cb**

Whataburger:

	C	F	Cb
#1 Original	590	25	62
#2 Double Meat	830	44	62
#3 Triple Meat	1080	63	62
#4 Jalapeno & Cheese	680	32	63
#5 Bacon & Cheese	750	37	62
#6 Double Meat Jr.	420	20	37
#7 Whataburger Jr.	310	11	37

Other Burgers & Sandwiches:

Avocado Bacon Burger	820	52	51
Chop House Cheddar Burger	1110	69	61
Green Chili Double	980	57	61
Grilled Chkn Sandwich	430	13	45
Honey BBQ Chicken Strip S'wich	870	39	90

Whatachick'n:

Bites: 6 pieces, without sauce	450	22	33
9 pieces without sauce	640	31	45
Sandwich	530	20	55
Strips, 3 pieces, w/out sce	530	28	42
Taco, Chicken Fajita, soft	340	11	31
French Fries: Small, 3 oz	280	14	35
Medium, 4.5 oz	420	21	52
Large, 6 oz	560	28	70
Onion Rings: Medium, 3.2 oz	300	17	32
Large, 4.8 oz	450	25	49

Salad: Without Dressing

Garden:

w/ Grilled Chicken	290	12	12
with Whatachick'n	400	20	22
without Chicken	160	10	10
Breakfast: Cinnamon Roll	430	10	79
Biscuits: Plain	290	16	32
with Gravy	470	29	46
Honey Butter Chicken	560	33	51

Biscuit Sandwiches:

with Bacon	470	29	32
with Sausage	630	45	32
On A Bun: with Bacon	350	15	34
with Sausage	520	31	34
Platters: with Bacon	580	36	36
with Sausage	740	52	36
Taquitos: with Cheese	350	19	28
with Bacon, Egg & Cheese	400	22	28
with Potato, Egg & Cheese	440	25	38

Desserts:

Chocolate Chunk Cookie	230	11	31
Hot Apple Pie, 3 oz	270	14	34
Malts: Chocolate, 20 oz	570	11	109
Vanilla, 20 oz	520	12	93
Shake, Chocolate, 20 oz	550	12	101

White Castle® (Sept '17)

C **F** **Cb**

Note: Nutritional Information varies from state to state. Please check instore

Sliders:

	C	F	Cb
Original Slider (1)	140	6	13

Bacon & Cheddar:

Crispy	290	16	21
Grilled	270	15	14
Bacon Cheese	220	14	13
BlackBean: with Honey Mustard	160	3.5	23
with Ranch	260	17	19
Cheddar Cheese	170	9	14
Cheese Slider: Single	160	9	14
Double	300	17	20
Chicken: and Waffles, Crispy	350	18	36
Savory Grilled	340	18	30
Breast	220	10	20
Ring	200	10	16
Savory Grilled Chicken	180	7	13
Fish	340	24	18
Surf & Turf	540	38	27
Veggie: with Ranch	270	18	21
with Sweet Thai Sauce	170	3.5	26
Sides: Clam Strips, medium	410	34	9
Cheese Fries, small	400	27	35

Chicken Rings:

6 rings, 5 oz	530	47	12
9 rings, 7.5 oz	790	71	18
Mozzarella Cheese Sticks, 3 sticks	460	33	26
Onion Chips, medium	930	65	73
Mac & Cheese Nibblers, medium	800	47	74

French Fries: Kids

French Fries: Kids	250	16	24
Small, 5.2 oz	330	21	32
Medium, 9.4 oz	600	39	57

Breakfast:

Sliders: Bacon, Egg & Cheese	210	12	13
Egg & Cheese	160	7	13
Ssg, Egg & Cheese	310	22	13

Waffle:

With Bacon, Egg & Cheese	350	22	27
With Sausage, Egg & Cheese	440	31	27

Toasted Sandwiches:

Bacon, Egg & Cheese	340	19	29
Egg & Cheese	230	9	29
Ssg, Egg & Cheese	380	23	29
Hash Round Nibblers: Small	340	25	23
Medium	560	42	39

Dessert:

On A Stick: Fudge Dipped Brownie	250	12	33
Fudge Dipped Cheesecake	180	10	21
Gooey Butter Cake	220	10	32

Updated Nutrition Data ~ www.CalorieKing.com
Persons with Diabetes ~ See Disclaimer (Page 22)

Wienerschnitzel® (Sept '17)

Hot Dogs: On Hot Dog Bun

	C	F	Cb
Chicago Dog	290	11	38
Chili Dog	260	12	31
Chili Cheese Dog	310	16	32
Deluxe Dog	250	10	32
Junkyard Dog	410	21	43
Kraut Dog	240	10	30
Mustard Dog	240	10	29
Relish Dog	250	10	32
Street Dog	310	16	31
Pretzel Bun Substitute, Add	80	1	15

Burgers:

Chili	320	14	28
Chili Cheeseburger	370	18	28

Specialties:

Corn Dogs: Regular (1)	230	13	21
Mini (6 pack)	300	18	24
Jalapeno Poppers, (6 pack)	300	16	31
Ranch Dressing	150	16	1
Polish Ssg S'wich	490	32	38

Sides:

Chili Cheese Fries: Regular	560	31	58
Bacon Ranch, regular	900	66	60
Triple Cheese, Double Bacon, reg.	900	66	39
French Fries: Small	310	16	38
Medium	440	23	54
Large	750	39	92
Po'taters: Small	390	27	33
Medium	670	47	56
Large	1110	78	94

Breakfast:

Biscuits: Egg, Bacon, Cheese	490	30	36
Egg, Sausage, Cheese	540	34	40
Burritos: Egg, Bacon, Cheese	370	19	29
Egg, Sausage, Cheese	460	28	33
French Toast Sticks	530	28	61
Syrup, 1 oz	120	0	31

Desserts:

Banana Split	820	24	148
Cones: Regular, Plain, 5 oz	250	9	41
Chocolate Dipped, 5 oz	450	27	50
Freezees: Choc. Strawb.	980	56	120
Oreo; M&M, Reese's, av.	630	25	99
Shakes, average all flavors	700	24	116
Sundaes:			
Caramel; Choc; Hot Fudge, av.	400	15	64
Strawberry	370	14	59
Mini Sundaes, average	190	6	33

Winchell's® (Sept '17)

Donuts: Per Donut

	C	F	Cb
Buttermilk Bars, Choc Iced/Glazed	420	19	61
Jelly Filled:			
Apple with Cinnamon Crumb	370	15	53
Raspberry with Glaze	390	13	61
Strawberry with Sugar	380	13	60
Old Fashioned, Glazed; Maple Iced	410	17	60
Raised Ring: Chocolate Iced	270	10	41
Sugared	230	9	34

WingStreet (Sept '17)

Chicken: Without Dipping Sauce

Bone Out Wings: Per Wing

	C	F	Cb
Buffalo, Mild	90	4	10
Garlic Parmesan	130	9	6
Honey BBQ	110	4	13
Ranch Rub	80	4	6

Traditional Bone In Wings: Per Wing

Buffalo, Medium/Hot	100	4.5	5
Garlic Parmesan	140	11	0.5
Spicy Garlic	120	8	3
Sides: Baked, hot/mild, av.	50	3.5	0
Breadstick (1)	140	4.5	19
Straight Cut Fries, with Ketchup	500	24	67
Stuffed Garlic Knot	80	3	11

Woody's Bar-B-Q® (Sept '17)

Starters:

	C	F	Cb
Breaded Wings (10)	700	47	13
Beef Chili Cheese Fries	805	38	63

Dinner Entrees: Without Sides

½ Chicken	840	56	0
Baby Back Combo	680	48	1
Baby Back Ribs	520	40	2
Beef Prime Rib	760	62	1
New York Strip	490	36	2
Pork Sampler	1010	62	4
Ribeye Steak	735	54	2

Sandwiches: Per Regular, without Sides

Beef	390	14	28
Pork	490	26	29

Wraps: Without Sides

Beef BBQ	380	13	31
Pork BBQ	440	21	31
Extras: BBQ Beans	170	8	20
Cobettes	80	1	18
French Fries	185	7	28
Garlic Toast	120	6	14
Green Beans	50	2.5	6
Okra	95	1	21
Squash	140	1	28

Fast - Foods & *Restaurants*

Yard House® (Jan '18)

Appetizers: With Sides & Sauce	C	F	Cb
Blue Crab Cakes	570	39	33
Buffalo Wings, Traditional	1020	68	10
California Roll	1000	56	97
Chicken Lettuce Wraps	1120	56	92
Chicken Nachos	2400	154	142
Fried Mac & Cheese	1520	103	109
Poke Nachos	910	63	52
Spinach Cheese Dip	1280	98	73
Snacks: Asado Taco (1)	240	13	16
Guacamole & Chips	480	32	44
Hot Spicy Edamame	100	5	8
Sweet Potato Fries	650	35	78
Burgers: Without Fries			
BBQ Bacon Cheddar Burger	1170	78	51
Black Truffle Chseburger	920	57	49
Kurobuta Pork Burger	850	50	54
Fries, 1 Serving	490	28	54
House Favorites: With Sides & Sauce			
Fish & Chips	1840	142	98
Mac & Cheese, w/ Chicken, full	1860	124	113
Nashville Hot Chicken	1460	68	142
Parmesan Crusted Pork Loin	1130	45	81
Spicy Jambalaya Pasta, full	1420	81	104
Pizza: Margherita	900	33	107
The Carnivore	1450	80	101
Seafood: With Sides & Sauce			
Ginger Crusted Salmon	1070	63	85
Lobster Garlic Noodles	1030	57	76
Soups:			
Chicken Tortilla, bowl	980	75	45
Clam Chowder, bowl	360	23	26
Salads: Full Entree Size, with Dressing			
Cobb Chicken Salad	980	66	31
Kale, Grilled Shrimp Caesar Salad	690	48	27

For Complete Nutritional Data ~ see CalorieKing.com

Yoshinoya® (Jan '18)

Entrees: As Served			
Angus Steak Bowl: Regular	570	11	97
Large	850	17	144
Beef Bowl: Regular	730	27	91
Large	1040	38	131
With Vegetables: Regular	650	20	95
Large	960	29	141
Teriyaki Chicken Bowl:			
Regular, without Skin	740	15	110
Large, without Skin	1090	21	156
Grilled Tilapia: with Rice & Slaw	570	13	91
with Rice, Veggies & Teriyaki Sce	590	12	100
Sides, Clam Chowder Soup	210	7	34
Kid's Meals: Beef	350	11	48
Teriyaki Chicken without skin	340	6	53

For Complete Nutritional Data ~ see CalorieKing.com

Zaxby's® (Jan '18)

Zappertizers: With Menu Set Sauce	C	F	Cb
Fried Mushrooms	590	46	39
Onion Rings & Cheddar Bites	690	42	58
Tater Chips: with Ranch Sauce	880	64	70
with Onion Rings	820	57	69
Zalads: With Texas Toast, Without Dressing			
Blackened Blue	540	27	32
Buffalo Blue	690	37	43
Fried Cobb Zalad	820	46	42
Fried House Zalad	700	38	41
Garden House Zalad	400	24	31
Grilled Cobb Zalad	680	35	34
Grilled House Zalad	560	28	33
Dressings: Per 1.2 oz Serving			
Blue Cheese	180	19	2
Caesar	90	8	2
Honey French	150	12	9
Mediterranean	140	14	4
Ranch	160	16	2
Sandwich Meals: With Menu Set Components			
Cajun Club	1040	49	92
Chicken Finger	1190	64	106
Chicken Salad	990	58	90
Grilled Chicken	900	38	97
Kickin' Chicken	1130	57	102
Nibblerz	1340	69	131
Zaxby's Club	1300	75	101
Wings & Fingers: With Sweet & Spicy Sauce			
Boneless: 5 Wings	410	19	37
10 Wings	810	37	73
20 Wings	1620	74	146
Traditional: 5 Wings	340	20	10
10 Wings	670	39	20
20 Wings	1340	78	40
Chicken Finger: 1 Finger	120	5	8
5 Fingers	600	23	42
10 Fingers	1210	47	85
20 Fingers	2420	93	180
Sides:			
Crinkle Fries: Regular, 5 oz	370	16	50
Large, 8 oz	590	36	86
Texas Toast:			
1 Slice, 1.5 oz	150	7	19
Basket, 4.5 oz	460	22	56
Kidz Meals:			
Kiddie Finger, 8.5 oz	720	41	63
Kidz Nibbler, 7.5 oz	670	31	78
Kiddie Cheese, 8.5 oz	840	46	91

Zero Sub's® ~ *see CalorieKing.com*

Fats & Cholesterol Guide

Notes on Cholesterol

- **Cholesterol** is a white waxy substance produced mainly by our liver. It is also found in animal food products. Plant foods have no cholesterol.

- **Cholesterol is essential to life.** It is a structural part of every body cell wall and is the building block for vitamin D, sex hormones, and bile acids which help in the digestion of dietary fats. **Cholesterol is also vital for a healthy brain** (which contains some 20% of total body cholesterol).

- **The body makes sufficient cholesterol** for its needs and does not rely on cholesterol in the diet. Dietary fats have a major influence on blood cholesterol levels. (See next page)

- **A high blood cholesterol level increases** the risk of atherosclerosis - the thickening of arteries that can reduce or block blood flow to the heart, brain, eyes, kidneys, sex organs and other body parts.

  This in turn increases the risk of heart attack, stroke, blindness, kidney failure, impotence and other blood circulatory problems.

  Other risk factors which increase the risk of atherosclerosis include high blood pressure, smoking, obesity and uncontrolled diabetes.

BLOOD CHOLESTEROL

CHECK YOUR RISK!

Total Cholesterol Level (mg/dl) ▼		Risk of Heart Attack ▼
240 and above	~	**High Risk**
200 - 239	~	**Borderline/High**
Below 200	~	**Desirable**

- **Know your cholesterol level, particularly if there is a family history of heart disease or stroke. If your level is high, see your doctor.**

- **All adults should have their cholesterol, HDL and triglycerides tested at least every 5 years.**

▲ **Atherosclerosis can clog arteries and impede blood flow to the heart or other body organs.**

▼ **A thrombus (blood clot) can form on unstable, festering atherosclerotic plaque and rapidly block blood flow. A heart attack or stroke can result.**

Fats & Cholesterol Guide

The amount and type of dietary fat has the greatest influence on blood cholesterol levels.

Fats in food are a mixture of 3 basic types: saturated, monounsaturated, and polyunsaturated. Animal fats are mainly saturated while plant oils and fish oils are mainly mono- and polyunsaturated.

Saturated fats have subgroups known as long-chain, medium-chain, and short-chain fats. Most of the long chain fats raise blood cholesterol, and increase the risk of blood clots and thrombosis leading to artery blockage.

Long-chain saturated fats are found mainly in full-cream milk, cheese, butter, cream, fatty meats and sausages, and processed foods.

Medium-chain fats (MCT) have little effect on LDL-cholesterol but may raise "good" HDL. *Note: Coconut oil has some MCT but is mainly saturated fat – so limit use.*

Monounsaturated fats tend to more selectively lower 'bad' LDL cholesterol and maintain the protective 'good' HDL cholesterol in the bloodstream – but only if they replace saturated fats in the diet. Foods rich in monounsaturates include canola and olive oils, canola margarine, peanuts, and avocados.

Polyunsaturated fats consist of two main classes. **Omega-6** polyunsaturates tend to lower blood cholesterol. Rich sources include safflower, sunflower and corn oils.

Omega-3 polyunsaturated fats can lower blood cholesterol; significantly lower blood triglycerides; and reduce the rise of thrombosis, heart arrythmmia, and artery spasm.

Best practical omega-3 sources include canola oil and margarine, soybean oil and fish.

A balanced intake of the two omega classes is important for optimal health. For most Americans, slightly increasing omega-3 intake would help attain a more ideal balance.

Trans fats from hydrogenated vegetable oils and shortenings should also be avoided. They are common in commercial baked and fried food products such as cakes, muffins, pastries, doughnuts, fried snacks and french fries.

DIETARY FATS COMPARISON

■ Saturated Fat   ▨ Monounsaturated Fat
Polyunsaturated Fats:
▨ Linoleic (Omega-6)   ■ Alpha-Linolenic (Omega-3)

OILS — PERCENTAGE CONTENT

OIL	Saturated Fat	Monounsaturated Fat	Linoleic (Omega-6)	Alpha-Linolenic (Omega-3)
CANOLA OIL	7	63	20	10
LINSEED/FLAX OIL	9	19	17	55
SAFFLOWER OIL	9	14	77	
GRAPESEED OIL	10	22	68	
SUNFLOWER OIL	11	23	66	
CORN OIL	14	32	52	2
OLIVE OIL	14	76		10
SOYBEAN OIL	15	23	54	8
PEANUT OIL	19	45	34	2
COTTONSEED OIL	26	16	58	
PALM OIL	51	39		10

SPREADS & FATS
Saturated Fat includes 'Trans Fats'   ☐ WATER CONTENT

	Saturated Fat	Monounsaturated	Linoleic	Alpha-Linolenic	Water Content
LIGHT MARGARINE	14	14	21		51
CANOLA MARGARINE	18	45	12	6	19
POLYUNSATURATED MARG	24	20	36		20
BUTTER	57		18	2	24
LARD	41	47			12
BEEF FAT	44	37	4		15

GOOD SOURCES OF OMEGA-3 FATS

Plant Sources	Omega-3 Fats (Grams)
Canola Oil, 1 Tbsp, ½ fl.oz	1.5g
Flaxseed Oil, 1 Tbsp	8g
Soybean Oil, 1 Tbsp	1.2g
Canola Margarine, 1 Tbsp, ½ oz	1g
Soybeans, cooked, ½ cup, 4 oz	0.5g
Walnuts, ½ oz	0.5g

FISH - *Per 4 oz Serving*

High Content: Salmon (Chinook), Tuna,	3g
Trout (Lake), Sardines, Herring, Mackerel	3g
Medium Content:	
Salmon, (Pink/Red/Coho), 4 oz	2g

Fair Content: *Per 4 oz Serving*
Bass, Catfish, Cod, Grouper, Hake, Halibut, Kingfish, Perch, Pollock, Shark, Trout (Rainbow), Tuna, Crab, Oysters, Blue Mussels, Shrimp, Squid } 0.5-1g

How Much Is Needed?

As little as 1-2 grams daily of omega-3 fats may benefit general health. High doses of fish-oil supplements should only be taken as directed by your Healthcare provider.

Dietary Cholesterol

Cholesterol in food varies in its effect on blood cholesterol level (BCL) from person to person. Much depends on the amount and type of fat and fiber eaten at the same meal.

Any elevating effect of dietary cholesterol on BCL is more likely to occur when the diet is high in saturated fat. Little elevation, if any, generally occurs when dietary fats are balanced in favor of mono- and poly-unsaturated fats (including omega-3 fats).

Example: While fish does contain cholesterol, the omega-3 fats can prevent any increase in BCL. Conversely, a meal containing no cholesterol but rich in saturated fat may result in a significant increase in BCL - as well as impairing artery wall functions.

Consequently, the need to be overly concerned about dietary cholesterol is being de-emphasized in favor of simply limiting total fat, saturated fat, and trans fat in particular – and substituting unsaturated fats (including omega-3 fats).

Note: Persons with familial (genetic) hyper-cholesterolemia should limit cholesterol; and ideally follow a plant-based diet.

The liver usually cuts back its own cholesterol production in response to cholesterol in the diet. Many people can consume high-cholesterol foods without concern.

However, it is difficult to identify just who is at risk - the so-called 'hyper-responders'. Because over 50% of Americans have a BCL above ideal levels, it may be prudent to limit cholesterol intake to less than 300mg daily, as well as to adopt a heart-healthy diet.

This limitation still allows the inclusion of most foods that are regularly eaten – even the overly maligned egg.

Avocados (like all plant foods) contain no cholesterol. Their fats are mainly monounsaturated and can lower blood cholesterol.

CHOLESTEROL COUNTER

Cholesterol is found only in foods of animal origin. Plant foods contain no cholesterol.

	Cholesterol mg
Meat - Average all types:	
Lean Meat, cooked, 120g	100
Fatty Meat, cooked, 120g	100
Fat, thick strip, 60g	40

Note: While lean meat and fat have similar amounts of cholesterol, choose lean meat to limit fat intake.

	Cholesterol mg
Chicken/Turkey, average, 120g	100
Organ Meats: Liver, fried, 4 oz	500
Brains, beef, pan fried, 3 oz	1700
Sausages: Frankfurter, 40g	25
Salami, 2 slices, 55g	40
Bacon: 3 slices, cooked, 30g	20
Fish: Fish fillets, average, ckd, 120g	70
Tuna/Salmon, canned, 100g	50
Scallops, 9 medium, 3 oz	30
Prawns, raw, 100g	110
Oysters, raw, 6 medium, 85g	45
Crayfish, Crab, cooked, 100g	70
Eggs (Chicken), 1 large	210
1 medium	180
Egg White, *Scramblers*	0
Milk/Yoghurt: Whole, 1 cup, 250ml	30
Light/low-fat Milk (1%), 1 cup	10
Skim/Non-fat, 1 cup	10
Soy Milk, Tofu, Tempeh	0
Cheese: Natural/Hard/Cream, 30g	30
Cottage, low-fat, 2 Tbsp, 40g	5
Cream Cheese, 30g	25
Fats: Butter, 1 Tbsp, 20g	45
Margarine, Oils (vegetable)	0
Mayonnaise, 1 Tbsp	10
Cream: Heavy, whipping, 2 Tbsp, 40g	40
Light/Sour, 2 Tbsp	10
Ice Cream: Full-fat (10-11%), 100ml/50g	20
Low-fat (less than 4%), 50g	5
Fruit, Vegetables, Avocados	0
Nuts, Seeds, Grains	0
Coffee, Tea, Beer, Wine	0

For Comprehensive Food Listings ~ see www.CalorieKing.com

Blood Cholesterol ~ Diet Hints

DIETARY HINTS TO LOWER BLOOD CHOLESTEROL

1. **Maintain a healthy weight.**
   If overweight, lose weight with a sensible, low-fat meal plan and daily exercise.

2. **Reduce saturated fat intake by:**

   (a) eating less dairy fat. Choose low-fat or fat-reduced varieties of milk, yogurt, soy drinks, cheese, and ice cream.

   (b) replacing saturated fats with fats and oils rich in monounsaturated and polyunsaturated fats. Choose vegetable oils such as extra-virgin olive, canola and soybean. Avoid solid frying fats.

   Note: *Promise Active* and *Benecol* spreads contain plant stanol esters which can lower total and LDL cholesterol.

   (c) eating less fat from meat and poultry. Choose lean cuts of meat and skinless chicken. Go easy on lunch meats, salami and fatty sausages. Enjoy fish.

   (d) eating less saturated and trans fats from baked and fried fast-foods. Avoid deep-fried foods. Avoid donuts, cakes, pastries and cookies unless made with healthier fats and oils.

3. **Increase your soluble fiber intake.**
   Foods rich in soluble fiber include beans, lentils, chickpeas, hummus, nuts, seeds, psyllium-seed husks and psyllium-fiber supplements. Oat bran, rice bran and barley are also good sources, as are fruit, vegetables and avocados.
   (See Fiber Guide - Page 264-269).

4. **Eat more soy bean products such as:**
   soy drinks, tofu, tempeh (cultured soy beans), soy flour, soy vegetarian foods and edamame (fresh green soybeans).

   Soy protein in place of animal protein can significantly decrease high blood cholesterol levels as well as 'bad' LDL cholesterol and blood triglycerides while 'good' HDL cholesterol is maintained. For best results, eat at least 25g of soy protein per day (from 3-4 servings).

5. **Eat more fruit, vegetables, and whole grains** in place of high-fat foods. Aim for 2 fruits and 5 servings of vegetables per day. They also contain valuable antioxidants. The fat of avocados (and most nuts) is mainly unsaturated and can lower blood cholesterol levels.

6. **Limit cholesterol to 300mg per day.**
   (Extra Notes ~ See Previous Page)

7. **Avoid brewed unfiltered coffee**
   (espresso; plunger-style). Several cups per day may raise blood cholesterol. Filtered coffee is fine.

8. **Spread your food intake over the day.**
   Have 5-6 small meals per day rather than just 2-3 large meals. Nibbling, versus gorging, favors lower blood cholesterol.

ALCOHOL – WINE

Alcohol is a mixed bag. Moderate amounts of 1-2 drinks daily appear to reduce the risk of heart attack and ischemic stroke in older persons.

However, larger amounts increase the risk of high blood pressure, obesity, heart failure and hemorrhagic stroke, and can aggravate hypertriglyceridemia: as well as many other health hazards. (See Alcohol Guide – Page 23)

The speculative benefits of moderate alcohol intake have been overstated in the media. The overriding harmful effects of excess alcohol do not allow its recommendation for any aspects of health promotion.

Fruit, Vegetables & Tea Also Protect:

Red wine and red grapes (more so than white) contain antioxidants which may help protect cholesterol in the blood from becoming oxidized.

Many fruits, vegetables, grains, nuts and tea also contain protective antioxidants.

Fats in the diet affect more than blood cholesterol levels. They can also strongly influence blood clot formation and thrombosis, as well as blood flow and ultimate oxygen delivery to body parts and organs. While advanced atherosclerosis can impede blood flow to the heart and other organs, it is thrombosis (complete blockage by blood clots) or arterial spasm which commonly results in a heart attack or stroke.

Plant and fish oils rich in omega-3 fats lessen the risk of blood clots, thrombus formation, and artery spasm by reducing platelet stickiness and adhesion to artery walls. This also reduces inflammation of the artery wall lining. This in turn reduces the risk of atherosclerotic plaque becoming unstable and reactive.

Omega-3 fats also improve blood flow by reducing blood viscosity and increasing the flexibility of red blood cells that need to flex and twist on themselves in order to squeeze through tiny narrow capillaries often half their diameter.

A diet high in saturated fats (longer chain) has the opposite effect by stiffening red blood cell membranes and increasing blood viscosity, thereby hindering blood flow.

Stiff red blood cells may also form aggregates that resemble coin stacks. In narrow blood vessels, this further impedes blood flow and impairs oxygen release through the much-lessened surface area of red blood cell membranes exposed to blood.

Note: Smoking, lack of exercise, and stress can have similar adverse effects on thrombosis, red blood cell flexibility, and blood flow.

▲ *Picture of Healthy Blood Flow*

Flexible red blood cells twist and slide through tiny capillaries - often half the diameter of red blood cells.

▲ *A Not-So-Healthy Picture!*

Red blood cells have lost their flexibility and ability to twist and slip through capillaries. They are stacked up, thereby impeding blood flow.

A diet high in saturated fats can contribute to this picture - as can smoking, lack of exercise, and stress.

Fiber Guide

Introduction

`Fiber`

Fiber is the general term for those parts of plant food that we cannot digest (although bacteria in the large bowel partly digests fiber through fermentation). It is not found in foods of animal origin (meats, dairy products).

Fiber promotes intestinal health, bowel regularity, can benefit diabetes and blood cholesterol levels, and may help prevent colon cancer. High-fiber foods also assist weight control.

Most Americans don't eat enough fiber – less than 20 grams/day – instead of a healthier 25 to 35 grams/day.

A fiber-rich diet assists the growth of friendly gut microbes that can benefit our metabolism, weight and blood glucose levels – as well as hunger, mood and our immune system.

Types of Fiber

Plant foods contain a mixture of different fibers in varying proportions. Insoluble and soluble fiber categories are based on their solubility in water. All types of fiber are beneficial to the body.

♦ Insoluble fibers (cellulose, hemi-celluloses, lignin) make up the structural parts of plant cell walls.

Best food sources are wheat bran, corn bran, rice bran, wholegrain cereals and breads, beans and peas, nuts, seeds, and the skins of fruits and vegetables.

These fibers absorb many times their own weight in water. They create a soft bulk and hasten the passage of waste products through the intestines.

They promote bowel regularity, and aid in the prevention and treatment of uncomplicated forms of **constipation, diverticulosis and hemorrhoids.**

The risk of colon cancer may also be reduced by fiber's diluting effect on potentially harmful substances.

♦ Soluble fibers **(pectin, gums, mucilages)** are found mainly within plant cells, soy milk (whole bean) and products.

Best Sources of Soluble Fiber:

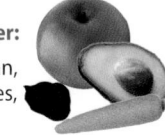

Fruits and vegetables, oat bran, barley, beans and peas, prunes, psyllium and flax seed.

These fibers form a gel which slows both stomach emptying and the absorption of sugars from the intestines. **This helps to control blood sugar levels.**

Weight control is also aided by the slower emptying of the stomach and the feeling of **fullness provided by soluble fiber.**

Soluble fiber can also lower blood cholesterol by binding bile acids and excreting them. More body cholesterol must then be broken down to supply bile acids for emulsification of dietary fats. **Rice bran, while not high in soluble fiber, can also lower blood cholesterol.**

♦ **Resistant starch** is that part of starchy foods (approx. 10%) which is tightly bound by fiber and resists normal digestion. Friendly bacteria in the large bowel ferment and change the resistant starch into short-chain fatty acids, which are important to bowel health and may protect against colon cancer.

Starchy foods include bread, cereals, rice, pasta, potatoes and legumes.

Fiber & Weight Control

Fiber can assist weight control in several ways. Fiber-rich foods such as fresh fruit and vegetables, potatoes and wholegrain bread contain few calories for their large volume (due to their low-fat, high-water content).

Their bulk fills the stomach and satisfies the appetite much sooner than fiber-depleted foods. The extra chewing time also contributes to satiety, and gives the stomach time to register a feeling of fullness. Excessive calories are less likely to be consumed.

Fiber-depleted foods and drinks are more concentrated in calories; e.g. fats, sugar, candy, soft drinks, fruit juices, alcohol. They require little or no chewing. Large amounts with excessive calories can be consumed before the appetite is satisfied.

Example: Whereas one fresh apple might satisfy the appetite, an apple juice drink with the equivalent sugars and calories of 2-3 apples only minimally satisfies the appetite. (See illustration below.)

High-fiber foods fill the stomach. Fewer calories are consumed.

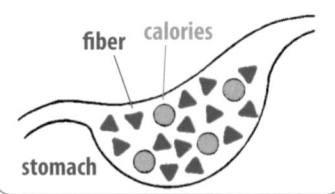

Low-fiber foods are more concentrated in calories. More food must be eaten to fill the stomach.

EFFECTS OF REMOVING FIBER FROM FOOD

2-3 pieces of fresh fruit produces 1 glass of fruit juice. The removal of fiber concentrates the sugar and calories.

FIBER REMOVED

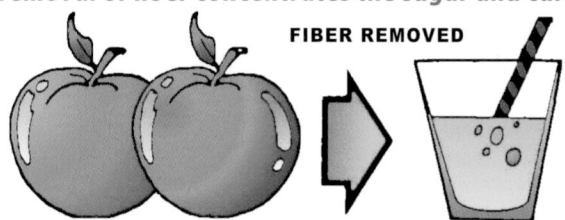

FRESH FRUIT	(Comparison)	FRUIT JUICE
High Fiber	←	Negligible Fiber
Low Calorie Density	←	High Calorie Density
Long Eating Time	←	No Eating Time (Drink)
Satisfies Hunger	←	Does Not Satisfy Hunger
Sugar Slowly Absorbed	←	Sugar More Quickly Absorbed
Less Insulin Required	←	More Insulin Required
Supports Gut Microbes	←	Few Benefits to Microbes

Fiber Guide ~ Constipation

Constipation

Constipation can reasonably be defined as a failure to have a bowel movement at least every second day – and just as importantly, without straining or pain.

Typically, constipated stools are too hard, too narrow and too small.

The **main cause** is simply a lack of dietary fiber. Other contributing factors include insufficient fluids, too little exercise, emotional stress, gastrointestinal disease, lack of proper dentition to chew high-fiber foods, and some medications (e.g. some antacids, antidepressants, pain medications).

Note: Check with your doctor to rule out any underlying medical problem – especially if you have a change in bowel habits in middle-age or later years.

DESIRABLE FIBER INTAKE

Adults: **25-35gm per day**
Children (under 18): **Age + 5gm**
Example: 6-year old (6 + 5)= **11gm**

SAMPLE FOOD QUANTITIES
For 35 Grams of Fiber/Day

	Fiber
Breakfast Cereal (higher-fiber)	5g
plus 4 slices wholegrain Bread	6g
plus 3 servings fresh Fruit	9g
plus 1 medium Potato (w. skin)	⎫
or 1 cup Brown Rice	⎬ 4g
or ½ cup wholegrain Pasta	⎭
plus 3-4 servings Veggies/Salad	6g
plus 1 cup Bean Soup	⎫
or ¼ cup Baked/Soy Beans	⎪
or ½ cup Corn/Peas/Lentils	⎬ 5g
or 1¼ oz Almonds (natural)	⎪
or 3 medium Figs	⎭

HINTS TO INCREASE FIBER AND AVOID CONSTIPATION

❶ Breakfast is an important contributor to daily fiber intake. Eat high-fiber breakfast cereals (bran-based cereals, oatmeal etc.). Add 1-2 tablespoons of unprocessed bran.

Dried fruits, chopped nuts, soy grits, and seeds are also excellent additions to cereals.

Note: A gradual increase in fiber will prevent bloating, gas or pain. People intolerant to bran may benefit from psyllium-based fiber supplements and cereals.

❷ Drink adequate water daily. Fiber works by absorbing many times its own weight in water.

❸ Eat wholegrain breads, or fiber-enriched breads. They have over double the fiber of regular white bread.

❹ Enjoy fruit as fresh fruit with skin rather than as fruit juice. Enjoy wholegrain pasta, barley, brown rice, nuts and seeds.

❺ Eat more vegetables, salads and legumes – especially cooked beans, lentils, potatoes with skins, avocado, broccoli, brussels sprouts, cabbage, carrots, celery, and peas.

❻ Add bran (barley/rice/wheat) or soy grits to soups, casseroles, yogurt, desserts, cookies, cakes. Also use whole-meal flour or soy flour in place of white flour. Use nuts, seeds, and ground linseed.

❼ Snack on fresh or dried fruits, carrot or celery sticks, popcorn, nuts or seeds, wholegrain crackers, high-fiber bars (low-fat). Limit amounts if overweight.

❽ Exercise regularly to strengthen abdominal muscles and stimulate the gut. Keep up water intake, especially in warm weather.

❾ Avoid indiscriminate and regular use of harsh laxatives. They can overstimulate the intestinal muscles and may make normal bowel activity impossible. It may take several weeks to restore normal bowel function.

FOODS WITH ZERO FIBER
- **Dairy Products (Milk, Cheese, etc)**
- **Meats, Poultry, Fish, Eggs**
- **Fats/Oils, Sugar/Syrups**
  (Only foods of plant origin contain fiber.)

Fiber ~ Fiber (grams)

Breakfast Cereals   **Fiber**

General Mills:
Basic 4, 1 cup, 2 oz	3
Cheerios (Honey Nut; Multigrain), 1 c., 1 oz	2
Fiber One, $^1/_2$ cup, 1.1 oz	14
Multi-Bran Chex, 1 cup, 2 oz	7
Oatmeal Crisp Almond, 1 cup, 2 oz	4
Raisin Nut Bran, $1^1/_4$ cup, 2 oz	6
Total, average all types, $^3/_4$ cup, 1 oz	3
Wheat Chex, 1 cup, 2 oz	6
Wheaties $^3/_4$ cup, 1 oz	3

Health Valley:
Amaranth Flakes, $^3/_4$ cup, 1 oz	3
Crunches & Flakes, $^3/_4$ cup, 1.9 oz	4
Fiber 7 Flakes, $^3/_4$ cup, 1 oz	7
Golden Flax, $^3/_4$ cup, 1.9 oz	6
Granola (Low-Fat), $^3/_4$ cup, 2 oz	6
Healthy Fiber Flakes, $^3/_4$ cup, 1.1 oz	4
Oat Bran Flakes, all types, $^3/_4$ cup, 1 oz	2
Oat Bran O's, $^3/_4$ cup, 1 oz	3
Real Oat Bran, $^1/_2$ cup, 1.7 oz	5

Kellogg's:
All-Bran, $^1/_2$ cup, 1.1 oz	10
All-Bran w. Extra Fiber, $^1/_2$ cup, 1 oz	13
All-Bran Bran Buds, $^1/_3$ cup, 1.1 oz	13
Corn Flakes, Fruit Loops, Smacks 1 cup, 1 oz	1
Cocoa/Rice Krispies Treats, $1^1/_4$ cup, 1 oz	0
Complete: Wheat Flakes, $^3/_4$ c., 1 oz	5
Oat Bran Flakes, $^3/_4$ cup, 1.1 oz	4
Corn Pops, 1 cup, 1.1 oz	0
Cracklin' Oat Bran, $^3/_4$ cup, 1.7oz	6
FiberPlus Antioxidants:	
Berry Yogurt Crunch, 1 c., 1.9 oz	10
Cinnamon Oat Crunch $^3/_4$ c., 1.1 oz	9
Frosted Mini Wheats, 24 bisc., 2 oz	5
Granola w. Raisins, $^2/_3$ cup, 2.1 oz	3
Raisin Bran, 1 cup, 2.1 oz	7
Smart Start, Strong Heart,	
Cinnamon Raisin, 1 cup, 1.8 oz	4
Special K, 1 cup, 1.1 oz	0.5

Breakfast Cereals (Cont)

Kashi:
GoLEAN Cereal, 1 cup, 1.8 oz	10
GoLEAN Crunch!, 1 cup, 1.9 oz	8
GoLEAN Bars, avg. (1)	6
Good Friends: Original, 1 cup, 1.9 oz	12
Cinna-Raisin Crunch, 1 cup, 1.8 oz	8
Heart to Heart, $^3/_4$ cup, 1.2 oz	5
7 Whole Grain Pilaf, $^1/_2$ cup, cooked, 5 oz	7
7 Whole Grain Puffs, 1 cup, 0.7 oz	1

Quaker:
Cap'n Crunch, $^3/_4$ cup, 1 oz	1
100% Natural Granola,	
avg., $^1/_2$ cup, 1.8 oz	3
Crunchy Corn Bran, 1 cup, 1 oz	5
Life Cereal, $^3/_4$ cup, 1.1 oz	2
Oat Bran, $^1/_2$ cup, 1.4 oz	6
Oatmeal, average, 1 packet	3

Post:
100% Bran, $^1/_3$ cup, 1 oz	9
Alpha Bits, 1 cup, 1 oz	2
Blueberry Morning, 1 cup, 1.9 oz	5
Cranberry Almond Crunch, 1 cup, 1.8 oz	3
Fruit & Bran, 1 cup, 1.9 oz	6
Grape-Nuts, $^1/_2$ cup, 2 oz	7
Great Grains, $^2/_3$ cup, 1.9 oz	5
Honey Bunches of Oats, $^3/_4$ cup, 1.1 oz	2
Shredded Wheat & Bran, $^1/_2$ cup, 2 oz	8

Brans & Supplements, Metamucil
Oat Bran: 1 Tbsp (level)	1
$^1/_3$ cup, ($5^1/_3$ Tbsp), 1 oz	5
Rice Bran, raw. $^1/_3$ cup, 1 oz	6
Wheat Bran, Unprocessed:	
Raw, 1 Tbsp	1.5
2 Tbsp (level), $^1/_4$ oz	3
$^1/_4$ cup, (4 Tbsp), $^1/_2$ oz	6
Wheat Germ, Raw, $^1/_4$ cup, 1 oz	4
Psyllium Seed Husks, 2 Tbsp	8
Fibersure, 1 heaping tsp	5
Metamucil: Orange, 1 rnd Tbsp, 11g	3
Fiber Wafers (2)	6

Hot Cereals, Oatmeal
Bulgur (cracked Wheat), ckd, 1 cup	8
Corn/Hominy Grits, dry, 3 Tbsp, 1 oz	0.5
Cream of Wheat, cooked, $^3/_4$ cup	1
Oatmeal (uncooked $^1/_3$ cup), ckd, $^2/_3$ cup	3

Fiber Counter

Breads & Crackers

	Fiber
Bread: White, 1 slice, 1 oz	0.6
Whole-wheat, 1 slice, 1 oz	1.5
Wholegrain, 1 slice, 1 oz	2
Rye, Pumpernickel, 1 oz	1.5
Bagel/Roll/Bun, 1 medium, 2 oz	1.5
Pita, whole wheat, 6.5" pocket	4.5
Crackers: Graham, average, 2	0.4
Saltine, 4 crackers	0.4
Crispbreads, average, 2	4
Matzo, 1 board, 1 oz	1
Rice Cakes, average, 1 cake	0.3
Tortilla: Regular, 6"	0.5
Whole-wheat, 6"	1.3

Barley, Pasta, Rice & Flours

	Fiber
Barley, pearled, raw, 1/4 cup, 1.7 oz	8
Rice:	
White, cooked, 1 cup	0.6
Brown, cooked, 1 cup	3.5
Rice-A-Roni, average, 1 cup, prepared	1.5
Spaghetti/Noodles: Cooked, 1 cup	2
Whole-Wheat, cooked, 1 cup	4
Flour: Wheat, All-purpose, 1 cup, 4.5 oz	3.5
Whole-Wheat, 1 cup, 4.5 oz	15
Cornmeal, stone ground, 1 cup, 4.5 oz	13
Carob Flour, 1 cup, 3.5 oz	41
Rye Flour, 1 cup, 3.5 oz	15
Soy Flour: Defatted, 1 cup, 3.5 oz	17
Full-fat, raw, 1 cup, 3 oz	8
Soy Meal, defatted, 1 cup, 4.5 oz	14

Frozen Entrees & Dinners

Average All Brands: Per Serving

	Fiber
Beans/Chili base, average	6-10
Potato/Pasta base, average	4-6
Vegetable base, average	3
Meat/Chicken base, average	2-3
Pizzas, 1/4 large, average	3
Vegetarian Soy Burgers, 1 pattie	4

Soups

	Fiber
Chicken Noodle, 1 cup	0.5
Tomato Soup, average, 1 cup	0.5
Vegetable Soup, average, 1 cup	3
Health Valley: Per 1 Cup	
Black Bean; Minestrone	8
Tomato	1
5 Bean Vegetable; Lentil & Carrots	10
Mushroom Barley; Vegetable	4
Split Pea	8
Progresso, High Fiber, all flavors, 1 cup	7

Fast Foods & Restaurants

	Fiber
Hamburgers: Small, average	1.5
Large/Whopper, average	2.5
Hot Dog, Regular	1.5
French Fries: Small serving, 2.5 oz	2.5
Regular/Medium, 3.5 oz	3.5
Chicken Nuggets, 6 pack	0.5
Chicken Sandwich, average	2
Taco, average	4
Sundaes, Shakes, Soft Drinks	0
Arby's, Classic Roast Beef Sandwich	1
Denny's: Grilled Chicken Salad, no bread	4
Classic Burger, no fries	4
Club Sandwich, no fries	2
Grilled Chicken Sandwich, no fries	4
Domino's: 12", Classic/Thin, 1 slice	1
Deep Dish, 1 slice	3
Feast Pizza, Classic/Thin, 1 slice	2
McDonald's: Big Mac	3
Hamburger; Quarter Pounder	3
Egg McMuffin	2
Grilled Chicken Caesar Salad	3
Pizza Hut: Per 1 Slice, Medium	
Pan Pizza: Cheese, Pepperoni	1
Supreme	2
Thin 'n Crispy, Supreme	2
Hand-Tossed, average all varieties	2
Subway: Sandwich, white roll, av.	4
With Honey Wheat Roll, average	3
Salads, average	4

Cakes, Cookies, Snack Bars

	Fiber
Apple/Fruit Pie, 1 serving, 4 oz	2
Cake: With plain flour, 1 serving, 3.4 oz	1.5
With whole-wheat flour, 1 serving	3
Carrot Cake, 4 oz	4
Cookies, oatmeal, (3 small/1 large)	1
Donuts, medium, 1.7 oz	0.7
Fruit Cake, 1 serving, 1.5 oz	2
Fig Bars, 1 cookie, 0.5 oz	0.7
Muffins, Oat Bran (2 small, 1 large), 4 oz	5
Granola Bars, average, 1 bar	2
Atkins Advantage Bars, average	7
Clif Bars, 2.5 oz	5
Curves, Chocolate Peanut Bar, 1 oz	5
Fi-Bar Chewy & Nutty, 1 bar	1
Fiber One (Gen. Mills), 1.4 oz bar	9
FiberPlus, all bars, 1.2 oz	9
Health Valley: Fruit/Granola Bars	3
Cereal Bars	1
Luna Bars, avg., 1.7 oz	3
Special K, Protein Meal Bar, 1.6 oz	5

Fiber Counter

Chocolate, Chips, Popcorn

	Fiber
Cheese Balls/Curls/Twists	1
Chocolate, Hard Candy, 1 oz	0
Chocolate with nuts/fruit, 2 oz bar	1.5
Mars Bar, 1.8 oz	1
Potato Chips; corn chips, 1 oz	1
Popcorn, 3 cups	3
Pretzels, Twists (6)	1

Nuts, Seeds

	Fiber
Almonds: Natural, 25 nuts, 1 oz	3.5
Blanched (skins removed), 1 oz	3
Cashews, Filberts, Pecans, 1 oz	1.7
Peanuts, Mixed Nuts, Coconut, 1 oz	2.5
Peanut Butter, 2 Tbsp, 1 oz	2
Pistachio Nuts, dried, shelled, 1 oz	3
Walnuts, Black/English, dried, 1 oz	2
Seeds: Amaranth, 2^1/$_2$ Tbsp, 1 oz	3.5
Flax Seeds, 3 Tbsp, 1 oz	7
Psyllium Seed Husks, 5 Tbsp, 1 oz	20
Quinoa Seeds, 3 Tbsp, 1 oz	1.7
Sesame Seeds, whole, 1 oz	3.4
Sesame Butter/Tahini, 2 Tbsp, 1.1 oz	1.4
Sunflower kernels, ^{1}/$_4$ cup, 1 oz	3.8
Teff Seeds, 1 oz	3.8

Fruit – Fresh

	Fiber
Apples: 1 medium, 5^1/$_2$ oz (whole)	
with skin + core	3.7
with skin, no core	3.2
without skin, no core	1.7
Apricots, 2 medium, 4 oz	1.5
Avocado, average, ^{1}/$_2$ medium	6
Banana, 1 medium, 6 oz (w. skin)	3
Blueberries, raw, ^{1}/$_2$ cup, 2.5 oz	1.7
Cherries, sweet, raw, 8 fruits, 1.6 oz	1
Grapefruit, average, ^{1}/$_2$ fruit, 10 oz	1.4
Grapes, 1 medium bunch, seedless, 7 oz	2
Kiwifruit, 1 medium, 2.7 oz	2.3
Mango, 1 medium, 11 oz (whole)	1.6
Melons, Cantaloupe, 4 oz (edible)	1
Nectarine, 1 medium, 4 oz	1.9
Olives, average all types, 7 jumbo, 2 oz	1.5
Oranges, 1 medium (7-8 oz w. skin)	
5^1/$_2$ oz (peeled)	3.8
Passionfruit, 2 medium, 2.5 oz	5
Peaches, 1 large, 6 oz	2
Pears, raw, 1 medium, 6 oz	4.5
Pineapple, 1 slice, 3 oz	1.2
Plums, 2 medium, 6 oz	1.8
Strawberries, 6 medium/3 large, 2 oz	1
Watermelon, 4 oz (edible)	0.5

Fruit – Dried, Juice

	Fiber
Dried Fruit: Apricots, 8 halves, 1 oz	2.2
Dates (3 med); Raisins (2 Tbsp), 1 oz	1.5
Figs, 3 medium, 1^1/$_2$ oz	5
Prunes, 4 medium, 1 oz	2
Fruit Juice: Orange/Apple etc, 1 glass	<0.5
Prune Juice, 5 oz	1.4
Carrot Juice, 8 oz	1.8

Vegetables

	Fiber
Asparagus, 4 medium spears	1.3
Bean Sprouts, ^{1}/$_2$ cup, 2 oz	1
Beans: Snap/Green, ^{1}/$_2$ cup, 2 oz	2
Baked Beans in Tom Sce, ^{1}/$_2$ c, 4.5 oz	5
Dried Beans, ckd, average, ^{1}/$_2$ cup	7
Beets, ckd, slices, ^{1}/$_2$ cup, 3 oz	1.7
Broccoli, cooked, ^{1}/$_2$ cup, 3 oz	2.4
Brussels Sprouts, ckd, ^{1}/$_2$ cup, 3 oz	3.5
Cabbage: White, ckd, ^{1}/$_2$ cup, 2.5 oz	1
Red, ckd, ^{1}/$_2$ cup, 2.5 oz	1
Carrots, 1 medium (7^1/$_2$"), ^{1}/$_2$ cup, 3 oz	2.5
Cauliflower, cooked, 3 flowerets, 2 oz	1.5
Celery, raw, diced, 1 cup, 3.5 oz	1.6
Chickpeas (Garbanzos), ckd, ^{1}/$_2$ c., 3 oz	6.5
Corn: Kernels, cooked, ^{1}/$_2$ cup, 2^1/$_2$ oz	2.5
Corn on the Cob, 1 ear, 5 oz	4
Cucumber/Lettuce/Mushrooms, 2 oz	0.5
Eggplant, raw, sliced, ^{1}/$_2$ cup, 1.5 oz	2
Lentils, cooked, ^{1}/$_2$ cup, 3.5 oz	8
Mixed Vegetables, frozen, cooked, ^{1}/$_2$ cup	3
Onions: Raw, 1 medium, 4 oz	1.5
Spring Onions, chop., ^{1}/$_4$ cup, 1 oz	0.7
Peas: Green, raw, ^{1}/$_2$ cup, 2.5 oz	3.7
Cowpeas (Black-eyed), ckd, ^{1}/$_2$ cup	10
Split Peas, cooked, ^{1}/$_2$ cup, 3.5 oz	8
Peppers, sweet, raw, 1 large, 6 oz	3
Potatoes: 1 medium, with skin, 5 oz	4
1 medium, without skin	2.5
^{1}/$_2$ cup mashed, 3.5 oz	1.5
French Fries, small, 2.6 oz	3
Spinach, cooked, ^{1}/$_2$ cup, 3 oz	2.2
Squash: Summer, cooked, ^{1}/$_2$ cup, 3 oz	2.5
Winter, cooked, ^{1}/$_2$ cup, 3.5 oz	2.4
Tomatoes: 1 medium, 4.5 oz	1.5
Tomato Sauce, 1 cup	0.3
Soybean Products: Miso, ^{1}/$_2$ c., 5 oz	7.4
Tempeh, cooked, 1 piece, 3 oz	3
Tofu, ^{1}/$_2$ cup, 4.4 oz	0.4

Salads:

	Fiber
Side Salad, average	1
Bean Salad, ^{1}/$_2$ cup	5
Coleslaw, ^{1}/$_2$ cup	1
Potato Salad, ^{1}/$_2$ cup	2

Protein Guide

General Notes

- **Protein has many important body functions.** It builds and repairs muscle, and is the basis of our body's organs, hormones, enzymes, and antibodies to fight infection.

- **Protein is also an emergency fuel** in the absence of sufficient carbohydrate and fats. For this reason, weight loss should be gradual so as to preserve protein levels in muscle, the heart and other body organs.

- **It is easy to obtain sufficient protein,** even if vegetarian. **Plant proteins are not inferior to animal proteins.** In fact, eating more soy and other plant proteins, and less animal protein, may help to build stronger bones and prevent osteoporosis, and may help to control blood cholesterol levels.

- **When changing to a vegetarian diet,** include soybeans, and other beans, soy milk drinks (calcium-enriched), lentils, tofu, tempeh, nuts and wholegrain breads and cereals. Milk, yogurt, cheese and eggs can enhance nutrient intake.

Protein & Muscle

- Although muscles are built of protein, protein is not a special fuel for working muscle cells – carbohydrates and fats are.

- In fact, a diet high in protein (and fat) and low in carbohydrate can significantly reduce the performance of endurance sports athletes. **Carbohydrates** are the best fuel for muscles exercised for long periods.

- Any **extra protein** required by athletes and body-builders can easily be obtained from the extra food eaten to satisfy hunger and energy needs.

- Remember, **excessive protein** intake will not build bigger muscles. Any excess is converted and stored as fat. Excess protein can also strain the kidneys, which excrete the waste products of protein metabolism.

Elderly people (and dieters) must eat sufficient food to ensure adequate protein intake.

Inadequate protein leads to a drop in immune response with greater susceptibility to illness and infections. Muscle strength and muscle mass also drop.

Protein needs are easily met with sensible eating. Athletes who eat enough food for their energy needs can obtain sufficient protein.

RECOMMENDED DAILY PROTEIN INTAKE
~ HEALTHY RANGE ~
(Lower figure is RDA)

		PROTEIN
Children:	1-3 yrs	13g-26g
	4-8 yrs	19g-38g
	9-13 yrs	34g-64g
Males:	14-18 yrs	52g-120g
	19+	56g-120g
Females:	14+	46g-110g
Pregnancy:		71g-120g
Breastfeeding:		71g-120g

Note: On lower-calorie diets, aim for higher amounts of protein within the Healthy Range.

Pro ~ Protein (grams)

Meat

	Pro
Bacon, 3 medium slices	6
Ground Beef Patty, lean, cooked, 3 oz	21
Ham: Luncheon, 2 slices, 1½ oz	7
Roasted, 2 pieces, 3 oz	18
Lamb chop, broiled, 3 oz	22
Liver, cooked, 3 oz	23
Pastrami, 3 slices, 1¾ oz	10
Pork, cooked, lean, 3 oz	24
Roast Beef, lean, 2 slices, 3 oz	24
Sausages: Bologna, 2 sl., 2 oz	7
Braunschweiger, 2 sl., 2 oz	8
Pork link, thick, 2 oz	6
Frankfurter, 1⅓ oz	5
Salami, hard, 3 slices, 1 oz	7
Steak: Average all cuts, lean (no fat)	
Small (4 oz raw/3 oz cooked)	23
Medium (6 oz raw/4¼ oz cooked)	34
Large (10 oz raw/7¼ oz cooked)	57
Veal cutlet, 1 medium	23
Vegetarian, 1 pattie	13

Chicken/Turkey: *Without Skin*

Chicken, cooked: Breast, Roasted, 4 oz	36
Leg/Thigh, Roasted, 2 oz	14
½ Whole Chicken	60
Drumstick, Rstd, 1 med., 3 oz	13
Turkey: Light meat, cooked, 3 oz	28
Dark meat, lean, 3 oz	24

Fish

Fresh Fish: *Per 4 oz, cooked*	
Cod, Flounder/Sole, Pollock	28
Catfish, Haddock, Halibut, M/Mahi	28
Ocean Perch, Swordf., Orange Roughy	28
Canned Fish: Tuna, Light, 3 oz	25
White, 3 oz	23
Salmon, pink, 3 oz	17
Salmon, red, 3 oz	17
Sardines, 3 whole (3"), 1¼ oz	9
Anchovies, 1 can, 1½ oz	13
Shellfish: Crabmeat, 3 oz	17.5
Clams, raw, 4 large/9 sml, 3 oz	11
Crayfish, cooked, 3 oz	20
Lobster, cooked, 3 oz	17
Oysters, raw, 6 medium, 3 oz	7
Scallops, 2 lge/5 small, 1 oz	5
Shrimp, raw, 6 large, 1½ oz	8.5
Fish Products: Fish Sticks, 4 sticks	10
Fish Portions, in batter, 4 oz	13
Gefilte Fish, 1 medium ball, 2 oz	8

Eggs

	Pro
1 Large Egg, whole	6
Egg Yolk	3
Egg White	3
Omelet: Plain, 2 eggs	13
Ham & cheese	17
Egg Substitutes, (liquid):	
Egg Beaters, ¼ cup, 2 oz	4.5
Better 'n Eggs/Scramblers, ¼ cup, 2 oz	6

Milk, Yogurt, Ice Cream

Milk: Whole: 2%, 1 cup	8
Low-Fat (1%); Fat-Free, 1 cup	8.5
Chocolate Milk, 1 cup	8
Thick Shake: Chocolate, 10 oz	9
Vanilla, 10 oz	11
Soymilk, (fortified), average, 1 cup	7
Soy Dream, Enriched, shelf-stable, 1 cup	7
Yogurt, average all brands:	
Plain, 6 oz	8
Fruit flavors, 6 oz	7
Chobani, Greek, Plain, 6 oz	14
Soy, fruit flavors, 6 oz	7
Ice Cream: Rich, ½ cup	2
Regular, Vanilla, ½ cup	2.5
Sherbet, ½ cup	1
Custard, baked, ½ cup	7

Cheese

Hard Cheeses, average, 1 oz	7
Cottage Cheese, ½ cup	13
Cream Cheese, avg., 1 oz	2
Ricotta, part skim, ½ cup	14

Bread, Bagels, Biscuits

Bread: *With enriched flour*	
1 slice, 1 oz	2
4 thin slices, 4 oz	8
4 thick slices, 6 oz	1.2
Bagel, plain 2 oz	6
Biscuits, 1 oz	2
Pita Bread, 1 pita, 1½ oz	4
Pumpernickel, 1 slice, 1 oz	3

Infant/Baby Foods

	Pro
Infant Formula Milk:	
Enfamil/Gerber/Similac,	
Regular/Low Iron , 5 fl.oz	2.2
Isomil/Nursoy/ProSobee,	3
Baby Cereals: *Average all brands*	
Dry, 4 Tbsp, ½ oz	1
Jars, with fruit, 4½ oz	1

Protein Counter

Breakfast Cereals	**Pro**
Hot Cereals ~ *Cooked:*	
Bulgur, cooked, 1 cup, 5 oz	9
Oatmeal: Reg., non-fortified, 1 cup	6
Instant, fortified, avg., 1 pkt	4
Quaker, all flavors, 1/2 cup	5
Corn/Hominy Grits: 1 cup	3
Quaker: Reg., 3 Tbsp, 1 oz	2
Instant White, 1 packet	2
Cream of Wheat, 1 cup	4
Brands ~ *Ready-To-Eat*	
General Mills:	
Cheerios, Original, 1 cup, 1 oz	3
Chex, Corn, 1 cup, 1.1 oz	2
Kix, Original, 1 1/4 cups, 1 oz	2
Lucky Charms, Original, 3/4 cup, 1 oz	2
Total, Raisin Bran, 1 cup, 1.8 oz	3
Wheaties, 3/4 cup, 1 oz	2
Health Valley:	
Amaranth Flakes, 1 1/4 cups, 2 oz	6
Bran Flakes, with Raisins, 1 cup, 1.8 oz	5
Corn Crunch-Ems, 1 cup, 1 oz	2
Oat Bran Flakes, with Raisins, 1 cup, 1.9 oz	5
Rice Crunch-Ems, 1 1/4 cups, 1 oz	2
Kashi:	
Good Friends, 1 cup, 1.9 oz	5
GoLean Crunch!, 1 cup, 1.9 oz	9
7 Whole Grain Flakes, 1 cup, 1.75 oz	6
Kellogg's:	
All-Bran, Original, 1/2 cup, 1 oz	4
Apple Jacks, 1 cup, 1 oz	1
Corn Flakes, 1 cup, 1 oz	2
Low-fat Granola	
with Raisins 2/3 cup, 2.1 oz	5
Product 19, 1 cup, 1 oz	3
Rice Krispies, 1 1/4 cup, 1.2 oz	2
Smart-Start Strong Heart, 1 c., 1.75 oz	4
Special K: All flavors, 1 c., 1.1 oz	2
Protein, 3/4 cup, 1.1 oz	10
Post:	
Grape Nuts, Original, 1/2 cup, 2 oz	8
Raisin Bran, 1 cup, 2 oz	5
Quaker:	
Corn Bran Crunch, 3/4 cup, 1 oz	2
Granola, 1/2 cup, 1.7 oz	5
Honey Graham Oh's, 3/4 cup, 1 oz	1
Life, Original, 3/4 cup, 1.1 oz	3

Brans & Wheatgerm	**Pro**
Oat Bran, raw, 1 Tbsp	2
Rice Bran, raw, 2 Tbsp	1
Wheat Bran, unprocessed, 2 T.	1
Wheat Germ, 2 Tbsp, 1/2 oz	4
Grains & Flours, Yeast	
Amaranth, 1/2 cup, 3.4 oz	14
Barley, 1/2 cup, 3.2 oz	12
Buckwheat Flour, Whole-groat, 1 cup	15
Carob Flour, 1 cup, 3.6 oz	5
Corn Flour, 1 cup, 4 oz	11
Corn Meal, 1 cup, 4 1/2 oz	8
Flour: White, 1 cup, 5.6 oz	9
Wholegrain, 1 cup, 4 1/4 oz	16
Millet, wholegrain, 1 cup, 3 1/2 oz	12
Rye Flour: Dark, 1 cup, 4 1/2 oz	18
Light, 1 cup, 3 1/2 oz	9
Soy Flour, full fat, 1 cup, 3 oz	29
Yeast: Brewers, 2 Tbsp, 1/2 oz	8
Nutritional Yeast Flakes *(Red Star),*	
1 heaping Tbsp, 1/2 oz	8
Rice, Spaghetti, Macaroni	
Rice: Brown/White, average	
1 cup cooked, 6 1/2 oz	5
Spaghetti/Macaroni/Noodles (enriched):	
Cooked, 1 cup, 4 1/2 oz	7
Canned: in Tomato Sce, 1/2 cup	2
with Meatballs, 1 cup, 8 oz	10
Macaroni & Cheese, 1 cup, 9 oz	8
Soups	
With Noodles/Vegetables, 1 cup	3
With Meat/Beans/Peas, 1 cup	8
Fruit	
Fresh/Canned:	
Average, all types,	
1 medium/2 small fruit	1
Avocado, 1/2 medium	2
Dried Fruit: Apricots, 8 halves, 1 oz	1
Dates, 6 dates, 2 oz	1.5
Figs, 4 medium figs, 2 oz	2
Prunes, 5 medium, 1 1/2 oz	1
Raisins, 1 oz	1
Fruit Juice: Average, 1 cup	0.5
Prune Juice, 6 fl.oz	1
Tomato Juice, 1 cup, 8 fl.oz	1.5

Vegetables — Pro

Beans: Snap/green, $^1/_2$ cup, 2 oz	1
Dried: Average all types, cooked, $^1/_2$ cup	7
Baked Beans, $^1/_2$ cup 4$^1/_2$ oz	5
Bean Sprouts, mung, 1 c., 4 oz	3
Broccoli, 3 raw, $^1/_2$ cup, 1$^1/_2$ oz	1.5
Cabbage; Cauliflower, raw, 1 c. 3 oz	1.5
Corn: Raw, $^1/_2$ cup kernels, 3 oz	2.5
1 ear trimmed to 3$^1/_2$"	2
Lentils, cooked, $^1/_2$ cup 3$^1/_2$ oz	9
Mushrooms, raw, $^1/_2$ c., sliced	1
Peas: Green, raw, $^1/_2$ c., 2$^1/_2$ oz	4
Split Peas, cooked, 1 cup, 7 oz	16
Potatoes: *Cooked:*	
1 medium, with skin, 5 oz	3.3
without skin, 4 oz	2.3
French Fries, small, 2.6 oz	2
Potato Salad, $^1/_2$ cup, 4 oz	3.5
Pumpkin, $^1/_2$ cup mashed, 4.3 oz	1
Seaweed, kelp, 1 oz	<1
Spinach, cooked, $^1/_2$ cup, 3 oz	2.7
Squash, ckd, all types, $^1/_2$ cup	1
Tomatoes, 1 medium, 4$^1/_2$ oz	1
Vegetables, mixed, ckd, 1 cup	2.5
Soybeans, cooked, $^1/_2$ cup, 3 oz	14

Tofu, Tempeh, Miso

Tofu, raw, firm, $^1/_2$ cup, 4$^1/_2$ oz	10
Tempeh, $^1/_2$ cup, 3 oz	16
Miso, $^1/_2$ cup, 5 oz	16
Miso Soup, 1 cup	3
Soybean Protein *(TVP),* 1 oz	18

Cakes, Pastries, Pies

(Made with enriched flour)	
Carrot w. cream cheese frosting, 4 oz	4
Cheesecake, 1 piece, 4 oz	6
Chocolate, 1 piece, 2 oz	2
Fruitcake, 1 piece, 3 oz	4
Plain, 1 piece, 3 oz	4
Croissant, plain, 2 oz	5
Danish Pastry, 1 pastry, 2$^1/_4$ oz	4
Donuts, average, 2 oz	4
Muffins, average, 1 med., 1$^1/_2$ oz	3
Pancakes, 4" diam., two, 2 oz	4
Pies: Fruit, 1 piece, 5$^1/_2$ oz	4
Pecan, 1 piece, 5 oz	7
Puddings, average, $^1/_2$ cup, 4$^1/_2$ oz	4
Waffles, 1 large, 2$^1/_2$ oz	7

Peanut Butter — Pro

Regular: 2 Tbsp, 1.1 oz	8
Peter Pan Plus, 2 Tbsp, 1.1 oz	8

Sugar, Honey, Jam

Sugar: White	0
Brown, 1 Tbsp	0
Molasses: Light/Med., 1 Tbsp	0
Blackstrap, 1 Tbsp, $^3/_4$ oz	0
Corn Syrup, 1 Tbsp, $^3/_4$ oz	0
Honey, Jams, Jelly	0

Candy, Chocolate, Carob

Candy, sugar-based	0
Chocolate: Plain, 2 oz bar	4
with nuts, 2 oz bar	6
Carob, plain, 2 oz	6

Cookies, Crackers, Chips

Cookies, average, 4 cookies	2
Crackers, Graham, 2$^1/_2$" sq., (2)	1
Rice Cakes, average, one	1
Corn/Potato Chips, 1 oz	2

Nuts:

Almonds, shelled, 20-25 nuts	6
Brazil Nuts, 7-8 medium nuts, 1 oz	4
Cashews, 12-16 nuts, 1 oz	5
Macadamias, 1 oz	2
Peanuts, dry rsted, 40 nuts, 1 oz	6
Pecans, 24 halves, 1 oz	2
Walnuts, 15 halves, 1 oz	4

Seeds:

Sesame Seeds, dry, 1 Tbsp	2
Pumpkin Kernels, dry, hulled, 1 oz	7
Sunflower Seeds, dried, hulled, 1 oz	6
Tahini, 1 Tbsp, $^1/_2$ oz	2.5

Granola & Food/Protein Bars

Granola Bars, average, 1 bar, 2 oz	2
Anytime Health,	
Meal Repl. Bars, 80g	20
Snack Bars, 50g	12
Balance Bars, Original, average all, 1.76 oz	14
Bariatrix, Proti-Bars (1), 1.4 oz	15
Dr Soy, Protein Bars, 1.76 oz	10
GeniSoy, Protein Bar, 1.6 oz	15
Jenny Craig, Bars, av., 1.8 oz	5
Met-Rx, "Big 100", av., 3.5 oz	27
Myoplex 30, all flavors, 3 oz	30
Optifast 800, all flavors, 2 oz	14
PowerBar, Energize, 2 oz	6
Slim-Fast, Protein Meal Bars, 1.7 oz	10
Special K: Protein Meal, 1.6 oz	10
Protein Snack, 0.9 oz	4

Protein Counter

High Protein Drinks   **Pro**

Anytime, Health,	
Whey Prot. Isolate, all flav., 1 oz	25
Atkins, Shakes, 11 fl.oz	18
Boost, High Protein, 8 fl.oz bottle	15
Carnation, B'fast Essentials, 11 fl.oz	10
Curves, Protein Drink, 2 scoops, dry	15
dotFIT, First String,	
Choc., 2 scps, 2.65 oz	21
Ensure, Plus, 8 fl.oz bottle	13
Gatorade, Protein Recovery Shake, 11 oz	20
GeniSoy, Protein Shake, 1 scoop, 1.2 oz	14
Met-Rx, Meal Replacement, RTD	40
Myoplex, Original Nutrition Shake, 1 pkt	42
Optifast 800, prepared, 8 fl oz	14
Slim-Fast Shakes: Meal, 10 oz can	10
High Protein Meal, 10 fl.oz bottle	20
Special K₂O, Protein Water, 16 fl.oz	5
Weider, Mass 1000, 4 scoops, 7 oz	34

Coffee, Tea, Soda

Coffee, Coffee Substitutes, 1 cup, 8 fl.oz	0
Coffee, with 2 oz milk, 1 cup, 8 fl.oz	2
Caffe latte, large, 16 fl.oz	12
Cappuccino, large, 16 fl.oz	8
Frappuccino, average, 16 fl.oz	6
Hot Chocolate, with milk, 1 cup, 8 fl.oz	8
Soft Drinks/Soda	0
Tea, all types	0

Beer, Wine, Spirits

Beer, 12 fl.oz	1
Wines, red/white, 1 glass	0
Spirits/Liquor	0

Fast-Foods/Burgers

Pancakes, average all outlets, 3	8
Shakes, Chocolate, 16 fl.oz	12
Sundaes, Average all outlets	7
Arby's:	
Chopped Farmhouse Salad, Crispy Chicken	30
Roast Beef Sandwich: Classic	23
Max	45
Burger King: Big Fish Sandwich	18
Double Bacon Cheeseburger	17
Whopper Sandwich	22

Fast Foods/Burgers (Cont)   **Pro**

Carl's Jr:	
Charbroiled Chicken Club Sandwich	36
Famous Star Hamburger with Cheese	28
Super Star Hamburger with Cheese	48
Domino's Pizza: Hand Tossed (12")	
Feast, Ultimate Pepperoni, 1 slice	11
Legend: Buffalo Chicken, 1 slice	13
Honolulu Hawaiian, 1 slice	8
KFC: Original Breast	36
Extra Crispy Tenders, 3 strips	33
Grilled, Breast	40
McDonald's: Big Mac	25
Cheeseburger	15
Chicken McNuggets (6)	13
Crispy Chicken Classic Sandwich	24
Filet-O-Fish	15
Hamburger	12
Quarter Pounder with Cheese	30
French Fries: Small, 2.5 oz	3
Large, 5.4 oz	6
Salad, with Chicken, average	26
Shake, McCafe, average, 12 fl.oz	12
Breakfast: Egg McMuffin	18
Bacon, Egg & Cheese McGriddles	19
Sausage Burrito	12
Sausage McMuffin with Egg	21
Pizza Hut: Per Medium, 1 slice, ⅛ Pizza	
Thin 'n Crispy, Supreme	10
Pan Pizzas, average	11
Hand Tossed: Pepperoni Lover's	12
Ultimate Cheese Lover's	10
Subway : 6" Subs with standard toppings, no oil	
Applewood Pulled Pork	25
Meatball Marinara	21
Spicy Italian	20
Subway Melt	23
Turkey Jalapeno Melt	21
Taco Bell: Bean Burrito	15
Cheesy Gordita Crunch	20
Chicken Quesadilla	27
Chicken/Steak Chalupas	16
Steak Burrito Supreme	20
Taco Supreme	9
Wendy's:	
Asiago Ranch Chicken Club	38
Dave's ¼ lb Single Burger	30
Jr Hamburger	14

High Blood Pressure

Many American adults have hypertension (high blood pressure), and are unaware of it. It is generally symptomless, so **have your blood pressure checked annually** – particularly if it runs in the family.

Untreated hypertension overworks the heart, damages arteries and promotes atherosclerosis. This in turn greatly increases the risk of heart disease, stroke, blindness, kidney disease and impotence. The earlier hypertension is detected, the sooner it can be brought under control.

BLOOD PRESSURE CLASSIFICATION

For Adults Age 18 & Older ~ Not Acutely ill or on Medication (American Heart Association)

	DIASTOLIC		SYSTOLIC
Normal ➤	Below 80	and	Below 120
Prehypertension ➤	80-89	or	120-139
Hypertension:			
Stage 1 ➤	90-99	or	140-159
Stage 2 ➤	100 or more	or	160 or more

Treating Hypertension

Prehypertension (in the chart above) means you don't have high blood pressure now but are likely to develop it in the future.

You can take steps to lessen the risk by adopting healthy lifestyle habits such as:
- reducing sodium intake
- eating adequate fruit and vegetables
- losing weight if overweight
- limiting alcohol to 2 drinks or less daily
- quitting smoking
- exercising regularly, managing stress.

Stage 1 hypertension can often be treated with the above lifestyle changes.

Stage 2 hypertension usually requires drug therapy. However, salt restriction, abstaining from alcohol, and the above lifestyle changes will improve the success of drug therapy, and enable smaller drug doses to be prescribed.

HYPERTENSION DAMAGES ARTERIES & PROMOTES ATHEROSCLEROSIS

STROKE (Brain) *Artery blockage or rupture*

NECK ARTERIES *Artherosclerosis can limit blood flow to brain*

HEART ATTACK *Coronary artery blockage*

STROKE
KNOW THE WARNING SIGNS

Stroke is a medical emergency! If you notice one or more of these signs, call 9-1-1 or your doctor immediately.

These signs may be signalling a possible stroke or transient ischemic attack:

- **Sudden weakness** or numbness in your face, arm, or leg on one side of your body.
- **Sudden confusion,** trouble speaking or understanding. Slurred speech.
- **Sudden trouble seeing,** in one or both eyes
- **Sudden trouble walking,** dizziness, loss of balance or coordination.
- **Sudden severe headache** - 'a bolt out of the blue' – with no apparent cause.

Extra Info: www.stroke.org

Salt & Sodium Guide

Salt & Sodium

- **Sodium is a mineral element** most commonly found in salt (sodium chloride). It also occurs naturally in much smaller amounts in animal and plant foods, and water – normally sufficient for our needs without having to add salt to our diet.

- **Sodium is required** for nerve and muscle function, as well as to balance the amount of fluid in our tissues and blood. Sodium acts like a sponge to attract and hold fluids in body tissues.

- **Excess sodium** can cause water retention, and increase the risk of developing hypertension. Very high salt intake may also increase the risk of stomach cancer.

- **Too little sodium** may cause low blood pressure (hypotension), and decrease blood flow to the heart, brain and kidneys – especially during exercise. (A certain blood volume is required to sustain the blood pressure needed for adequate blood flow in the capillaries).

Salt-Sensitive Persons

- **Normally, our kidneys** excrete excess dietary sodium. The thirst we feel after a salty meal is the body calling for water to dilute the sodium, and enable the kidneys to flush out excess sodium.

- However, **'salt - sensitive'** persons (up to 70% of adults) tend to retain excess sodium (above approximately 3000mg daily) instead of excreting it. Such persons are more likely to develop hypertension and would benefit most from sodium restriction. Assume you are susceptible if there is a family history of hypertension.

- **Although not everyone will benefit, all Americans are being asked to moderate their salt and sodium intake** as a public health measure – particularly because so many do not know whether or not they have hypertension, and also because we do not know just who is salt-sensitive.

SAFE SODIUM LEVELS

The American Heart Association recommends a **maximum sodium intake of 1500mg per day** for adults with normal blood pressure.

Persons with hypertension and kidney ailments are usually restricted to as little as **1000mg sodium per day**. Your doctor will discuss the correct sodium level for you.

FINDING HIDDEN SODIUM

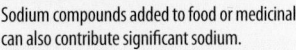

On average, **less than one third of our sodium intake comes from the salt shaker.** The rest is hidden in processed foods that have salt added during manufacture.

Sodium compounds added to food or medicinals can also contribute significant sodium.

Sodium bicarbonate in particular is widely used in antacid tablets (such as *Alka Seltzer*) and powders. Sodium bicarbonate contains 27% sodium by weight. Each gram has 270mg of sodium. Large amounts of sodium can be unwittingly consumed – up to 600mg per tablet. (See Antacids ~ Page 280)

Example: 2 *Alka-Seltzer* Tablets = 1000mg sodium

Other sodium compounds include monosodium glutamate (MSG), sodium ascorbate, sodium nitrite, and sodium citrate.

POTASSIUM BALANCES SODIUM

Potassium helps to balance sodium by helping the kidneys to excrete excess sodium. Fruit and vegetables are rich sources of potassium - another reason to ensure you have your 5-7 servings every day.

Nuts also provide potassium as well as magnesium and other heart-healthy nutrients and anti-oxidants. Eat them unsalted.

Note: This info is only for people with normal kidney function. Also not for persons on potassium-sparing diuretics.

ALCOHOL DANGER

Excessive alcohol intake contributes to hypertension. Susceptible persons should limit alcohol intake to 1-2 drinks per day.

Salt Sodium Guide

Sodium accounts for only 40% of the weight of salt (sodium chloride). Examples:

1 gram (1000mg) Salt has 400mg Sodium

1 teaspoon (5g) Salt has 2000mg Sodium

HINTS TO REDUCE SODIUM

- **Cut down use of the salt shaker.** Start with an easy 50% cut in sodium by using Lite Salt (*Morton*) or *Cardia* Salt. Then gradually cut back until you can leave the salt shaker off the table. Sea salt is still high in sodium.

- **Use fresh herbs,** and salt-free seasonings to add flavor to food.

- **Choose low-sodium,** sodium-free, and reduced-sodium products in place of regular, salted products.

- **Check food labels for sodium levels.** FDA Guidelines for sodium descriptors are:
  - **Reduced Sodium:** At least 25% less sodium than the original product
  - **Low Sodium:** 140 mg or less/serving
  - **Very Low Sodium:** 35mg or less/serving
  - **Sodium Free:** Less than 5mg/serving
  - **No Salt Added:** Made without the salt normally added, but still contains the sodium that is a natural part of the food

- **Use reduced-sodium breads,** butter and margarine. Regular varieties are considered high in sodium in view of their significant contribution to our diet.

- **Go easy on salty condiments and sauces** such as ketchup, mustard, soy sauce, spaghetti sauces, and salad dressings. Use low-sodium varieties.

- **Limit pizzas and salty fast-foods.** Check the *CalorieKing.com* food database.

- **Avoid salty snack foods** such as potato chips, corn chips, salted nuts, pretzels and cheesy-flavored snacks. **Choose unsalted** popcorn, nuts or seeds. Eat more fruit.

- **Don't salt children's food** to your taste.

- **Avoid antacids with** sodium bicarbonate (such as *Alka-Seltzer*). They are high in sodium. Look for low-sodium alternatives.

FOODS HIGH IN SODIUM

- Bread (4 slices/day), Bagels, Biscuits
- Cheese, Butter, Margarine
- Pickles, Sauerkraut, Olives
- Condiments, Sauces
- Salad Dressings
- Canned vegetables/salads/beans
- Deli Salads (with dressing)
- Frozen/Packaged Meals/Entrees
- Soups: Canned/dry; bouillon cubes
- Meats: Ham, bacon, sausage, luncheon meats, smoked meats
- Canned Fish (in brine/salt)
- Sea Salt, Garlic/Celery Salt
- Snack Foods (potato chips, pretzels)
- Tomato Juice (Canned), V8 Vegetable Juice
- Fast Foods: Pizza, Burgers, Chicken
- *Alka-Seltzer* Antacid

MODERATE SODIUM

- Meat, Fish, Poultry - Unprocessed
- Milk, Yogurt, Soy Drinks, Eggs
- Peanut Butter
- Breakfast Cereals (less than 200mg/serving)
- Chocolate Candy, Fruit/Nut Bars
- *Reduced Sodium & Low Sodium* Products

FOODS LOW IN SODIUM

- Products labelled *Very Low Sodium*, or *Sodium Free*
- Bread (No Salt Added)
- Fresh fruits and vegetables
- Canned and Dried Fruits
- Potatoes, Rice, Pasta
- Dried Beans & Lentils, Tofu
- Nuts & Seeds (unsalted)
- Corn & Popcorn (unsalted)
- Pepper, Spices, Herbs
- Jam, Honey, Syrup
- Candy, Gum
- Hard & Jelly Candy
- Coffee, Tea, Alcohol
- Fresh Fruit Juices, Water

Sodium Counter

Sodium ~ Sodium (mg)

Milk & Dairy Products

	Sodium
Milk: Whole/lowfat/skim, average	
1 glass, 8 fl.oz	120
Whole, low sodium, 1 cup	5
Choc Milk, 1 cup	130
Soy Milk, 8 fl.oz	30
Buttermilk, cultured, 8 fl.oz	250
Dry/Powder, skim, ¼ cup, 1 oz	110
Yogurt, with fruit average, 8 oz	130
Cheese: Bleu, 1 oz	330
Cottage Cheese, Creamed, ½ cup, 4 oz	450
Kraft: American, 2% milk, 1 sl., 0.7 oz	230
Philadelphia Cream Cheese Brick, Orig.,1 oz	105
Parmesan, 1 oz	425
Process Cheese., average,1 oz	430
Ricotta Cheese, ½ cup, 4 oz	110
Swiss, Deli Deluxe, 1 slice	40

Ice Cream, Frozen Yogurt

Icecream, average, ½ cup	50
Frozen Yogurt, ½ cup	50

Fats/Oils

Butter/Margarine:	
Regular, 2 Tbsp, 1 oz	230
Unsalted, reg., 2 Tbsp, 1 oz	5
Mayonnaise, avg., 2 Tbsp, 1 oz	160
Oils/Lard/Drippings	0
Cream, average, 1 Tbsp	5
Coffee-Mate: Powdered, 1 tsp	2
Liquid, 1 Tbsp	5

Eggs

Whole, 1 large	70
Omelet: 2 egg, plain	220
With 1 oz Cheddar Cheese	400
Egg Beaters: Original, 3 Tbsp	90
Flavors, average, 3 Tbsp	140

Meats

Meat, average all types, cooked	
Beef/Lamb/Veal/Pork, 4 oz	80
Corned Beef, cooked, 3 oz	800
Bacon, cooked, 2 slices, 0.5 oz	270
Ham, 3 oz	1100

Chicken & Turkey

Chicken/Turkey, cooked, unsalted, 4 oz	80
Stuffing Mixes, average., ½ cup	500

Sausages & Meats

	Sodium
Bologna, 1 oz	280
Frankfurter, 2 oz	640
Ham, chopped, 0.8 oz slice	290
Liverwurst (Braunschweiger), 1 oz	320
Pepperoni, 5 slices, 1 oz	570
Salami: Cooked, 1 oz	350
dry/hard, 1 oz	600
Sausage, 1 oz link	220
Pork, 2 oz patty	260
Spam: Classic, 2 oz	790
25% Less Sodium, 2 oz	580
Turkey Roll, 1 oz	160

Fish:

Fresh Fish: average, plain	
Cooked, 4 oz, without bone	60
Broiled w. butter, 4 oz	150
Breaded & fried, 4 oz	320
Fish fillets, batter-dipped 3 oz	350
Fish sticks, 1 oz stick	160
Gefilte Fish, with broth, 1 pce, 1.5 oz	220
Herring, pickled, 2 pces, 1 oz	260
Lobster, meat only, 4 oz	180
Oysters, fresh, 6 med., 3 oz	95
Salmon: Canned, 3 oz	460
No Salt Added, 3 oz	65
Smoked fish, average, 3 oz	650
Tuna: Canned, drained, 3 oz	160
Light, drained, 3 oz	200
No Added Salt, 3 oz	40
Spicy Flavored, 5 oz	260

Entrees & Meals

Frozen Meals, average	600-1300
Lean Cuisine, average	700
Stouffer's, For One, Beef Pot Roast	1570
Dinners, average	900-1200
Side Dishes, average	400-600
Pizza, frozen, ¼ large, 6 oz	800-1200
Microwave, Cup Meals	900-1200
Cup O'Noodles, average	1500

More Sodium Counts:
www.CalorieKing.com

Sodium Counter

Soups

	Sodium
Condensed: Average, 1 cup, 8 oz	800-1000
Low Sodium, average	70
Chicken Noodle, average, 1 cup	900
Bouillon Cube, average	950
Ramen Noodle Soup, av., 3 oz pkg	1500
Soup Cups, average	850
Soup Mixes, average, 1 cup	900

Condiments, Sauces, Dressings

A-1 Sauce, 1 Tbsp	280
Barbecue Sauce, 1 Tbsp	130
Bragg's Liquid Aminos, 1 tsp	220
Chili Sauce, 1 Tbsp	230
Ketchup: Tomato, 1 Tbsp	180
Low Sodium, 1 Tbsp	20
Mayonnaise, 1 Tbsp	80
Mustard, 1 tsp	70
Pizza Sauce, 1/2 cup	700
Salad Dressings, 2 Tbsp, 1 oz	160-400
Spaghetti Sauce, 1/2 cup	500
Soy Sauce: 1 Tbsp	900
Lite, 1 Tbsp	600
Sweet & Sour, 1/2 cup	250
Tabasco, 1 tsp	25
Vinegar, Lemon Juice	0
Worcestershire, 1 Tbsp	65
Tomato: Sauce, 1 cup	1200
Paste/Puree (salted), 1/2 cup	1000
No Salt Added, 1/2 cup	75

Salt & Salt Substitutes

Table Salt: 1 teaspoon, 6g	2400
Single Serve package, 1 g	400
Cardia Salt, 1 teaspoon	1080
Lite Salt, 1 teaspoon, 6g	1200
Morton, No Salt Substitute, 1 tsp	5
Garlic/Onion/Seasoned Salt, 1 tsp, 4g	1350
Garlic/Seasoned Salt 1 teaspoon, 4g	1300
Sea Salt, 1 teaspoon, 5g	2250

Seasonings, Herbs & Spices

Baking Powder, 1 tsp, 3g	340
Baking Soda (Sodium bicarb), 1 tsp, 3g	810
Accent, Flavor Enhancer, 1 tsp	680
Chili Powder, 1 tsp, 3g	25
Curry Powder	0
Lemon Pepper 1 tsp	340
Meat Tenderizer, 1 tsp, 5g	1750
MSG (Monosodium Glutamate), 5g	500
Mrs Dash, Blends/Marinades	0
Old Bay: Seasoning, 1 tsp, 2.4 oz	640
Seasoning, Less Sodium, 1 tsp, 2.4 oz	380
Pepper, Mustard (dry), 1 tsp	1
Yeast, Nutritional, 1 Tbsp	10

Breakfast Cereals

	Sodium
Kellogg's:	
All-Bran, Original, 1/2 cup, 1 oz	80
Special K, Original, 1 cup, 1.1 oz	210
Corn Flakes, 1 cup, 1 oz	200
Frosted Mini Wheats, Blueb./Strawb., (25)	0
Raisin Bran, 1 cup	210
Quaker:	
Corn Bran Crunch, 3/4 cup, 1 oz	210
Oh's, 3/4 cup, 1 oz	170
Puffed Rice/Wheat, 2 cups, 1 oz	1
Simply Granola, average, 1/2 cup, 1 oz	30
General Mills, Total, 3/4 cup, 1 oz	140
Oatmeal: Regular, 3/4 cup	1
Quaker, Instant Maple & Brown Sugar (1 pkt)	260

Breads, Bagels, Crackers

Bread: Thin Slice, average 1 oz	140
Thick Slice, 1.5 oz	210
Low Sodium, 1 oz	10
Bagels: Plain, medium, 2 oz	200
Large, take-out, average, 4 oz	550
Panera Bread, 3.8 oz	460
Biscuits, average, 1 oz	180
Bun/Roll: 1 medium, 1.5 oz	200
Large, 4 oz	560
Crackers: Saltine, 2 crackers	70
Low Salt, 2	25
Graham, 2 regular	50
Croissant, Plain, average, 2 oz	280
Rice Cakes, average	25
Ritz Crackers, Hint of Salt, 1 oz	60
Ry-Krisp, Crispbread, Sesame, 0.7 oz	70

Cookies, Cakes, Desserts

Cookies: Average, 2-3 cookies, 1 oz	100
Average, 1 cookie, 2.5 oz	180
Baked Custard, 1/2 cup	100
Brownie, 1.5 oz	130
Carrot Cake, 8 oz	650
Cheesecake, 7 oz	350
Cinnamon Sweet Roll, 2 oz	250
Danish, Apple/Fruit	250
Donut, average	150
Muffins: 1 medium, 2 oz	150
1 extra large, 4 oz	300
Pancakes, (4"), x 3	360
Fruit Pies, average, 7 oz	600
Pudding: Average, 1/2 cup	160
Jell-O Instant Pudding Mix, 1/4 pkg	360
Waffles: Home-made, 7", 2.5 oz	350
Frozen: Average, 1.2 oz	260
Aunt Jemima, Homestyle, av., 2.5 oz	480

Sodium Counter

Fruit & Juices | Sodium
Fresh Fruit, average all types, 1 serving — 1
Dried/Canned Fruit, 1/2 cup — 1
Fruit Juice: Fresh, squeezed, 6 fl.oz — 1
  Commercial, aver., 6 fl.oz — 20
Tomato Juice *(Campbell's)*, 8 fl.oz — 680
  Low Sodium (No Salt Added), 8 fl.oz — 140
V8 Vegetable *(Campbell's):*
  11.5 fl.oz bottle — 880
  Low Sodium, 5.5 fl.oz can — 80

Vegetables
Fresh/Frozen (No Salt Added): Per 1/2 Cup
Asparagus, Bean Sprouts, Corn — 3
Beets, Carrots, Celery, 1/2 cup — 40
Broccoli, Cabbage, Cauliflower — 10
Cucumber, Green Beans, Mushroom, Okra — 3
Onions, Peas, Potato, Pumpkin, Squash — 3
Peppers, Hot Chili, raw, each — 3
Spinach, Turnips, 1/2 cup, cooked — 40
Tomato, 1 medium, 5 oz — 10
Canned: Asparagus, 4 spears — 300
  Beans, baked in tomato sauce — 450
  Beets, 1/2 cup, 3 oz — 240
  Corn Kernels, 1/2 cup, 3 oz — 190
    Creamed, 1/2 cup, 4.5 oz — 330
  Mushrooms w. butter sce, 2oz — 550
  Peas, 1/2 cup, 3 oz — 250
  Sauerkraut, 1/2 cup, 4 oz — 750

Pickles, Olives
Olives: pickled: Green, 1 large — 90
  Ripe/black, 1 large — 40
Pickles: Bread & Butter, 4 slices, 1 oz — 200
  Dill, 1 pickle, 2.5oz — 900
  Sweet, 1 gherkin, 0.5 oz — 130

Soybean Products
Miso (Soy Paste), 1/4 c., 2.5 oz — 2500
Soybean Protein Isolate, 1 oz — 280
Tempeh, Natural, 1/2 cup, 3 oz — 5
Tofu, average, 1/2 cup, 4 oz — 5

Jam, Honey, Syrups
Jam/Jelly, 1 Tbsp — 2
Honey/Maple Syrup, 1 Tbsp — 1
Log Cabin, Syrup, 1 fl.oz — 35
  Lite, 1 fl.oz — 90

Peanut Butter
Peanut Butter: Regular, 2 Tbsp, 0.5 oz — 190
  Jif, Low Sodium, 2 Tbsp — 65
  Trader Joe's, Unsalted, 2 Tbsp — 5

Snacks, Nuts | Sodium
Cheese Balls/Curls, 1 oz — 280
Cheetos, 1 oz — 290
Corn/Tortilla Chips: average, 1 oz — 220
  Fritos, Lightly Salted, 1 oz — 80
Granola bars, average, 1 bar — 80
Nuts: Plain, unsalted, 1 oz — 1
  Lightly salted, 1 oz — 80
  Salted or Honey Roasted, 1 oz — 160
Popcorn: Plain (unsalted), 1 cup — 1
  Flavored, average, 1 cup — 60
  Salt added, 1 cup — 180
Potato Chips: Plain, 1 oz — 160
  Lay's, Lightly Salted, 1 oz — 85
  Flavored, average, 1 oz — 200
Pretzels: Regular, 3, 1 oz — 450
  Soft, salted, large — 1000

Candy, Chocolate
Chocolate, milk, 1 oz — 30
Fudge, chocolate, 1 oz — 55
Candy Bars, average, 1.5 oz — 60
Hard Candy, 1 oz — 10
Licorice, 1 oz — 30

Beverages, Alcohol
Coffee or Tea, 1 cup — 1
Cocoa: Dry, plain, 1 Tbsp — 0
  Mix, average, 1 envelope — 120
Quik, 2 tsp — 35
Soft Drinks, average, 8 fl.oz — 20
Mineral Water: Perrier, 8 fl.oz — 5
  Gatorade, Thirst Quencher, 8 fl.oz — 110
Red Bull: 8.4 fl.oz can — 105
  Sugar Free, 8.4 fl.oz — 200
Water, Average, 1 cup, 8 fl.oz — 5
Alcohol: Beer, average, 12 fl.oz — 15
  Wines, average, 4 fl.oz — 10
  Spirits (distilled), 1.5 fl.oz — 1

Antacids ~ Alka-Seltzer
Alka-Seltzer: *Per Tablet* | Sodium
  Original; Heartburn — 570
  Extra Strength — 590
  Lemon Lime — 500
  Gold — 310
Alka-Mints, chewable — 0
Bromo Seltzer, 3/4 capful — 760
Picot, 1 packet, 5g — 670
Rolaids, All types — 0
Tums, Regular/Extra Strength — 0

Cold & Flu ~ Alka-Seltzer Plus
Effervescents, average, 1 tablet — 480
Fast Crystal Packs; Liquid Gels — 0

Sodium Counter

Fast-Foods & Restaurants	Sodium
Burger King:	
Burgers: Cheeseburger	540
Double Bacon Cheeseburger	800
Hamburger	460
Whoppers: Original	910
With Cheese	1260
Whopper Jr. with Cheese	640
Chicken Sandwich, Original	1170
Sides: French Fries, medium, salted	570
Onion Rings, medium	1080
Breakfast, Ham, Egg & Cheese Croissan'wich	1080
Denny's:	
Burgers: Bacon Avocado Cheeseburger	1490
Spicy Sriracha	2100
Sandwiches: Club	2180
Prime Rib Philly Melt	2340
Dinner: Brooklyn Spaghetti & Meatballs	2480
Sirloin Steak	1260
Sides: Broccoli	20
French Fries, salted, 6 oz	110
Red-Skinned Potatoes	590
Soup: Chicken Noodle, 12 oz bowl	1130
Clam Chowder, 12 oz bowl	1870
Breakfast: Buttermilk Pancakes (2), w/ Marg.	1210
Moons Over My Hammy Omelette, w/ Hash	2560
Hearty Breakfast Skillet	2050
Sides: Hash Browns, 1 serving	410
Hearty Breakfast Sausage	840
Dessert, Apple Pie, 1 slice, 14 oz	750
Jack In The Box:	
Burgers: Bacon Untimate Cheeseburger	2190
Hamburger	680
Jumbo Jack with Cheese	1310
Sandwiches: H'style Ranch Chicken Club	1910
Sourdough Grilled Chiken Club	1490
KFC:	
Chicken Breast: Original	1140
Extra Crispy	1140
Grilled	730
Popcorn Nuggets,	
Family Tray	4670
Sandwich, Crispy Twister	1300
Tenders, Extra Crispy Tenders, Family Tray	310
Wings, HBBQ Hot (1)	270
Sides: Macaroni & Cheese	830
Mashed Potatoes with Gravy	530
Potato Wedges	810

Fast-Foods & Restaurants	Sodium
McDonalds:	
Burgers: Big Mac	970
Cheeseburger	680
Double	1050
Hamburger	490
Quarter Pounder with Cheese	1110
Chicken McNuggets: 6 pieces	540
Spicy Buffalo Sauce, 1 package, 0.8 oz	540
Sandwich, Buttermilk Crispy Chicken	900
French Fries: Small, 2.6 oz	130
Medium, 3.9 oz	190
Large, 5.9 oz	290
Ketchup, 1 package, 10g	90
Breakfast: Egg McMuffin	750
Big Breakfast, reg. size Biscuit	1560
Hash Browns, 2 oz	310
Hotcakes, with Syrup & Whipped Margarine	590
Sausage McGriddle	1030
Southern Style Chicken Biscuit, regular bisc.	1180
Desserts/Shakes: Hot Fudge Sundae	170
Strawberry McCafe Shake, 12 fl.oz	160
Pizza Hut:	
Pan Pizza: *Per 1/2 Medium Pizza, 4 Slices*	
Meat Lovers	2960
Cheese; Cock A Doodle Bacon	2000
Pepperoni Lover's	3080
Pepperoni; Buffalo State of Mind, av.	2420
Subway:	
6" Lowfat Sandwich: *W/ Set Menu Board Toppings, no oil*	
Chicken, oven roasted	610
Roast Beef	660
Subway Club	800
Sweet Onion Chicken Teriyaki	770
6" Sandwiches: *W/ Set Menu Board Toppings, no oil*	
Chicken Bacon Ranch Melt with Cheese	1050
Meatball Marinara	920
Spicy Italian	1490
12" Footlong ~ Double the above figures	
Taco Bell:	
Burritos: Combo, 8.2 oz	1380
Supreme, Chicken; Steak	1090
Chalupa Supreme, Chicken; Steak	530
Gordita Supreme, Steak	530
Nachos: BellGrande	1310
Supreme	860
Specialties, Cheese Quesadillas	980
Tacos: Chicken, Soft	480
Crunchy Supreme	340

Index Symbols - C

FAST-FOODS INDEX
~ PAGE 175 ~

Index D - I

FAST-FOODS INDEX
~ PAGE 175 ~

Index P - S

FAST-FOODS INDEX
~ PAGE 175 ~

Notes